T0181041

Respiratory Medicine

Series Editor:
Sharon I.S. Rounds

More information about this series at http://www.springer.com/series/7665

Vineet Bhandari
Editor

Bronchopulmonary Dysplasia

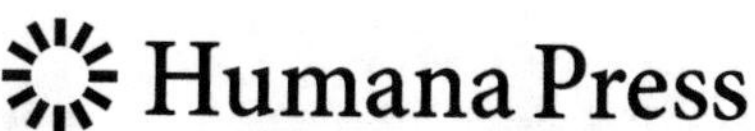

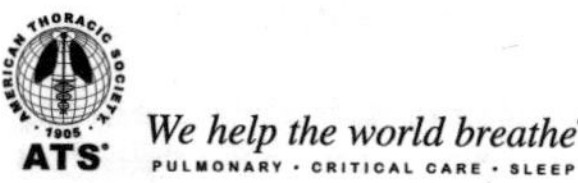

Editor
Vineet Bhandari, MBBS, MD, DM
Drexel University College of Medicine
Philadelphia, PA, USA

Department of Neonatology (Pediatrics)
St. Christopher's Hospital for Children/Hahnemann University Hospital/Temple University Hospital
Philadelphia, PA, USA

ISSN 2197-7372 ISSN 2197-7380 (electronic)
Respiratory Medicine
ISBN 978-3-319-80361-6 ISBN 978-3-319-28486-6 (eBook)
DOI 10.1007/978-3-319-28486-6

Springer Cham Heidelberg New York Dordrecht London

Softcover reprint of the hardcover 1st edition 2016

Printed on acid-free paper

Humana Press is a brand of Springer
Springer International Publishing AG Switzerland is part of Springer Science+Business Media (www.springer.com)

*Dedicated to the babies who constantly
remind us physicians and scientists
to continue to strive to help them
breathe easier.*

Preface

While I have edited two issues (*BPD: State of the Art—Seminars in Perinatology* August 2006;30:163–232 and *Progress in Experimental and Clinical BPD—Seminars in Perinatology* April 2013;37:59–138) dedicated to various aspects of *Bronchopulmonary Dysplasia (BPD)* previously, putting this book on BPD together was a unique opportunity that was offered to me. Since this is a topic near and dear to many neonatologists given the fact that babies in various phases of this disease can be found in most neonatal intensive care units (NICUs), compiling this book presented some interesting challenges. I wanted an international representation of authors for two reasons. One, BPD is a major problem (or becoming one, in some countries) as neonatologists are getting better at saving premature lives around the world, and two, I wanted to tap into the reservoir of international talent of physicians and scientists who have been tackling this problem and making some significant inroads in understanding the pathogenesis and/or providing clinical care and/or evaluating therapeutic options for this condition. My goal was to share the knowledge of the latest state-of-the-art information provided by this international collaborative exercise with those interested in this disease.

With the above in mind, I first divided the different areas of BPD into four categories highlighting *Basic Research*, *Translational Aspects*, *Clinical Aspects*, and *Novel Therapeutic Options*. Next, I distributed the chapters as noted in the table of contents and went about inviting authors who I felt would provide the latest information, as they were actively involved in that area of work. It was such a wonderful feeling when I was able to secure all my first choices of senior authors, in a fairly short time frame. I am extremely grateful to all of them—I consider them more friends, rather than colleagues—for their acceptance of the respective chapters allotted to them and have them delivered to me by the deadline. I am also grateful to the coauthors for working with their mentors and to all of them for their patience as we went through the editing process. The authors hail from the USA, Germany, France, Canada, Spain, Australia, Finland, and South Korea. I hope all of them will enjoy reading the completed product and appreciate the complementary nature of their contributions.

Putting this book together would have been impossible without the support of the Springer team. I would like to express my heartfelt gratitude to Michael Griffin for all his hard work in dotting the "i's" and crossing the "t's" (or more precisely, checking on affiliations, permissions, as well as locating "missing" figures and tables).

I sincerely hope that this book will provide an excellent reference to an international audience for those wishing to stay up to date with BPD. This should (I hope) spur more research into preventing, curing, or at the very least, ameliorating this devastating disease of immaturity. This would not only improve the short-term outcomes for the babies we care for, but in the long run, also decrease the respiratory and neurodevelopmental consequences that impact their health and impose such a significant financial burden on these infants (and their parents) during childhood, adolescence, and even reaching up to adulthood.

Philadelphia, PA Vineet Bhandari

Contents

Part I BPD: Basic Research

1 **Hyperoxia in the Pathogenesis of Bronchopulmonary Dysplasia** 3
Anantha K. Harijith and Vineet Bhandari

2 **Invasive Mechanical Ventilation in the Pathogenesis of Bronchopulmonary Dysplasia** 27
Lauren M. Ramos, Tanbir Najrana, and Juan Sanchez-Esteban

3 **Pre and Postnatal Inflammation in the Pathogenesis of Bronchopulmonary Dysplasia** 55
Kirsten Glaser and Christian P. Speer

4 **Mycoplasma in Bronchopulmonary Dysplasia** 79
Rose M. Viscardi

5 **Chronic Obstructive Pulmonary Disease Following Bronchopulmonary Dysplasia** 93
Alice Hadchouel and Christophe Delacourt

Part II BPD: Translational Aspects

6 **Genetics of Bronchopulmonary Dysplasia** 109
Pascal M. Lavoie

7 **Biomarkers of Bronchopulmonary Dysplasia** 129
Wesley Jackson and Matthew M. Laughon

8 **Pathology of Bronchopulmonary Dysplasia** 149
Monique E. De Paepe

Part III BPD: Clinical Aspects

9 Bronchopulmonary Dysplasia: Definitions and Epidemiology 167
Eduardo Bancalari and Nelson Claure

10 Oxygen Modulation and Bronchopulmonary Dysplasia: Delivery Room and Beyond 183
Isabel Torres-Cuevas, María Cernada, Antonio Nuñez, and Maximo Vento

11 Noninvasive Ventilation for the Prevention of Bronchopulmonary Dysplasia 199
Louise S. Owen, Brett J. Manley, Vineet Bhandari, and Peter G. Davis

12 Nutrition in Bronchopulmonary Dysplasia: In the NICU and Beyond 223
Richard A. Ehrenkranz and Fernando R. Moya

13 Radiology of Bronchopulmonary Dysplasia: From Preterm Birth to Adulthood 243
Outi Tammela and Päivi Korhonen

14 Pulmonary Hypertension in Bronchopulmonary Dysplasia 259
Charitharth Vivek Lal and Namasivayam Ambalavanan

15 Pulmonary Function in Survivors of Bronchopulmonary Dysplasia 281
Jennifer S. Landry and Simon P. Banbury

Part IV BPD: Novel Therapeutic Options

16 Stem Cells for the Prevention of Bronchopulmonary Dysplasia 299
Won Soon Park

17 Less Invasive Surfactant Administration (LISA) for the Prevention of Bronchopulmonary Dysplasia 315
Wolfgang Göpel, Angela Kribs, and Egbert Herting

18 Anti-inflammatory Agents for the Prevention of Bronchopulmonary Dysplasia 325
Sneha Taylor and Virender K. Rehan

Index 345

Contributors

Namasivayam Ambalavanan, MBBS, MD, FAAP Division of Neonatology, Department of Pediatrics, University of Alabama, Birmingham, AL, USA

Women and Infant Center, University of Alabama, Birmingham, AL, USA

Childrens Hospital of Alabama, Birmingham, AL, USA

Simon P. Banbury, BSc, PhD Psychology Department, C3 Human Factors Consulting, Quebec City, QC, Canada

Eduardo Bancalari, MD Division of Neonatology, Department of Pediatrics, University of Miami School of Medicine, Miami, FL, USA

Vineet Bhandari, MBBS, MD, DM Department of Neonatology (Pediatrics), Drexel University College of Medicine, St. Christopher's Hospital for Children, Philadelphia, PA, USA

Hahnemann University Hospital, Philadelphia, PA, USA

Temple University Hospital, Philadelphia, PA, USA

María Cernada, MD Health Research Institute La Fe, Neonatal Research Group, Valencia, Spain

Nelson Claure, MSc, PhD Division of Neonatology, Department of Pediatrics, University of Miami School of Medicine, Miami, FL, USA

Peter G. Davis, MD, MBBS Royal Women's Hospital, Neonatal Services and Newborn Research Centre

Department of Obstetrics and Gynaecology, University of Melbourne, Melbourne, VIC, Australia

Monique E. De Paepe, MD Department of Pathology, Women and Infants Hospital of Rhode Island, Providence, RI, USA

Christophe Delacourt, MD, PhD Pediatric Pulmonology, Necker-Enfants Malades Hospital, Paris, France

INSERM, Créteil, France

Paris-Descartes University, Sorbonne Paris Cité, Paris, France

Richard A. Ehrenkranz, MD Department of Pediatrics/Section of Neonatal-Perinatal Medicine, Yale University School of Medicine, New Haven, CT, USA

Kirsten Glaser, MD University Children's Hospital, University of Würzburg, Würzburg, Bavaria, Germany

Wolfgang Göpel, MD Department of Pediatrics, University Hospital Schleswig Holstein, Campus Lübeck, Lübeck, Germany

Alice Hadchouel, MD, PhD Pediatric Pulmonology, Necker-Enfants Malades Hospital, Paris, France

INSERM, Créteil, France

Paris-Descartes University, Sorbonne Paris Cité, Paris, France

Anantha K. Harijth, MD, MRCP (UK) Department of Pediatrics, Children's Hospital at University of Illinois Chicago, Chicago, IL, USA

Egbert Herting, MD, PhD Department of Pediatrics, University Hospital Schleswig Holstein, Campus Lübeck, Lübeck, Germany

Wesley Jackson, MD Division of Neonatal-Perinatal Medicine, University of North Carolina at Chapel Hill, Chapel Hill, NC, USA

Päivi Korhonen, MD, PhD Department of Pediatrics, Tampere University Hospital, Tampere, Finland

Angela Kribs, MD Department of Pediatrics, University Hospital Cologne, Cologne, Germany

Charitharth Vivek Lal, MBBS, FAAP Division of Neonatology, Department of Pediatrics, University of Alabama, Birmingham, AL, USA

Women and Infant Center, University of Alabama, Birmingham, AL, USA

Childrens Hospital of Alabama, Birmingham, AL, USA

Jennifer S. Landry, MD, MSc, FRCP(C) Montreal Chest Institute, McGill University Health Center, Montréal, QC, Canada

Matthew M. Laughon, MD, MPH Division of Neonatal-Perinatal Medicine, University of North Carolina at Chapel Hill, Chapel Hill, NC, USA

Pascal M. Lavoie, MDCM, PhD, FRCPC Child and Family Research Institute, Vancouver, BC, Canada

Division of Neonatology, Department of Pediatrics, University of British Columbia, Vancouver, BC, Canada

Department of Pediatrics, Division of Neonatology, Children's and Women's Health Centre of British Columbia, Vancouver, BC, Canada

Brett J. Manley, MBBS (Hons), PhD Royal Women's Hospital, Neonatal Services and Newborn Research Centre

Department of Obstetrics and Gynaecology, University of Melbourne, Melbourne, VIC, Australia

Fernando R. Moya, MD Betty Cameron Children's Hospital, Wilmington, NC, USA

Tanbir Najrana, PhD Department of Pediatrics, Neonatal-Perinatal Medicine, Women and Infants Hospital of Rhode Island, The Warren Alpert Medical School of Brown University, Providence, RI, USA

Antonio Nuñez, MD Health Research Institute La Fe, Neonatal Research Group, Valencia, Spain

Louise S. Owen, MBChB, MRCPCH, FRACP, MD Royal Women's Hospital, Neonatal Services and Newborn Research Centre

Department of Obstetrics and Gynaecology, University of Melbourne, Melbourne, VIC, Australia

Won Soon Park, MD, PhD Department of Pediatrics, Sungkyunkwan University School of Medicine, Samsung Medical Center, Kangnam Gu, Seoul, South Korea

Lauren M. Ramos, MD Department of Pediatrics, Neonatal-Perinatal Medicine, Women and Infants Hospital of Rhode Island, The Warren Alpert Medical School of Brown University, Providence, RI, USA

Virender K. Rehan, MD, MRCP (UK), MRCPI (Dublin) Department of Neonatology, Pediatrics, Harbor-UCLA Medical Center, Torrance, CA, USA

Juan Sanchez-Esteban, MD Department of Pediatrics, Neonatal-Perinatal Medicine, Women and Infants Hospital of Rhode Island, The Warren Alpert Medical School of Brown University, Providence, RI, USA

Christian P. Speer, MD, FRCPE University Children's Hospital, University of Würzburg, Würzburg, Bavaria, Germany

Outi Tammela, MD, PhD Department of Pediatrics, Tampere University Hospital, Tampere, Finland

Sneha Taylor, MBBS, MD, FAAP Department of Neonatology, Pediatrics, Harbor-UCLA Medical Center, Torrance, CA, USA

Isabel Torres-Cuevas, PharmD, MSc Health Research Institute La Fe, Neonatal Research Group, Valencia, Spain

Maximo Vento, MD, PhD Division of Neonatology, University and Polytechnic Hospital La Fe, Valencia, Spain

Rose M. Viscardi, MD Department of Pediatrics, University of Maryland School of Medicine, Baltimore, MD, USA

Part I
BPD: Basic Research

Chapter 1
Hyperoxia in the Pathogenesis of Bronchopulmonary Dysplasia

Anantha K. Harijith and Vineet Bhandari

Introduction

Bronchopulmonary dysplasia (BPD) is a disease that is multifactorial in origin secondary to genetic and environmental factors including exposure to invasive mechanical ventilation, ante- and post-natal infections, and hyperoxia [1]. Among the aforementioned environmental factors, the contribution of hyperoxia to the pathogenesis of BPD is well established [2–5]. Compulsive evidence of the role of hyperoxia in the causation of BPD was demonstrated in a clinical study by Deulofeut et al. who found decreased incidence of BPD in infants born at <1250 g when they were treated with target oxygen saturation of 85–92 % compared to a similar cohort of infants who had a target oxygen saturation of 92–100 % [6]. A major clinical study that studied the efficacy and safety of supplemental therapeutic oxygen in infants was the Supplemental Therapeutic Oxygen for Prethreshold Retinopathy of Prematurity (STOP-ROP) trial. The STOP-ROP trial randomized infants to two target groups—one with a lower saturation of 89–94 % and the other with a higher level of 96–99 % [7]. The trial found that use of supplemental oxygen at saturations of 96–99 % did not cause additional progression of prethreshold ROP but higher rates of pneumonia and BPD. Those infants with underlying lung disease targeted

A.K. Harijith, MD, MRCP (UK) (✉)
Department of Pediatrics, Children's Hospital at University of Illinois Chicago, 840 S Wood St., Chicago, IL, 60612, USA
e-mail: harijith@uic.edu

V. Bhandari, MBBS, MD, DM
Department of Neonatology (Pediatrics), Drexel University College of Medicine, St. Christopher's Hospital for Children, 160 East Erie Avenue, Philadelphia, PA, 19134, USA

Hahnemann University Hospital, Philadelphia, PA, USA

Temple University Hospital, Philadelphia, PA, USA
e-mail: vineet.bhandari@drexelmed.edu

V. Bhandari (ed.), *Bronchopulmonary Dysplasia*, Respiratory Medicine,
DOI 10.1007/978-3-319-28486-6_1

to the higher oxygen saturation range were more likely to be hospitalized and in need of supplemental oxygen and diuretic therapy at 3 months of age. Other clinical studies have also found that chronic exposure to high oxygen saturations can injure the lungs of preterm infants [6, 8].

Transition from in utero life from a relative hypoxic environment into room air at birth in itself is a relatively hyperoxic event, even for a term infant with mature lungs. In case of a preterm infant with less mature lungs, the transition to ex utero environment takes a toll on lung development. The structurally and functionally immature lungs of preterm infants are inadequately prepared to oxygenate the body in room air. This necessitates administration of elevated levels of O_2 to prevent hypoxia, exacerbating the magnitude of the injury from hyperoxic exposure. Clinical evidence of the harmful effects of hyperoxia to the newborn developing lung has emerged recently, as detailed below.

Pathology of New BPD

Advances in medicine along with the use of newer therapies, such as prenatal steroids, exogenous surfactant, and “gentle” ventilation strategies, have increased the survival of infants of younger gestational age. This increase in survival rates of extreme preterm newborns has resulted in an increase in the number of children with BPD and associated respiratory pathologies. It has been noted that along with the improvement in survival the morphology of BPD has changed to what is described as the “new” BPD. “New” BPD occurring in very preterm infants (mean gestational age of less than 28 weeks) is characterized by alveolar hypoplasia and abnormal vascular organization [9, 10]. There is minimal to no fibrosis of lung tissue. This represents an impairment in the saccular stage of lung development due to interference, or an interruption, in the stage of rapid alveolar and distal vascular development of the lung [9, 11]. It has also been argued that BPD represents altered developmental programming of the lung due to external factors. The exact mechanisms leading to the impaired or altered programing of lung development are unclear. Hence, there is an urgent need to understand how prematurity and related exposure to O_2 contribute to the pathogenesis of BPD and morbidity later in life.

Hyperoxia-Induced Animal Models of BPD

Newborn animal models have helped us to understand the effects of exposure to hyperoxia in the developing lung, resulting in histopathologic findings similar to those observed in BPD of the human neonate [2, 12–14]. Newborn animal models of BPD survive at least twice as long as adults in hyperoxia and are noted to have a significantly later onset of inflammation [15, 16]. Along with monocytes/macrophages and lymphocytes, stromal, epithelial, and endothelial cells can release significant amount of chemokines. Experiments in adult animal species showed that exposure to high levels of O_2 leads to pulmonary endothelial and epithelial cell injury, followed by pulmonary edema and hemorrhage impairing lung function [17–19]. However, some interesting observations have been made regarding the differences in response to hyperoxia in newborn and adult animals [15–17, 20]. Upon exposure to hyperoxia, 100 % of the adult mice die within 3–7 days, whereas most newborn pups survive beyond 1 week [12, 21]. This difference is probably due to the developmental regulation of the response to hyperoxia. This sensitivity to hyperoxia in adult animals has been attributed, in part, to rapid death of microvascular endothelial and alveolar type I epithelial cells [22, 23] leading to respiratory insufficiency.

Newborn mouse models of BPD with alveolar simplification have been developed by exposure of neonatal mice to 85–100 % O_2 following birth [14, 24, 25]. Similarly, in another model of preterm ventilated baboons, it was demonstrated that the percentage of O_2 exposure plays a role in alveolar simplification and the overall outcome [26]. Preterm baboons exposed to 100 % O_2 for 11 days developed severe lung injury and BPD-like lung morphology, whereas animals exposed to a lower level of 30 % O_2 had minimal lung damage.

Premature baboons delivered at equivalent to approximately 30 weeks of gestation (75 % of gestation) in humans and ventilated with the minimum required O_2 to maintain normal arterial oxygen concentrations had significantly less damage than those ventilated with 100 % O_2 [26]. However, baboons delivered at a stage comparable to 26 weeks of gestation (67 % of gestation) in humans and managed with the minimum necessary mechanical ventilation and supplemental O_2 still developed BPD-like lung morphology characterized by alveolar hypoplasia and variable saccular wall fibrosis [13]. Hyperoxia appears to worsen the severity of lung injury in animal models of BPD. Lung injury is likely to occur with lower amounts of supplemental O_2 at earlier stages of lung development.

Reports of BPD in infants <1000 g birth weight with minimal initial O_2 supplementation and ventilatory support suggest that high level of O_2 supplementation is not an absolute requirement for the development of BPD [9, 27–29]. It is a combination of the immature stage of lung development and some degree of (relative) hyperoxia that induces the pathology of BPD. However, supplemental O_2 exposure remains as one of the main inciting agents for the development of BPD.

Mechanism of Lung Injury Secondary to Hyperoxia

Causation of BPD is primarily attributed to the premature exposure to high concentration of O_2 and the production of cytotoxic reactive oxygen species (ROS) and reactive nitrogen species (RNS) that injure developing lungs [30, 31]. Studies in animal models have demonstrated that hyperoxia initially induces focal endothelial cell injury and, with continued exposure, necrosis of epithelial cells [32, 33]. Pulmonary microvascular endothelial cells undergo rapid necrosis, leaving areas of denuded capillary basement membrane. Disruption of the alveolar–capillary basement membrane leads to exudation of fluid into the alveoli, adversely affecting gas exchange as well as the pulmonary mechanics [34]. Premature infants born during the stage of primary septation have disruption of rapid alveolar formation following exposure to hyperoxia. Primary septation of early air spaces occurs during the saccular phase (24–36 weeks gestational age) and the secondary septation and true alveolar development in the alveolar stage at approximately 36 weeks of gestation extending through 2 to perhaps, 8 years of age [14, 35–37].

In the normal intrauterine development, hypoxia-inducible factor 1 alpha (HIF-1α) produced in the hypoxic environment increases production of vascular endothelial growth factor (VEGF), which is involved in facilitating appropriate formation of the pulmonary and alveolar vasculature [38]. Premature exposure to hyperoxia results in the degradation of HIF-1α followed by decreased VEGF levels and interruption of pulmonary vascular development. Studies have shown that the disrupted vascularization adversely impacts alveolar formation. Thebaud et al. have demonstrated that development of the pulmonary vasculature drives alveolar development [39]. Vadivel et al. showed that inhibition of VEGF interrupted vascular development and blunted alveolar formation [40]. The same authors demonstrated that intratracheal administration of an adenovirus encoding for a stable form of HIF-1α increased HIF-1α and VEGF in the lung tissue. This improved alveolar growth and capillary formation in a neonatal rat model of hyperoxia-induced alveolar arrest. Another study utilized mice expressing a stable form of HIF-1α demonstrated increased alveolar formation during the early prenatal period [41].

Oxygen-induced injury is primarily mediated through both ROS and RNS [42–44]. It is well established that ROS, when produced in moderation, plays a physiological role in mediating intracellular signaling pathways involved in normal cell growth and differentiation as well as cytotoxic responses during host defense [45]. ROS function physiologically as signaling molecules mediating various growth-related responses including angiogenesis. ROS-driven angiogenesis can be regulated by endogenous antioxidant enzymes such as superoxide dismutase (SOD) and thioredoxin. NADPH oxidase (Nox) is the major source of ROS in endothelial cells (ECs). Nox is composed of proteins Nox1, Nox2, Nox4, Nox5, p22phox, p47phox, and the small G-protein Rac1 [46]. In addition to hypoxia and ischemia, NADPH oxidase is activated by various growth factors including VEGF and angiopoietin-1. VEGF stimulates EC proliferation and migration primarily through the VEGF receptor type 2 (VEGFR2, Flk1/KDR) [47]. ROS derived from Nox is involved in VEGFR2 autophosphorylation, leading to induction of transcription factors and genes involved in angiogenesis. Another angiogenic agent known to enhance hyperoxia-induced lung injury is angiopoietin-2 [48, 49]. Increased levels of angiopoietin-2 have been associated with increased BPD and/death in human preterm neonates [50].

Oxidative stress occurs when the production of ROS exceeds the antioxidant capacity of the cell resulting in cellular and tissue injury via lipid peroxidation, DNA damage, and protein oxidation [43]. ROS is generated both by the mitochondrial system and by the NADPH oxidase systems in lung tissue upon exposure to hyperoxia. Lung ECs generate ROS initially followed by inflammatory cells. It has been shown that both necrosis and apoptosis occur simultaneously in the same cell types upon hyperoxia exposure. It is assumed that both apoptotic and necrotic pathways of cell death might be induced in hyperoxia [51–55].

Studies in human neonates have shown a decrease in levels of antioxidants and an increase in oxidative damage to pulmonary proteins in the epithelial lining fluid or plasma of ventilated oxygen-dependent preterm infants in comparison to those infants who were not oxygen dependent [56–58]. The nutritional state of the newborn and exposure to antenatal corticosteroids also play a role in early-life sensitivity to oxygen [59–64].

ROS generated in excess such as the superoxide anion (O_2^-) reacts with nitric oxide (NO) generated in the vascular endothelium forming peroxynitrite. Peroxynitrite reacts to form additional RNS including nitrogen dioxide ($NO_2^{\bullet}$), dinitrogen trioxide (N_2O_3), nitrosoperoxycarbonate ($ONOOCO_2^-$), and carbonate radical ($O{=}C(O^{\bullet})O^-$). RNS reacts with lipids, thiols, amino acid residues, DNA bases, and low-molecular weight antioxidants while depleting the activity of NO [65]. NO is a key mediator of vascular smooth muscle tone and cell signaling [66].

It is known that alveolar type II epithelial cells are more resistant to hyperoxic injury and participate in repair of the injured lung [67]. Hyperoxia not only triggers increased production of ROS and RNS activating cytotoxic pathways but also protective pathways such as that of the transcription factor nuclear factor-erythroid 2-related factor 2 (Nrf2). Nrf2 is known to regulate the inducible gene expression of antioxidant enzymes, critical in detoxifying oxygen-mediated generation of ROS [68, 69]. Nrf2 knockout mice exhibit aggravated lung injury and the absence of upregulation of antioxidant enzymes in response to hyperoxia [70]. Assessment of the role of Nrf2 activation in the neonatal lung has improved our understanding of endogenous antioxidant responses. Under normal conditions, Nrf2 is sequestered by Keap1, and oxidative stress leads to activation and degradation of Keap1 [71–73]. Nrf2 released from Keap1 translocates to the nucleus and activates antioxidant response elements which modulate antioxidant genes. Nrf2 hence plays a key role in activating antioxidant mechanisms necessary for cell survival [68, 72]. Newborn $Nrf2^{-/-}$ mice have more lung injury and impaired alveolarization due to hyperoxia exposure [74, 75]. In fact, in human subjects, a single nucleotide polymorphism in the Nrf2 promoter region in humans has been identified to increase the risk of acute lung injury [76]. Newborn mice overexpressing mitochondrial manganese SOD (MnSOD) or extracellular SOD (ecSOD) in alveolar type II epithelial cells, and exposed to hyperoxia, had preservation of postnatal lung development [77, 78]. Impaired mitochondrial function promotes alveolar simplification in newborn mice, mimicking the impact of exposure to hyperoxia [79]. P53, a known tumor suppressor protein, protects cells from damage by modulating the transcription of genes that inhibit cell proliferation, promote DNA repair, and facilitate apoptosis of damaged cells. Studies have revealed that p53 can affect the maintenance of mitochondrial homeostasis [80], but whether p53 signaling contributes to neonatal lung disease remains to be determined.

Animal studies have demonstrated that hyperoxia exposure increases airway epithelial layer thickness [81] and airway smooth muscle area [82]. O'Reilly et al. examined the long-term effects of neonatal exposure to hyperoxia in mice and found that at 10 months postnatal age neonatal mice exposed to 65 % O_2 for 21 days from birth demonstrated increased airway smooth muscle, but no differences were noted in the bronchiolar epithelium or collagen deposition [83]. Mice exposed to moderate hyperoxia (40 % O_2) for 7 days demonstrated increased airway reactivity and increased airway smooth muscle compared to room air [84]. Hyperoxia exposure may contribute to neonatal lung injury and airway hyperreactivity by disruption of nitric oxide (NO)-cyclic guanosine monophosphate (cGMP) signaling and elevated arginase activity [85]. Thus, hyperoxia causes both alveolar growth impairment and airway remodeling in a dose dependent manner.

Been et al. in a systemic meta-analysis looking at incidence of childhood wheezing disorders found an increased risk (30–90 %) of wheezing in preterm compared to term infants. Extreme preterm infants were at the highest risk, with a three times greater incidence of wheezing disorders compared to term infants [86]. Higher risk of BPD in extreme preterms (<27 weeks) is well established, but a recent study examined respiratory symptoms in moderately premature infants (gestational age 32–37 weeks) and showed an increased risk of wheezing and airway disease as late as 5 years of age in former premature infants, indicating that even these relatively healthier premature infants are impacted by respiratory morbidities [87].

The airway epithelium serves as a first line of defense for the airway by playing a key role in the initiation of immunoprotective and inflammatory responses. Pulmonary epithelial cells when exposed to pathogens and subsequently to hyperoxia showed augmented injury characterized by increased alveolar neutrophils, histological injury, and epithelial barrier permeability [88]. Further disruption of this layer leads to increased barrier disruption, pulmonary permeability, and infiltration of inflammatory mediators into the alveoli leading to airway inflammation and remodeling [89].

Hyperoxia is associated with an inflammatory response in the acute phase of exposure in the immature lung [2, 18, 90] resulting in a significant macrophage and polymorphonuclear cell (PMN) infiltration, which results in interstitial edema aggravating injury to endothelial and epithelial cells [89]. ROS is produced by immune cell infiltrates, particularly neutrophils that result in increased mitochondrial stress and activation of apoptotic pathways. This leads to lung injury and airway remodeling in premature infants at risk of developing BPD. Tracheal aspirates and bronchoalveolar lavage (BAL) fluid from preterm infants have been shown to have significantly increased levels of proinflammatory mediators [91]. Increased mast cell and eosinophil infiltration into lungs have also been noted in infants with BPD [92, 93].

Molecular Mechanisms of Hyperoxia-Induced Lung Cell Injury and Cell Death

Hyperoxia-induced inflammation is partly due to ROS and RNS triggered inflammatory response and due to cell death triggered inflammation. A proposed mechanism delineating the known pathways to hyperoxia-induced lung injury is shown in Fig. 1.1. In addition to generation of ROS, activation of key caspases and

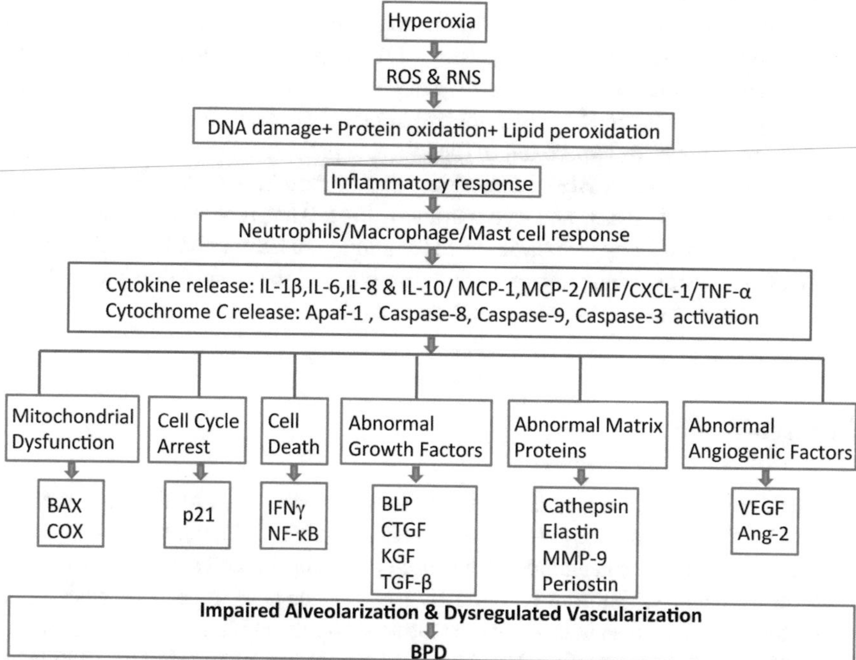

Fig. 1.1 Exposure to hyperoxia leads to expression of reactive oxygen species (ROS) and reactive nitrogen species (RNS). This causes DNA damage, protein oxidation, and lipid peroxidation which are manifested as an inflammatory response as well as a neutrophils/macrophage/mast cell response. This is followed by release of cytokines, cytochrome C, and caspases, thus leading to mitochondrial dysfunction, cell cycle arrest, cell death, abnormal growth factors, abnormal matrix proteins, or abnormal angiogenic factor production. This in turn can lead to inappropriate expression of bcl-2-like protein 4 (BAX), cyclooxygenase (COX), protein 21, interferon gamma (IFNγ), nuclear factor-kappa B (NF-κB), bombesin-like peptide (BLP), connective tissue growth factor (CTGF), keratinocyte growth factor (KGF), transforming growth factor beta (TGF-β), cathepsin, elastin, matrix matelloprotease 9 (MMP-9), periostin, vascular endothelial growth factor (VEGF), and angiopoietin 2 (Ang-2). A combination of aforementioned cascading events leads to impaired alveolarization and dysregulated vasularization, causing bronchopulmonary dysplasia (BPD). *IL* interleukin, *MCP* monocyte chemoattractant protein, *MIF* macrophage migration inhibitory factor, *CXCL* chemokine (C-X-C motif) ligand, *TNF* tumor necrosis factor

components of the extrinsic/death receptor and intrinsic/mitochondrial cell death pathways along with other cytokines appears to underlie the molecular mechanisms of hyperoxia-induced lung cell injury and cell death.

Caspases and Components of the Cell Death Pathway

Caspase-8 is activated downstream of the extrinsic pathway triggered by surface "death receptors" such as Fas binding to Fas ligand, and tumor necrosis factor (TNF) receptor 1. In addition, a key role in modulating cell death is played by NF-κB- the redox sensitive transcription factor, protein kinase B/Akt, and the members of the Bcl-2 gene family (comprising of three groups: antiapoptotic Bcl-2 and Bcl-xL, proapoptotic Bax-type proteins, and proapoptotic BH3-domain-only family members) [52]. Mitochondrial dysfunction signals cell death through the intrinsic pathway in response to hyperoxia. In the intrinsic pathway, Caspase-9 activation is preceded by activation of BH3 domain-only family members such as Bid, Bax-type proteins (Bax, Bak, Bok), and cytochrome *c* [94]. The mitochondrial-dependent pathway is relevant in hyperoxia-induced lung injury, as mitochondria maintain the levels of adenosine triphosphate (ATP) through cellular respiration and release death-promoting factors, such as cytochrome *c* [52].

Interleukin-1

Interleukin-1 (IL-1) along with the three known constituents of the IL-1 family, IL-1α, IL-1β, IL-1 receptor antagonist (IL-1RA), and IL-1 receptors (IL-1R) could play a role in hyperoxia induced lung injury leading to BPD. Newborn rabbits exposed to hyperoxia showed elevated IL-1 by 2–4 days of hyperoxia, peaking at 6–10 days [95]. Changes in IL-1β were paralleled by the evidence of a rise in histologic evidence of inflammation [95]. Transgenic mice overexpressing IL-1β in lung epithelial cells led to a BPD phenotype in neonatal mice [96].

IL-6

IL-6 acts as an autocrine, paracrine, and exocrine inflammatory hormone and is secreted by stimulated monocyte/macrophages, fibroblasts, epithelial, and endothelial cells [97]. The tracheal aspirates of IL-6 levels in the premature baboon model of BPD, on days 9–10 and 16–44, were significantly increased when compared with those at 48–72 h [13]. IL-6 showed a significant elevation in mice treated with IL-1 demonstrating a downstream response [97]. Neonatal mice exposed to hyperoxia had a significant increase in lung mRNA for IL-6 after 7 days of exposure [15] and those mice with increased lung IL-6 levels had increased mortality on hyperoxia exposure [98].

Dexamethasone treatment reduced the levels of IL-6 in newborn rats exposed to 48 h of hyperoxia (95 $\%O_2$) [99].

IL-8/Cytokine-Induced Neutrophil Chemoattractant-1

IL-8 protein levels were significantly increased and correlated with infiltration of the neutrophils in the BAL fluid [95]. Upregulation of cytokine-induced neutrophil chemoattractant-1 (CINC-1) in premature rat lungs [100] and newborn rabbits [95] was noted following exposure to prolonged hyperoxia (10 days) [101].

IL-1β, 6, and 8 are expressed significantly in the acute phase response to injury. These proinflammatory agents are elevated very early following exposure to hyperoxia in the human preterm population who ultimately develop BPD [102].

IL-10

IL-10 acts as an anti-inflammatory agent as it suppresses activation of macrophages and dendritic cells. This suppresses the secretion of cytokines and the ability of those cells to function as accessory cells for T-cell and NK-cell stimulation [97]. Serum and tracheal aspirate IL-10 levels were found decreased in those infants who developed BPD [102].

Keratinocyte Growth Factor

Tracheal aspirate keratinocyte growth factor (KGF) concentrations were elevated in survivors without BPD, compared to those who developed BPD [103].

Monocyte Chemoattractant Protein-1

Monocyte chemoattractant protein-1 (MCP-1) is one of the ligands for CCR2 and it acts as a chemoattractant for monocytes, lymphocytes, and basophils. It is produced by a variety of cells in response to inflammatory stimuli [97]. MCP-1 levels were increased in tracheal aspirates of very low birth weight infants who developed BPD [104]. Anti-MCP-1 treatment given to newborn rats exposed to hyperoxia at birth ameliorated injury to developing lungs [105].

Matrix Metalloproteinase 9

Studies have come up with divergent findings on matrix metalloproteinase 9 (MMP9). MMP9 expression was found to be decreased in neonatal rat lungs exposed to hyperoxia in one study [106], whereas another reported an increase [107]. MMP9 was increased in the lungs of the baboon model of BPD [108]. MMP9 null mutant neonatal mice were protected from hyperoxia-induced lung injury [109], but in the IL-1β transgenic model of BPD, lack of MMP9 worsened the BPD phenotype [110]. Most of the preterm human studies have shown that hyperoxia leads to increased MMP9 levels in the lung and is associated with BPD [111, 112].

Interferon Gamma

Increased level of interferon gamma (IFNγ) following hyperoxia plays a role in mediating neonatal lung injury. This was found to be MMP-9 dependent. Increased concentrations of the downstream targets of IFNγ chemokine (C-X-C motif) ligands (CXCL10 and CXCL11) were noted in baboon and human lungs with BPD. This showed that IFNγ and its downstream targets may contribute to the final common pathway of hyperoxia-induced injury in the developing lung and in human BPD [113, 114].

Treatment of newborn mice with cyclooxygenase-2 inhibitors ameliorated hyperoxia-induced lung injury, which was due to reduction in the endoplasmic reticulum (ER) stress response [115]. Mitogen-activated protein kinases (MAPKs) contribute to activation of ER stress responses [116], and thus MAPKs serve as a link between oxidant injury and cellular stress responses.

Transforming Growth Factor Beta

Transforming growth factor beta (TGFβ) signaling was potentiated by hyperoxia and it was evident that primary alveolar type II cells were more susceptible to TGFβ-induced apoptosis. Lung growth and compliance were significantly impaired in pups exposed to 85 % O_2, accompanied by dysregulated expression and localization of TGFβ receptor (ALK-1, ALK-3, ALK-6, and the TGF-beta type II receptor) and Smad (Smads 1, 3, and 4) proteins [117]. Li et al. have shown that the effects of hyperoxia were mediated via the c-jun N-terminal kinase (JNK) pathway. Increased expression of TGF-β1 by epithelial cells on exposure to hyperoxia was noted and inhibition of JNK signaling significantly improved the spontaneously impaired alveolarization in room air and decreased mortality on exposure to hyperoxia in lung epithelial cell targeted TGF-β1-overexpressing mice [118]. This was confirmed in another study where it was shown that increased TGFβ1 expression in newborn mice lungs led to increased mortality, macrophage and immature monocyte infiltration, apoptotic cell death specifically in type II alveolar epithelial cells (AECs) accompanied by impaired alveolarization, and dysregulated angiogenic molecular markers [119].

Tumor Necrosis Factor Alpha

Human neonates who developed BPD showed increased levels of tumor necrosis factor alpha (TNFα) in the tracheal aspirates [102]. Lung tissue of neonatal rat and mice pups exposed to hyperoxia also showed an increase in TNFα [15].

Macrophage Migration Inhibiting Factor

It is now known that macrophage migration inhibiting factor (MIF) plays a significant role in lung maturation and a protective role in newborn lung disease [120]. The lungs of pups genetically deficient in MIF demonstrated lower levels of VEGF and corticosterone. A lack or an excess of MIF in the developing lung leads to impaired pulmonary architecture. In neonatal murine models partial recovery of the pulmonary phenotype was demonstrated in the wild-type BPD model treated with the MIF agonist, as well as the MIF transgenic (TG) mice treated with the MIF antagonist [121]. These data point to the careful regulatory balance exerted by MIF in the developing lung and response to hyperoxia and support. Angiopoietins 1, 2 and their receptor Tie2 could play a potential role in the MIF-regulated response in room air and upon hyperoxia exposure in the neonatal lung [122].

VEGF

Though widely expressed in tissues, the highest amount of this dimeric glycoprotein is present in lung tissue [97]. It has been shown in various animal models that VEGF and its receptors increase in normal animal lung development; however, its pathophysiological role in neonatal respiratory failure is not yet entirely clear [123]. In humans, a bimodal distribution of VEGF levels has been noted with proportionately higher levels measured within the first 12 h of life followed by another rise at 3–4 weeks of gestational age. VEGF acts through specific transmembrane receptor tyrosine kinase (RTK) receptors; such as VEGFR1/Flt-1 and KDR/Flk-1/VEGFR2 [97]. VEGF, by promoting endothelial cell growth and remodeling, plays a significant role in the appropriate development of alveolar tissue. Premature human infants who recover without BPD have progressively increasing VEGF levels over time, whereas babies who developed BPD had decreased VEGF levels [124]. Hyperoxia causes microvascular injury and VEGF plays a role in the repair and remodeling process and its levels are often increased disproportionately. In an animal model of BPD using premature fetal baboons delivered at 125 days (term is 140 days) and treated with oxygen and mechanical ventilation as needed for 14 days, the expression of VEGF mRNA and protein was markedly decreased along with the expression of VEGFR1 by 40 % while VEGFR2 mRNA expression was unchanged [97, 123].

A role for mitochondrial oxidants initiating BAX- or BAK-dependent alveolar epithelial cell death contributing to hyperoxia-induced lung injury has been demonstrated [125].

Mechanisms of increased ROS generation by changes in oxygen pressure from 150 to 300 mmHg are unclear, but hyperoxia stimulates signaling pathways mediated by Rac1 [126], MAP kinases [127], PI3 kinase-Akt [128], cytoskeletal redistribution [46], and formation of lipid rafts [129] that contribute to NOX-dependent and independent ROS formation leading to lung injury. In addition, lipid peroxides can form as a result of hyperoxia. These peroxides damage the inner mitochondrial membrane, release cytochrome C and cellular apoptosis. This can contribute to disruption of postnatal alveolar development, inflammation, and potentially fibrosis [130, 131]. In addition, major transcription factors regulated by ROS are HIF, Nrf2, and AP-1 [89, 132, 133], as discussed earlier.

Bombesin-Like Peptide

A variety of exogenously administered agents downregulate the toxicity induced by hyperoxia by modulating local cell death responses [97]. Increased numbers of pulmonary neuroendocrine cells containing Bombesin-like peptide (BLP) have been reported to occur in human infants with BPD [134, 135]. Urine BLP levels correlated with the development of BPD in both the animal model and humans [134, 136]. Using a baboon model, postnatal administration of anti-BLP antibody attenuated features of hyperoxia-induced lung injury [134].

Hepatocyte Growth Factor

Exposure of neonatal rats to hyperoxia upregulated expression of lung hepatocyte growth factor (HGF) [137]. While anti-HGF treatment led to a simplified alveolar structure in neonatal rat pups in room air [137], other investigators reported that recombinant HGF partially protected against the inhibition of alveolarization and improved lung function in a hyperoxia-induced neonatal mice model of BPD. Lower levels of HGF in tracheal aspirate were associated with more severe lung disease in preterm human newborns [138].

Sphingosine-1-Phosphate

Harijith et al. found that sphingosine-1-phosphate (S1P) synthesized in the lung tissue following hyperoxia promotes alveolar simplification. Hyperoxia promotes increased sphingosine kinase 1 (SphK-1) expression which catalyzes increased formation of S1P from sphingosine. Sphingosine kinase-1 knockout neonatal mice showed significant protection against hyperoxia-induced lung injury [139].

Melatonin

Melatonin (MT) is a pleiotropic molecule secreted by the pineal gland as a circadian rhythm transducer. MT has multiple antioxidant effects exerted through actions on different pathways [140]. MT is a direct antioxidant as it presents scavenger properties against ROS. It activates different intracellular signaling pathways triggered by G-proteins, calcium–calmodulin complex, and nuclear factor-kappa B (NF-kB) and upregulates the expression of antioxidants, particularly glutathione peroxidase (GPx), glutathione reductase (GRx), SOD, and catalase (CAT) [140]. In a clinical trial, MT administered to 110 preterm newborns with RDS was associated with significantly lower ventilator settings and circulating levels of IL-6, IL-8, and TNFα compared to untreated controls [141]. Data on long-term respiratory outcomes and the incidence of BPD in preterm newborns are not known [142].

Superoxide Dismutase

SOD is considered an enzyme crucial to maintain lung function. Studies in animal and cellular models showed that the absence of SOD3 activity induces severe lung injury during hyperoxia, whereas SOD2 overexpression in type II alveolar cells is associated with prolonged survival in a hyperoxic environment [78, 143]. SOD3 administration in animal models reduced hyperoxic lung injury and the need for mechanical ventilation [144–147]. In animal models, exogenously administered SOD got rapidly incorporated into different lung cell types following endotracheal administration [146]. Endotracheal administration of recombinant human SOD (rhSOD) helped to reduce lung injury in preterm newborns receiving mechanical ventilation for RDS [148, 149]. In a trial, 26 newborns with birth weight <1250 g were randomized to receive placebo, low-dose, or high-dose rhSOD within 30 min after the first surfactant. SOD levels in serum, tracheal aspirates, and urine significantly increased in the treatment group with respect to the placebo group [148]. The lung protective effect of the treatment was dose dependent and tracheal aspirates of SOD-treated newborns showed lower levels of markers of acute lung injury such as neutrophil chemotactic activity and albumin concentration. But the brief increase in SOD following a single administration of SOD did not affect the risk of BPD and hence a regimen of repeated endotracheal administration of SOD was subsequently studied [149]. In this randomized controlled trial, a cohort of 36 preterm newborn with birth weight <1300 g were given placebo, low, or high dose of endotracheal rhSOD within 2 h of surfactant treatment and every 48 h as long as the infant remained on mechanical ventilation, up to seven doses. In spite of giving multiple doses, no differences in the rate of BPD were detected [149, 150]. In a follow-up report, the subgroup of rhSOD-treated infants born before 27 weeks of gestational age had a 55 % reduction in wheezing episodes, emergency department visits, and a 44 % reduction in hospitalization compared to the gestational age-matched untreated infants [150].

Summary and Conclusions

Hyperoxia plays a significant role in the pathogenesis of BPD which is a condition of multifactorial origin. The STOP-ROP trial provided evidence that infants exposed to hyperoxia had a significantly higher rate of BPD. "New" BPD occurring in extreme preterm infants is characterized by alveolar simplification due to impairment in the saccular stage of lung development. Developmental regulation of protective mechanisms in the lung is probably responsible for increased survival of newborns in hyperoxia at the same time contributing to the development of BPD. An understanding of the mechanisms involved in the pathogenesis of BPD is essential to identify therapeutic targets in BPD. Animal models exposed to hyperoxia have served as good models for this purpose. Oxygen-induced injury, which is primarily mediated through both ROS and RNS, causes endothelial cell necrosis affecting angiogenesis leading to impaired alveolar formation. Multiple cytotoxic pathways are affected. The caspase-8 mediated extrinsic pathway of apoptosis activated triggers Fas binding to Fas ligand, and TNF receptor 1. Interleukin system involving IL-1, -6, -8 and -10 is elevated along with an increase in MCP-1, MMP9, and IFNγ. However, hyperoxia potentiated activation of TGFβ signaling was accompanied by dysregulated expression and localization of TGFβ receptor and Smad proteins. This followed activation of the JNK pathway. Inhibition of JNK signaling significantly improved the spontaneously impaired alveolarization in room air and decreased mortality on exposure to hyperoxia in TGFβ1 TG mice. MIF plays a significant role in lung maturation, the deficiency of which was associated with lower levels of VEGF and corticosterone. VEGF plays a crucial role in the development of alveolar tissue, by promoting endothelial cell growth and remodeling. VEGF acts through specific transmembrane RTK receptors. In humans, a bimodal distribution of VEGF levels has been noted, but its pathophysiological role in neonatal respiratory failure is unclear. A role for mitochondrial oxidants initiating BAX- or BAK-dependent alveolar epithelial cell death contributing to hyperoxia-induced lung injury has been demonstrated. Experimental therapy with SOD has not been successful in humans.

Promoting protective pathways as mediated by Nrf-2, suppression of ROS producing pathways by inhibitors of sphingosine kinase-1, or modulation of MIF pathways are among the few novel potential therapeutic targets. Further research is needed to elucidate the mechanisms of hyperoxic lung injury and BPD so that effective therapies could be instituted.

Acknowledgements Supported, in part, by grants HL-085103 from the NIH/NHLBI and The Hartwell Foundation to VB.

Conflict of interest None.

References

1. Bhandari V. Drug therapy trials for the prevention of bronchopulmonary dysplasia: current and future targets. Front Pediatr. 2014;2:76. doi:10.3389/fped.2014.00076. eCollection 2014. PMID: 25121076.
2. Bhandari V. Hyperoxia-derived lung damage in preterm infants. Semin Fetal Neonatal Med. 2010;15(4):223–9. doi:10.1016/j.siny.2010.03.009. Epub 2010 Apr 28.PMID: 20430708.
3. Buczynski BW, Yee M, Martin KC, Lawrence BP, O'Reilly MA. Neonatal hyperoxia alters the host response to influenza A virus infection in adult mice through multiple pathways. Am J Physiol Lung Cell Mol Physiol. 2013;305(4):L282–90. doi:10.1152/ajplung.00112.2013. Epub 2013 Jun 7. PMID: 23748535.
4. Jobe AH, Kallapur SG. Long term consequences of oxygen therapy in the neonatal period. Semin Fetal Neonatal Med. 2010;15(4):230–5. doi:10.1016/j.siny.2010.03.007. Epub 2010 May 10. PMID: 20452844.
5. Velten M, Heyob KM, Rogers LK, Welty SE. Deficits in lung alveolarization and function after systemic maternal inflammation and neonatal hyperoxia exposure. J Appl Physiol (1985). 2010;108(5):1347–56. doi:10.1152/japplphysiol.01392.2009. Epub 2010 Mar 11. PMID: 20223995.
6. Deulofeut R, Critz A, Adams-Chapman I, Sola A. Avoiding hyperoxia in infants < or = 1250 g is associated with improved short- and long-term outcomes. J Perinatol. 2006;26(11):700–5. Epub 2006 Oct 12. PMID: 17036032.
7. The STOP-ROP Multicenter Study Group. Supplemental therapeutic oxygen for prethreshold retinopathy of prematurity (STOP-ROP), a randomized, controlled trial. I: Primary outcomes. Pediatrics. 2000;105(2):295–310. PMID: 10654946.
8. Tin W, Milligan DW, Pennefather P, Hey E. Pulse oximetry, severe retinopathy, and outcome at one year in babies of less than 28 weeks gestation. Arch Dis Child Fetal Neonatal Ed. 2001;84(2):F106–10. PMID: 11207226.
9. Jobe AJ. The new BPD: an arrest of lung development. Pediatr Res. 1999;46(6):641–3. PMID: 10590017.
10. Abman SH. Bronchopulmonary dysplasia: "a vascular hypothesis". Am J Respir Crit Care Med. 2001;164(10 Pt 1):1755–6. PMID: 11734417.
11. Coalson JJ. Pathology of bronchopulmonary dysplasia. Semin Perinatol. 2006;30(4):179–84. PMID: 16860157.
12. Bonikos DS, Bensch KG, Northway Jr WH. Oxygen toxicity in the newborn. The effect of chronic continuous 100 percent oxygen exposure on the lungs of newborn mice. Am J Pathol. 1976;85(3):623–50. PMID: 998734.
13. Coalson JJ, Winter VT, Siler-Khodr T, Yoder BA. Neonatal chronic lung disease in extremely immature baboons. Am J Respir Crit Care Med. 1999;160(4):1333–46. PMID: 10508826.

14. Berger J, Bhandari V. Animal models of bronchopulmonary dysplasia. The term mouse models. Am J Physiol Lung Cell Mol Physiol. 2014;307(12):L936–47. doi:10.1152/ajplung.00159.2014. Epub 2014 Oct 10. PMID: 25305249.
15. Johnston CJ, Wright TW, Reed CK, Finkelstein JN. Comparison of adult and newborn pulmonary cytokine mRNA expression after hyperoxia. Exp Lung Res. 1997;23(6):537–52. PMID: 9358235.
16. Frank L. Developmental aspects of experimental pulmonary oxygen toxicity. Free Radic Biol Med. 1991;11(5):463–94. PMID: 1769607.
17. Frank L, Bucher JR, Roberts RJ. Oxygen toxicity in neonatal and adult animals of various species. J Appl Physiol Respir Environ Exerc Physiol. 1978;45(5):699–704. PMID: 730565.
18. Clark JM, Lambertsen CJ. Pulmonary oxygen toxicity: a review. Pharmacol Rev. 1971;23(2):37–133. PMID: 4948324.
19. Robinson FR, Casey HW, Weibel ER. Animal model: oxygen toxicity in nonhuman primates. Am J Pathol. 1974;76(1):175–8. PMID: 4210278.
20. D'Angio CT, Johnston CJ, Wright TW, Reed CK, Finkelstein JN. Chemokine mRNA alterations in newborn and adult mouse lung during acute hyperoxia. Exp Lung Res. 1998;24(5):685–702. PMID: 9779377.
21. Bhandari V, Choo-Wing R, Lee CG, Yusuf K, Nedrelow JH, Ambalavanan N, Malkus H, Homer RJ, Elias JA. Developmental regulation of NO-mediated VEGF-induced effects in the lung. Am J Respir Cell Mol Biol. 2008;39(4):420–30. doi:10.1165/rcmb.2007-0024OC. Epub 2008 Apr 25. PMID: 18441284.
22. Adamson IY, Bowden DH, Wyatt JP. Oxygen poisoning in mice. Ultrastructural and surfactant studies during exposure and recovery. Arch Pathol. 1970;90(5):463–72. PMID: 5476243.
23. Bowden DH, Adamson IY, Wyatt JP. Reaction of the lung cells to a high concentration of oxygen. Arch Pathol. 1968;86(6):671–5. PMID: 5701641.
24. Warner BB, Stuart LA, Papes RA, Wispé JR. Functional and pathological effects of prolonged hyperoxia in neonatal mice. Am J Physiol. 1998;275(1 Pt 1):L110–7.
25. Yee M, Chess PR, McGrath-Morrow SA, Wang Z, Gelein R, Zhou R, Dean DA, Notter RH, O'Reilly MA. Neonatal oxygen adversely affects lung function in adult mice without altering surfactant composition or activity. Am J Physiol Lung Cell Mol Physiol. 2009;297(4):L641–9. doi:10.1152/ajplung.00023.2009. Epub 2009 Jul 17. PMID: 19617311.
26. Delemos RA, Coalson JJ, Gerstmann DR, Kuehl TJ, Null Jr DM. Oxygen toxicity in the premature baboon with hyaline membrane disease. Am Rev Respir Dis. 1987;136(3):677–82. PMID: 3307571.
27. Bancalari E. Changes in the pathogenesis and prevention of chronic lung disease of prematurity. Am J Perinatol. 2001;18(1):1–9. PMID: 11321240.
28. Rojas MA, Gonzalez A, Bancalari E, Claure N, Poole C, Silva-Neto G. Changing trends in the epidemiology and pathogenesis of neonatal chronic lung disease. J Pediatr. 1995;126(4):605–10. PMID: 7699543.
29. Charafeddine L, D'Angio CT, Phelps DL. Atypical chronic lung disease patterns in neonates. Pediatrics. 1999;103(4 Pt 1):759–65. PMID: 10103299.
30. Chess PR, D'Angio CT, Pryhuber GS, Maniscalco WM. Pathogenesis of bronchopulmonary dysplasia. Semin Perinatol. 2006;30(4):171–8. PMID:16860156.
31. Northway Jr WH, Rosan RC. Radiographic features of pulmonary oxygen toxicity in the newborn: bronchopulmonary dysplasia. Radiology. 1968;91(1):49–58. PMID: 4871379.
32. Horowitz S. Pathways to cell death in hyperoxia. Chest. 1999;116(1 Suppl):64S–7. PMID: 10424596.
33. O'Reilly MA. DNA damage and cell cycle checkpoints in hyperoxic lung injury: braking to facilitate repair. Am J Physiol Lung Cell Mol Physiol. 2001;281(2):L291–305. PMID: 11435201.
34. Thickett DR, Armstrong L, Christie SJ, Millar AB. Vascular endothelial growth factor may contribute to increased vascular permeability in acute respiratory distress syndrome. Am J Respir Crit Care Med. 2001;164(9):1601–5. PMID: 11719296.

35. Davis RP, Mychaliska GB. Neonatal pulmonary physiology. Semin Pediatr Surg. 2013;22(4):179–84. doi:10.1053/j.sempedsurg.2013.10.005. Epub 2013 Oct 16.
36. Joshi S, Kotecha S. Lung growth and development. Early Hum Dev. 2007;83(12):789–94. Epub 2007 Oct 1.
37. Smith LJ, McKay KO, van Asperen PP, Selvadurai H, Fitzgerald DA. Normal development of the lung and premature birth. Paediatr Respir Rev. 2010;11(3):135–42. doi:10.1016/j.prrv.2009.12.006. Epub 2010 Jan 25. Review. PMID: 20692626.
38. Groenman F, Rutter M, Caniggia I, Tibboel D, Post M. Hypoxia-inducible factors in the first trimester human lung. J Histochem Cytochem. 2007;55(4):355–63. Epub 2006 Dec 22. PMID: 17189520.
39. Thébaud B, Ladha F, Michelakis ED, Sawicka M, Thurston G, Eaton F, Hashimoto K, Harry G, Haromy A, Korbutt G, Archer SL. Vascular endothelial growth factor gene therapy increases survival, promotes lung angiogenesis, and prevents alveolar damage in hyperoxia-induced lung injury: evidence that angiogenesis participates in alveolarization. Circulation. 2005;112(16):2477–86. PMID: 1623050.
40. Vadivel A, Alphonse RS, Ionescu L, Machado DS, O'Reilly M, Eaton F, Haromy A, Michelakis ED, Thébaud B. Exogenous hydrogen sulfide (H2S) protects alveolar growth in experimental O2-induced neonatal lung injury. PLoS One. 2014;9(3):e90965. doi:10.1371/journal.pone.0090965. eCollection 2014. PMID: 24603989.
41. Huang Y, Kapere Ochieng J, Kempen MB, Munck AB, Swagemakers S, van Ijcken W, Grosveld F, Tibboel D, Rottier RJ. Hypoxia inducible factor 3α plays a critical role in alveolarization and distal epithelial cell differentiation during mouse lung development. PLoS One. 2013;8(2):e57695. doi:10.1371/journal.pone.0057695. Epub 2013 Feb 25. Erratum in: PLoS One. 2015;10(3):e0119359. PMID: 23451260.
42. Wilborn AM, Evers LB, Canada AT. Oxygen toxicity to the developing lung of the mouse: role of reactive oxygen species. Pediatr Res. 1996;40(2):225–32. PMID: 8827770.
43. Weinberger B, Laskin DL, Heck DE, Laskin JD. Oxygen toxicity in premature infants. Toxicol Appl Pharmacol. 2002;181(1):60–7. PMID: 12030843.
44. Saugstad OD. Oxygen and oxidative stress in bronchopulmonary dysplasia. J Perinat Med. 2010;38(6):571–7. doi:10.1515/JPM.2010.108. Epub 2010 Aug 31. PMID: 20807008.
45. Vento M, Escobar J, Cernada M, Escrig R, Aguar M. The use and misuse of oxygen during the neonatal period. Clin Perinatol. 2012;39(1):165–76. doi:10.1016/j.clp.2011.12.014. Epub 2012 Jan 9. PMID: 22341544.
46. Pendyala S, Usatyuk PV, Gorshkova IA, Garcia JG, Natarajan V. Regulation of NADPH oxidase in vascular endothelium: the role of phospholipases, protein kinases, and cytoskeletal proteins. Antioxid Redox Signal. 2009;11(4):841–60. doi:10.1089/ARS.2008.2231. PMID: 18828698.
47. Ushio-Fukai M, Nakamura Y. Reactive oxygen species and angiogenesis: NADPH oxidase as target for cancer therapy. Cancer Lett. 2008;266(1):37–52. doi:10.1016/j.canlet.2008.02.044. Epub 2008 Apr 10. PMID: 18406051.
48. Bhandari V, Choo-Wing R, Lee CG, Zhu Z, Nedrelow JH, Chupp GL, Zhang X, Matthay MA, Ware LB, Homer RJ, Lee PJ, Geick A, de Fougerolles AR, Elias JA. Hyperoxia causes angiopoietin 2-mediated acute lung injury and necrotic cell death. Nat Med. 2006;12(11):1286–93. Epub 2006 Nov 5. PMID: 17086189.
49. Bhandari V, Elias JA. The role of angiopoietin 2 in hyperoxia-induced acute lung injury. Cell Cycle. 2007;6(9):1049–52. Epub 2007 May 2. PMID: 17438375.
50. Aghai ZH, Faqiri S, Saslow JG, Nakhla T, Farhath S, Kumar A, Eydelman R, Strande L, Stahl G, Leone P, Bhandari V. Angiopoietin 2 concentrations in infants developing bronchopulmonary dysplasia: attenuation by dexamethasone. J Perinatol. 2008;28(2):149–55. Epub 2007 Nov 22. PMID: 18033304.
51. Barazzone C, White CW. Mechanisms of cell injury and death in hyperoxia: role of cytokines and Bcl-2 family proteins. Am J Respir Cell Mol Biol. 2000;22(5):517–9. PMID: 10783120.

52. Pagano A, Barazzone-Argiroffo C. Alveolar cell death in hyperoxia-induced lung injury. Ann N Y Acad Sci. 2003;1010:405–16. PMID: 15033761.
53. Mantell LL, Horowitz S, Davis JM, Kazzaz JA. Hyperoxia-induced cell death in the lung—the correlation of apoptosis, necrosis, and inflammation. Ann N Y Acad Sci. 1999;887:171–80. PMID: 10668473.
54. O'Reilly MA, Staversky RJ, Huyck HL, Watkins RH, LoMonaco MB, D'Angio CT, Baggs RB, Maniscalco WM, Pryhuber GS. Bcl-2 family gene expression during severe hyperoxia induced lung injury. Lab Invest. 2000;80(12):1845–54. PMID:11140697.
55. Wang X, Ryter SW, Dai C, Tang ZL, Watkins SC, Yin XM, Song R, Choi AM. Necrotic cell death in response to oxidant stress involves the activation of the apoptogenic caspase-8/bid pathway. J Biol Chem. 2003;278(31):29184–91. Epub 2003 May 15. PMID: 12754217.
56. Collard KJ, Godeck S, Holley JE, Quinn MW. Pulmonary antioxidant concentrations and oxidative damage in ventilated premature babies. Arch Dis Child Fetal Neonatal Ed. 2004;89(5):F412–6. PMID: 15321959.
57. Gladstone Jr IM, Levine RL. Oxidation of proteins in neonatal lungs. Pediatrics. 1994;93(5):764–8. PMID: 8165075.
58. Smith CV, Hansen TN, Martin NE, McMicken HW, Elliott SJ. Oxidant stress responses in premature infants during exposure to hyperoxia. Pediatr Res. 1993;34(3):360–5. PMID: 8134179.
59. Sosenko IR, Frank L. Nutritional influences on lung development and protection against chronic lung disease. Semin Perinatol. 1991;15(6):462–8. PMID: 1803523.
60. Frank L, Lewis PL, Garcia-Pons T. Intrauterine growth-retarded rat pups show increased susceptibility to pulmonary O2 toxicity. Pediatr Res. 1985;19(3):281–6. PMID: 3982889.
61. Frank L, Roberts RJ. Effects of low-dose prenatal corticosteroid administration on the premature rat. Biol Neonate. 1979;36(1–2):1–9. PMID: 476207.
62. Walther FJ, Jobe AH, Ikegami M. Repetitive prenatal glucocorticoid therapy reduces oxidative stress in the lungs of preterm lambs. J Appl Physiol (1985). 1998;85(1):273–8. PMID: 9655786.
63. Vento M, Aguar M, Escobar J, Arduini A, Escrig R, Brugada M, Izquierdo I, Asensi MA, Sastre J, Saenz P, Gimeno A. Antenatal steroids and antioxidant enzyme activity in preterm infants: influence of gender and timing. Antioxid Redox Signal. 2009;11(12):2945–55. doi:10.1089/ars.2009.2671. PMID: 19645572.
64. Wemhöner A, Ortner D, Tschirch E, Strasak A, Rüdiger M. Nutrition of preterm infants in relation to bronchopulmonary dysplasia. BMC Pulm Med. 2011;11:7. doi:10.1186/1471-2466-11-7. PMID: 21291563.
65. O'Donnell VB, Eiserich JP, Chumley PH, Jablonsky MJ, Krishna NR, Kirk M, Barnes S, Darley-Usmar VM, Freeman BA. Nitration of unsaturated fatty acids by nitric oxide-derived reactive nitrogen species peroxynitrite, nitrous acid, nitrogen dioxide, and nitronium ion. Chem Res Toxicol. 1999;12(1):83–92. PMID: 9894022.
66. Guzik TJ, West NE, Pillai R, Taggart DP, Channon KM. Nitric oxide modulates superoxide release and peroxynitrite formation in human blood vessels. Hypertension. 2002;39(6):1088–94. PMID: 12052847.
67. Adamson IY, Bowden DH. The type 2 cell as progenitor of alveolar epithelial regeneration. A cytodynamic study in mice after exposure to oxygen. Lab Invest. 1974;30(1):35–42. PMID: 4812806.
68. Cho HY, Reddy SP, Kleeberger SR. Nrf2 defends the lung from oxidative stress. Antioxid Redox Signal. 2006;8(1–2):76–87. PMID: 16487040.
69. Cho HY, Reddy SP, Debiase A, Yamamoto M, Kleeberger SR. Gene expression profiling of NRF2-mediated protection against oxidative injury. Free Radic Biol Med. 2005;38(3):325–43. PMID: 15629862.
70. Cho HY, Jedlicka AE, Reddy SP, Kensler TW, Yamamoto M, Zhang LY, Kleeberger SR. Role of NRF2 in protection against hyperoxic lung injury in mice. Am J Respir Cell Mol Biol. 2002;26(2):175–82. PMID: 11804867.

71. Reddy NM, Kleeberger SR, Cho HY, Yamamoto M, Kensler TW, Biswal S, Reddy SP. Deficiency in Nrf2-GSH signaling impairs type II cell growth and enhances sensitivity to oxidants. Am J Respir Cell Mol Biol. 2007;37(1):3–8. Epub 2007 Apr 5. PMID: 17413030.
72. Cho HY, Gladwell W, Wang X, Chorley B, Bell D, Reddy SP, Kleeberger SR. Nrf2-regulated PPAR{gamma} expression is critical to protection against acute lung injury in mice. Am J Respir Crit Care Med. 2010;182(2):170–82. doi:10.1164/rccm.200907-1047OC. Epub 2010 Mar 11. PMID: 20224069.
73. Zhang J, Ohta T, Maruyama A, Hosoya T, Nishikawa K, Maher JM, Shibahara S, Itoh K, Yamamoto M. BRG1 interacts with Nrf2 to selectively mediate HO-1 induction in response to oxidative stress. Mol Cell Biol. 2006;26(21):7942–52. Epub 2006 Aug 21. PMID: 16923960.
74. Cho HY, van Houten B, Wang X, Miller-DeGraff L, Fostel J, Gladwell W, Perrow L, Panduri V, Kobzik L, Yamamoto M, Bell DA, Kleeberger SR. Targeted deletion of nrf2 impairs lung development and oxidant injury in neonatal mice. Antioxid Redox Signal. 2012;17(8):1066–82. doi:10.1089/ars.2011.4288. Epub 2012 Apr 18. PMID: 22400915.
75. McGrath-Morrow S, Lauer T, Yee M, Neptune E, Podowski M, Thimmulappa RK, O'Reilly M, Biswal S. Nrf2 increases survival and attenuates alveolar growth inhibition in neonatal mice exposed to hyperoxia. Am J Physiol Lung Cell Mol Physiol. 2009;296(4):L565–73. doi:10.1152/ajplung.90487.2008. Epub 2009 Jan 16. PMID: 19151108.
76. Marzec JM, Christie JD, Reddy SP, Jedlicka AE, Vuong H, Lanken PN, Aplenc R, Yamamoto T, Yamamoto M, Cho HY, Kleeberger SR. Functional polymorphisms in the transcription factor NRF2 in humans increase the risk of acute lung injury. FASEB J. 2007;21(9):2237–46. Epub 2007 Mar 23. PMID: 17384144.
77. Auten RL, O'Reilly MA, Oury TD, Nozik-Grayck E, Whorton MH. Transgenic extracellular superoxide dismutase protects postnatal alveolar epithelial proliferation and development during hyperoxia. Am J Physiol Lung Cell Mol Physiol. 2006;290(1):L32–40. Epub 2005 Aug 12. PMID: 16100289.
78. Wispé JR, Warner BB, Clark JC, Dey CR, Neuman J, Glasser SW, Crapo JD, Chang LY, Whitsett JA. Human Mn-superoxide dismutase in pulmonary epithelial cells of transgenic mice confers protection from oxygen injury. J Biol Chem. 1992;267(33):23937–41. PMID: 1385428.
79. Ratner V, Starkov A, Matsiukevich D, Polin RA, Ten VS. Mitochondrial dysfunction contributes to alveolar developmental arrest in hyperoxia-exposed mice. Am J Respir Cell Mol Biol. 2009;40(5):511–8. doi:10.1165/rcmb.2008-0341RC. Epub 2009 Jan 23. PMID: 19168698.
80. Matoba S, Kang JG, Patino WD, Wragg A, Boehm M, Gavrilova O, Hurley PJ, Bunz F, Hwang PM. p53 regulates mitochondrial respiration. Science. 2006;312(5780):1650–3. Epub 2006 May 25. PMID: 16728594.
81. Hershenson MB, Aghili S, Punjabi N, Hernandez C, Ray DW, Garland A, Glagov S, Solway J. Hyperoxia-induced airway hyperresponsiveness and remodeling in immature rats. Am J Physiol. 1992;262(3 Pt 1):L263–9. Erratum in: Am J Physiol 1993;265(2 Pt 1):section L followi. PMID: 1550249.
82. Denis D, Fayon MJ, Berger P, Molimard M, De Lara MT, Roux E, Marthan R. Prolonged moderate hyperoxia induces hyperresponsiveness and airway inflammation in newborn rats. Pediatr Res. 2001;50(4):515–9. PMID: 11568296.
83. O'Reilly M, Hansbro PM, Horvat JC, Beckett EL, Harding R, Sozo F. Bronchiolar remodeling in adult mice following neonatal exposure to hyperoxia: relation to growth. Anat Rec (Hoboken). 2014;297(4):758–69. doi:10.1002/ar.22867. Epub 2014 Jan 17. PMID: 24443274.
84. Wang H, Jafri A, Martin RJ, Nnanabu J, Farver C, Prakash YS, MacFarlane PM. Severity of neonatal hyperoxia determines structural and functional changes in developing mouse airway. Am J Physiol Lung Cell Mol Physiol. 2014;307(4):L295–301. doi:10.1152/ajplung.00208.2013. Epub 2014 Jun 20. PMID: 24951774.
85. Ali NK, Jafri A, Sopi RB, Prakash YS, Martin RJ, Zaidi SI. Role of arginase in impairing relaxation of lung parenchyma of hyperoxia-exposed neonatal rats. Neonatology. 2012;101(2):106–15. doi:10.1159/000329540. Epub 2011 Sep 23. PMID: 21952491.

86. Been JV, Lugtenberg MJ, Smets E, van Schayck CP, Kramer BW, Mommers M, Sheikh A. Preterm birth and childhood wheezing disorders: a systematic review and meta-analysis. PLoS Med. 2014;11(1):e1001596. doi:10.1371/journal.pmed.1001596. eCollection 2014 Jan. Review. PMID: 2449240.
87. Vrijlandt EJ, Kerstjens JM, Duiverman EJ, Bos AF, Reijneveld SA. Moderately preterm children have more respiratory problems during their first 5 years of life than children born full term. Am J Respir Crit Care Med. 2013;187(11):1234–40. doi:10.1164/rccm.201211-2070OC. PMID: 2352593.
88. Aggarwal NR, D'Alessio FR, Tsushima K, Files DC, Damarla M, Sidhaye VK, Fraig MM, Polotsky VY, King LS. Moderate oxygen augments lipopolysaccharide-induced lung injury in mice. Am J Physiol Lung Cell Mol Physiol. 2010;298(3):L371–81. doi:10.1152/ajplung.00308.2009. Epub 2009 Dec 24. PMID: 20034961.
89. Bhandari V. Molecular mechanisms of hyperoxia-induced acute lung injury. Front Biosci. 2008;13:6653–61. PMID: 18508685, Review.
90. Konsavage WM, Zhang L, Wu Y, Shenberger JS. Hyperoxia-induced activation of the integrated stress response in the newborn rat lung. Am J Physiol Lung Cell Mol Physiol. 2012;302(1):L27–35. doi:10.1152/ajplung.00174.2011. Epub 2011 Oct 7. PMID: 21984568.
91. Ambalavanan N, Carlo WA, D'Angio CT, McDonald SA, Das A, Schendel D, Higgins RD, Eunice Kennedy Shriver National Institute of Child Health and Human Development Neonatal Research Network. Cytokines associated with bronchopulmonary dysplasia or death in extremely low birth weight infants. Pediatrics. 2009;123(4):1132–41. doi:10.1542/peds.2008-0526. PMID: 19336372.
92. Bhattacharya S, Go D, Krenitsky DL, Huyck HL, Solleti SK, Lunger VA, Metlay L, Srisuma S, Wert SE, Mariani TJ, Pryhuber GS. Genome-wide transcriptional profiling reveals connective tissue mast cell accumulation in bronchopulmonary dysplasia. Am J Respir Crit Care Med. 2012;186(4):349–58. doi:10.1164/rccm.201203-0406OC. Epub 2012 Jun 21. PMID: 22723293.
93. Broström EB, Katz-Salamon M, Lundahl J, Halldén G, Winbladh B. Eosinophil activation in preterm infants with lung disease. Acta Paediatr. 2007;96(1):23–8. PMID: 17187598.
94. Joza N, Kroemer G, Penninger JM. Genetic analysis of the mammalian cell death machinery. Trends Genet. 2002;18(3):142–9. PMID: 11858838.
95. D'Angio CT, LoMonaco MB, Chaudhry SA, Paxhia A, Ryan RM. Discordant pulmonary proinflammatory cytokine expression during acute hyperoxia in the newborn rabbit. Exp Lung Res. 1999;25(5):443–65. PMID: 10483526.
96. Bry K, Whitsett JA, Lappalainen U. IL-1beta disrupts postnatal lung morphogenesis in the mouse. Am J Respir Cell Mol Biol. 2007;36(1):32–42. Epub 2006 Aug 3. PMID: 16888287.
97. Bhandari V, Elias JA. Cytokines in tolerance to hyperoxia-induced injury in the developing and adult lung. Free Radic Biol Med. 2006;41(1):4–18. Epub 2006 Feb 17. PMID: 16781448.
98. Choo-Wing R, Nedrelow JH, Homer RJ, Elias JA, Bhandari V. Developmental differences in the responses of IL-6 and IL-13 transgenic mice exposed to hyperoxia. Am J Physiol Lung Cell Mol Physiol. 2007;293(1):L142–50. Epub 2007 Mar 30. PMID: 17400600.
99. Lindsay L, Oliver SJ, Freeman SL, Josien R, Krauss A, Kaplan G. Modulation of hyperoxia-induced TNF-alpha expression in the newborn rat lung by thalidomide and dexamethasone. Inflammation. 2000;24(4):347–56. PMID: 10850856.
100. Wagenaar GT, ter Horst SA, van Gastelen MA, Leijser LM, Mauad T, van der Velden PA, de Heer E, Hiemstra PS, Poorthuis BJ, Walther FJ. Gene expression profile and histopathology of experimental bronchopulmonary dysplasia induced by prolonged oxidative stress. Free Radic Biol Med. 2004;36(6):782–801. PMID: 14990357.
101. Deng H, Mason SN, Auten Jr RL. Lung inflammation in hyperoxia can be prevented by antichemokine treatment in newborn rats. Am J Respir Crit Care Med. 2000;162(6):2316–23. PMID: 11112157.
102. Thompson A, Bhandari V. Pulmonary biomarkers of bronchopulmonary dysplasia. Biomark Insights. 2008;3:361–73. PMID: 19430584.

103. Danan C, Franco ML, Jarreau PH, Dassieu G, Chailley-Heu B, Bourbon J, Delacourt C. High concentrations of keratinocyte growth factor in airways of premature infants predicted absence of bronchopulmonary dysplasia. Am J Respir Crit Care Med. 2002;165(10):1384–7. PMID: 12016100.
104. Baier RJ, Majid A, Parupia H, Loggins J, Kruger TE. CC chemokine concentrations increase in respiratory distress syndrome and correlate with development of bronchopulmonary dysplasia. Pediatr Pulmonol. 2004;37(2):137–48. PMID: 14730659.
105. Vozzelli MA, Mason SN, Whorton MH, Auten Jr RL. Antimacrophage chemokine treatment prevents neutrophil and macrophage influx in hyperoxia-exposed newborn rat lung. Am J Physiol Lung Cell Mol Physiol. 2004;286(3):L488–93. Epub 2003 Feb 14. PMID: 12588706.
106. Hosford GE, Fang X, Olson DM. Hyperoxia decreases matrix metalloproteinase-9 and increases tissue inhibitor of matrix metalloproteinase-1 protein in the newborn rat lung: association with arrested alveolarization. Pediatr Res. 2004;56(1):26–34. Epub 2004 May 5. PMID: 15128910.
107. Radomski A, Sawicki G, Olson DM, Radomski MW. The role of nitric oxide and metalloproteinases in the pathogenesis of hyperoxia-induced lung injury in newborn rats. Br J Pharmacol. 1998;125(7):1455–62. PMID: 9884073.
108. Tambunting F, Beharry KD, Hartleroad J, Waltzman J, Stavitsky Y, Modanlou HD. Increased lung matrix metalloproteinase-9 levels in extremely premature baboons with bronchopulmonary dysplasia. Pediatr Pulmonol. 2005;39(1):5–14. PMID: 15521085.
109. Chetty A, Cao GJ, Severgnini M, Simon A, Warburton R, Nielsen HC. Role of matrix metalloprotease-9 in hyperoxic injury in developing lung. Am J Physiol Lung Cell Mol Physiol. 2008;295(4):L584–92. doi:10.1152/ajplung.00441.2007. Epub 2008 Jul 25. PMID: 18658276.
110. Lukkarinen H, Hogmalm A, Lappalainen U, Bry K. Matrix metalloproteinase-9 deficiency worsens lung injury in a model of bronchopulmonary dysplasia. Am J Respir Cell Mol Biol. 2009;41(1):59–68. doi:10.1165/rcmb.2008-0179OC. Epub 2008 Dec 18. PMID: 19097983.
111. Cederqvist K, Sorsa T, Tervahartiala T, Maisi P, Reunanen K, Lassus P, Andersson S. Matrix metalloproteinases-2, -8, and -9 and TIMP-2 in tracheal aspirates from preterm infants with respiratory distress. Pediatrics. 2001;108(3):686–92. PMID: 11533337.
112. Sweet DG, Curley AE, Chesshyre E, Pizzotti J, Wilbourn MS, Halliday HL, Warner JA. The role of matrix metalloproteinases -9 and -2 in development of neonatal chronic lung disease. Acta Paediatr. 2004;93(6):791–6. PMID: 15244229.
113. Harijith A, Choo-Wing R, Cataltepe S, Yasumatsu R, Aghai ZH, Janér J, Andersson S, Homer RJ, Bhandari V. A role for matrix metalloproteinase 9 in IFNγ-mediated injury in developing lungs: relevance to bronchopulmonary dysplasia. Am J Respir Cell Mol Biol. 2011;44(5):621–30. doi:10.1165/rcmb.2010-0058OC. Epub 2011 Jan 7. PMID: 21216975.
114. Sharif O, Krishnan PV, Thekdi AD, Gordon SC. Acute hepatitis B in an urban tertiary care hospital in the United States: a cohort evaluation. J Clin Gastroenterol. 2013;47(9):e87–90. doi:10.1097/MCG.0b013e31828a383c. PMID: 23470641.
115. Choo-Wing R, Syed MA, Harijith A, Bowen B, Pryhuber G, Janér C, Andersson S, Homer RJ, Bhandari V. Hyperoxia and interferon-γ-induced injury in developing lungs occur via cyclooxygenase-2 and the endoplasmic reticulum stress-dependent pathway. Am J Respir Cell Mol Biol. 2013;48(6):749–57. doi:10.1165/rcmb.2012-0381OC. PMID: 23470621.
116. Darling NJ, Cook SJ. The role of MAPK signalling pathways in the response to endoplasmic reticulum stress. Biochim Biophys Acta. 2014;1843(10):2150–63. doi:10.1016/j.bbamcr.2014.01.009. Epub 2014 Jan 15. Review. PMID: 2444027.
117. Alejandre-Alcázar MA, Kwapiszewska G, Reiss I, Amarie OV, Marsh LM, Sevilla-Pérez J, Wygrecka M, Eul B, Köbrich S, Hesse M, Schermuly RT, Seeger W, Eickelberg O, Morty RE. Hyperoxia modulates TGF-beta/BMP signaling in a mouse model of bronchopulmonary dysplasia. Am J Physiol Lung Cell Mol Physiol. 2007;292(2):L537–49. Epub 2006 Oct 27. PMID: 17071723.
118. Li Z, Choo-Wing R, Sun H, Sureshbabu A, Sakurai R, Rehan VK, Bhandari V. A potential role of the JNK pathway in hyperoxia-induced cell death, myofibroblast transdifferentiation

and TGF-β1-mediated injury in the developing murine lung. BMC Cell Biol. 2011;12:54. doi:10.1186/1471-2121-12-54. PMID: 22172122.
119. Sureshbabu A, Syed MA, Boddupalli CS, Dhodapkar MV, Homer RJ, Minoo P, Bhandari V. Conditional overexpression of TGFβ1 promotes pulmonary inflammation, apoptosis and mortality via TGFβR2 in the developing mouse lung. Respir Res. 2015;16:4. doi:10.1186/s12931-014-0162-6. PMID: 25591994.
120. Kevill KA, Bhandari V, Kettunen M, Leng L, Fan J, Mizue Y, Dzuira JD, Reyes-Mugica M, McDonald CL, Baugh JA, O'Connor CL, Aghai ZH, Donnelly SC, Bazzy-Asaad A, Bucala RJ. A role for macrophage migration inhibitory factor in the neonatal respiratory distress syndrome. J Immunol. 2008;180(1):601–8. PMID: 18097062.
121. Sun H, Choo-Wing R, Fan J, Leng L, Syed MA, Hare AA, Jorgensen WL, Bucala R, Bhandari V. Small molecular modulation of macrophage migration inhibitory factor in the hyperoxia-induced mouse model of bronchopulmonary dysplasia. Respir Res. 2013;14:27. doi:10.1186/1465-9921-14-27. PMID: 23448134.
122. Sun H, Choo-Wing R, Sureshbabu A, Fan J, Leng L, Yu S, Jiang D, Noble P, Homer RJ, Bucala R, Bhandari V. A critical regulatory role for macrophage migration inhibitory factor in hyperoxia-induced injury in the developing murine lung. PLoS One. 2013;8(4):e60560. doi:10.1371/journal.pone.0060560. Print 2013. PMID: 23637753.
123. Meller S, Bhandari V. VEGF levels in humans and animal models with RDS and BPD: temporal relationships. Exp Lung Res. 2012;38(4):192–203. doi:10.3109/01902148.2012.663454. Epub 2012 Mar 6. PMID: 22394267.
124. D'Angio CT, Maniscalco WM. The role of vascular growth factors in hyperoxia-induced injury to the developing lung. Front Biosci. 2002;7:d1609–23. Epub 2002 Jul 1. PMID: 12086914.
125. Budinger GR, Mutlu GM, Urich D, Soberanes S, Buccellato LJ, Hawkins K, Chiarella SE, Radigan KA, Eisenbart J, Agrawal H, Berkelhamer S, Hekimi S, Zhang J, Perlman H, Schumacker PT, Jain M, Chandel NS. Epithelial cell death is an important contributor to oxidant-mediated acute lung injury. Am J Respir Crit Care Med. 2011;183(8):1043–54. doi:10.1164/rccm.201002-0181OC. Epub 2010 Oct 19. PMID: 20959557.
126. Brueckl C, Kaestle S, Kerem A, Habazettl H, Krombach F, Kuppe H, Kuebler WM. Hyperoxia-induced reactive oxygen species formation in pulmonary capillary endothelial cells in situ. Am J Respir Cell Mol Biol. 2006;34(4):453–63. Epub 2005 Dec 15. PMID: 16357365.
127. Zhang X, Shan P, Sasidhar M, Chupp GL, Flavell RA, Choi AM, Lee PJ. Reactive oxygen species and extracellular signal-regulated kinase 1/2 mitogen-activated protein kinase mediate hyperoxia-induced cell death in lung epithelium. Am J Respir Cell Mol Biol. 2003;28(3):305–15. PMID: 12594056.
128. Truong SV, Monick MM, Yarovinsky TO, Powers LS, Nyunoya T, Hunninghake GW. Extracellular signal-regulated kinase activation delays hyperoxia-induced epithelial cell death in conditions of Akt downregulation. Am J Respir Cell Mol Biol. 2004;31(6):611–8. Epub 2004 Aug 12. PMID: 15308507.
129. Singleton PA, Pendyala S, Gorshkova IA, Mambetsariev N, Moitra J, Garcia JG, Natarajan V. Dynamin 2 and c-Abl are novel regulators of hyperoxia-mediated NADPH oxidase activation and reactive oxygen species production in caveolin-enriched microdomains of the endothelium. J Biol Chem. 2009;284(50):34964–75. doi:10.1074/jbc.M109.013771. Epub 2009 Oct 15. PMID: 19833721.
130. Hilgendorff A, Reiss I, Ehrhardt H, Eickelberg O, Alvira CM. Chronic lung disease in the preterm infant. Lessons learned from animal models. Am J Respir Cell Mol Biol. 2014;50(2):233–45. doi:10.1165/rcmb.2013-0014TR. PMID: 24024524, Review.
131. Madurga A, Mizíková I, Ruiz-Camp J, Morty RE. Recent advances in late lung development and the pathogenesis of bronchopulmonary dysplasia. Am J Physiol Lung Cell Mol Physiol. 2013;305(12):L893–905. doi:10.1152/ajplung.00267.2013. Epub 2013 Nov 8. Review. PMID: 24213917.

132. Cho KA, Suh JW, Lee KH, Kang JL, Woo SY. IL-17 and IL-22 enhance skin inflammation by stimulating the secretion of IL-1β by keratinocytes via the ROS-NLRP3-caspase-1 pathway. Int Immunol. 2012;24(3):147–58. doi:10.1093/intimm/dxr110. Epub 2011 Dec 29. PMID: 22207130.
133. Lee PJ, Choi AM. Pathways of cell signaling in hyperoxia. Free Radic Biol Med. 2003;35(4):341–50. PMID: 12899937, Review.
134. Sunday ME, Yoder BA, Cuttitta F, Haley KJ, Emanuel RL. Bombesin-like peptide mediates lung injury in a baboon model of bronchopulmonary dysplasia. J Clin Invest. 1998;102(3):584–94. PMID: 9691095.
135. Subramaniam M, Bausch C, Twomey A, Andreeva S, Yoder BA, Chang L, Crapo JD, Pierce RA, Cuttitta F, Sunday ME. Bombesin-like peptides modulate alveolarization and angiogenesis in bronchopulmonary dysplasia. Am J Respir Crit Care Med. 2007;176(9):902–12. Epub 2007 Jun 21. PMID: 17585105.
136. Cullen A, Van Marter LJ, Allred EN, Moore M, Parad RB, Sunday ME. Urine bombesin-like peptide elevation precedes clinical evidence of bronchopulmonary dysplasia. Am J Respir Crit Care Med. 2002;165(8):1093–7. PMID: 11956050.
137. Padela S, Cabacungan J, Shek S, Belcastro R, Yi M, Jankov RP, Tanswell AK. Hepatocyte growth factor is required for alveologenesis in the neonatal rat. Am J Respir Crit Care Med. 2005;172(7):907–14. Epub 2005 Jun 30. PMID: 15994466.
138. Lassus P, Heikkilä P, Andersson LC, von Boguslawski K, Andersson S. Lower concentration of pulmonary hepatocyte growth factor is associated with more severe lung disease in preterm infants. J Pediatr. 2003;143(2):199–202. PMID: 12970632.
139. Harijith A, Ebenezer DL, Natarajan V. Reactive oxygen species at the crossroads of inflammasome and inflammation. Front Physiol. 2014;5:352. doi:10.3389/fphys.2014.00352. eCollection 2014. PMID: 25324778.
140. Rodriguez C, Mayo JC, Sainz RM, Antolín I, Herrera F, Martín V, Reiter RJ. Regulation of antioxidant enzymes: a significant role for melatonin. J Pineal Res. 2004;36(1):1–9. PMID: 14675124.
141. Gitto E, Reiter RJ, Amodio A, Romeo C, Cuzzocrea E, Sabatino G, Buonocore G, Cordaro V, Trimarchi G, Barberi I. Early indicators of chronic lung disease in preterm infants with respiratory distress syndrome and their inhibition by melatonin. J Pineal Res. 2004;36(4):250–5. PMID: 15066049.
142. Kinsella JP, Greenough A, Abman SH. Bronchopulmonary dysplasia. Lancet. 2006;367(9520):1421–31. PMID: 16650652.
143. Carlsson LM, Jonsson J, Edlund T, Marklund SL. Mice lacking extracellular superoxide dismutase are more sensitive to hyperoxia. Proc Natl Acad Sci USA. 1995;92(14):6264–8. PMID: 7603981.
144. Turrens JF, Crapo JD, Freeman BA. Protection against oxygen toxicity by intravenous injection of liposome-entrapped catalase and superoxide dismutase. J Clin Invest. 1984;73(1):87–95. PMID: 6690485.
145. Padmanabhan RV, Gudapaty R, Liener IE, Schwartz BA, Hoidal JR. Protection against pulmonary oxygen toxicity in rats by the intratracheal administration of liposome-encapsulated superoxide dismutase or catalase. Am Rev Respir Dis. 1985;132(1):164–7. PMID: 4014861.
146. Davis JM, Rosenfeld WN, Sanders RJ, Gonenne A. Prophylactic effects of recombinant human superoxide dismutase in neonatal lung injury. J Appl Physiol (1985). 1993;74(5):2234–41. PMID: 8335553.
147. Barnard ML, Baker RR, Matalon S. Mitigation of oxidant injury to lung microvasculature by intratracheal instillation of antioxidant enzymes. Am J Physiol. 1993;265(4 Pt 1):L340–5. PMID: 8238368.
148. Rosenfeld WN, Davis JM, Parton L, Richter SE, Price A, Flaster E, Kassem N. Safety and pharmacokinetics of recombinant human superoxide dismutase administered intratracheally to premature neonates with respiratory distress syndrome. Pediatrics. 1996;97(6 Pt 1):811–7. PMID: 8657519.

149. Davis JM, Rosenfeld WN, Richter SE, Parad MR, Gewolb IH, Spitzer AR, Carlo WA, Couser RJ, Price A, Flaster E, Kassem N, Edwards L, Tierney J, Horowitz S. Safety and pharmacokinetics of multiple doses of recombinant human CuZn superoxide dismutase administered intratracheally to premature neonates with respiratory distress syndrome. Pediatrics. 1997;100(1):24–30. PMID: 9200356.
150. Davis JM, Parad RB, Michele T, Allred E, Price A, Rosenfeld W, North American Recombinant Human CuZnSOD Study Group. Pulmonary outcome at 1 year corrected age in premature infants treated at birth with recombinant human CuZn superoxide dismutase. Pediatrics. 2003;111(3):469–76. PMID: 12612223.

Chapter 2
Invasive Mechanical Ventilation in the Pathogenesis of Bronchopulmonary Dysplasia

Lauren M. Ramos, Tanbir Najrana, and Juan Sanchez-Esteban

Introduction

Many premature infants born with underdeveloped lungs are exposed to excessive, non-physiological levels of stretch. Invasive mechanical ventilation is life saving for preterm infants with respiratory failure. However, mechanical ventilation uses positive pressure that may result in ventilator-induced lung injury (VILI). It is estimated that around 30 % of patients born before 32 weeks of gestation will develop bronchopulmonary dysplasia (BPD) [1]. BPD is a chronic lung disease characterized by alveolar hypoplasia and impaired pulmonary vascular development [2]. BPD is a devastating condition that disrupts not only normal lung development but is also associated with long-term neurodevelopmental sequelae [3]. Although the etiology of BPD is multifactorial, resulting from the interaction between genetic and environmental factors [4], invasive mechanical ventilation plays a central role. In this chapter, we will review the contribution of invasive mechanical ventilation to the pathogenesis of BPD. First, we will describe how mechanical ventilation promotes lung inflammation and injury. We will then review the biomechanical determinants and mechanotransduction in VILI. Next, we will review the signaling pathways modulating the critical stage of alveolar development and disruption by mechanical ventilation. Finally, we will go over animal models of invasive mechanical ventilation.

L.M. Ramos, MD • T. Najrana, PhD • J. Sanchez-Esteban, MD (✉)
Department of Pediatrics, Neonatal-Perinatal Medicine, Women and Infants Hospital of Rhode Island, The Warren Alpert Medical School of Brown University, 101 Dudley Street, Providence, RI 02905, USA
e-mail: LauRamos@wihri.org; TNajrana@wihri.org; jsanchezesteban@wihri.org

V. Bhandari (ed.), *Bronchopulmonary Dysplasia*, Respiratory Medicine,
DOI 10.1007/978-3-319-28486-6_2

Role of Mechanical Ventilation in Causing Lung Inflammation and Injury

The pathogenesis of BPD is multifactorial. However, inflammation secondary to mechanical injury plays a central role. Numerous studies have demonstrated that invasive mechanical ventilation induces lung injury [5–7]. Overdistension of the lung damages resident cells and disrupts the alveolar–capillary barrier with subsequent release of proinflammatory cytokines, increase in permeability, and influx of neutrophils and macrophages to the lung [8]. In the next section, we will review how positive pressure ventilation promotes inflammation and lung injury (VILI). It is difficult to completely tease out the contribution of mechanical distention alone to the pathogenesis of lung injury, given that the majority of premature infants exposed to mechanical ventilation also receive moderate amount of oxygen. Moreover, many premature infants might have been exposed in utero to chorioamnionitis and therefore are more susceptible to lung injury after birth [9].

Mechanical Injury of Lung Resident Cells

In order to understand the effects of invasive mechanical ventilation on the generation of inflammation in the lung, it is important to review the contribution of individual cells to lung injury using in vitro model systems.

Alveolar Type II Epithelial Cells (AECII) Type II epithelial cells are key components of the alveolar structure. Physiological mechanical stimulation of alveolar type II cells is important for surfactant secretion [10] and surfactant protein gene expression [11]. However, alveolar type II epithelial cells can also be exposed to overstretch, and therefore to injury secondary to mechanical ventilation. Previous in vitro studies in adult rat type II epithelial cells have demonstrated that excessive stretch can induce apoptosis [12, 13] and cell membrane stress failure [14] resulting in cell death [15]. In addition, cyclic stretch of adult type II cells can also promote inflammation by stimulating release of interleukin-8 (IL-8) [16, 17] and monocyte chemoattractant protein-1 (MCP-1) [18]. Studies from our laboratory have showed that excessive stretch of rat fetal type II cells isolated on embryonic day 19 (E19) of gestation (transition from canalicular to saccular stages of lung development) induces necrosis, apoptosis, proliferation, and inflammation [19]. Moreover, other investigations have also shown that type II epithelial cells are an important source of chemokines that orchestrate leukocyte migration to the peripheral lung during stimulation with lipopolysaccharide (LPS) [20]. These studies support a role for type II cells in the pathogenesis of BPD by releasing proinflammatory cytokines after injury induced by mechanical ventilation.

Alveolar Type I Epithelial Cells (AEC1) AEC1 appear in the late canalicular period and increase in number during the saccular and alveolar stages of lung development. Given that they cover much of the distal epithelium of the lung, AEC1 are at risk for injury mediated by mechanical ventilation. However, the contribution of type

I cells to the pathogenesis of BPD is not clearly defined, probably because of the difficulty in isolating AEC1 cells in vitro [21]. Nevertheless, recent studies have found that these cells produce tumor necrosis factor-alpha (TNF-α), IL-1beta (IL-1β), and IL-6 after exposure to LPS [22]. In fact, some authors believe that AEC1 are a more important source of proinflammatory cytokines than AEC2 [23]. Moreover, the receptor for advanced glycation endproducts (RAGE), found only on AEC1 in the lung, may also participate in inflammation and alveolar simplification. AEC1 are important to maintain adequate fluid balance in the alveolus via the tight junctions [24]. These junctions could be affected by mechanical injury leading to pulmonary edema [25].

Fibroblasts Fibroblasts are critical for lung development and repair [26]. Fibroblasts can also secrete cytokines and trigger an inflammatory response [27]. Given that interstitial cells are directly exposed to mechanical injury, we investigated whether lung fibroblasts participate in lung injury secondary to mechanical stretch. Fetal mouse lung fibroblasts isolated during the saccular stage of lung development were exposed to 20 % cyclic stretch to simulate mechanical injury. Our data showed that mechanical stretch increased necrosis and apoptosis in these cells. In addition, there was increased release of proinflammatory cytokines and chemokines IL-1β, MCP-1, regulated on activation, normal T-cell expressed and secreted (RANTES), IL-6, keratinocyte chemoattractant (KC), and TNF-α [28]. These studies suggest that mesenchymal cells could be an important source of proinflammatory cytokines and chemokines after exposure to mechanical ventilation.

Endothelial Cells Similar to alveolar epithelium, vascular endothelial cells can sense mechanical signals during mechanical ventilation. It has been demonstrated that endothelial cells exposed to 15–20 % distention increase production of the proinflammatory cytokines IL-8 and MCP-1 [29]. Furthermore, excessive mechanical stretch also alters endothelial cell barrier properties contributing to increase in alveolar–capillary permeability and pulmonary edema [30].

Macrophages Lung macrophages exposed to 12 % cyclic strain, to mimic mechanical ventilation, released inflammatory mediators such as TNF-α, IL-8, IL-6, matrix metalloproteinase-9 (MMP-9), and nuclear factor-kappa light-chain-enhancer of activated B cells (NF-κB). Synergistic proinflammatory effects of mechanical stretch and bacterial endotoxin were observed, supporting the concept that mechanical ventilation is particularly deleterious in infected lungs [31].

In summary, these in vitro studies indicate that pulmonary resident cells may play a critical role in the initiation of the inflammatory cascade by sensing mechanical signals mediated by mechanical ventilation and triggering the release of proinflammatory cytokines (Fig. 2.1).

Alterations in Alveolar–Capillary Permeability

The increase in alveolar–capillary permeability is present during the early stages of mechanical injury [8]. Protein leakage into the lung of preterm infants has been observed soon after the initiation of mechanical ventilation [32]. There are

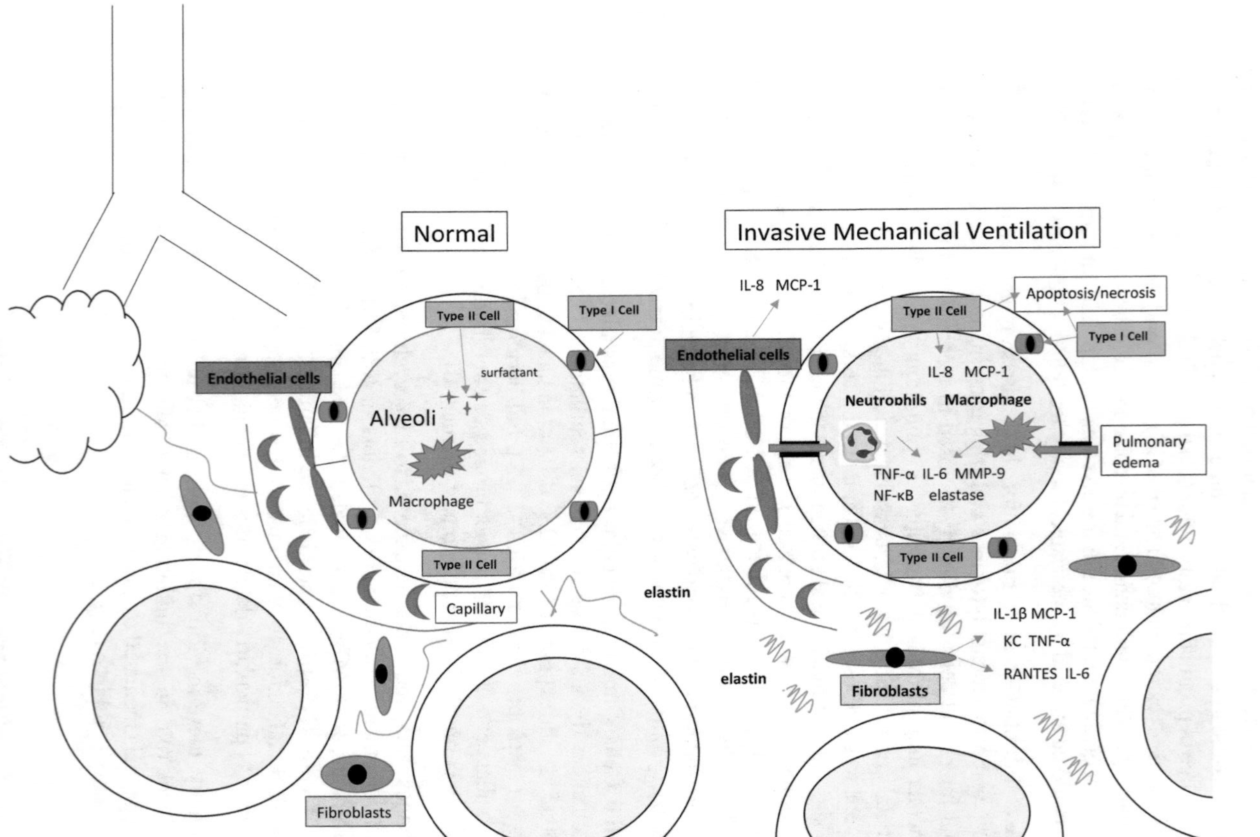

Fig. 2.1 Invasive mechanical ventilation can damage lung resident cells, such as type II and type I epithelial cells, fibroblasts, endothelial cells, and macrophages, with subsequent release of proinflammatory cytokines. In addition, overdistension of the lung can disrupt the alveolar–capillary barrier causing an increase in permeability, followed by pulmonary edema, and further recruitment of neutrophils and macrophages to the lung. *IL* interleukin, *MCP-1* monocyte chemoattractant protein-1, *TNF-α* tumor necrosis factor alpha, *MMP-9* matrix metalloproteinase-9, *NF-κB* nuclear factor kappa-light-chain-enhancer of acti-

experimental evidences to support damage to the alveolar–capillary barrier induced by mechanical injury [7]. Major alterations in pulmonary epithelial and endothelial permeability have been reported in isolated lungs and intact animals exposed to mechanical ventilation. For example, increased vascular permeability and subsequent alveolar edema occurred with a peak inspiratory pressure as low as 13 cm H_2O in isolated perfused rat lungs [33]. Likewise, microvascular permeability injury was also demonstrated in intact animals [34]. Positive pressure ventilation in lambs resulted in altered alveolar permeability to small solutes using clearance of aerosolized ^{99m}Tc-DTPA as a marker [35]. Electron microscope studies provided clear evidence for the major abnormalities in the epithelial and endothelial cells that resulted in increased permeability during VILI. Damage of alveolar type I epithelial cells was observed in rabbits ventilated with a peak inspiratory pressure of 20 cm H_2O for 6 h [36]. In these studies, some endothelial cells were detached from their basement membrane, resulting in the formation of intracapillary blebs. There were also occasional breaks in endothelial cells. More prolonged exposure to injurious stress produced alveolar epithelial pathology ranging from inter and intracellular gap formations with denuded basement membranes to extensive cell destruction [37]. The blood–gas barrier of rabbit lungs exposed to high capillary pressures revealed not only epithelial gaps and endothelial lesions but also basement membrane breaks. Although increase in microvascular transmural pressure may contribute to pulmonary edema, these electron microscopy findings strongly support that changes in the permeability of the alveolar–capillary barrier are a main determinant of ventilator-induced pulmonary edema [7].

Influx of Neutrophils and Macrophages to the Lung and Their Contribution to the Inflammatory Response

Increase in pulmonary vascular permeability and subsequent influx of neutrophils and macrophages into the lung occur soon after initiation of mechanical ventilation [32, 38]. As discussed before, the initial influx of inflammatory cells is probably initiated by lung resident cells, as demonstrated in isolated and perfused rat lung exposed to mechanical injury [39]. However, neutrophils and macrophages recruited to the lung play a critical role in pulmonary inflammation by producing inflammatory mediators, recruiting more inflammatory cells, and therefore amplifying the inflammatory response (Fig. 2.1). There are many studies demonstrating the influx of leukocytes into the lung in response to mechanical ventilation [40, 41]. Woo and Hedley-Whyte [42] observed that overinflation of lungs in open-chest dog models produced edema and accumulation of leukocytes and macrophages in the alveoli. Similar findings were observed in piglets ventilated at high tidal volumes [43] and in premature monkeys exposed to mechanical ventilation. However, neutrophil influx occurs earlier during the inflammatory response followed by macrophages [41]. These data are consistent with bronchoalveolar lavage studies in premature infants exposed to mechanical ventilation where neutrophils were detected at 3–4 days, whereas macrophages were predominantly observed after 10 days [44].

Migration to the lung and activation of neutrophils and macrophages are mediated largely via proinflammatory cytokines. Tracheal aspirates of premature infants with BPD show an increase of chemoattractant factors such as IL-8, IL-6, TNFα, IL-1, IL-16, complement component 5a (C5a), lipoxygenase products, leukotriene B4, elastin fragments, fibronectin, MCP, macrophage inflammatory protein (MIP), etc. [38, 45]. Among them, IL-8 and perhaps IL-6 seem to have important roles in the initial recruitment of inflammatory cells to the lung, given that elevation of these cytokines was found to precede the influx of neutrophils in tracheal aspirates from preterm infants who developed BPD [38, 46]. It has been shown experimentally that ventilation strategies with high or low volumes have an impact on the release of proinflammatory cytokines [39, 47]. Moreover, several animal models of BPD have demonstrated that invasive mechanical ventilation increases the level of proinflammatory cytokines [40, 48–51]. On the other hand, low levels of anti-inflammatory cytokines, such as IL-10, were observed in the bronchoalveolar lavage of patients with BPD [52]. In vitro studies from our laboratory have shown that mechanical injury of fetal epithelial cells and fibroblasts increases the release of proinflammatory cytokines and decreases the release of IL-10. Preincubation of these cells with IL-10 prior to stretch reduced apoptosis and the release of proinflammatory cytokines [19, 28]. These studies indicate that an imbalance between proinflammatory and anti-inflammatory cytokines, favoring proinflammatory cytokines, could be critical to promote lung injury [38].

In addition to releasing proinflammatory cytokines, neutrophils and macrophages produce potent proteases, especially elastase, which is believed to play an important role in the damage of the extracellular matrix (ECM) and impairment of alveolarization observed in patients with BPD [53]. Transforming growth factor-beta (TGF-β) is induced in the lung after injury to limit the inflammatory response and to regulate tissue repair [54]. However, in the presence of persistent injury, this process could be abnormal, resulting in severe pulmonary fibrosis [55]. It has been demonstrated that overexpression of TGF-β resulted in significant fibrosis with extensive deposition of ECM proteins such as collagen, fibronectin, and elastin [56]. TGF-β is produced mainly by macrophages, and elevated levels of TGF-β in the bronchoalveolar lavage of premature infants are predictive and associated with BPD [57, 58].

Biomechanical Determinants of VILI

Under normal conditions, the lung is exposed to a variety of mechanical forces such as mechanical strain and shear stress. *Mechanical strain* occurs when a force is applied to an elastic tissue causing stretch or distortion. These forces are generated to overcome the elastic recoil of the lung during normal breathing. During lung injury, the magnitude of these forces is increased. A second form of mechanical distortion is *shear stress*, generated when fluids such as blood or air move across a cell surface, generating a force parallel to the plasma membrane that produces a tangential distortion of the cell. Such shearing forces occur in the conducting airways, due to airflow, and in the vascular systems as a consequence of blood flow [59].

VILI is the result of complex interactions among various forces acting on lung structures during mechanical ventilation [60]. In a broad sense, the concept of VILI can be defined at the whole organ, cellular, or molecular levels. There are various forms of VILI, including volutrauma (caused by overdistension of the lung), atelectrauma (by repeated opening/closing of the lung), and biotrauma (by release of inflammatory mediators). Studies by Dreyfuss and Saumon in the late 1990s [7] clearly showed that lungs are injured if they are inflated to volumes that exceed total lung capacity (*volutrauma*) [5]. This concept has been tested in preterm lambs, where as few as six manual inflations of 35–40 mL/kg compromised the subsequent response to surfactant administration [61]. Likewise, preterm lambs ventilated with a tidal volume of 20 mL/kg before surfactant treatment had more acute lung injury than lambs ventilated with 5 or 10 mL/kg [62]. Similarly, lung injury can occur if lungs are ventilated below a normal functional residual capacity (FRC) (*atelectrauma*) resulting in cyclic opening and closing of the lung and injury. During positive-pressure ventilation, the distal lung can undergo rapid and cyclic transitions from being small and flooded at the end of expiration to being large and air-filled at the end of inspiration. This transition can generate significant shear stress forces and lung injury at the alveolar surface as the edema fluid redistributes and the alveolar volume changes. In the surfactant-deficient lung, ventilation at low lung volumes caused release of cytokines in vivo and in isolated lungs [47] and during intermittent mandatory ventilation; use of inadequate PEEP to maintain an appropriate FRC also increased lung injury [63]. On the other hand, recruitment of lung volumes to increase FRC protected against VILI and reduced the need for high levels of inspired oxygen [64]. Therefore, these studies clearly show that in premature infants on mechanical ventilation, the use of optimum tidal volume in combination with "ideal" PEEP would minimize lung injury.

There are several factors, from the biomechanical point of view, to explain injury of the lung. First, the lung of premature infants is not uniformly ventilated; there are areas of normal ventilation alternating with poorly aerated or even completely collapsed lung units. Therefore, the less injured areas of the lung are preferentially recruited during positive-pressure ventilation with the subsequent risk of injury from overexpansion. In addition, the resistance to lung expansion is not uniform. This heterogeneity in lung impedance results in shear stress being generated between neighboring, interdependent units that operate at different volumes [65]. Moreover, there is also injury to small airways and distal lung caused by the repeated opening and closure and by stress on the lining cells by the movement of air–liquid interfaces with respiration [66].

How does the lung respond to prevent/minimize lung injury? One of the mechanisms is by the *reorganization of the cell's stress-bearing elements* formed by elastin and collagen network of the ECM, integrins, and cytoskeleton. During mechanical ventilation, epithelial cells, basement membrane, and endothelial cells are exposed to mechanical deformation, and as a result, there is an increase in basement membrane surface area and a change in the shape of epithelial and endothelial cells. The cellular change is generally accompanied by the reorganization of the cell's stress-bearing elements. Therefore, this deformation-induced remodeling of the stress-bearing elements is critical to prevent cellular stress failure. Another important mechanism is by *vesicular lipid trafficking* to and from the plasma membrane. This lipid trafficking serves to regulate cell surface area and plasma membrane tension and ultimately helps to prevent plasma membrane stress failure [67–69].

Despite all these preventive mechanisms, excessive mechanical forces can injure the plasma membrane [37, 70]. It has been calculated that "a typical plasma membrane can sustain strains of only 1–3 % before it breaks" [71]. Several studies have examined the biophysical determinants of plasma membrane stress failure in cultured alveolar epithelial cells and found a correlation with strain amplitude and strain rate [15, 68, 72]. The ability to restore membrane integrity after cell wounding is essential for cell survival. One of the mechanisms is by "self-sealing" whereby hydrophobic interactions between phospholipids and water would drive lipid flow toward the free edges of a defect [73, 74]. Another mechanism is mediated by calcium. Small disruptions trigger calcium-dependent exocytosis of vesicles near the wound site, lower plasma membrane tension, and thereby facilitate wound closure [75]. For larger defects, vesicular endomembranes present in the lysosomes are transported and fused to the membrane defect via a rise in cytosolic Ca^{2+} [76–78].

Alveolar Epithelial Barrier Function The epithelial barrier is composed of tight junctions connected to the actin cytoskeleton via occludin or zonula occludens. It has been shown that mechanical strain of alveolar epithelial cells, mimicking mechanical ventilation with high tidal volumes, resulted in actin-mediated cell contraction with subsequent increased paracellular permeability [79]. This process is regulated by the family of Rho GTPases RhoA, Rac-1, and Cdc42 and mediated by Ca^{2+}/calmodulin-dependent phosphorylation of myosin light chain (MLC) kinase with consequent contraction of the actin–myosin complex and breakdown of intercellular junctions [80, 81]. In addition to maintaining the integrity of the epithelial barrier by the tight junctions, the cells need mechanisms to reabsorb the fluids present in the interstitium and alveolar spaces after lung injury mediated by mechanical ventilation [82]. This process is mediated by active transport of Na^+ through amiloride-sensitive cation channels (ENaC) present in the apical cell membranes and the Na^+/K^+-ATPases localized mainly in the basolateral cell membrane [83–86]. It has been shown that mechanical ventilation with higher tidal volumes leads to decreased alveolar fluid reabsorption [87], probably due to a decrease in Na^+/K^+-ATPase activity [88].

Alveolar Epithelial Plasma Membrane Stress Failure As discussed before, cells experience plasma membrane stress failure when the matrix to which they adhere undergoes large deformations and this is a frequent mechanism for necrotic cell death [89]. Data from animal models clearly demonstrate that ventilation with high distending pressures causes tissue destruction [7, 90]. This was tested in ex vivo mechanically ventilated rat lungs. They found that the number of subpleural cells with membrane defects rises with increasing tidal volumes and duration of ventilation. In addition, they found that over 60 % of injured cells were able to repair the plasma membrane defects [70]. In vitro studies from our laboratory also found that

20 % stretch of fetal epithelial cells increased release of lactate dehydrogenase (LDH) by 50 % when compared to control, unstretched cells [91] supporting the concept that overdistension of the membrane can cause cell death by necrosis.

Stress Failure of Endothelial and Epithelial Barriers Not only can the plasma membrane break, but also the contact between cells [14, 92]. If such a disruption happens to the pulmonary endothelial and epithelial barrier, this could cause a loss of compartmentalization. As a result, local proinflammatory mediators can spread in the systemic circulation [93–95]. In addition, loss of the barriers will also allow white blood cells to enter the lungs and promote inflammation. Therefore, exposure to mechanical force produces alveolar epithelial pathology ranging from inter and intracellular gap formations, denudation of the basement membrane, and cell destruction [7, 36, 96]. The current hypothesis is that disruption of the integrity of the endothelial cellular barrier occurs via cytoskeletal rearrangement and generation of tensile forces within the cell [97]. These changes result in cellular contraction with subsequent interruption of intercellular adhesion complexes and the creation of gaps between neighboring cells, or through cells, that allow the exudation of fluid, macromolecules, and leukocytes into the interstitium and ultimately into alveolar spaces [98–101].

Mechanotransduction in Ventilator-Induced Lung Injury (Fig. 2.2)

Mechanotransduction refers to the processes through which cells sense and respond to mechanical stimuli by converting them to biochemical signals that elicit specific cellular responses [102]. The degree and magnitude of mechanical deformation observed with injurious forms of ventilation probably do not occur normally in nature. Therefore, it is unlikely that evolutionary mechanisms have been specifically developed to deal with the overdistension that can occur with mechanical ventilation. Consequently, the inflammatory response generated by mechanical ventilation might "borrow" mechanoreceptors and signal transduction pathways from other more established signaling systems [60, 103] An example is the epidermal growth factor receptor (EGFR). Mechanical signals through this receptor are important for lung development [104]. However, EGFR also participates in mechanical ventilation-induced lung injury [105].

Mechanoreceptors

1. Stretch-activated Ion channels
2. Integrins–focal adhesions–cytoskeleton

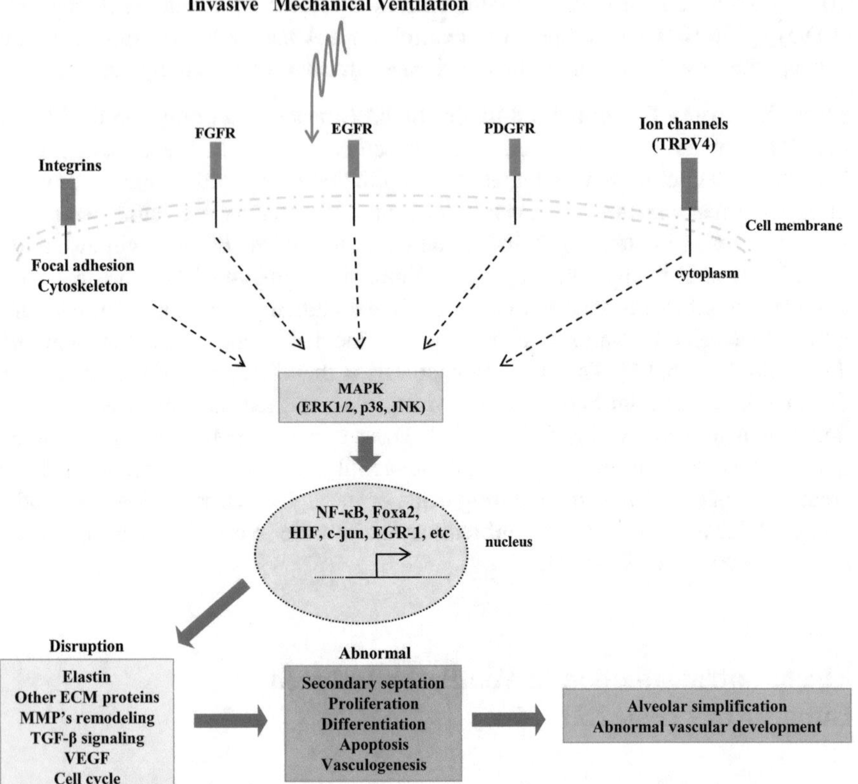

Fig. 2.2 Mechanoreceptors and signaling pathways activated by invasive mechanical ventilation that lead to abnormal alveolar development. Abbreviations: *FGFR* fibroblast growth factor receptor, *EGFR* epidermal growth factor receptor, *PDGFR* platelet-derived growth factor receptor, *TRPV* transient receptor potential vanilloids, *MAPK* mitogen-activated protein kinases, *ERK* extracellular signal-regulated kinases, *JNK* c-Jun N-terminal kinases, *NF-κB* nuclear factor kappa-light-chain-enhancer of activated B cells, *Foxa2* forkhead box A2, *EGR* early growth response, *HIF* hypoxia-inducible factors, *ECM* extracellular matrix, *MMP* matrix metalloproteinase, *TGFβ* transforming growth factor beta, *VEGF* vascular endothelial growth factor

Stretch-Activated Ion Channels

It has been demonstrated that physical forces applied to the plasma membrane of the cells can increase the permeability for ions [106, 107]. Ion channels can be activated either by direct opening of the channel by strain or as a consequence of forces transmitted to the channel via membrane-associated proteins [108]. Previous studies in alveolar epithelial cells have shown that Na^+ pump activity increases in proportion to the magnitude of stretch [60]. Moreover, cation channels seem to mediate the inflammatory response generated in the lung after mechanical stretch. Parker et al. [109] found that the increased microvascular permeability by mechanical injury was abolished by gadolinium (a stretch-activated nonselective cation channels inhibitor), suggesting that stretch-activated cation channels may initiate the increase in permeability induced by mechanical ventilation. Waters et al. [110] also showed that Na^+-K^+-ATPase activity was significantly increased in murine lung epithelial cells exposed to mechanical stretch. These studies suggest that stretch-activated cation channels may also regulate Na^+-K^+-ATPase activity, a factor that may play an important role in lung edema clearance.

Calcium channels are also important mechanoreceptors in lung injury. Boitano et al. demonstrated that mechanical stretch of airway epithelial cells opened the voltage-gated Ca^{2+} channels [111]. Transient receptor potential vanilloids (TRPV) channels have gained recent attention as key modulators of lung injury. TRPV4 in particular is a Ca^{2+}-permeable cation channel known to play an important role in osmotic and mechanical sensing [112]. In adult lungs, TRPV4 is expressed in the capillaries of septal walls and in alveolar type I cells. TRPV4 agonists produced blebs or breaks in the endothelial and epithelial layers of the alveolar wall and increased lung endothelial permeability [113] In addition to regulating the integrity of the lung alveolar capillary endothelium [114–116] and maintenance of the airway epithelial barrier function [117], TRPV4 has been recently implied as a key mediator of inflammation. TRPV4 inhibitors have potent anti-inflammatory effects by limiting neutrophil and macrophage infiltration, and blunting proinflammatory cytokine and chemokine production [118]. Moreover, recent studies from our laboratory have shown that TRPV4 is expressed in the fetal lung and may play an important role in the transduction of mechanical signals in the distal epithelium by modulating inflammation via p38 and extracellular signal regulated kinases (ERK) pathways [119]. All together, these data suggest that TRPV4 blockade may represent a therapeutic approach to decrease pulmonary edema and inflammation in lungs exposed to mechanical ventilation.

Integrins–Focal Adhesions–Cytoskeleton

Integrins, focal adhesion plaques, and the cytoskeleton are the probable key structures in sensing mechanical signals [120]. Integrins belong to a family of transmembrane receptors that cluster in focal adhesion plaques [121]. Their main role is to anchor cells to the basement membrane and ECM [122]. The cytoplasmic portion of integrins is in close contact with proteins such as vinculin, paxillin, talin, Src kinase, and focal adhesion kinase, which serve as adapter molecules for anchoring the cytoskeleton microfilaments and microtubules to the plasma membrane [122, 123]. Conformational changes of integrins, such as those induced by mechanical strain, lead to the activation of focal adhesion kinase and the mitogen-activated protein kinase (MAPK) pathway [124–126]. Previous studies from our laboratory in isolated fetal epithelial cells showed that mechanical strain induces conformational changes of integrin $\alpha6\beta1$ and releases EGFR ligands via ADAM 17 [127].

Other models propose that the cytoskeleton itself senses cellular deformation. Stretch-induced deformation of the actin filaments and microtubules can activate intracellular signaling pathways similar to those induced by stimulation of focal adhesion kinase [128, 129].

Evidence also indicates that cell matrix and adhesion molecules may be important in mediating the inflammatory response characteristic of VILI. It has been shown that magnetic twisting applied to beads coated with collagen, but not to control beads, increased transcription of inflammatory genes such as TNF-α and TGF-β, suggesting that both the magnitude and specific cell–matrix connections are important determinants of the airway epithelial response to mechanical forces [60, 108].

Mechanotransducers and Signaling Pathways Related to VILI

Growth Factor Receptors There is evidence to suggest that receptor tyrosine kinases can serve as mechanotransducers [130]. It has been demonstrated that mechanical forces can activate platelet-derived growth factor (PDGF) receptor in vascular smooth muscle cells [131] and fetal rat lung cells [132]. Moreover, compressive stress of airway epithelial cells [133] or mechanical strain of fetal epithelial cells [127, 134] activates EGFR via release of EGFR ligands by an autocrine/paracrine mechanism.

Intracellular Signaling Pathways A growing body of evidence indicates that MAPK plays an important role in transducing mechanical signals to the nucleus [120]. MAPK signaling pathways regulate essential cellular functions, such as cell proliferation, inflammation [135], and programmed cell death [136]. Activation of ERK, c-Jun N-terminal kinases (JNK), and p38 has been observed in various cell types exposed to mechanical stretch [126, 137–140]. Uhlig et al. [141] showed that ERK and JNK are phosphorylated in rat lungs following injurious mechanical ventilation. Protein kinase A, a cAMP-dependent kinase, has been shown to be increased in mechanically ventilated animals [142] and in cultured fetal type II epithelial cells exposed to stretch [143].

The adherens junction and gap junction seem to be also important in mechanotransduction [144]. Ko and coworkers demonstrated that mechanical forces applied to adherens junctions in fibroblasts activate stretch-sensitive calcium channels and increase actin polymerization [135] In addition, mechanical stretch-induced intercellular Ca^{2+} signaling in airway epithelial cells [145, 146]. The intercellular calcium propagation was mediated via gap junctions [147]. Considering the importance of integrity of alveolar epithelium in maintaining the barrier function in the lung, cell–cell interaction may play an important role in mechanotransduction, especially during mechanical ventilation [107].

Transcription Factors One of the most important mediators of inflammation is NF-κB, which plays a critical role in the generation of proinflammatory cytokines in response to mechanical injury. NF-κB contains a DNA "shear-stress" response element in the promoter region and binds to IL-6, IL-8, IL-1β, and TNF-α promoter sequences [60, 148]. A number of in vitro and ex vivo studies have shown that NF-κB is upregulated in response to stretch [149–151]. NF-κB activation was observed in the tracheal secretions of premature infants exposed to mechanical ventilation. Furthermore, stimulation of NF-κB was associated with elevated levels of TNFα, IL-8, prolonged mechanical ventilation, and BPD [152, 153].

Gene Expression Several studies have addressed gene expression profiling in VILI. Copland et al. found upregulation of transcription factors (early growth response-1 or EGR-1 and c-Jun), stress proteins (heat shock protein-70 or HSP-70), and inflammatory mediators (IL-1β) after 30 min of high tidal volume ventilation in rats [154]. Microarray analysis of isolated perfused mouse lungs ventilated with high tidal volumes revealed upregulation of genes related to growth factors, cellular communication, cytoskeletal function, proinflammatory cytokines and genes for immune/defense response, signal transduction pathways, and apoptosis [155–157]. Transcription analyses of lung samples from ventilated premature baboons, mouse, and rat models of BPD identified several highly conserved genes in response to mechanical ventilation. These included elastin (ELN), gastrin-releasing polypeptide (GRP), and connective tissue growth factor (CTGF) [158].

Signaling Pathways Modulating Alveolar Development and Disruption by Mechanical Ventilation (Fig. 2.2)

In order to understand the potential impact of mechanical ventilation on lung development, it is important first to review the molecular mechanisms regulating late stages of lung development and, specifically, alveolar formation. Extremely low birth weight (ELBW) infants are born at the transition from the canalicular to the saccular stages of lung development. At this time, the histology of the distal lung is characterized by clusters of widened air space called saccules. The walls of these sacs, the primary septae, are closely associated with the capillary network. At the same time, the cuboidal epithelial cells begin to differentiate into the alveolar epithelial type 1 and type 2 cells (AEC1 and AEC2). During alveolarization, the saccules are subdivided by the ingrowth of ridges or crests known as secondary septae. Both myofibroblast and endothelial cells migrate to these crests, and a scaffold of matrix proteins is deposited, enriched in elastin at the tip [159]. These later stages of lung development require a precise temporal and spatial coordination of multiple signaling pathways, making this process susceptible to disruption by mechanical ventilation [160, 161].

Alveolar Septation

Alveolar septation involves substantial tissue growth and remodeling, including the deposit of elastin and other proteins and ECM remodeling [160]. Elastin deposition at the tip of the primary septa plays a critical role in secondary septation or alveolarization. Myofibroblasts produce elastin from tropoelastin by the enzyme lysyl oxidase. The essential role for elastin in alveolar development was demonstrated in genetically modified mice. Deletion of the elastin gene impaired distal airway development with fewer and dilated distal air sacs and attenuated tissue septa [162]. Myofibroblasts differentiation and elastin production are regulated by platelet-derived growth factor-α (PDGF-α). Knockout mice lacking PDGF-α show loss of alveolar myofibroblasts and associated elastin fiber deposits, resulting in a significant compromise in alveolar formation [163, 164]. Retinoic acid (RA) and fibroblast growth factor (FGF) are also key controllers of elastin formation. RA enhances the expression of PDGFA/PDGFRα [165] and tropoelastin [166], and increases the total number of alveoli [167, 168]. FGF signaling is also important for alveolarization. Secondary septation is compromised in mice lacking FGFR3 and FGFR4 [169]. Moreover, FGF18 promotes myofibroblast expression of tropoelastin, lysyl oxidase, and microfibril proteins such as fibrillins and fibulins that act as scaffold for elastin assembly [170].

Elastin was found to be increased in ventilated infants who died from BPD [171, 172]. Elastic fibers were described as thickened, tortuous, and irregularly distributed [173]. Moreover, increased elastase activity was observed in guinea pigs exposed to mechanical ventilation [174] and in infants who developed BPD [175]. Therefore, exaggerated elastase activity can result in destruction of mature cross-linked elastic fibers, reduction of proteins that regulate elastic fiber assembly and disordered pulmonary elastic deposition, as described in preterm lambs and newborn mice exposed to mechanical ventilation [176, 177]. Disruption of other ECM proteins such as hyaluronan, laminin, etc. has been also attributed to elastase hyperactivity [178, 179]. Taken together, these studies indicate that elastolytic damage may contribute to reduced secondary septation and alveolarization and explain altered lung elastin deposition and defective septation observed in patients with BPD [180, 181].

In addition to elastin, deposition of other components of the ECM, such as collagen, fibronectin, and proteoglycans is important for alveolar septation [160]. Postmortem studies in newborn infants with BPD found a damaged collagen network with thickened collagenous saccular walls and a wide interstitium with increased quantity and size of collagen fibers [182].

Remodeling of the ECM is also critical for alveolar septation. MMPs play a central role in this process. MMP-1, MMP-2, and MMP-9 are expressed during alveolarization in humans and mice [183, 184]. Mice lacking MMP-2 show abnormal saccular development [185]. However, enhanced proteolytic activity also appears to be detrimental to the developing lung. Overexpression of MMP-2, MMP-8, and MMP-9 has been identified in airway secretions of infants with BPD [186]. A similar pattern was found in the bronchoalveolar lavage fluid in baboon models of BPD [187, 188]. Therefore, a perturbation of a fine balance of ECM remodeling by MMPs induced by mechanical ventilation could have a negative impact on alveolar septation.

TGF-β plays an important role in lung development by regulating cell survival and ECM production and remodeling [189]. It has been shown that transient decrease in TGF-β activity alters cell proliferation and inhibits septation [190]. In contrast, overexpression of TGF-β1 in the neonatal mouse lung induces histological changes observed in BPD, such as enlarged alveolar sacs, poor secondary septation, thick and hypercellular septa, and abnormal capillary development [168, 191, 192]. High levels of TGF-β have been detected in airway secretions from preterm infants with BPD [58]. Moreover, TGF-β signaling is disrupted in animal models of BPD. Mechanical ventilation increases the expression of TGF-β in preterm lambs [193], and neutralization of the abnormal TGF-β activity improves alveologenesis and microvascular development in the injured developing lung [194]. The mechanism by which an increase of TGF-β activity alters alveologenesis is not clearly defined although previous studies indicate that it could be mediated in part by enhancing apoptosis and decreasing proliferation of AEC2 cells [195]. Thus, the balance of TGF-β signaling appears to be critical to alveolar development.

Regulation of Cell Proliferation, Differentiation, and Apoptosis

Tissue remodeling during later stages of lung development requires well-coordinated regulation of cell proliferation and apoptosis [168]. Proliferation and differentiation of the distal epithelium play a critical role in alveolar septation. As discussed before, at the transition from canalicular to saccular stages, cuboidal epithelium begins to differentiate into alveolar type II and type I cells. Both cell types are critical in the signaling pathways regulating alveolar formation. For example, deletion of the transcription factor Foxa2, required for alveolar type II cell differentiation [196], caused extensive airspace enlargement and altered septation [197]. Moreover, mice null for T1α, an alveolar type I cell marker, showed abnormal distal lung cell proliferation, and narrower and irregular air spaces [198]. These studies support that both type II and type I cells are important for alveologenesis.

Several growth factors have been shown to promote proliferation and differentiation of epithelial cells. FGF7 (keratinocyte growth factor) for example, has a potent stimulatory effect on proliferation and maturation of type II cells [199]. FGF7 has also been shown to prevent lung epithelial injury induced by mechanical ventilation [200]. Insulin growth factor (IGF) also promotes alveolar development [201]. Heparin-binding EGF (HB-EGF) has been shown to induce type II cell differentiation and a modulator of cell proliferation [127, 134].

Studies in the premature baboon model of BPD [202] and newborn rats [203] have demonstrated that mechanical ventilation causes cell cycle arrest at the G1–G2 phase by affecting cyclin and Cdk expression. Both mesenchymal and epithelial cells were equally affected. In vitro studies from our laboratory also found that mechanical strain inhibits cell proliferation in fetal rat lung cells [91]. This effect could be mediated via the EGFR since decrease of proliferation mediated by mechanical stretch was absent in fibroblasts isolated from EGFR knockout mice [204]. Given the critical role of cellular proliferation in alveolar formation, these studies support the concept that proliferative arrest secondary to mechanical ventilation may cause a reduction in alveolarization resulting in alveolar simplification.

Apoptosis is also important for normal lung development and specifically for remodeling of the distal lung [205]. However, an imbalance between proliferation and apoptosis can compromise alveolar development. Studies by Bland's group observed a fivefold increase in the number of terminal deoxynucleotidyl transferase dUTP nick end labeling (TUNEL)-stained cells with a corresponding increase in active caspase-3 protein in the lungs of pups exposed to mechanical ventilation without a significant effect on cell proliferation, as assessed by proliferating cell nuclear antigen (PCNA) staining of lung sections. These findings, which are similar to those previously reported for 4-day-old pups that received mechanical ventilation with 40 % O_2 for 24 h [180], suggest that cyclic stretch of the lung during development increases apoptosis and causes septal loss leading to defective alveolar formation [177].

Vascular Endothelial Growth Factor

Vascular Endothelial Growth Factor (VEGF) is critical not only for angiogenesis [206] but also for alveolarization [207, 208]. Administration of VEGF inhibitors impaired pulmonary vascular growth and secondary septation [207, 209] VEGF expression is decreased in patients with BPD. Histology of these patients shows rarefied and dilated peripheral vessels, fewer air–blood barriers, and a decreased airspace–parenchyma ratio [210, 211]. VEGF is a downstream target of hypoxia-inducible factors (HIFs). Deletion of HIF-2 reduces VEGF levels and leads to early death due to respiratory failure [212]. Relative hyperoxic conditions associated with preterm birth could potentially lead to decreased expression of HIF [213]. In addition, premature infants exposed to mechanical ventilation also received a moderate amount of oxygen. All of this could inhibit HIF with the subsequent decrease in VEGF expression and disruption of lung vascular growth and alveolar septation [208]. VEGF is decreased in the preterm baboon model of BPD [214]. Mechanical ventilation of newborn mice reduces VEGF expression and results in lung structural abnormalities consistent with BPD [181]. Moreover, overexpression of VEGF in newborn rats increases survival, promotes lung angiogenesis, and prevents hyperoxia-induced alveolar damage [215].

Animal Models of Invasive Mechanical Ventilation

Animal models of invasive mechanical ventilation have provided insights into the mechanisms of VILI [168, 216, 217] Studies in preterm baboon at the saccular stage have shown that mechanical ventilation with moderate degree of hyperoxia induces inflammation, by releasing proinflammatory cytokines and recruiting inflammatory cells to the lung, and impairs alveolar and vascular development [49,

214, 218]. Similar findings were observed in chronically ventilated preterm lambs [40]. Even a short period of mechanical ventilation was sufficient to induce inflammation, demonstrated by an increase of the proinflammatory cytokines such as IL-1β, IL-6, MCP, etc. [48]. High tidal volume ventilation at the alveolar stage in rats and mice also promoted inflammation [50, 51, 219]. Some limitations of these models are the inclusion of hyperoxia injury in addition to mechanical stretch caused by the ventilators. To specifically address the component of mechanical strain in lung injury, Bland's group [177] exposed 6-day-old mice to mechanical ventilation without hyperoxia and found that stretch alone can inhibit alveolar septation and angiogenesis and increase apoptosis and lung elastin, which was distributed throughout alveolar walls rather than at septal tips. In another model, Harding's group [220] investigated the injurious effects of mechanical ventilation per se in the immature lung using a technique to ventilate the lungs of the ovine fetus with an intact placenta. After 24 h of mechanical ventilation of preterm lungs at the saccular stage, lung parenchyma and bronchioles were severely injured; tissue space and myofibroblast density were increased, collagen and elastin fibers were deformed and secondary crest density was reduced. Bronchioles contained debris and their epithelium was injured and thickened. In this model, mechanical ventilation did not upregulate genes involved in the production of proinflammatory cytokines [220]. In a similar model, injury caused by mechanical ventilation increased EGR-1 and expression of pro- and anti-inflammatory cytokines within 1 h. Mechanical injury induced granulocyte/macrophage colony-stimulating factor and matured monocytes to alveolar macrophages by 24 h [48]. Also, and as previously discussed, mechanical ventilation for 24 h without oxygen in a 7-day rat model led to cell cycle arrest [203]. In summary, these models show that mechanical injury without hyperoxia replicate some of the hallmarks typical of BPD such as inflammation, impairment of alveolarization, altered elastin deposit, and abnormal vasculogenesis.

Conclusions

In conclusion, overdistension of the lung can damage lung resident cells and disrupt the alveolar–capillary barrier with subsequent release of proinflammatory cytokines, increase in permeability, and influx of neutrophils and macrophages to the lung. In addition to inducing an inflammatory response, invasive mechanical ventilation can also have a negative impact on important signaling pathways regulating alveolar development, such as secondary septation, cell proliferation, differentiation, apoptosis, and vasculogenesis. The final consequence is alveolar simplification and abnormal vascular development observed in the histology of patients with BPD. Therefore, aggressive extubation and the use of noninvasive modes of ventilation [221], would be considered beneficial and have been shown to have a positive impact on the incidence of this devastating disease in premature infants.

References

1. Trembath A, Laughon MM. Predictors of bronchopulmonary dysplasia. Clin Perinatol. 2012;39(3):585–601.
2. Jobe AH, Bancalari E. Bronchopulmonary dysplasia. Am J Respir Crit Care Med. 2001;163(7):1723–9.
3. Skidmore MD, Rivers A, Hack M. Increased risk of cerebral palsy among very low-birthweight infants with chronic lung disease. Dev Med Child Neurol. 1990;32(4):325–32.
4. Bhandari A, Bhandari V. Biomarkers in bronchopulmonary dysplasia. Paediatr Respir Rev. 2013;14(3):173–9.
5. Jobe AH, Ikegami M. Mechanisms initiating lung injury in the preterm. Early Hum Dev. 1998;53(1):81–94.
6. Clark RH, Gerstmann DR, Jobe AH, Moffitt ST, Slutsky AS, Yoder BA. Lung injury in neonates: causes, strategies for prevention, and long-term consequences. J Pediatr. 2001;139(4):478–86.
7. Dreyfuss D, Saumon G. Ventilator-induced lung injury: lessons from experimental studies. Am J Respir Crit Care Med. 1998;157(1):294–323.
8. Speer CP. Inflammation and bronchopulmonary dysplasia: a continuing story. Semin Fetal Neonatal Med. 2006;11(5):354–62.
9. Kramer BW, Kallapur S, Newnham J, Jobe AH. Prenatal inflammation and lung development. Semin Fetal Neonatal Med. 2009;14(1):2–7.
10. Wirtz HR, Dobbs LG. Calcium mobilization and exocytosis after one mechanical stretch of lung epithelial cells. Science. 1990;250(4985):1266–9.
11. Sanchez-Esteban J, Cicchiello LA, Wang Y, et al. Mechanical stretch promotes alveolar epithelial type II cell differentiation. J Appl Physiol. 2001;91(2):589–95.
12. Edwards YS, Sutherland LM, Power JH, Nicholas TE, Murray AW. Cyclic stretch induces both apoptosis and secretion in rat alveolar type II cells. FEBS Lett. 1999;448(1):127–30.
13. Hammerschmidt S, Kuhn H, Grasenack T, Gessner C, Wirtz H. Apoptosis and necrosis induced by cyclic mechanical stretching in alveolar type II cells. Am J Respir Cell Mol Biol. 2004;30(3):396–402.
14. Vlahakis NE, Hubmayr RD. Invited review: plasma membrane stress failure in alveolar epithelial cells. J Appl Physiol. 2000;89(6):2490–6. discussion 2497.
15. Tschumperlin DJ, Oswari J, Margulies AS. Deformation-induced injury of alveolar epithelial cells. Effect of frequency, duration, and amplitude. Am J Respir Crit Care Med. 2000;162(2 Pt 1):357–62.
16. Vlahakis NE, Schroeder MA, Limper AH, Hubmayr RD. Stretch induces cytokine release by alveolar epithelial cells in vitro. Am J Physiol. 1999;277(1 Pt 1):L167–73.
17. Yamamoto H, Teramoto H, Uetani K, Igawa K, Shimizu E. Cyclic stretch upregulates interleukin-8 and transforming growth factor-beta1 production through a protein kinase C-dependent pathway in alveolar epithelial cells. Respirology. 2002;7(2):103–9.
18. Hammerschmidt S, Kuhn H, Sack U, et al. Mechanical stretch alters alveolar type II cell mediator release toward a proinflammatory pattern. Am J Respir Cell Mol Biol. 2005;33(2):203–10.
19. Lee HS, Wang Y, Maciejewski BS, et al. Interleukin-10 protects cultured fetal rat type II epithelial cells from injury induced by mechanical stretch. Am J Physiol Lung Cell Mol Physiol. 2008;294(2):L225–32.
20. Thorley AJ, Ford PA, Giembycz MA, Goldstraw P, Young A, Tetley TD. Differential regulation of cytokine release and leukocyte migration by lipopolysaccharide-stimulated primary human lung alveolar type II epithelial cells and macrophages. J Immunol. 2007;178(1):463–73.
21. Rozycki HJ. Potential contribution of type I alveolar epithelial cells to chronic neonatal lung disease. Front Pediatr. 2014;2:45.

22. Wong MH, Chapin OC, Johnson MD. LPS-stimulated cytokine production in type I cells is modulated by the renin-angiotensin system. Am J Respir Cell Mol Biol. 2012;46(5):641–50.
23. Wong MH, Johnson MD. Differential response of primary alveolar type I and type II cells to LPS stimulation. PLoS One. 2013;8(1):e55545.
24. Schneeberger EE, Lynch RD. The tight junction: a multifunctional complex. Am J Physiol Cell Physiol. 2004;286(6):C1213–28.
25. Dipaolo BC, Davidovich N, Kazanietz MG, Margulies SS. Rac1 pathway mediates stretch response in pulmonary alveolar epithelial cells. Am J Physiol Lung Cell Mol Physiol. 2013;305(2):L141–53.
26. McGowan SE, Torday JS. The pulmonary lipofibroblast (lipid interstitial cell) and its contributions to alveolar development. Annu Rev Physiol. 1997;59:43–62.
27. Gahler A, Stallmach T, Schwaller J, Fey MF, Tobler A. Interleukin-8 expression by fetal and neonatal pulmonary cells in hyaline membrane disease and amniotic infection. Pediatr Res. 2000;48(3):299–303.
28. Hawwa RL, Hokenson MA, Wang Y, Huang Z, Sharma S, Sanchez-Esteban J. IL-10 inhibits inflammatory cytokines released by fetal mouse lung fibroblasts exposed to mechanical stretch. Pediatr Pulmonol. 2011;46(7):640–9.
29. Okada M, Matsumori A, Ono K, et al. Cyclic stretch upregulates production of interleukin-8 and monocyte chemotactic and activating factor/monocyte chemoattractant protein-1 in human endothelial cells. Arterioscler Thromb Vasc Biol. 1998;18(6):894–901.
30. Birukov KG, Jacobson JR, Flores AA, et al. Magnitude-dependent regulation of pulmonary endothelial cell barrier function by cyclic stretch. Am J Physiol Lung Cell Mol Physiol. 2003;285(4):L785–97.
31. Pugin J, Dunn I, Jolliet P, et al. Activation of human macrophages by mechanical ventilation in vitro. Am J Physiol. 1998;275(6 Pt 1):L1040–50.
32. Jaarsma AS, Braaksma MA, Geven WB, van Oeveren W, Bambang Oetomo S. Activation of the inflammatory reaction within minutes after birth in ventilated preterm lambs with neonatal respiratory distress syndrome. Biol Neonate. 2004;86(1):1–5.
33. Omlor G, Niehaus GD, Maron MB. Effect of peak inspiratory pressure on the filtration coefficient in the isolated perfused rat lung. J Appl Physiol (1985). 1993;74(6):3068–72.
34. Dreyfuss D, Soler P, Basset G, Saumon G. High inflation pressure pulmonary edema. Respective effects of high airway pressure, high tidal volume, and positive end-expiratory pressure. Am Rev Respir Dis. 1988;137(5):1159–64.
35. Ramanathan R, Mason GR, Raj JU. Effect of mechanical ventilation and barotrauma on pulmonary clearance of 99mtechnetium diethylenetriamine pentaacetate in lambs. Pediatr Res. 1990;27(1):70–4.
36. John E, McDevitt M, Wilborn W, Cassady G. Ultrastructure of the lung after ventilation. Br J Exp Pathol. 1982;63(4):401–7.
37. Dreyfuss D, Basset G, Soler P, Saumon G. Intermittent positive-pressure hyperventilation with high inflation pressures produces pulmonary microvascular injury in rats. Am Rev Respir Dis. 1985;132(4):880–4.
38. Speer CP. Inflammation and bronchopulmonary dysplasia. Semin Neonatol. 2003;8(1):29–38.
39. Tremblay L, Valenza F, Ribeiro SP, Li J, Slutsky AS. Injurious ventilatory strategies increase cytokines and c-fos m-RNA expression in an isolated rat lung model. J Clin Invest. 1997;99(5):944–52.
40. Albertine KH, Jones GP, Starcher BC, et al. Chronic lung injury in preterm lambs. Disordered respiratory tract development. Am J Respir Crit Care Med. 1999;159(3):945–58.
41. Jackson JC, Chi EY, Wilson CB, Truog WE, Teh EC, Hodson WA. Sequence of inflammatory cell migration into lung during recovery from hyaline membrane disease in premature newborn monkeys. Am Rev Respir Dis. 1987;135(4):937–40.

42. Woo SW, Hedley-Whyte J. Macrophage accumulation and pulmonary edema due to thoracotomy and lung over inflation. J Appl Physiol. 1972;33(1):14–21.
43. Tsuno K, Miura K, Takeya M, Kolobow T, Morioka T. Histopathologic pulmonary changes from mechanical ventilation at high peak airway pressures. Am Rev Respir Dis. 1991;143(5 Pt 1):1115–20.
44. Merritt TA, Stuard ID, Puccia J, et al. Newborn tracheal aspirate cytology: classification during respiratory distress syndrome and bronchopulmonary dysplasia. J Pediatr. 1981;98(6): 949–56.
45. Groneck P, Gotze-Speer B, Oppermann M, Eiffert H, Speer CP. Association of pulmonary inflammation and increased microvascular permeability during the development of bronchopulmonary dysplasia: a sequential analysis of inflammatory mediators in respiratory fluids of high-risk preterm neonates. Pediatrics. 1994;93(5):712–8.
46. Munshi UK, Niu JO, Siddiq MM, Parton LA. Elevation of interleukin-8 and interleukin-6 precedes the influx of neutrophils in tracheal aspirates from preterm infants who develop bronchopulmonary dysplasia. Pediatr Pulmonol. 1997;24(5):331–6.
47. Muscedere JG, Mullen JB, Gan K, Slutsky AS. Tidal ventilation at low airway pressures can augment lung injury. Am J Respir Crit Care Med. 1994;149(5):1327–34.
48. Hillman NH, Polglase GR, Pillow JJ, Saito M, Kallapur SG, Jobe AH. Inflammation and lung maturation from stretch injury in preterm fetal sheep. Am J Physiol Lung Cell Mol Physiol. 2011;300(2):L232–41.
49. Coalson JJ, Winter VT, Siler-Khodr T, Yoder BA. Neonatal chronic lung disease in extremely immature baboons. Am J Respir Crit Care Med. 1999;160(4):1333–46.
50. Wu S, Capasso L, Lessa A, et al. High tidal volume ventilation activates Smad2 and upregulates expression of connective tissue growth factor in newborn rat lung. Pediatr Res. 2008;63(3):245–50.
51. Kroon AA, Wang J, Huang Z, Cao L, Kuliszewski M, Post M. Inflammatory response to oxygen and endotoxin in newborn rat lung ventilated with low tidal volume. Pediatr Res. 2010;68(1):63–9.
52. Jones CA, Cayabyab RG, Kwong KY, et al. Undetectable interleukin (IL)-10 and persistent IL-8 expression early in hyaline membrane disease: a possible developmental basis for the predisposition to chronic lung inflammation in preterm newborns. Pediatr Res. 1996;39(6):966–75.
53. Bland RD. Neonatal chronic lung disease in the post-surfactant era. Biol Neonate. 2005; 88(3):181–91.
54. Bartram U, Speer CP. The role of transforming growth factor beta in lung development and disease. Chest. 2004;125(2):754–65.
55. Sime PJ, Marr RA, Gauldie D, et al. Transfer of tumor necrosis factor-alpha to rat lung induces severe pulmonary inflammation and patchy interstitial fibrogenesis with induction of transforming growth factor-beta1 and myofibroblasts. Am J Pathol. 1998;153(3):825–32.
56. Sime PJ, Xing Z, Graham FL, Csaky KG, Gauldie J. Adenovector-mediated gene transfer of active transforming growth factor-beta1 induces prolonged severe fibrosis in rat lung. J Clin Invest. 1997;100(4):768–76.
57. Kotecha S, Wangoo A, Silverman M, Shaw RJ. Increase in the concentration of transforming growth factor beta-1 in bronchoalveolar lavage fluid before development of chronic lung disease of prematurity. J Pediatr. 1996;128(4):464–9.
58. Lecart C, Cayabyab R, Buckley S, et al. Bioactive transforming growth factor-beta in the lungs of extremely low birthweight neonates predicts the need for home oxygen supplementation. Biol Neonate. 2000;77(4):217–23.
59. Schumacker PT. Straining to understand mechanotransduction in the lung. Am J Physiol Lung Cell Mol Physiol. 2002;282(5):L881–2.
60. Dos Santos CC, Slutsky AS. Invited review: mechanisms of ventilator-induced lung injury: a perspective. J Appl Physiol (1985). 2000;89(4):1645–55.
61. Bjorklund LJ, Ingimarsson J, Curstedt T, et al. Manual ventilation with a few large breaths at birth compromises the therapeutic effect of subsequent surfactant replacement in immature lambs. Pediatr Res. 1997;42(3):348–55.

62. Wada K, Jobe AH, Ikegami M. Tidal volume effects on surfactant treatment responses with the initiation of ventilation in preterm lambs. J Appl Physiol (1985). 1997;83(4):1054–61.
63. Michna J, Jobe AH, Ikegami M. Positive end-expiratory pressure preserves surfactant function in preterm lambs. Am J Respir Crit Care Med. 1999;160(2):634–9.
64. Dreyfuss D, Saumon G. Role of tidal volume, FRC, and end-inspiratory volume in the development of pulmonary edema following mechanical ventilation. Am Rev Respir Dis. 1993;148(5):1194–203.
65. Mead J, Takishima T, Leith D. Stress distribution in lungs: a model of pulmonary elasticity. J Appl Physiol. 1970;28(5):596–608.
66. Vlahakis NE, Hubmayr RD. Cellular stress failure in ventilator-injured lungs. Am J Respir Crit Care Med. 2005;171(12):1328–42.
67. Vlahakis NE, Schroeder MA, Pagano RE, Hubmayr RD. Deformation-induced lipid trafficking in alveolar epithelial cells. Am J Physiol Lung Cell Mol Physiol. 2001;280(5):L938–46.
68. Vlahakis NE, Schroeder MA, Pagano RE, Hubmayr RD. Role of deformation-induced lipid trafficking in the prevention of plasma membrane stress failure. Am J Respir Crit Care Med. 2002;166(9):1282–9.
69. Fisher JL, Levitan I, Margulies SS. Plasma membrane surface increases with tonic stretch of alveolar epithelial cells. Am J Respir Cell Mol Biol. 2004;31(2):200–8.
70. Gajic O, Lee J, Doerr CH, Berrios JC, Myers JL, Hubmayr RD. Ventilator-induced cell wounding and repair in the intact lung. Am J Respir Crit Care Med. 2003;167(8):1057–63.
71. Bloom M, Evans E, Mouritsen OG. Physical properties of the fluid lipid-bilayer component of cell membranes: a perspective. Q Rev Biophys. 1991;24(3):293–397.
72. Tschumperlin DJ, Margulies SS. Equibiaxial deformation-induced injury of alveolar epithelial cells in vitro. Am J Physiol. 1998;275(6 Pt 1):L1173–83.
73. Benz R, Zimmermann U. The resealing process of lipid bilayers after reversible electrical breakdown. Biochim Biophys Acta. 1981;640(1):169–78.
74. Lipowsky R. The conformation of membranes. Nature. 1991;349(6309):475–81.
75. Togo T, Krasieva TB, Steinhardt RA. A decrease in membrane tension precedes successful cell-membrane repair. Mol Biol Cell. 2000;11(12):4339–46.
76. Terasaki M, Miyake K, McNeil PL. Large plasma membrane disruptions are rapidly resealed by Ca2+–dependent vesicle-vesicle fusion events. J Cell Biol. 1997;139(1):63–74.
77. McNeil PL, Vogel SS, Miyake K, Terasaki M. Patching plasma membrane disruptions with cytoplasmic membrane. J Cell Sci. 2000;113(Pt 11):1891–902.
78. Bi GQ, Alderton JM, Steinhardt RA. Calcium-regulated exocytosis is required for cell membrane resealing. J Cell Biol. 1995;131(6 Pt 2):1747–58.
79. DiPaolo BC, Lenormand G, Fredberg JJ, Margulies SS. Stretch magnitude and frequency-dependent actin cytoskeleton remodeling in alveolar epithelia. Am J Physiol Cell Physiol. 2010;299(2):C345–53.
80. Garcia JG, Davis HW, Patterson CE. Regulation of endothelial cell gap formation and barrier dysfunction: role of myosin light chain phosphorylation. J Cell Physiol. 1995;163(3):510–22.
81. Goeckeler ZM, Wysolmerski RB. Myosin light chain kinase-regulated endothelial cell contraction: the relationship between isometric tension, actin polymerization, and myosin phosphorylation. J Cell Biol. 1995;130(3):613–27.
82. Hochberg I, Abassi Z, Azzam ZS. Patterns of alveolar fluid clearance in heart failure. Int J Cardiol. 2008;130(2):125–30.
83. Goodman BE, Fleischer RS, Crandall ED. Evidence for active Na+ transport by cultured monolayers of pulmonary alveolar epithelial cells. Am J Physiol. 1983;245(1):C78–83.
84. Basset G, Bouchonnet F, Crone C, Saumon G. Potassium transport across rat alveolar epithelium: evidence for an apical Na+-K+ pump. J Physiol. 1988;400:529–43.
85. Matalon S, Benos DJ, Jackson RM. Biophysical and molecular properties of amiloride-inhibitable Na+ channels in alveolar epithelial cells. Am J Physiol. 1996;271(1 Pt 1):L1–22.
86. Sznajder JI, Olivera WG, Ridge KM, Rutschman DH. Mechanisms of lung liquid clearance during hyperoxia in isolated rat lungs. Am J Respir Crit Care Med. 1995;151(5):1519–25.

87. Frank JA, Gutierrez JA, Jones KD, Allen L, Dobbs L, Matthay MA. Low tidal volume reduces epithelial and endothelial injury in acid-injured rat lungs. Am J Respir Crit Care Med. 2002;165(2):242–9.
88. Lecuona E, Saldias F, Comellas A, Ridge K, Guerrero C, Sznajder JI. Ventilator-associated lung injury decreases lung ability to clear edema in rats. Am J Respir Crit Care Med. 1999;159(2):603–9.
89. Uhlig S. Ventilation-induced lung injury and mechanotransduction: stretching it too far? Am J Physiol Lung Cell Mol Physiol. 2002;282(5):L892–6.
90. Webb HH, Tierney DF. Experimental pulmonary edema due to intermittent positive pressure ventilation with high inflation pressures. Protection by positive end-expiratory pressure. Am Rev Respir Dis. 1974;110(5):556–65.
91. Sanchez-Esteban J, Wang Y, Cicchiello LA, Rubin LP. Cyclic mechanical stretch inhibits cell proliferation and induces apoptosis in fetal rat lung fibroblasts. Am J Physiol Lung Cell Mol Physiol. 2002;282(3):L448–56.
92. West JB. Invited review: pulmonary capillary stress failure. J Appl Physiol (1985). 2000;89(6):2483–9. discussion 2497.
93. Haitsma JJ, Uhlig S, Goggel R, Verbrugge SJ, Lachmann U, Lachmann B. Ventilator-induced lung injury leads to loss of alveolar and systemic compartmentalization of tumor necrosis factor-alpha. Intensive Care Med. 2000;26(10):1515–22.
94. Murphy DB, Cregg N, Tremblay L, et al. Adverse ventilatory strategy causes pulmonary-to-systemic translocation of endotoxin. Am J Respir Crit Care Med. 2000;162(1):27–33.
95. Verbrugge SJ, Sorm V, van 't Veen A, Mouton JW, Gommers D, Lachmann B. Lung overinflation without positive end-expiratory pressure promotes bacteremia after experimental Klebsiella pneumoniae inoculation. Intensive Care Med. 1998;24(2):172–7.
96. Dreyfuss D, Soler P, Saumon G. Mechanical ventilation-induced pulmonary edema. Interaction with previous lung alterations. Am J Respir Crit Care Med. 1995;151(5): 1568–75.
97. dos Santos CC, Slutsky AS. The contribution of biophysical lung injury to the development of biotrauma. Annu Rev Physiol. 2006;68:585–618.
98. Neal CR, Michel CC. Transcellular openings through frog microvascular endothelium. Exp Physiol. 1997;82(2):419–22.
99. Michel CC, Neal CR. Openings through endothelial cells associated with increased microvascular permeability. Microcirculation. 1999;6(1):45–54.
100. Elliott AR, Fu Z, Tsukimoto K, Prediletto R, Mathieu-Costello O, West JB. Short-term reversibility of ultrastructural changes in pulmonary capillaries caused by stress failure. J Appl Physiol (1985). 1992;73(3):1150–8.
101. Feng D, Nagy JA, Hipp J, Pyne K, Dvorak HF, Dvorak AM. Reinterpretation of endothelial cell gaps induced by vasoactive mediators in guinea-pig, mouse and rat: many are transcellular pores. J Physiol. 1997;504(Pt 3):747–61.
102. Wang N, Tytell JD, Ingber DE. Mechanotransduction at a distance: mechanically coupling the extracellular matrix with the nucleus. Nat Rev Mol Cell Biol. 2009;10(1):75–82.
103. Wajant H, Muhlenbeck F, Scheurich P. Identification of a TRAF (TNF receptor-associated factor) gene in *Caenorhabditis elegans*. J Mol Evol. 1998;47(6):656–62.
104. Huang Z, Wang Y, Nayak PS, Dammann CE, Sanchez-Esteban J. Stretch-induced fetal type II cell differentiation is mediated via ErbB1-ErbB4 interactions. J Biol Chem. 2012;287(22):18091–102.
105. Bierman A, Yerrapureddy A, Reddy NM, Hassoun PM, Reddy SP. Epidermal growth factor receptor (EGFR) regulates mechanical ventilation-induced lung injury in mice. Transl Res. 2008;152(6):265–72.
106. Spieth PM, Bluth T, Gama De Abreu M, Bacelis A, Goetz AE, Kiefmann R. Mechanotransduction in the lungs. Minerva Anestesiol. 2014;80(8):933–41.
107. Han B, Lodyga M, Liu M. Ventilator-induced lung injury: role of protein-protein interaction in mechanosensation. Proc Am Thorac Soc. 2005;2(3):181–7.
108. Fredberg JJ, Kamm RD. Stress transmission in the lung: pathways from organ to molecule. Annu Rev Physiol. 2006;68:507–41.

109. Parker JC, Ivey CL, Tucker JA. Gadolinium prevents high airway pressure-induced permeability increases in isolated rat lungs. J Appl Physiol (1985). 1998;84(4):1113–8.
110. Waters CM, Ridge KM, Sunio G, Venetsanou K, Sznajder JI. Mechanical stretching of alveolar epithelial cells increases Na(+)-K(+)-ATPase activity. J Appl Physiol (1985). 1999;87(2): 715–21.
111. Boitano S, Sanderson MJ, Dirksen ER. A role for Ca(2+)-conducting ion channels in mechanically-induced signal transduction of airway epithelial cells. J Cell Sci. 1994;107(Pt 11):3037–44.
112. Yin J, Kuebler WM. Mechanotransduction by TRP channels: general concepts and specific role in the vasculature. Cell Biochem Biophys. 2010;56(1):1–18.
113. Alvarez DF, King JA, Weber D, Addison E, Liedtke W, Townsley MI. Transient receptor potential vanilloid 4-mediated disruption of the alveolar septal barrier: a novel mechanism of acute lung injury. Circ Res. 2006;99(9):988–95.
114. Stevens T. Functional and molecular heterogeneity of pulmonary endothelial cells. Proc Am Thorac Soc. 2011;8(6):453–7.
115. Herold S, Gabrielli NM, Vadasz I. Novel concepts of acute lung injury and alveolar-capillary barrier dysfunction. Am J Physiol Lung Cell Mol Physiol. 2013;305(10):L665–81.
116. Cioffi DL, Lowe K, Alvarez DF, Barry C, Stevens T. TRPing on the lung endothelium: calcium channels that regulate barrier function. Antioxid Redox Signal. 2009;11(4):765–76.
117. Sidhaye VK, Schweitzer KS, Caterina MJ, Shimoda L, King LS. Shear stress regulates aquaporin-5 and airway epithelial barrier function. Proc Natl Acad Sci USA. 2008;105(9): 3345–50.
118. Balakrishna S, Song W, Achanta S, et al. TRPV4 inhibition counteracts edema and inflammation and improves pulmonary function and oxygen saturation in chemically induced acute lung injury. Am J Physiol Lung Cell Mol Physiol. 2014;307(2):L158–72.
119. Nayak PS, Wang Y, Najrana T, et al. Mechanotransduction via TRPV4 regulates inflammation and differentiation in fetal mouse distal lung epithelial cells. Respir Res. 2015;16:60.
120. Pugin J. Molecular mechanisms of lung cell activation induced by cyclic stretch. Crit Care Med. 2003;31(4 Suppl):S200–6.
121. Hynes RO. Integrins: bidirectional, allosteric signaling machines. Cell. 2002;110(6): 673–87.
122. Zamir E, Geiger B. Molecular complexity and dynamics of cell-matrix adhesions. J Cell Sci. 2001;114(Pt 20):3583–90.
123. Ilic D, Damsky CH, Yamamoto T. Focal adhesion kinase: at the crossroads of signal transduction. J Cell Sci. 1997;110(Pt 4):401–7.
124. Seko Y, Takahashi N, Tobe K, Kadowaki T, Yazaki Y. Pulsatile stretch activates mitogen-activated protein kinase (MAPK) family members and focal adhesion kinase (p125(FAK)) in cultured rat cardiac myocytes. Biochem Biophys Res Commun. 1999;259(1):8–14.
125. Aikawa R, Komuro I, Yamazaki T, et al. Rho family small G proteins play critical roles in mechanical stress-induced hypertrophic responses in cardiac myocytes. Circ Res. 1999;84(4):458–66.
126. Wang JG, Miyazu M, Matsushita E, Sokabe M, Naruse K. Uniaxial cyclic stretch induces focal adhesion kinase (FAK) tyrosine phosphorylation followed by mitogen-activated protein kinase (MAPK) activation. Biochem Biophys Res Commun. 2001;288(2):356–61.
127. Wang Y, Huang Z, Nayak PS, et al. Strain-induced differentiation of fetal type II epithelial cells is mediated via the integrin alpha6beta1-ADAM17/tumor necrosis factor-alpha-converting enzyme (TACE) signaling pathway. J Biol Chem. 2013;288(35):25646–57.
128. Shafrir Y, Forgacs G. Mechanotransduction through the cytoskeleton. Am J Physiol Cell Physiol. 2002;282(3):C479–86.
129. Gillespie PG, Walker RG. Molecular basis of mechanosensory transduction. Nature. 2001;413(6852):194–202.
130. Chen KD, Li YS, Kim M, et al. Mechanotransduction in response to shear stress. Roles of receptor tyrosine kinases, integrins, and Shc. J Biol Chem. 1999;274(26):18393–400.

131. Hu Y, Bock G, Wick G, Xu Q. Activation of PDGF receptor alpha in vascular smooth muscle cells by mechanical stress. FASEB J. 1998;12(12):1135–42.
132. Liu M, Liu J, Buch S, Tanswell AK, Post M. Antisense oligonucleotides for PDGF-B and its receptor inhibit mechanical strain-induced fetal lung cell growth. Am J Physiol. 1995;269(2 Pt 1):L178–84.
133. Tschumperlin DJ, Dai G, Maly IV, et al. Mechanotransduction through growth-factor shedding into the extracellular space. Nature. 2004;429(6987):83–6.
134. Wang Y, Maciejewski BS, Soto-Reyes D, Lee HS, Warburton D, Sanchez-Esteban J. Mechanical stretch promotes fetal type II epithelial cell differentiation via shedding of HB-EGF and TGF-alpha. J Physiol. 2009;587(Pt 8):1739–53.
135. Ko KS, Arora PD, McCulloch CA. Cadherins mediate intercellular mechanical signaling in fibroblasts by activation of stretch-sensitive calcium-permeable channels. J Biol Chem. 2001;276(38):35967–77.
136. Chang L, Karin M. Mammalian MAP kinase signalling cascades. Nature. 2001;410(6824): 37–40.
137. Oudin S, Pugin J. Role of MAP kinase activation in interleukin-8 production by human BEAS-2B bronchial epithelial cells submitted to cyclic stretch. Am J Respir Cell Mol Biol. 2002;27(1):107–14.
138. Correa-Meyer E, Pesce L, Guerrero C, Sznajder JI. Cyclic stretch activates ERK1/2 via G proteins and EGFR in alveolar epithelial cells. Am J Physiol Lung Cell Mol Physiol. 2002;282(5):L883–91.
139. Quinn D, Tager A, Joseph PM, Bonventre JV, Force T, Hales CA. Stretch-induced mitogen-activated protein kinase activation and interleukin-8 production in type II alveolar cells. Chest. 1999;116(1 Suppl):89S–90.
140. Sanchez-Esteban J, Wang Y, Gruppuso PA, Rubin LP. Mechanical stretch induces fetal type II cell differentiation via an epidermal growth factor receptor-extracellular-regulated protein kinase signaling pathway. Am J Respir Cell Mol Biol. 2004;30(1):76–83.
141. Uhlig U, Haitsma JJ, Goldmann T, Poelma DL, Lachmann B, Uhlig S. Ventilation-induced activation of the mitogen-activated protein kinase pathway. Eur Respir J. 2002;20(4): 946–56.
142. Russo LA, Rannels SR, Laslow KS, Rannels DE. Stretch-related changes in lung cAMP after partial pneumonectomy. Am J Physiol. 1989;257(2 Pt 1):E261–8.
143. Wang Y, Maciejewski BS, Lee N, et al. Strain-induced fetal type II epithelial cell differentiation is mediated via cAMP-PKA-dependent signaling pathway. Am J Physiol Lung Cell Mol Physiol. 2006;291(4):L820–7.
144. Ko K, Arora P, Lee W, McCulloch C. Biochemical and functional characterization of intercellular adhesion and gap junctions in fibroblasts. Am J Physiol Cell Physiol. 2000;279(1): C147–57.
145. Sanderson MJ, Charles AC, Dirksen ER. Mechanical stimulation and intercellular communication increases intracellular Ca2+ in epithelial cells. Cell Regul. 1990;1(8):585–96.
146. Hansen M, Boitano S, Dirksen ER, Sanderson MJ. Intercellular calcium signaling induced by extracellular adenosine 5′-triphosphate and mechanical stimulation in airway epithelial cells. J Cell Sci. 1993;106(Pt 4):995–1004.
147. Boitano S, Dirksen ER, Evans WH. Sequence-specific antibodies to connexins block intercellular calcium signaling through gap junctions. Cell Calcium. 1998;23(1):1–9.
148. Blackwell TS, Christman JW. The role of nuclear factor-kappa B in cytokine gene regulation. Am J Respir Cell Mol Biol. 1997;17(1):3–9.
149. Lentsch AB, Czermak BJ, Bless NM, Van Rooijen N, Ward PA. Essential role of alveolar macrophages in intrapulmonary activation of NF-kappaB. Am J Respir Cell Mol Biol. 1999;20(4):692–8.
150. McRitchie DI, Isowa N, Edelson JD, et al. Production of tumour necrosis factor alpha by primary cultured rat alveolar epithelial cells. Cytokine. 2000;12(6):644–54.
151. Schwartz MD, Moore EE, Moore FA, et al. Nuclear factor-kappa B is activated in alveolar macrophages from patients with acute respiratory distress syndrome. Crit Care Med. 1996;24(8):1285–92.

152. Cheah FC, Winterbourn CC, Darlow BA, Mocatta TJ, Vissers MC. Nuclear factor kappaB activation in pulmonary leukocytes from infants with hyaline membrane disease: associations with chorioamnionitis and Ureaplasma urealyticum colonization. Pediatr Res. 2005;57(5 Pt 1):616–23.
153. Bourbia A, Cruz MA, Rozycki HJ. NF-kappaB in tracheal lavage fluid from intubated premature infants: association with inflammation, oxygen, and outcome. Arch Dis Child Fetal Neonatal Ed. 2006;91(1):F36–9.
154. Copland IB, Martinez F, Kavanagh BP, et al. High tidal volume ventilation causes different inflammatory responses in newborn versus adult lung. Am J Respir Crit Care Med. 2004;169(6):739–48.
155. Dolinay T, Kaminski N, Felgendreher M, et al. Gene expression profiling of target genes in ventilator-induced lung injury. Physiol Genomics. 2006;26(1):68–75.
156. Siegl S, Uhlig S. Using the one-lung method to link p38 to pro-inflammatory gene expression during overventilation in C57BL/6 and BALB/c mice. PLoS One. 2012;7(7):e41464.
157. Gharib SA, Liles WC, Klaff LS, Altemeier WA. Noninjurious mechanical ventilation activates a proinflammatory transcriptional program in the lung. Physiol Genomics. 2009;37(3):239–48.
158. Kompass KS, Deslee G, Moore C, McCurnin D, Pierce RA. Highly conserved transcriptional responses to mechanical ventilation of the lung. Physiol Genomics. 2010;42(3):384–96.
159. Morrisey EE, Hogan BL. Preparing for the first breath: genetic and cellular mechanisms in lung development. Dev Cell. 2010;18(1):8–23.
160. Bourbon J, Boucherat O, Chailley-Heu B, Delacourt C. Control mechanisms of lung alveolar development and their disorders in bronchopulmonary dysplasia. Pediatr Res. 2005;57 (5 Pt 2):38R–46.
161. Bourbon JR, Boucherat O, Boczkowski J, Crestani B, Delacourt C. Bronchopulmonary dysplasia and emphysema: in search of common therapeutic targets. Trends Mol Med. 2009;15(4):169–79.
162. Wendel DP, Taylor DG, Albertine KH, Keating MT, Li DY. Impaired distal airway development in mice lacking elastin. Am J Respir Cell Mol Biol. 2000;23(3):320–6.
163. Bostrom H, Willetts K, Pekny M, et al. PDGF-A signaling is a critical event in lung alveolar myofibroblast development and alveogenesis. Cell. 1996;85(6):863–73.
164. Lindahl P, Karlsson L, Hellstrom M, et al. Alveogenesis failure in PDGF-A-deficient mice is coupled to lack of distal spreading of alveolar smooth muscle cell progenitors during lung development. Development. 1997;124(20):3943–53.
165. Liebeskind A, Srinivasan S, Kaetzel D, Bruce M. Retinoic acid stimulates immature lung fibroblast growth via a PDGF-mediated autocrine mechanism. Am J Physiol Lung Cell Mol Physiol. 2000;279(1):L81–90.
166. Liu B, Harvey CS, McGowan SE. Retinoic acid increases elastin in neonatal rat lung fibroblast cultures. Am J Physiol. 1993;265(5 Pt 1):L430–7.
167. Massaro GD, Massaro D. Postnatal treatment with retinoic acid increases the number of pulmonary alveoli in rats. Am J Physiol. 1996;270(2 Pt 1):L305–10.
168. Hadchouel A, Franco-Montoya ML, Delacourt C. Altered lung development in bronchopulmonary dysplasia. Birth Defects Res A Clin Mol Teratol. 2014;100(3):158–67.
169. Weinstein M, Xu X, Ohyama K, Deng CX. FGFR-3 and FGFR-4 function cooperatively to direct alveogenesis in the murine lung. Development. 1998;125(18):3615–23.
170. Chailley-Heu B, Boucherat O, Barlier-Mur AM, Bourbon JR. FGF-18 is upregulated in the postnatal rat lung and enhances elastogenesis in myofibroblasts. Am J Physiol Lung Cell Mol Physiol. 2005;288(1):L43–51.
171. Husain AN, Siddiqui NH, Stocker JT. Pathology of arrested acinar development in postsurfactant bronchopulmonary dysplasia. Hum Pathol. 1998;29(7):710–7.
172. Thibeault DW, Mabry SM, Ekekezie II, Truog WE. Lung elastic tissue maturation and perturbations during the evolution of chronic lung disease. Pediatrics. 2000;106(6):1452–9.
173. Margraf LR, Tomashefski Jr JF, Bruce MC, Dahms BB. Morphometric analysis of the lung in bronchopulmonary dysplasia. Am Rev Respir Dis. 1991;143(2):391–400.

174. Merritt TA. Oxygen exposure in the newborn guinea pig lung lavage cell populations, chemotactic and elastase response: a possible relationship to neonatal bronchopulmonary dysplasia. Pediatr Res. 1982;16(9):798–805.
175. Merritt TA, Cochrane CG, Holcomb K, et al. Elastase and alpha 1-proteinase inhibitor activity in tracheal aspirates during respiratory distress syndrome. Role of inflammation in the pathogenesis of bronchopulmonary dysplasia. J Clin Invest. 1983;72(2):656–66.
176. Pierce RA, Albertine KH, Starcher BC, Bohnsack JF, Carlton DP, Bland RD. Chronic lung injury in preterm lambs: disordered pulmonary elastin deposition. Am J Physiol. 1997;272(3 Pt 1):L452–60.
177. Mokres LM, Parai K, Hilgendorff A, et al. Prolonged mechanical ventilation with air induces apoptosis and causes failure of alveolar septation and angiogenesis in lungs of newborn mice. Am J Physiol Lung Cell Mol Physiol. 2010;298(1):L23–35.
178. Alnahhas MH, Karathanasis P, Kriss VM, Pauly TH, Bruce MC. Elevated laminin concentrations in lung secretions of preterm infants supported by mechanical ventilation are correlated with radiographic abnormalities. J Pediatr. 1997;131(4):555–60.
179. Murch SH, MacDonald TT, Walker-Smith JA, Levin M, Lionetti P, Klein NJ. Disruption of sulphated glycosaminoglycans in intestinal inflammation. Lancet. 1993;341(8847):711–4.
180. Bland RD, Ertsey R, Mokres LM, et al. Mechanical ventilation uncouples synthesis and assembly of elastin and increases apoptosis in lungs of newborn mice. Prelude to defective alveolar septation during lung development? Am J Physiol Lung Cell Mol Physiol. 2008;294(1):L3–14.
181. Bland RD, Mokres LM, Ertsey R, et al. Mechanical ventilation with 40% oxygen reduces pulmonary expression of genes that regulate lung development and impairs alveolar septation in newborn mice. Am J Physiol Lung Cell Mol Physiol. 2007;293(5):L1099–110.
182. Thibeault DW, Mabry SM, Ekekezie II, Zhang X, Truog WE. Collagen scaffolding during development and its deformation with chronic lung disease. Pediatrics. 2003;111(4 Pt 1): 766–76.
183. Masumoto K, de Rooij JD, Suita S, Rottier R, Tibboel D, de Krijger RR. Expression of matrix metalloproteinases and tissue inhibitors of metalloproteinases during normal human pulmonary development. Histopathology. 2005;47(4):410–9.
184. Schulz CG, Sawicki G, Lemke RP, Roeten BM, Schulz R, Cheung PY. MMP-2 and MMP-9 and their tissue inhibitors in the plasma of preterm and term neonates. Pediatr Res. 2004;55(5):794–801.
185. Kheradmand F, Rishi K, Werb Z. Signaling through the EGF receptor controls lung morphogenesis in part by regulating MT1-MMP-mediated activation of gelatinase A/MMP2. J Cell Sci. 2002;115(Pt 4):839–48.
186. Cederqvist K, Sorsa T, Tervahartiala T, et al. Matrix metalloproteinases-2, -8, and -9 and TIMP-2 in tracheal aspirates from preterm infants with respiratory distress. Pediatrics. 2001;108(3):686–92.
187. Altiok O, Yasumatsu R, Bingol-Karakoc G, et al. Imbalance between cysteine proteases and inhibitors in a baboon model of bronchopulmonary dysplasia. Am J Respir Crit Care Med. 2006;173(3):318–26.
188. Yasumatsu R, Altiok O, Benarafa C, et al. SERPINB1 upregulation is associated with in vivo complex formation with neutrophil elastase and cathepsin G in a baboon model of bronchopulmonary dysplasia. Am J Physiol Lung Cell Mol Physiol. 2006;291(4):L619–27.
189. Teichert-Kuliszewska K, Kutryk MJ, Kuliszewski MA, et al. Bone morphogenetic protein receptor-2 signaling promotes pulmonary arterial endothelial cell survival: implications for loss-of-function mutations in the pathogenesis of pulmonary hypertension. Circ Res. 2006;98(2):209–17.
190. Colarossi C, Chen Y, Obata H, et al. Lung alveolar septation defects in Ltbp-3-null mice. Am J Pathol. 2005;167(2):419–28.
191. Vicencio AG, Lee CG, Cho SJ, et al. Conditional overexpression of bioactive transforming growth factor-beta1 in neonatal mouse lung: a new model for bronchopulmonary dysplasia? Am J Respir Cell Mol Biol. 2004;31(6):650–6.

192. Gauldie J, Galt T, Bonniaud P, Robbins C, Kelly M, Warburton D. Transfer of the active form of transforming growth factor-beta 1 gene to newborn rat lung induces changes consistent with bronchopulmonary dysplasia. Am J Pathol. 2003;163(6):2575–84.
193. Bland RD, Xu L, Ertsey R, et al. Dysregulation of pulmonary elastin synthesis and assembly in preterm lambs with chronic lung disease. Am J Physiol Lung Cell Mol Physiol. 2007;292(6):L1370–84.
194. Nakanishi H, Sugiura T, Streisand JB, Lonning SM, Roberts Jr JD. TGF-beta-neutralizing antibodies improve pulmonary alveologenesis and vasculogenesis in the injured newborn lung. Am J Physiol Lung Cell Mol Physiol. 2007;293(1):L151–61.
195. Zhao Y, Gilmore BJ, Young SL. Expression of transforming growth factor-beta receptors during hyperoxia-induced lung injury and repair. Am J Physiol. 1997;273(2 Pt 1):L355–62.
196. Wan H, Xu Y, Ikegami M, et al. Foxa2 is required for transition to air breathing at birth. Proc Natl Acad Sci USA. 2004;101(40):14449–54.
197. Wan H, Kaestner KH, Ang SL, et al. Foxa2 regulates alveolarization and goblet cell hyperplasia. Development. 2004;131(4):953–64.
198. Ramirez MI, Millien G, Hinds A, Cao Y, Seldin DC, Williams MC. T1alpha, a lung type I cell differentiation gene, is required for normal lung cell proliferation and alveolus formation at birth. Dev Biol. 2003;256(1):61–72.
199. Chelly N, Mouhieddine-Gueddiche OB, Barlier-Mur AM, Chailley-Heu B, Bourbon JR. Keratinocyte growth factor enhances maturation of fetal rat lung type II cells. Am J Respir Cell Mol Biol. 1999;20(3):423–32.
200. Welsh DA, Summer WR, Dobard EP, Nelson S, Mason CM. Keratinocyte growth factor prevents ventilator-induced lung injury in an ex vivo rat model. Am J Respir Crit Care Med. 2000;162(3 Pt 1):1081–6.
201. Epaud R, Aubey F, Xu J, et al. Knockout of insulin-like growth factor-1 receptor impairs distal lung morphogenesis. PLoS One. 2012;7(11):e48071.
202. Das KC, Ravi D. Altered expression of cyclins and cdks in premature infant baboon model of bronchopulmonary dysplasia. Antioxid Redox Signal. 2004;6(1):117–27.
203. Kroon AA, Wang J, Kavanagh BP, et al. Prolonged mechanical ventilation induces cell cycle arrest in newborn rat lung. PLoS One. 2011;6(2):e16910.
204. Giordani VM, DeBenedictus CM, Wang Y, Sanchez-Esteban J. Epidermal growth factor receptor (EGFR) contributes to fetal lung fibroblast injury induced by mechanical stretch. J Recept Signal Transduct Res. 2014;34(1):58–63.
205. Scavo LM, Ertsey R, Chapin CJ, Allen L, Kitterman JA. Apoptosis in the development of rat and human fetal lungs. Am J Respir Cell Mol Biol. 1998;18(1):21–31.
206. Stenmark KR, Abman SH. Lung vascular development: implications for the pathogenesis of bronchopulmonary dysplasia. Annu Rev Physiol. 2005;67:623–61.
207. Jakkula M, Le Cras TD, Gebb S, et al. Inhibition of angiogenesis decreases alveolarization in the developing rat lung. Am J Physiol Lung Cell Mol Physiol. 2000;279(3):L600–7.
208. Vadivel A, Alphonse RS, Etches N, et al. Hypoxia-inducible factors promote alveolar development and regeneration. Am J Respir Cell Mol Biol. 2014;50(1):96–105.
209. Le Cras TD, Markham NE, Tuder RM, Voelkel NF, Abman SH. Treatment of newborn rats with a VEGF receptor inhibitor causes pulmonary hypertension and abnormal lung structure. Am J Physiol Lung Cell Mol Physiol. 2002;283(3):L555–62.
210. Bhatt AJ, Pryhuber GS, Huyck H, Watkins RH, Metlay LA, Maniscalco WM. Disrupted pulmonary vasculature and decreased vascular endothelial growth factor, Flt-1, and TIE-2 in human infants dying with bronchopulmonary dysplasia. Am J Respir Crit Care Med. 2001;164(10 Pt 1):1971–80.
211. Thibeault DW, Mabry SM, Norberg M, Truog WE, Ekekezie II. Lung microvascular adaptation in infants with chronic lung disease. Biol Neonate. 2004;85(4):273–82.
212. Compernolle V, Brusselmans K, Acker T, et al. Loss of HIF-2alpha and inhibition of VEGF impair fetal lung maturation, whereas treatment with VEGF prevents fatal respiratory distress in premature mice. Nat Med. 2002;8(7):702–10.

213. Grover TR, Asikainen TM, Kinsella JP, Abman SH, White CW. Hypoxia-inducible factors HIF-1alpha and HIF-2alpha are decreased in an experimental model of severe respiratory distress syndrome in preterm lambs. Am J Physiol Lung Cell Mol Physiol. 2007;292(6): L1345–51.
214. Maniscalco WM, Watkins RH, Pryhuber GS, Bhatt A, Shea C, Huyck H. Angiogenic factors and alveolar vasculature: development and alterations by injury in very premature baboons. Am J Physiol Lung Cell Mol Physiol. 2002;282(4):L811–23.
215. Thebaud B, Ladha F, Michelakis ED, et al. Vascular endothelial growth factor gene therapy increases survival, promotes lung angiogenesis, and prevents alveolar damage in hyperoxia-induced lung injury: evidence that angiogenesis participates in alveolarization. Circulation. 2005;112(16):2477–86.
216. Bhandari V. Postnatal inflammation in the pathogenesis of bronchopulmonary dysplasia. Birth Defects Res A Clin Mol Teratol. 2014;100(3):189–201.
217. Hilgendorff A, Reiss I, Ehrhardt H, Eickelberg O, Alvira CM. Chronic lung disease in the preterm infant. Lessons learned from animal models. Am J Respir Cell Mol Biol. 2014;50(2):233–45.
218. Tambunting F, Beharry KD, Waltzman J, Modanlou HD. Impaired lung vascular endothelial growth factor in extremely premature baboons developing bronchopulmonary dysplasia/chronic lung disease. J Investig Med. 2005;53(5):253–62.
219. Cannizzaro V, Zosky GR, Hantos Z, Turner DJ, Sly PD. High tidal volume ventilation in infant mice. Respir Physiol Neurobiol. 2008;162(1):93–9.
220. Brew N, Hooper SB, Zahra V, Wallace M, Harding R. Mechanical ventilation injury and repair in extremely and very preterm lungs. PLoS One. 2013;8(5):e63905.
221. Bhandari V. The potential of non-invasive ventilation to decrease BPD. Semin Perinatol. 2013;37(2):108–14.

Chapter 3
Pre and Postnatal Inflammation in the Pathogenesis of Bronchopulmonary Dysplasia

Kirsten Glaser and Christian P. Speer

Introduction

Neonatal strategies and therapeutic advances with improved survival from respiratory distress syndrome (RDS) have altered the nature of bronchopulmonary dysplasia (BPD), but have not changed its incidence in extremely premature preterm infants [1–3]. Lung pathology of preterm infants with "old" BPD—originally described by Northway and colleagues—was characterized by severe lung injury comprising inflammation, protein-rich lung edema, extensive airway epithelial metaplasia, peribronchial fibrosis, and marked airway and pulmonary vascular smooth muscle hypertrophy [1, 4]. In contrast, "new" BPD in the post-surfactant era is characterized by alveolar simplification, dysmorphic capillaries, and severe disturbance of vascular and airway smooth muscle cell development [5–7]. In vitro and in vivo data have clearly demonstrated that pre and postnatal inflammation contributes to its pathogenesis. Intra-amniotic infection and inflammation have been associated with an increased risk for the development of fetal and neonatal systemic inflammatory response syndrome and the development of diseases of prematurity, such as RDS and BPD [8–10]. In addition, various postnatal factors such as mechanical ventilation, oxygen toxicity, and neonatal infections may perpetuate or amplify an injurious inflammatory response in the airways and interstitium [2, 10–13]. Endotoxin-mediated priming of the fetal lung is an important pathogenetic factor in the initiation of the inflammatory reaction, and additional adverse conditions may act as a "second strike" amplifying or aggravating the inflammatory response [14]. Cytokines, chemokines, growth factors, and other substances may

K. Glaser, MD (✉) • C.P. Speer, MD, FRCPE
University Children's Hospital, University of Würzburg,
Josef-Schneider-Str. 2, Würzburg, Bavaria 97080, Germany
e-mail: Glaser_K@ukw.de; Speer_C@ukw.de

V. Bhandari (ed.), *Bronchopulmonary Dysplasia*, Respiratory Medicine,
DOI 10.1007/978-3-319-28486-6_3

orchestrate a complex interplay of sustained and dysregulated inflammation in prematurity-associated lung injury [2, 12, 15, 16]. Immaturity and dysfunction of innate immune cells and impairments in the termination of inflammation may contribute to perpetuated inflammation [17–20], which may subsequently affect normal alveolarization and pulmonary vascular development [6, 21, 22]. Current efforts focus on pharmacological interventions of adverse intrauterine and postnatal infection [23, 24], prevention of postnatal iatrogenic injurious events [3, 25–28], and implementation of new biomarkers of inflammation that might help to identify infants at risk [15, 29, 30]. The role of genetic predisposition has been subject of clinical studies and in vitro trials [31–33]. This chapter summarizes the current pathogenetic concepts of pre and postnatal inflammatory mechanisms, referred to as "multiple-hit theory," contributing to the development of BPD.

Prenatal Risk Factors of Adverse Pulmonary Inflammation

Chorioamnionitis

Histologic chorioamnionitis (CA) is an inflammatory condition of the placenta involving amnion, choriodecidua, and/or chorionic plate in response to microbial invasion or pathological processes [34]. Various microorganisms residing in the maternal rectovaginal tract may invade the amniotic cavity and may cause intra-amniotic inflammation and subsequent induction of preterm labor [34, 35]. Elevated concentrations of pro-inflammatory cytokines have been identified in amniotic fluid of high-risk pregnancies [35]. Increased concentrations of pro-inflammatory cytokines in human amniotic fluid and fetal cord blood have been repetitively shown to be independent risk factors of BPD [12, 36, 37]. Incidence and prevalence of CA appear to be inversely related to gestational age with the highest risk in very immature preterm infants <28 weeks of gestation [9, 35, 38–40]. Severity of CA may vary significantly and may depend on the duration of in utero infection [35, 38, 40]. Most pathogens associated with CA are of low virulence implying subclinical courses in many cases. In general, anaerobic, aerobic, and atypical bacteria contribute to the list, such as *Ureaplasma* species (spp.), and *Mycoplasma hominis*, *Fusobacterium* spp., *Streptococcus* spp., *Bacteroides* spp., and *Prevotella* spp. [34, 41]. Little is known about polymicrobial immunomodulation and pathogen synergy. In preterm infants who develop BPD, *Ureaplasma* spp. are the most common microorganisms isolated from the amniotic fluid, cord blood, and respiratory tract [12, 42]. Relevant epidemiological and experimental data suggest an association of perinatal *Ureaplasma* infection, and increased risk of fetal inflammatory response syndrome (FIRS) and BPD [16, 38, 42, 43].

The term "chorioamnionitis" is inconsistently used among clinicians and across epidemiologic studies. Definition of CA may refer to histologic examination, based on microscopic evidence of inflammation of the membranes [34], as well as clinical data, based on clinical manifestations of local or systemic inflammation, such as fever, tachycardia, elevated maternal inflammation parameters, uterine tenderness, foul-smelling vaginal discharge, and fetal tachycardia [44]. Both microbial colonization of placental tissue and histologic evidence of placental and umbilical cord vessel inflammation have been shown to be associated with spontaneous preterm birth, especially at earlier gestational ages, contributing itself to prematurity-associated neonatal morbidities [35, 36, 40]. Attempts to assess a gestation-independent effect of CA on neonatal outcome have presented inconclusive results for BPD, and the correlation has been somewhat controversial [10, 45, 46]. Clinical CA has been identified as an independent risk factor for RDS in premature infants, whereas histological CA seems to confer a beneficial effect on the incidence of RDS [46–48]. This maturational effect in turn seems to contribute to a heightened susceptibility of the lung to postnatal injury [8, 45, 46, 49]. Data for histological CA are consistent with a maturational effect of prenatal exposure to inflammation on lung development as shown in an animal model [50]. However, in the same animal model, pulmonary maturation induced by fetal inflammation is followed by significantly disturbed structural development of the lung [51]. A recent meta-analysis of 59 studies involving more than 15,000 infants confirmed an association of histologic CA and the development of BPD [52]. A subanalysis of 17 studies adjusting results for gestational age and birth weight, documented less accentuated, but still significant estimates [52]. However, the authors found substantial heterogeneity across the studies as well as evidence of confounding publication bias. In the Alabama Preterm Birth Study, no association between CA and BPD was observed, although umbilical cord blood cultures positive for *Ureaplasma* spp. significantly increased the risk for BPD [38]. A cohort study, including 789 infants <30 weeks of gestation, yielded a reduced risk of BPD in infants with histologic CA plus umbilical vasculitis and a trend toward reduced incidence in infants with histologic CA alone [39]. A nested case–control study found a protective effect of histologic CA in the absence of postnatal sepsis and prolonged ventilation, but demonstrated an increased risk of BPD for infants with histologic CA, who experienced mechanical ventilation and postnatal sepsis [53]. Finally, a recent cohort study including 301 infants <32 weeks of gestation pointed to a lower response to surfactant replacement therapy and a prolonged need for mechanical ventilation in infants exposed to histologic CA [54]. The reduced response to exogenous surfactant was associated with a higher risk of developing BPD [54]. Those data might underline the impact of CA in concert with adverse pro-inflammatory conditions, such as hyperoxia, hypoxia, or mechanical ventilation [53, 55]. Priming of the fetal lung by endotoxin [lipopolysaccharide (LPS)] may be another orchestrating factor. Animal experiments indicate that LPS injection may initiate placental and pulmonary inflammation reflected by increased expression of pro-inflammatory cytokines and chemokines, recruitment of polymorphonuclear cells (PMNs) and monocytes, and impaired alveolar and microvascular development [50, 51]. In sheep and mice models, amnionitis-induced pulmonary maturation was followed by significantly disturbed structural development of the lung [51, 56].

In conclusion, CA clearly increases the likelihood of very premature preterm birth with the latter being the most important risk factor for the development of BPD. Moreover, CA may induce a chronic inflammatory process driving the immature

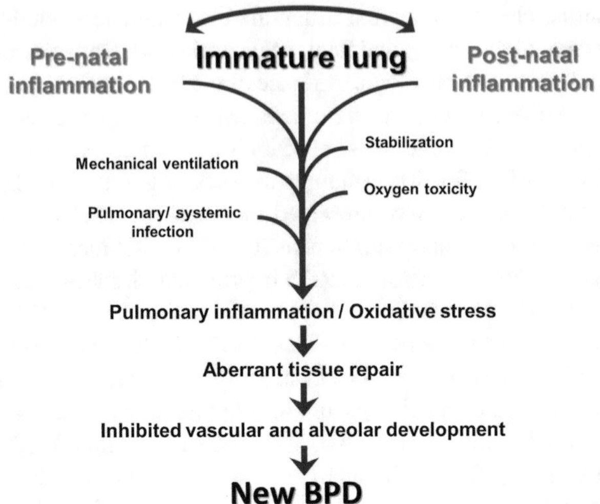

Fig. 3.1 Illustration of the complex interplay of pre and postnatal pro-inflammatory conditions contributing to perpetuated adverse lung inflammation, impaired alveolarization, and simplified pulmonary microvasculature in the structurally and immunologically immature lungs of premature preterm infants. According to our current state of knowledge, "new BPD" may result from inflammation-induced lung injury and impaired lung development during a window of vulnerability. Individual infants may be particularly susceptible to sustained lung inflammation and BPD due to predisposing genetic factors

lung, making it more susceptible to postnatal injuries. An adverse condition, such as mechanical ventilation, may act as a "second strike" amplifying the inflammatory response (Fig. 3.1) [14]. Correlation between CA and neonatal morbidities may be challenging due to a number of antenatal and postnatal confounding factors, such as imprecise diagnoses of CA, RDS, and BPD, variability of study populations, higher prevalence of antenatal steroids and surfactant replacement therapy nowadays, polymicrobial immunomodulation and pathogen synergy, the individual fetal response, oxygen toxicity, mechanical ventilation, and neonatal infection [16, 35, 40, 46, 52].

Fetal Inflammatory Response Syndrome

Intrauterine inflammation may induce a fetal inflammatory response, characterized histologically by funisitis with PMN infiltration of the chorionic vessels or umbilical cord and biochemically by elevated umbilical cord concentrations of pro-inflammatory cytokines, chemokines, matrix metalloproteinases (MMPs), and angiogenic factors such as vascular endothelial growth factor (VEGF) [46, 57]. FIRS has been implicated in the development of diseases of prematurity, such as BPD, by induction of cytokines and augmentation of deleterious effects, including free radical and excitatory amino acid release [16, 58]. Increased concentrations of pro-inflammatory cytokines in fetal cord blood were identified as independent risk factors for BPD [12, 58]. A pronounced infiltration of inflammatory cells, an increased expression of cytokines and markers of endothelial activation, as well as a large number of apoptotic airway cells were observed in lung tissues of human fetuses with funisitis [59, 60]. Of note, fetal exposure to severe maternal chorioamnionitis might not necessarily result in an inflammatory response of an individual fetus. In contrast, a rather smoldering or nearly inapparent amniotic infection/inflammation might induce a severe fetal reaction [46]. We are currently unable to identify a fetus at risk of subsequent development of adverse neonatal sequelae following exposure to prenatal inflammation [61].

Postnatal Risk Factors Inducing or Amplifying Neonatal Lung Inflammation

Infection

Neonatal sepsis is associated with considerable acute and long-term morbidity, especially in preterm infants [62–64]. Early-onset sepsis (EOS), associated with acquisition of microorganisms by transplacental or ascending infection, is most commonly caused by *group B Streptococci* and *Escherichia coli* with decreasing incidence due to the implementation of a prenatal screening and treatment protocol for *group B Streptococci* [62]. Nosocomial late-onset sepsis (LOS) is mainly caused by bacterial infections from coagulase-negative *Staphylococci*, *S. aureus*, or gram-negative bacteria [65, 66]. Highest incidence rates are documented in very immature preterm infants due to increased susceptibility and more frequent invasive procedures [63, 64, 67]. Both EOS and LOS have been identified as individual risk factors of BPD [12, 37, 66]. Of note, infants with *S. epidermidis* sepsis may be at higher risk for the development of BPD than others [68]. Conversely, both histological and clinical CA have been associated with increased risk of EOS in extremely premature preterm infants [69, 70], underlying the pathogenetic role of intrauterine inflammation on the development of BPD. Histologic CA might be protective against LOS [9, 69, 71].

Mechanical Ventilation

A considerable number of in vitro studies and animal experiments have confirmed that any kind of mechanical ventilation may be injurious to airways and lung tissue, provoking a stretch-induced injurious cascade [11, 26, 72]. However, certain ventilatory strategies may cause more damage than others. Volutrauma, rather than barotrauma, has been implicated as the primary determinant of lung injury. Overdistension of the lungs or cyclic opening and closing of lung units cause bronchial epithelial disruption and the release of pro-inflammatory mediators with subsequent leukocyte influx [14, 72, 73]. In animal models, the severity of inflammatory reaction was related to ventilatory strategies characterized by high peak and lack of positive end-expiratory pressure [72]. In a murine model of BPD, inflammation-induced alterations and structural lung damage were strongly related to developmental stages with the saccular stage of lung development being particularly vulnerable [74]. These data are consistent with the clinical observation that extremely premature preterm infants <28 weeks of gestation (saccular stage) are at highest risk for inflammation-induced BPD, whereas preterm infants born >32 weeks of gestation (early alveolar stage) are at much lower risk [5]. Current neonatal strategies attempt to minimize the need for endotracheal intubation and intermittent positive pressure ventilation and favor continuous positive airway pressure (CPAP)-based strategies [25, 75, 76]. However, more and more extremely low-birth weight (ELBW) infants exposed to no or minimal barotrauma and to relatively low levels of supplemental oxygen may develop respiratory deterioration at a postnatal age of 1–2 weeks [26, 77]. Correspondingly, in newborn rat lungs, even low tidal volume ventilation was shown to induce acute phase cytokines and CXC chemokines, with expression of pro-inflammatory cytokines and chemokines being amplified by oxygen and oxygen combined with LPS pre-treatment [78]. In a previous study in a rat model, LPS challenge had already been shown to result in significantly increased levels of pro-inflammatory cytokines in bronchoalveolar lavage fluid (BALF) despite "less injurious" ventilation strategies [79]. Those data may underline the relevant pathogenetic role of pro-inflammatory priming on the downhill progression to BPD (Fig. 3.1). An initial "hit" may be followed by a "second strike" aggravating lung inflammation [5, 16, 78].

Hyperoxia and Hypoxia

Transition from the fetal normotoxic in utero environment to postnatal room air represents a sudden exposure of the structurally and functionally immature lungs of premature preterm infants to a relatively "hyperoxic" environment. On the contrary, episodes of hypoxia or fluctuating oxygen saturations most often due to apnea of prematurity adversely affect lung development, both directly and by iatrogenic oxygen supplementation [80]. A considerable number of studies confirmed injurious effects of perinatal supplemental oxygen administration on pulmonary development [13, 80]. Subsequently, optimum target ranges of oxygen saturation in extremely premature preterm infants have been reassessed [3, 27, 28]. Profound deficiency in antioxidant enzyme activity may leave very immature preterm infants at high risk of suffering from potential detrimental effects of hyperoxia and hyperoxemia [81]. In animal models, hyperoxia has been shown to be a strong and independent inductor of various mediators involved in pulmonary inflammation in preterm and term neonates [80]. In premature rat lungs, hyperoxia affected a complex orchestra of genes involved in inflammation, extracellular matrix turnover, coagulation and other events, and induced influx of inflammatory cells in pulmonary tissue [82].

Moreover, hyperoxia resulted in progressive lung disease demonstrating many features of the BPD phenotype [82]. Current knowledge of hypoxia-derived pulmonary inflammation is limited. Data from a rat model of acute hypoxia-induced lung injury point to enhanced LPS-induced pulmonary inflammation due to cytokines, excessive neutrophil accumulation, and increased vascular permeability [83].

Molecular Mechanisms of Adverse Pulmonary Inflammation Contributing to BPD

Cellular and Humoral Mediators of Inflammation

Priming and activation of PMNs and mononuclear cells [peripheral blood mononuclear cells (PBMCs)] are essential stages of the early immune response to invading microorganisms or tissue damage [12, 19, 20, 84]. Several studies revealed significantly higher and persisting numbers of neutrophils and macrophages in BALFs of preterm infants who developed BPD compared to infants who recovered from RDS [85–87]. In experimental and clinical BPD, the cellular inflammatory response is characterized by a neutrophil and later mononuclear-cell influx into the airways immediately after initiation of mechanical ventilation [37, 85, 87]. This reaction is paralleled by a decrease in the number of circulating neutrophils and has been correlated with pulmonary edema formation reflecting injury to the alveolar–capillary unit [86, 88, 89]. Circulating neutrophils and monocytes become rapidly activated within 1–3 h after initiation of mechanical ventilation [90]. Most likely, activation of neutrophils is followed by adherence to the endothelium of the pulmonary vascular system and initiation of pro-inflammatory events. Apoptosis of inflammatory neutrophils and their timely removal by resident macrophages is critical to the resolution of inflammation. However, a relevant number of studies documented altered neonatal phagocyte function, a reduced phagocytosis of apoptotic tissue cells, and prolonged survival of neonatal PMNs [17, 18, 20]. Those impairments in the termination of inflammation may contribute to prolonged and perpetuated inflammation [19]. In a rat model of lung inflammation, apoptotic cells induced inflammatory and fibrotic pulmonary responses [91]. Neonatal neutrophils surviving spontaneous apoptosis were shown to exhibit augmented inflammatory function reflected by enhanced secretion of interleukin (IL-) 8 and macrophage inflammatory protein (MIP)-1β [20]. Besides PMNs, alveolar and pulmonary tissue macrophages play a central role in lung inflammation by orchestrating the inflammatory response via cytokine release [19]. In lung tissues of preterm infants who had died during the early stages of RDS, the interstitial density of $CD68^+$ macrophages and neutrophils was at least 10- to 15-fold higher than in stillborn infants of equivalent age [92]. Moreover, connective tissue mast cells have been shown to accumulate in the lungs of preterm infants with BPD [93], and data from baboon model of neonatal lung disease point to a critical role of autoreactive T cells [94].

Cellular and Endothelial Interaction

A relevant number of adhesion molecules, such as intercellular adhesion molecules (ICAMs) and vascular cell adhesion molecules (VCAMs), promote attachment of inflammatory cells to the endothelium [95]. In infants with BPD, increased concentrations of selectins and ICAMs were detected in airway secretions and circulation, reflecting enhanced shedding in response to inflammation [96]. Moreover, significant upregulation of ICAM-1 on endothelial cord cells and increased serum levels of soluble ICAM-1 were shown in preterm infants exposed to chorioamnionitis [96]. These data may point to an effective recruitment of circulating neutrophils and monocytes into the airways and pulmonary tissue of preterm infants.

Chemotactic and Chemokinetic Factors

Recruitment of inflammatory cells is mainly promoted by chemokines, thus playing a central role in regulating pulmonary inflammation [97]. Chemokines are classified into four families (C, CC, CXC, and CX_3C) with the CC family being activators of monocytes and macrophages, lymphocytes, eosinophils, and basophils [98]. In lung inflammation, IL-8 (CXCL8) may be the most important chemotactic factor for recruitment of monocytes and neutrophils to the site of inflammation [99]. A role for CC chemokines in the pathogenesis of acute and chronic lung disease was suggested by animal and clinical studies [100]. The application of a selective chemokine receptor antagonist was shown to inhibit neutrophil influx into the rat lung, to suppress pulmonary inflammation, and to enhance lung growth [101]. Increased concentrations of members of the CC family, monocyte chemoattractant protein (MCP-) 1 and MIP-1α, were found in ventilated premature preterm infants suffering from acute lung injury and correlated with BPD [92, 102]. Moreover, increased tracheal aspirate concentrations of MCP-1, MCP-2, MCP-3, and MIP-1β were identified as independent risk factors for RDS and BPD [97]. Expression of additional chemoattractants, such as C5a, IL-8, IL-16, lipoxygenase products, leukotriene B_4, elastin fragments, metalloproteases, and fibronectin, were also increased in infants with BPD compared to those who recovered from RDS [12, 37].

Pro- and Anti-inflammatory Cytokines

Pro-inflammatory cytokines, such as tumor necrosis factor (TNF-)α, IL-1, and IL-6, play a crucial role in early inflammation, mediating up and/or downregulation of genes and transcription factors [15]. Pro-inflammatory cytokines are synthezised by various inflammatory and pulmonary cells upon stimulation by hyperoxia, LPS, other bacterial cell wall constituents, and biophysical factors, such as volu and barotrauma [37]. Increased protein levels and high mRNA expression of pro-inflammatory

TNF-α and IL-1β have been detected in respiratory fluids, bronchoalveolar and pulmonary cells, and, moreover, in the systemic circulation of preterm infants with RDS and evolving BPD pointing towards a disturbed balance of pro- and anti-inflammatory factors [12, 15, 37]. Macrophage-derived TNF-α is considered to contribute significantly to the pro-inflammatory reaction being a known trigger of various inflammatory mediators in alveolar cells [12]. Moreover, IL-1β is a central pro-inflammatory cytokine found in the amniotic fluid in chorioamnionitis [103] that has been shown to significantly disturb lung morphogenesis in a fetal mouse model [104, 105]. The influx of TNF-α positive macrophages in pulmonary tissues of preterm infants who had died of severe RDS was found to be associated with severe destruction of pulmonary interstitium [106]. In a bi-transgenic mouse model, perinatal overexpression of IL-1β in pulmonary epithelial cells was shown to induce increased TNF-α and IL-6 expression and profound tissue injury similar to BPD [104, 107]. In vitro findings suggest that IL-1β may induce epithelial IL-8 expression, with nuclear transcription factor-kappa B (NF-κB) being involved. Lung macrophage activation with subsequent IL-1β production and NF-κB activation was found to contribute significantly to arrested lung development in a fetal mouse model of BPD [108]. NF-κB activation was found in airway neutrophils and macrophages and in tracheobronchial secretions from infants with RDS, considered essential in LPS-induced cellular inflammation [109, 110]. On the contrary, NF-κB was recently shown to promote physiological angiogenesis and alveolarization in the developing lung by regulating the angiogenic mediator VEGF receptor-2 [111]. The authors hypothesize that these interrelations might explain how glucocorticoids, being potent inhibitors of NF-κB activation, accelerate the development of the surfactant system on the one hand, but inhibit angiogenesis and secondary septation during later lung development on the other [111].

Experimental and clinical data indicate that the profound pro-inflammation present in BPD may, in part, be attributed to inadequate anti-inflammatory cytokine responses, involving IL-4, IL-10, IL-11, IL-12, IL-13, IL-18, or IL-1 receptor antagonist [12, 37, 112]. IL-10 inhibits the release of pro-inflammatory mediators from monocytes and macrophages, enhances the release of anti-inflammatory mediators, and has been ascribed physiological relevance in the prevention and limitation of adverse inflammatory immune reactions [113]. Exposure of lung inflammatory cells of preterm infants to IL-10 in vitro resulted in reduced expression of pro-inflammatory cytokines [114]. However, cellular IL-10 mRNA was undetectable in most airway samples of preterm infants with BPD, but regularly found in term infants with respiratory failure [112]. In vitro IL-10 synthesis of neonatal monocytes was far below the level needed to inhibit a submaximal release of IL-8 from mononuclear cells [115]. An imbalance of pro- and anti-inflammatory cytokines, favoring pro-inflammatory immune responses, has been considered an important feature of BPD. Especially in preterm infants exposed to CA or affected by FIRS, insufficient inhibition of exaggerated fetal pro-inflammatory cytokine responses may increase the risk of BPD [29]. Prophylactic treatment of surfactant-depleted rabbits with aerosolized IL-1 receptor antagonist decreased inflammation and experimental lung injury [116].

Pattern Recognition Receptors

Activation of PMNs and PBMCs is mediated by pattern recognition receptors (PRRs), which recognize structurally stable microbial membrane components [117]. PRRs display a complex system of sentinel receptors including cell-associated receptors, such as Toll-like receptors (TLRs), nucleotide oligomerization domain (NOD)-like receptors, retinoic acid inducible gene (RIG)-like receptors, and C-type lectin receptors, as well as soluble recognition molecules, such as complement, collectins, ficolins, or pentraxins [117, 118]. Among these, TLRs represent the best characterized family, currently comprising 10 human receptors, expressed either on the plasma membrane (TLR1, 2, 4, 5, 6) or intracellularly on endoplasmic reticulum and endosomal membranes (TLR3, 7, 8, 9, 10) [117, 119, 120]. Recognizing peptidoglycans and LPS, respectively, TLR2 and TLR4 provide an innate immune response against the most common pathogens involved in CA and neonatal sepsis and have been associated with inflammatory disorders of prematurity [120–122]. Besides peptidoglycans and LPS, both recognize a wide range of endogenous ligands, termed danger-associated molecular patterns (DAMPs), such as heat shock proteins and breakdown products of fibronectin, heparin sulfate, and hyaluronic acid [123]. However, interactions of PAMPs with several TLR co-receptors, rather than directly with TLRs, provide a model of how chemically distinct structures induce cellular activation via the same TLRs [123, 124]. Ligand binding is followed by recruitment of IL-1 receptor-associated kinases (IRAKs) or TNF receptor-associated factor (TRAF-) 6 and subsequent activation of complex signaling cascades culminating in the upregulation of pro-inflammatory cytokines, co-stimulatory molecules, and chemokines [119, 125]. Five different adaptor proteins are known to be involved in TLR signaling [126]. Of these, myeloid differentiation factor 88 (MyD88) is the best characterized and seems to be essential in TLR signaling except for TLR3 [127]. Data from animal model as well as in vitro data provide evidence of a gestational-age dependent expression of TLRs and TLR-related molecules with significant increase from late gestation to term and even further into adulthood [120, 128–130]. In animal models of CA, LPS-induced cytokine synthesis directly correlated with TLR4 expression and subsequent activation of NF-κB [131, 132]. In neonatal PMNs, TLR4 stimulation by purified LPS correspondingly resulted in enhanced secretion of TNF-α, IL-1β, IL-6, and IL-8 [20, 133]. In terms of quality of cytokine response, a tendency toward the pro-inflammatory state potentially reflecting immaturity of the neonatal innate immune system has been discussed [120, 134].

TLR signaling is tightly controlled by a number of exo and endogenous regulatory molecules [119, 123], such as IRAK-M, which prevents NF-κB activation [135]. Exposure of alveolar macrophages to surfactant protein (SP-) A, a member of the collectin family, was found to upregulate IRAK-M in experimental lung inflammation [136]. The latter inhibits TLR-mediated NF-κB activity in vitro by binding MyD88, leading to significantly reduced LPS-induced TNF-α and IL-6 synthesis [135, 136]. A number of studies documented a decrease of NF-κB activation induced by surfactant preparations [137–139]. Beneficial effects of SP-A and SP-D were documented for modulation of TLR2 and TLR4, p38 mitogen-activated protein kinase, cytosolic calcium, cAMP, and peroxisome function [140]. However, primary deficiency of pulmonary surfactant in preterm infants is even aggravated in the event of inflammation due to secondary inactivation of SP [8].

Oxygen Radicals and Proteolytic Mediators

Exposure to high inspiratory oxygen concentrations causes direct oxidative cell damage due to increased production of reactive oxygen species (ROS) released by neutrophils and macrophages at sites of inflammation [80, 90]. Moreover, ROS are generated upon hyperoxia or reoxygenation by free iron and the cell bound xanthine–oxidase system. Free iron was detected in the vast majority of ventilated preterm infants with RDS [141]. Animal experiments confirm that oxidative stress may be a crucial event in the initiation of pulmonary inflammation [131], with oxygen radicals exerting direct toxic effects on broncho-alveolar structures, such as lipid peroxidation, inactivation of protective anti-proteases, and upregulation of MMPs [80, 81, 141]. Extremely premature preterm infants are particularly susceptible to hyperoxia-derived lung damage due to a profound deficiency in antioxidant enzyme activity [81]. Moreover, data from in vitro studies, animal experiments, and clinical observation in preterm infants point to an imbalance of proteases and protease inhibitors contributing to lung injury in BPD [142, 143]. Following elastolytic damage, increased concentrations of various markers of tissue destruction were detected in airway secretions and urine of preterm infants [12, 37]. Of note, elastase and neutral proteases were shown to prime macrophages for increased release of toxic oxygen metabolites [144]. At sites of inflammation, neutrophil and macrophage-released proteases, such as elastase, β-glucoronidase, myeloperoxidase, cathepsin, MMPs, and others, play an essential role in the destruction of the alveolar–capillary unit and in extracellular matrix remodeling [80]. Similarly, overexpression of MMPs might cause disruption of the extracellular matrix. High concentrations of MMPs were detected in airway secretions of infants with BPD [145]. Moreover, protective levels of tissue inhibitors of MMPs were rather low in infants with BPD [145], and blocking of MMP-9 was shown to reduce hyperoxia-derived lung injury in fetal mice [146]. However, in the context of overexpression of IL-1β in a bi-transgenic mouse model, MMP-9 played a protective role, and MMP-9 deficiency, on the contrary, further exaggerated perturbation of lung morphogenesis [147]. Very recently, genetic variants of antioxidant response elements were found to be associated with an increased risk for BPD [148].

Increased Alveolar Capillary Permeability

Inflammation and inflammatory mediators have detrimental effects on the microvascular integrity. Increased alveolar capillary permeability is a pathognomonic feature of early stages of lung inflammation and has been associated with a deterioration of lung function [12, 37]. A variety of lipid mediators, such as leukotrienes, prostacyclin, platelet-derived factor, and endothelin-1, detected in airways of infants with BPD, seem to directly affect the alveolar–capillary unit [149]. Within 1 h after initiation of mechanical ventilation, protein leakage into the alveoli and airways of preterm infants was documented [89]. Moreover, a drastic increase in albumin concentrations in airway secretions was reported at a postnatal age of 10–14 days in preterm infants who later developed BPD, significantly contributing to alveolar edema, inactivation of the surfactant system, and deterioration of lung function [86]. In magnetic resonance imaging studies, infants with BPD showed an increased lung water content and were susceptible to gravity-induced collapse of the lung [150]. In mechanically ventilated infants with RDS, a simultaneous activation of clotting, fibrinolysis, kinin–kalikrein system, and the complement system was observed [37], indicating that injury to the pulmonary vascular endothelium may subsequently promote neutrophil and platelet activation and may induce pulmonary as well as systemic inflammation and activation of the clotting system.

Alveolarization and Angiogenesis

Airway branching plays a central role in embryonic lung development. Alveolar simplification is the typical pathological finding in lung tissues from animal models and infants with BPD being caused by apoptosis of cells critical for alveolar and vessel formation [5]. Moreover, pathologic examinations reveal fewer small arteries and an abnormal distribution of vessels within the distal lungs [5, 7, 11]. Increasing evidence suggests that pulmonary blood vessels actively promote normal alveolar development and contribute to the maintenance of alveolar structures [6, 21]. Adverse stimuli inhibiting pulmonary angiogenesis may significantly disturb and disrupt secondary septation [6]. It is currently assumed that disruption of pulmonary angiogenesis results in impaired alveolarization characteristic of BPD [6]. In a rat model of neonatal lung injury, antenatal LPS administration resulted in arrest of alveolarization [22]. In preterm lambs, a similar, time- and dose-dependent effect was observed [151]. The severity of inflammation-induced lung injury may depend on the efficacy of the individual's immune response. Data from a neonatal baboon model of *Ureaplasma* infection showed more severe disturbance of lung morphology in animals that remained colonized with *Ureaplasma* spp. than in preterm baboons that eradicated the pathogen [152]. Of note, intra-amniotic LPS led to increased levels of the angiostatic chemoattractants interferon (IFN-) γ-inducible protein-10 and monokine, induced by IFN-γ, in preterm lamb lungs [153]. Data from the mouse model suggest that inflammation may induce abnormal angiogenesis in the developing preterm lung by upregulation of angiogenic CC chemokines, such as MIP-1a and MCP-1 in fetal lung tissue [154]. Moreover, LPS-induced disruption of lung branching was shown to depend on macrophage NF-kB activation [108]. Even inflammation in the absence of infection has been shown to result in structural remodeling of the lung, including altered extracellular matrix formation, as well as impaired alveolarization and angiogenesis. Data from baboon, mouse, and rabbit models of neonatal lung injury confirmed potentiated airway inflammation and cytokine expression following a combination of hyperoxia and mechanical ventilation [155–157].

Repair Mechanisms and Growth Factors

Inflammation-induced tissue injury may be followed by tissue repair which has only partially been studied in BPD. Lung injury and the associated inflammatory process appear to result in the induction of transforming growth factor (TGF)-β that limits inflammatory reactions and plays a key role in mediating tissue remodeling and repair [158]. As a counter player to fibroblast growth factor-β and IL-1β, both lowering elastin mRNA in human lung fibroblasts, TGF-β seems to increase elastin by transcriptional and posttranscriptional mechanisms [159]. Hyperoxia-induced increases in TGF-β may contribute to impaired and simplified alveolarization characteristic of BPD [160]. In preterm animals, increased expression of TGF-β inhibited normal lung development and promoted fibrosis [37]. It has been hypothesized that overexpression of TGF-β, as well as low or suboptimal levels of various pulmonary and vascular growth factors in preterm infants with BPD might add to the pathogenesis of "new BPD," being characterized by growth arrest of lung tissue and pulmonary vessels rather than by fibrosis [5, 7]. Among several angiogenic growth factors, VEGF is essential and critical for vascular development and exists in high concentrations in heavily vascularized tissues [6, 80]. It is a key regulator of angiogenesis and lung maturation coordinating airway branching and angiogenesis [161]. Perturbation of VEGF signaling has been implicated in impaired lung parenchymal development and long-term lung injury, demonstrating an essential role of intrapulmonary vascular structures on lung parenchymal development [2, 6, 7, 162]. While VEGF levels were shown to be significantly increased in newborn rabbits following exposure to prolonged hyperoxia, decreased VEGF levels, and VEGF signaling were reported in the same setting in a premature fetal baboon model of BPD [163]. Significantly lower levels of VEGF were found in preterm infants, who developed BPD, compared to infants who recovered from ventilator- and hyperoxia-induced lung injury [164]. Decreased VEGF signaling has been considered a potential mechanism in the pathogenesis of reduced pulmonary capillary volume and impaired alveolarization. In extremely preterm animals developing BPD, impaired expression of VEGF, its angiogenic receptors, and angiopoetin were shown to contribute to dysmorphic microvasculature and disrupted alveolarization [165, 166]. In newborn rats, treatment with recombinant human VEGF as well as VEGF gene therapy promoted angiogenesis indicating a potential preventive strategy [162, 165]. A reduced expression of connective tissue growth factor (CTGF), which is responsible for various downstream actions of TGF-β and second important key mediator in the induction of pulmonary fibrosis, was found in a sheep model of BPD [167]. Moreover, low concentrations of hypoxic-inducible factor, keratinocyte, and hepatocyte growth factors, all thought to participate in normal lung development and tissue regeneration after lung injury, were detected in infants with BPD [168, 169].

Genetic Predisposition to Inflammation

Individual infants may be particularly susceptible to sustained lung inflammation. Twin concordance studies have pointed to a relevant impact of genetic risk, and current research has focused on identifying genetic factors contributing to heightened risk of intrauterine infection, preterm birth, and inflammatory lung injury [31, 33]. Genetic predisposition might comprise, e.g., variability in cytokine and chemokine response, imbalance toward exaggerated pro-inflammatory responses, and polymorphisms in key regulators of pro-inflammatory signaling, antioxidants, and modulators of angiogenesis [33, 170]. Genetic polymorphisms may confer an increased risk of altered vaginal flora, ascending infections, and preterm birth [171]. Numerous studies documented an impact of single nucleotide polymorphisms, such as TNF-α, IL-1β, TGF-β1, and MCP-1 on BPD manifestation [172]. Moreover, mutations affecting synthesis and metabolism of surfactant proteins or Clara Cell Protein 10 might contribute to individual courses of disease [32, 173].

Emerging Strategies and Therapies

Despite growing understanding of the underlying inflammatory mechanisms of preterm lung injury, there is still no specific or effective treatment of BPD. Currently, there is promising data on stem cell therapy for preventing and treating neonatal lung injury [174–176]. However, any potential therapeutic strategy would be applied best, if we could identify preterm infants at highest risk [30, 61]. Current research focuses on the detection of new biomarkers [15, 30].

Conclusion

There is profound evidence that a complex interplay of pre and postnatal pro-inflammatory conditions, primarily comprising pre and postnatal infection, mechanical ventilation, and hyperoxia, initiates and perpetuates an adverse inflammation in the structural and functional immature lung of preterm infants (Fig. 3.1). An initial injury, also referred to as "first hit," activates early immune responses directed to pathogen clearance and/or tissue repair. Functional immaturity in early and late immune responses, in antioxidant enzymes and protease system, in key regulators of alveolar homeostasis, in growth factors of angiogenesis, and in repair mechanisms, may promote an injurious lung inflammation, characterized by rapid accumulation of neutrophils and macrophages in the airways and pulmonary tissues. An arsenal of inflammatory mediators might subsequently affect the alveolar capillary unit and tissue integrity with an imbalance of pro-inflammatory and anti-inflammatory mechanisms favoring pro-inflammation. Multiple pre and postnatal events, such as neonatal sepsis, may further aggravate the ongoing inflammation, as a "second" or "third hit." Altered TLR-mediated immune responses have been implicated in the pathogenesis of BPD, and lung damage has been related to the particularly vulnerable saccular stage of lung development. As a devastating consequence, normal alveolarization and vascular development may be compromised with lifelong consequences. However, while seeking strategies to prevent or ameliorate BPD in high-risk infants, we still need a deeper insight into the pathogenesis of inflammatory events. New biomarkers might help to identify those preterm infants being at highest risk and might allow for optimal application of novel therapies. So far, we do not know whether and to what extent, a preterm infant at risk will face the given sequence of adverse lung inflammation, since the orchestra of confounding pre and postnatal factors, genetic susceptibility, and "window of vulnerability" may differ from infant to infant.

References

1. Philip AG. Bronchopulmonary dysplasia: then and now. Neonatology. 2012;102(1):1–8.
2. Reyburn B, Martin RJ, Prakash YS, MacFarlane PM. Mechanisms of injury to the preterm lung and airway: implications for long-term pulmonary outcome. Neonatology. 2012;101(4): 345–52.
3. Hallman M, Curstedt T, Halliday HL, Saugstad OD, Speer CP. Better neonatal outcomes: oxygen, surfactant and drug delivery. Preface. Neonatology. 2013;103(4):316–9.
4. Northway Jr WH, Rosan RC, Porter DY. Pulmonary disease following respirator therapy of hyaline-membrane disease. Bronchopulmonary dysplasia. N Engl J Med. 1967;276(7): 357–68.
5. Jobe AH. The new bronchopulmonary dysplasia. Curr Opin Pediatr. 2011;23(2):167–72.
6. Thebaud B, Abman SH. Bronchopulmonary dysplasia: where have all the vessels gone? Roles of angiogenic growth factors in chronic lung disease. Am J Respir Crit Care Med. 2007;175(10):978–85.
7. Baker CD, Abman SH. Impaired pulmonary vascular development in bronchopulmonary dysplasia. Neonatology. 2015;107(4):344–51.
8. Speer CP. Neonatal respiratory distress syndrome: an inflammatory disease? Neonatology. 2011;99(4):316–9.
9. Garcia-Munoz Rodrigo F, Galan Henriquez G, Figueras Aloy J, Garcia-Alix Perez A. Outcomes of very-low-birth-weight infants exposed to maternal clinical chorioamnionitis: a multicentre study. Neonatology. 2014;106(3):229–34.
10. Thomas W, Speer CP. Chorioamnionitis is essential in the evolution of bronchopulmonary dysplasia—the case in favour. Paediatr Respir Rev. 2014;15(1):49–52.
11. Cullen AB, Cooke PH, Driska SP, Wolfson MR, Shaffer TH. The impact of mechanical ventilation on immature airway smooth muscle: functional, structural, histological, and molecular correlates. Biol Neonate. 2006;90(1):17–27.
12. Speer CP. Chorioamnionitis, postnatal factors and proinflammatory response in the pathogenetic sequence of bronchopulmonary dysplasia. Neonatology. 2009;95(4):353–61.
13. Vogel ER, Britt Jr RD, Trinidad MC, Faksh A, Martin RJ, MacFarlane PM, et al. Perinatal oxygen in the developing lung. Can J Physiol Pharmacol. 2015;93(2):119–27.
14. Thome U, Gotze-Speer B, Speer CP, Pohlandt F. Comparison of pulmonary inflammatory mediators in preterm infants treated with intermittent positive pressure ventilation or high frequency oscillatory ventilation. Pediatr Res. 1998;44(3):330–7.
15. Bose CL, Dammann CE, Laughon MM. Bronchopulmonary dysplasia and inflammatory biomarkers in the premature neonate. Arch Dis Child Fetal Neonatal Ed. 2008;93(6):F455–61.

16. Viscardi RM. Perinatal inflammation and lung injury. Semin Fetal Neonatal Med. 2012;17(1):30–5.
17. Speer CP, Gahr M, Wieland M, Eber S. Phagocytosis-associated functions in neonatal monocyte-derived macrophages. Pediatr Res. 1988;24(2):213–6.
18. Grigg JM, Savill JS, Sarraf C, Haslett C, Silverman M. Neutrophil apoptosis and clearance from neonatal lungs. Lancet. 1991;338(8769):720–2.
19. Kramer BW, Jobe AH, Ikegami M. Monocyte function in preterm, term, and adult sheep. Pediatr Res. 2003;54(1):52–7.
20. Nguyen CN, Schnulle PM, Chegini N, Luo X, Koenig JM. Neonatal neutrophils with prolonged survival secrete mediators associated with chronic inflammation. Neonatology. 2010;98(4):341–7.
21. Abman SH. Bronchopulmonary dysplasia: "a vascular hypothesis". Am J Respir Crit Care Med. 2001;164(10 Pt 1):1755–6.
22. Ueda K, Cho K, Matsuda T, Okajima S, Uchida M, Kobayashi Y, et al. A rat model for arrest of alveolarization induced by antenatal endotoxin administration. Pediatr Res. 2006;59(3):396–400.
23. Grigsby PL, Novy MJ, Sadowsky DW, Morgan TK, Long M, Acosta E, et al. Maternal azithromycin therapy for Ureaplasma intraamniotic infection delays preterm delivery and reduces fetal lung injury in a primate model. Am J Obstet Gynecol. 2012;207(6):475.e1–14.
24. Nair V, Loganathan P, Soraisham AS. Azithromycin and other macrolides for prevention of bronchopulmonary dysplasia: a systematic review and meta-analysis. Neonatology. 2014;106(4):337–47.
25. Morley CJ. CPAP and low oxygen saturation for very preterm babies? N Engl J Med. 2010;362(21):2024–6.
26. Martin RJ, Fanaroff AA. The preterm lung and airway: past, present, and future. Pediatr Neonatol. 2013;54(4):228–34.
27. Manja V, Lakshminrusimha S, Cook DJ. Oxygen saturation target range for extremely preterm infants: a systematic review and meta-analysis. JAMA Pediatr. 2015;169(4):332–40.
28. Saugstad OD. Delivery room management of term and preterm newly born infants. Neonatology. 2015;107(4):365–71.
29. Paananen R, Husa AK, Vuolteenaho R, Herva R, Kaukola T, Hallman M. Blood cytokines during the perinatal period in very preterm infants: relationship of inflammatory response and bronchopulmonary dysplasia. J Pediatr. 2009;154(1):39–43.e3.
30. Piersigilli F, Bhandari V. Biomarkers in neonatology: the new "omics" of bronchopulmonary dysplasia. J Matern Fetal Neonatal Med. 2015;10:1–7. [Epub ahead of print].
31. Hallman M, Marttila R, Pertile R, Ojaniemi M, Haataja R. Genes and environment in common neonatal lung disease. Neonatology. 2007;91(4):298–302.
32. Abman SH, Mourani PM, Sontag M. Bronchopulmonary dysplasia: a genetic disease. Pediatrics. 2008;122(3):658–9.
33. Lavoie PM, Dube MP. Genetics of bronchopulmonary dysplasia in the age of genomics. Curr Opin Pediatr. 2010;22(2):134–8.
34. Menon R, Taylor RN, Fortunato SJ. Chorioamnionitis—a complex pathophysiologic syndrome. Placenta. 2010;31(2):113–20.
35. Combs CA, Gravett M, Garite TJ, Hickok DE, Lapidus J, Porreco R, et al. Amniotic fluid infection, inflammation, and colonization in preterm labor with intact membranes. Am J Obstet Gynecol. 2014;210(2):125.e1–15.
36. Onderdonk AB, Delaney ML, DuBois AM, Allred EN, Leviton A, Extremely Low Gestational Age Newborns Study I. Detection of bacteria in placental tissues obtained from extremely low gestational age neonates. American Journal of Obstet Gynecol. 2008;198(1):110.e1–7.
37. Speer CP. Inflammation and bronchopulmonary dysplasia: a continuing story. Semin Fetal Neonatal Med. 2006;11(5):354–62.
38. Goldenberg RL, Andrews WW, Goepfert AR, Faye-Petersen O, Cliver SP, Carlo WA, et al. The Alabama Preterm Birth Study: umbilical cord blood *Ureaplasma urealyticum* and

Mycoplasma hominis cultures in very preterm newborn infants. Am J Obstet Gynecol. 2008;198(1):43.e1–5.

39. Lahra MM, Beeby PJ, Jeffery HE. Intrauterine inflammation, neonatal sepsis, and chronic lung disease: a 13-year hospital cohort study. Pediatrics. 2009;123(5):1314–9.
40. Lee Y, Kim HJ, Choi SJ, Oh SY, Kim JS, Roh CR, et al. Is there a stepwise increase in neonatal morbidities according to histological stage (or grade) of acute chorioamnionitis and funisitis?: effect of gestational age at delivery. J Perinat Med. 2015;43(2):259–67.
41. DiGiulio DB. Diversity of microbes in amniotic fluid. Semin Fetal Neonatal Med. 2012;17(1):2–11.
42. Viscardi RM. Ureaplasma species: role in neonatal morbidities and outcomes. Arch Dis Child Fetal Neonatal Ed. 2014;99(1):F87–92.
43. Lowe J, Watkins WJ, Edwards MO, Spiller OB, Jacqz-Aigrain E, Kotecha SJ, et al. Association between pulmonary ureaplasma colonization and bronchopulmonary dysplasia in preterm infants: updated systematic review and meta-analysis. Pediatr Infect Dis J. 2014;33:697–702.
44. Heller DS, Rimpel LH, Skurnick JH. Does histologic chorioamnionitis correspond to clinical chorioamnionitis? J Reprod Med. 2008;53(1):25–8.
45. Been JV, Zimmermann LJ. Histological chorioamnionitis and respiratory outcome in preterm infants. Arch Dis Child Fetal Neonatal Ed. 2009;94(3):F218–25.
46. Thomas W, Speer CP. Chorioamnionitis: important risk factor or innocent bystander for neonatal outcome? Neonatology. 2011;99(3):177–87.
47. Lee J, Oh KJ, Park CW, Park JS, Jun JK, Yoon BH. The presence of funisitis is associated with a decreased risk for the development of neonatal respiratory distress syndrome. Placenta. 2011;32(3):235–40.
48. Park CW, Park JS, Jun JK, Yoon BH. Mild to moderate, but not minimal or severe, acute histologic chorioamnionitis or intra-amniotic inflammation is associated with a decrease in respiratory distress syndrome of preterm newborns without fetal growth restriction. Neonatology. 2015;108(2):115–23.
49. Watterberg KL, Demers LM, Scott SM, Murphy S. Chorioamnionitis and early lung inflammation in infants in whom bronchopulmonary dysplasia develops. Pediatrics. 1996;97(2):210–5.
50. Kramer BW, Kallapur S, Newnham J, Jobe AH. Prenatal inflammation and lung development. Semin Fetal Neonatal Med. 2009;14(1):2–7.
51. Kramer BW, Ladenburger A, Kunzmann S, Speer CP, Been JV, van Iwaarden JF, et al. Intravenous lipopolysaccharide-induced pulmonary maturation and structural changes in fetal sheep. Am J Obstet Gynecol. 2009;200(2):195.e1–10.
52. Hartling L, Liang Y, Lacaze-Masmonteil T. Chorioamnionitis as a risk factor for bronchopulmonary dysplasia: a systematic review and meta-analysis. Arch Dis Child Fetal Neonatal Ed. 2012;97(1):F8–17.
53. Van Marter LJ, Dammann O, Allred EN, Leviton A, Pagano M, Moore M, et al. Chorioamnionitis, mechanical ventilation, and postnatal sepsis as modulators of chronic lung disease in preterm infants. J Pediatr. 2002;140(2):171–6.
54. Been JV, Rours IG, Kornelisse RF, Jonkers F, de Krijger RR, Zimmermann LJ. Chorioamnionitis alters the response to surfactant in preterm infants. J Pediatr. 2010;156(1):10–5. e1.
55. Inatomi T, Oue S, Ogihara T, Hira S, Hasegawa M, Yamaoka S, et al. Antenatal exposure to Ureaplasma species exacerbates bronchopulmonary dysplasia synergistically with subsequent prolonged mechanical ventilation in preterm infants. Pediatr Res. 2012;71(3):267–73.
56. Prince LS, Dieperink HI, Okoh VO, Fierro-Perez GA, Lallone RL. Toll-like receptor signaling inhibits structural development of the distal fetal mouse lung. Dev Dyn. 2005;233(2):553–61.
57. Buhimschi CS, Dulay AT, Abdel-Razeq S, Zhao G, Lee S, Hodgson EJ, et al. Fetal inflammatory response in women with proteomic biomarkers characteristic of intra-amniotic inflammation and preterm birth. BJOG. 2009;116(2):257–67.
58. Viscardi RM, Muhumuza CK, Rodriguez A, Fairchild KD, Sun CC, Gross GW, et al. Inflammatory markers in intrauterine and fetal blood and cerebrospinal fluid compartments

are associated with adverse pulmonary and neurologic outcomes in preterm infants. Pediatr Res. 2004;55(6):1009–17.
59. Schmidt B, Cao L, Mackensen-Haen S, Kendziorra H, Klingel K, Speer CP. Chorioamnionitis and inflammation of the fetal lung. Am J Obstet Gynecol. 2001;185(1):173–7.
60. May M, Marx A, Seidenspinner S, Speer CP. Apoptosis and proliferation in lungs of human fetuses exposed to chorioamnionitis. Histopathology. 2004;45(3):283–90.
61. Kim MA, Lee YS, Seo K. Assessment of predictive markers for placental inflammatory response in preterm births. PLoS One. 2014;9(10):e107880.
62. Stoll BJ, Hansen NI, Sanchez PJ, Faix RG, Poindexter BB, Van Meurs KP, et al. Early onset neonatal sepsis: the burden of group B Streptococcal and *E. coli* disease continues. Pediatrics. 2011;127(5):817–26.
63. Bersani I, Speer CP. Nosocomial sepsis in neonatal intensive care: inevitable or preventable? Z Geburtshilfe Neonatol. 2012;216(4):186–90.
64. Boghossian NS, Page GP, Bell EF, Stoll BJ, Murray JC, Cotten CM, et al. Late-onset sepsis in very low birth weight infants from singleton and multiple-gestation births. J Pediatr. 2013;162(6):1120–4, 4.e1.
65. Dong Y, Speer CP. Late-onset neonatal sepsis: recent developments. Arch Dis Child Fetal Neonatal Ed. 2015;100(3):F257–63.
66. Ohlin A, Bjorkman L, Serenius F, Schollin J, Kallen K. Sepsis as a risk factor for neonatal morbidity in extremely preterm infants. Acta Paediatr. 2015;104:1070–6.
67. Auriti C, Maccallini A, Di Liso G, Di Ciommo V, Ronchetti MP, Orzalesi M. Risk factors for nosocomial infections in a neonatal intensive-care unit. J Hosp Infect. 2003;53(1):25–30.
68. Anderson-Berry A, Brinton B, Lyden E, Faix RG. Risk factors associated with development of persistent coagulase-negative staphylococci bacteremia in the neonate and associated short-term and discharge morbidities. Neonatology. 2011;99(1):23–31.
69. Strunk T, Doherty D, Jacques A, Simmer K, Richmond P, Kohan R, et al. Histologic chorioamnionitis is associated with reduced risk of late-onset sepsis in preterm infants. Pediatrics. 2012;129(1):e134–41.
70. Ericson JE, Laughon MM. Chorioamnionitis: implications for the neonate. Clin Perinatol. 2015;42(1):155–65. ix.
71. Bersani I, Thomas W, Speer CP. Chorioamnionitis—the good or the evil for neonatal outcome? J Matern Fetal Neonatal Med. 2012;25 Suppl 1:12–6.
72. Hillman NH, Nitsos I, Berry C, Pillow JJ, Kallapur SG, Jobe AH. Positive end-expiratory pressure and surfactant decrease lung injury during initiation of ventilation in fetal sheep. Am J Physiol Lung Cell Mol Physiol. 2011;301(5):L712–20.
73. Copland IB, Martinez F, Kavanagh BP, Engelberts D, McKerlie C, Belik J, et al. High tidal volume ventilation causes different inflammatory responses in newborn versus adult lung. Am J Respir Crit Care Med. 2004;169(6):739–48.
74. Backstrom E, Hogmalm A, Lappalainen U, Bry K. Developmental stage is a major determinant of lung injury in a murine model of bronchopulmonary dysplasia. Pediatr Res. 2011;69(4):312–8.
75. Network SSGotEKSNNR, Finer NN, Carlo WA, Walsh MC, Rich W, Gantz MG, et al. Early CPAP versus surfactant in extremely preterm infants. N Engl J Med. 2010;362(21):1970–9.
76. Roberts CT, Davis PG, Owen LS. Neonatal non-invasive respiratory support: synchronised NIPPV, non-synchronised NIPPV or bi-level CPAP: what is the evidence in 2013? Neonatology. 2013;104(3):203–9.
77. Laughon M, Allred EN, Bose C, O'Shea TM, Van Marter LJ, Ehrenkranz RA, et al. Patterns of respiratory disease during the first 2 postnatal weeks in extremely premature infants. Pediatrics. 2009;123(4):1124–31.
78. Kroon AA, Wang J, Huang Z, Cao L, Kuliszewski M, Post M. Inflammatory response to oxygen and endotoxin in newborn rat lung ventilated with low tidal volume. Pediatr Res. 2010;68(1):63–9.
79. Ricard JD, Dreyfuss D, Saumon G. Production of inflammatory cytokines in ventilator-induced lung injury: a reappraisal. Am J Respir Crit Care Med. 2001;163(5):1176–80.

80. Bhandari V. Hyperoxia-derived lung damage in preterm infants. Semin Fetal Neonatal Med. 2010;15(4):223–9.
81. Saugstad OD. Oxidative stress in the newborn—a 30-year perspective. Biol Neonate. 2005;88(3):228–36.
82. Wagenaar GT, ter Horst SA, van Gastelen MA, Leijser LM, Mauad T, van der Velden PA, et al. Gene expression profile and histopathology of experimental bronchopulmonary dysplasia induced by prolonged oxidative stress. Free Radic Biol Med. 2004;36(6):782–801.
83. Vuichard D, Ganter MT, Schimmer RC, Suter D, Booy C, Reyes L, et al. Hypoxia aggravates lipopolysaccharide-induced lung injury. Clin Exp Immunol. 2005;141(2):248–60.
84. Urlichs F, Speer CP. Neutrophil function in preterm and term infants. NeoReviews. 2004;5(10):e417–29.
85. Ogden BE, Murphy SA, Saunders GC, Pathak D, Johnson JD. Neonatal lung neutrophils and elastase/proteinase inhibitor imbalance. Am Rev Respir Dis. 1984;130(5):817–21.
86. Groneck P, Gotze-Speer B, Oppermann M, Eiffert H, Speer CP. Association of pulmonary inflammation and increased microvascular permeability during the development of bronchopulmonary dysplasia: a sequential analysis of inflammatory mediators in respiratory fluids of high-risk preterm neonates. Pediatrics. 1994;93(5):712–8.
87. Merritt TA, Stuard ID, Puccia J, Wood B, Edwards DK, Finkelstein J, et al. Newborn tracheal aspirate cytology: classification during respiratory distress syndrome and bronchopulmonary dysplasia. J Pediatr. 1981;98(6):949–56.
88. Nupponen I, Pesonen E, Andersson S, Makela A, Turunen R, Kautiainen H, et al. Neutrophil activation in preterm infants who have respiratory distress syndrome. Pediatrics. 2002; 110(1 Pt 1):36–41.
89. Jaarsma AS, Braaksma MA, Geven WB, van Oeveren W, Bambang Oetomo S. Activation of the inflammatory reaction within minutes after birth in ventilated preterm lambs with neonatal respiratory distress syndrome. Biol Neonate. 2004;86(1):1–5.
90. Turunen R, Nupponen I, Siitonen S, Repo H, Andersson S. Onset of mechanical ventilation is associated with rapid activation of circulating phagocytes in preterm infants. Pediatrics. 2006;117(2):448–54.
91. Wang L, Scabilloni JF, Antonini JM, Rojanasakul Y, Castranova V, Mercer RR. Induction of secondary apoptosis, inflammation, and lung fibrosis after intratracheal instillation of apoptotic cells in rats. Am J Physiol Lung Cell Mol Physiol. 2006;290(4):L695–702.
92. Murch SH, Costeloe K, Klein NJ, MacDonald TT. Early production of macrophage inflammatory protein-1 alpha occurs in respiratory distress syndrome and is associated with poor outcome. Pediatr Res. 1996;40(3):490–7.
93. Bhattacharya S, Go D, Krenitsky DL, Huyck HL, Solleti SK, Lunger VA, et al. Genome-wide transcriptional profiling reveals connective tissue mast cell accumulation in bronchopulmonary dysplasia. Am J Respir Crit Care Med. 2012;186(4):349–58.
94. Rosen D, Lee JH, Cuttitta F, Rafiqi F, Degan S, Sunday ME. Accelerated thymic maturation and autoreactive T cells in bronchopulmonary dysplasia. Am J Respir Crit Care Med. 2006;174(1):75–83.
95. Sarelius IH, Glading AJ. Control of vascular permeability by adhesion molecules. Tissue Barriers. 2015;3(1–2):e985954.
96. D'Alquen D, Kramer BW, Seidenspinner S, Marx A, Berg D, Groneck P, et al. Activation of umbilical cord endothelial cells and fetal inflammatory response in preterm infants with chorioamnionitis and funisitis. Pediatr Res. 2005;57(2):263–9.
97. Baier RJ, Majid A, Parupia H, Loggins J, Kruger TE. CC chemokine concentrations increase in respiratory distress syndrome and correlate with development of bronchopulmonary dysplasia. Pediatr Pulmonol. 2004;37(2):137–48.
98. Zlotnik A, Yoshie O. The chemokine superfamily revisited. Immunity. 2012;36(5): 705–16.
99. Garcia-Ramallo E, Marques T, Prats N, Beleta J, Kunkel SL, Godessart N. Resident cell chemokine expression serves as the major mechanism for leukocyte recruitment during local inflammation. J Immunol. 2002;169(11):6467–73.

100. Smith RE. Chemotactic cytokines mediate leukocyte recruitment in fibrotic lung disease. Biol Signals. 1996;5(4):223–31.
101. Yi M, Jankov RP, Belcastro R, Humes D, Copland I, Shek S, et al. Opposing effects of 60% oxygen and neutrophil influx on alveologenesis in the neonatal rat. Am J Respir Crit Care Med. 2004;170(11):1188–96.
102. Baier RJ, Loggins J, Kruger TE. Monocyte chemoattractant protein-1 and interleukin-8 are increased in bronchopulmonary dysplasia: relation to isolation of *Ureaplasma urealyticum*. J Invest Med. 2001;49(4):362–9.
103. Yoon BH, Romero R, Jun JK, Park KH, Park JD, Ghezzi F, et al. Amniotic fluid cytokines (interleukin-6, tumor necrosis factor-alpha, interleukin-1 beta, and interleukin-8) and the risk for the development of bronchopulmonary dysplasia. Am J Obstet Gynecol. 1997;177(4): 825–30.
104. Bry K, Whitsett JA, Lappalainen U. IL-1beta disrupts postnatal lung morphogenesis in the mouse. Am J Respir Cell Mol Biol. 2007;36(1):32–42.
105. Hogmalm A, Bry M, Strandvik B, Bry K. IL-1beta expression in the distal lung epithelium disrupts lung morphogenesis and epithelial cell differentiation in fetal mice. Am J Physiol Lung Cell Mol Physiol. 2014;306(1):L23–34.
106. Murch SH, Costeloe K, Klein NJ, Rees H, McIntosh N, Keeling JW, et al. Mucosal tumor necrosis factor-alpha production and extensive disruption of sulfated glycosaminoglycans begin within hours of birth in neonatal respiratory distress syndrome. Pediatr Res. 1996;40(3):484–9.
107. Kolb M, Margetts PJ, Anthony DC, Pitossi F, Gauldie J. Transient expression of IL-1beta induces acute lung injury and chronic repair leading to pulmonary fibrosis. J Clin Invest. 2001;107(12):1529–36.
108. Blackwell TS, Hipps AN, Yamamoto Y, Han W, Barham WJ, Ostrowski MC, et al. NF-kappaB signaling in fetal lung macrophages disrupts airway morphogenesis. J Immunol. 2011;187(5):2740–7.
109. Cao L, Liu C, Cai B, Jia X, Kang L, Speer CP, et al. Nuclear factor-kappa B expression in alveolar macrophages of mechanically ventilated neonates with respiratory distress syndrome. Biol Neonate. 2004;86(2):116–23.
110. Cheah FC, Winterbourn CC, Darlow BA, Mocatta TJ, Vissers MC. Nuclear factor kappaB activation in pulmonary leukocytes from infants with hyaline membrane disease: associations with chorioamnionitis and *Ureaplasma urealyticum* colonization. Pediatr Res. 2005; 57(5 Pt 1):616–23.
111. Iosef C, Alastalo TP, Hou Y, Chen C, Adams ES, Lyu SC, et al. Inhibiting NF-kappaB in the developing lung disrupts angiogenesis and alveolarization. Am J Physiol Lung Cell Mol Physiol. 2012;302(10):L1023–36.
112. Jones CA, Cayabyab RG, Kwong KY, Stotts C, Wong B, Hamdan H, et al. Undetectable interleukin (IL)-10 and persistent IL-8 expression early in hyaline membrane disease: a possible developmental basis for the predisposition to chronic lung inflammation in preterm newborns. Pediatr Res. 1996;39(6):966–75.
113. Sabat R, Grutz G, Warszawska K, Kirsch S, Witte E, Wolk K, et al. Biology of interleukin-10. Cytokine Growth Factor Rev. 2010;21(5):331–44.
114. Kwong KY, Jones CA, Cayabyab R, Lecart C, Khuu N, Rhandhawa I, et al. The effects of IL-10 on proinflammatory cytokine expression (IL-1beta and IL-8) in hyaline membrane disease (HMD). Clin Immunol Immunopathol. 1998;88(1):105–13.
115. Davidson D, Miskolci V, Clark DC, Dolmaian G, Vancurova I. Interleukin-10 production after pro-inflammatory stimulation of neutrophils and monocytic cells of the newborn. Comparison to exogenous interleukin-10 and dexamethasone levels needed to inhibit chemokine release. Neonatology. 2007;92(2):127–33.
116. Narimanbekov IO, Rozycki HJ. Effect of IL-1 blockade on inflammatory manifestations of acute ventilator-induced lung injury in a rabbit model. Exp Lung Res. 1995;21(2):239–54.
117. Takeuchi O, Akira S. Pattern recognition receptors and inflammation. Cell. 2010;140(6): 805–20.

118. Medzhitov R. Recognition of microorganisms and activation of the immune response. Nature. 2007;449(7164):819–26.
119. Akira S. TLR signaling. Curr Top Microbiol Immunol. 2006;311:1–16.
120. Glaser K, Speer CP. Toll-like receptor signaling in neonatal sepsis and inflammation: a matter of orchestration and conditioning. Expert Rev Clin Immunol. 2013;9(12):1239–52.
121. O'Hare FM, William Watson R, Molloy EJ. Toll-like receptors in neonatal sepsis. Acta Paediatr. 2013;102(6):572–8.
122. Kemp MW. Preterm birth, intrauterine infection, and fetal inflammation. Front Immunol. 2014;5:574.
123. Akira S, Uematsu S, Takeuchi O. Pathogen recognition and innate immunity. Cell. 2006;124(4):783–801.
124. Lee CC, Avalos AM, Ploegh HL. Accessory molecules for Toll-like receptors and their function. Nat Rev Immunol. 2012;12(3):168–79.
125. Yamamoto M, Takeda K. Current views of toll-like receptor signaling pathways. Gastroenterol Res Pract. 2010;2010:240365.
126. Jenkins KA, Mansell A. TIR-containing adaptors in Toll-like receptor signalling. Cytokine. 2010;49(3):237–44.
127. Medzhitov R, Preston-Hurlburt P, Kopp E, Stadlen A, Chen C, Ghosh S, et al. MyD88 is an adaptor protein in the hToll/IL-1 receptor family signaling pathways. Mol Cell. 1998;2(2):253–8.
128. Harju K, Glumoff V, Hallman M. Ontogeny of Toll-like receptors Tlr2 and Tlr4 in mice. Pediatr Res. 2001;49(1):81–3.
129. Hillman NH, Moss TJ, Nitsos I, Kramer BW, Bachurski CJ, Ikegami M, et al. Toll-like receptors and agonist responses in the developing fetal sheep lung. Pediatr Res. 2008;63(4):388–93.
130. Zhang J, Zhou J, Xu B, Chen C, Shi W. Different expressions of TLRs and related factors in peripheral blood of preterm infants. Int J Clin Exp Med. 2015;8(3):4108–14.
131. Kramer BW, Kramer S, Ikegami M, Jobe AH. Injury, inflammation, and remodeling in fetal sheep lung after intra-amniotic endotoxin. Am J Physiol Lung Cell Mol Physiol. 2002;283(2):L452–9.
132. Harju K, Ojaniemi M, Rounioja S, Glumoff V, Paananen R, Vuolteenaho R, et al. Expression of toll-like receptor 4 and endotoxin responsiveness in mice during perinatal period. Pediatr Res. 2005;57(5 Pt 1):644–8.
133. Contrino J, Krause PJ, Slover N, Kreutzer D. Elevated interleukin-1 expression in human neonatal neutrophils. Pediatr Res. 1993;34(3):249–52.
134. Kollmann TR, Levy O, Montgomery RR, Goriely S. Innate immune function by Toll-like receptors: distinct responses in newborns and the elderly. Immunity. 2012;37(5):771–83.
135. Wesche H, Gao X, Li X, Kirschning CJ, Stark GR, Cao Z. IRAK-M is a novel member of the Pelle/interleukin-1 receptor-associated kinase (IRAK) family. J Biol Chem. 1999;274(27):19403–10.
136. Nguyen HA, Rajaram MV, Meyer DA, Schlesinger LS. Pulmonary surfactant protein A and surfactant lipids upregulate IRAK-M, a negative regulator of TLR-mediated inflammation in human macrophages. Am J Physiol Lung Cell Mol Physiol. 2012;303(7):L608–16.
137. Wu YZ, Medjane S, Chabot S, Kubrusly FS, Raw I, Chignard M, et al. Surfactant protein-A and phosphatidylglycerol suppress type IIA phospholipase A2 synthesis via nuclear factor-kappaB. Am J Respir Crit Care Med. 2003;168(6):692–9.
138. Raychaudhuri B, Abraham S, Bonfield TL, Malur A, Deb A, DiDonato JA, et al. Surfactant blocks lipopolysaccharide signaling by inhibiting both mitogen-activated protein and IkappaB kinases in human alveolar macrophages. Am J Respir Cell Mol Biol. 2004;30(2):228–32.
139. Kerecman J, Mustafa SB, Vasquez MM, Dixon PS, Castro R. Immunosuppressive properties of surfactant in alveolar macrophage NR8383. Inflamm Res. 2008;57(3):118–25.
140. Bersani I, Kunzmann S, Speer CP. Immunomodulatory properties of surfactant preparations. Expert Rev Anti Infect Ther. 2013;11(1):99–110.

141. Gerber CE, Bruchelt G, Stegmann H, Schweinsberg F, Speer CP. Presence of bleomycin-detectable free iron in the alveolar system of preterm infants. Biochem Biophys Res Commun. 1999;257(1):218–22.
142. Speer CP, Ruess D, Harms K, Herting E, Gefeller O. Neutrophil elastase and acute pulmonary damage in neonates with severe respiratory distress syndrome. Pediatrics. 1993;91(4):794–9.
143. Altiok O, Yasumatsu R, Bingol-Karakoc G, Riese RJ, Stahlman MT, Dwyer W, et al. Imbalance between cysteine proteases and inhibitors in a baboon model of bronchopulmonary dysplasia. Am J Respir Crit Care Med. 2006;173(3):318–26.
144. Speer CP, Pabst MJ, Hedegaard HB, Rest RF, Johnston Jr RB. Enhanced release of oxygen metabolites by monocyte-derived macrophages exposed to proteolytic enzymes: activity of neutrophil elastase and cathepsin G. J Immunol. 1984;133(4):2151–6.
145. Cederqvist K, Sorsa T, Tervahartiala T, Maisi P, Reunanen K, Lassus P, et al. Matrix metalloproteinases-2, -8, and -9 and TIMP-2 in tracheal aspirates from preterm infants with respiratory distress. Pediatrics. 2001;108(3):686–92.
146. Chetty A, Cao GJ, Severgnini M, Simon A, Warburton R, Nielsen HC. Role of matrix metalloprotease-9 in hyperoxic injury in developing lung. Am J Physiol Lung Cell Mol Physiol. 2008;295(4):L584–92.
147. Lukkarinen H, Hogmalm A, Lappalainen U, Bry K. Matrix metalloproteinase-9 deficiency worsens lung injury in a model of bronchopulmonary dysplasia. Am J Respir Cell Mol Biol. 2009;41(1):59–68.
148. Sampath V, Garland JS, Helbling D, Dimmock D, Mulrooney NP, Simpson PM, et al. Antioxidant response genes sequence variants and BPD susceptibility in VLBW infants. Pediatr Res. 2015;77(3):477–83.
149. Speer CP. Pulmonary inflammation and bronchopulmonary dysplasia. J Perinatol. 2006;26 Suppl 1:S57–62. discussion S3–4.
150. Adams EW, Harrison MC, Counsell SJ, Allsop JM, Kennea NL, Hajnal JV, et al. Increased lung water and tissue damage in bronchopulmonary dysplasia. J Pediatr. 2004;145(4):503–7.
151. Kramer BW, Moss TJ, Willet KE, Newnham JP, Sly PD, Kallapur SG, et al. Dose and time response after intraamniotic endotoxin in preterm lambs. Am J Respir Crit Care Med. 2001;164(6):982–8.
152. Yoder BA, Coalson JJ, Winter VT, Siler-Khodr T, Duffy LB, Cassell GH. Effects of antenatal colonization with *ureaplasma urealyticum* on pulmonary disease in the immature baboon. Pediatr Res. 2003;54(6):797–807.
153. Kallapur SG, Jobe AH, Ikegami M, Bachurski CJ. Increased IP-10 and MIG expression after intra-amniotic endotoxin in preterm lamb lung. Am J Respir Crit Care Med. 2003;167(5): 779–86.
154. Miller JD, Benjamin JT, Kelly DR, Frank DB, Prince LS. Chorioamnionitis stimulates angiogenesis in saccular stage fetal lungs via CC chemokines. Am J Physiol Lung Cell Mol Physiol. 2010;298(5):L637–45.
155. Varughese R, Nayak JL, LoMonaco M, O'Reilly MA, Ryan RM, D'Angio CT. Effects of hyperoxia on tumor necrosis factor alpha and Grobeta expression in newborn rabbit lungs. Lung. 2003;181(6):335–46.
156. Wilson MR, Choudhury S, Takata M. Pulmonary inflammation induced by high-stretch ventilation is mediated by tumor necrosis factor signaling in mice. Am J Physiol Lung Cell Mol Physiol. 2005;288(4):L599–607.
157. Brew N, Hooper SB, Allison BJ, Wallace MJ, Harding R. Injury and repair in the very immature lung following brief mechanical ventilation. Am J Physiol Lung Cell Mol Physiol. 2011;301(6):L917–26.
158. Bartram U, Speer CP. The role of transforming growth factor beta in lung development and disease. Chest. 2004;125(2):754–65.
159. Kuang PP, Zhang XH, Rich CB, Foster JA, Subramanian M, Goldstein RH. Activation of elastin transcription by transforming growth factor-beta in human lung fibroblasts. Am J Physiol Lung Cell Mol Physiol. 2007;292(4):L944–52.

160. Zhao Y, Gilmore BJ, Young SL. Expression of transforming growth factor-beta receptors during hyperoxia-induced lung injury and repair. Am J Physiol. 1997;273(2 Pt 1):L355–62.
161. Hines EA, Sun X. Tissue crosstalk in lung development. J Cell Biochem. 2014;115(9): 1469–77.
162. Kunig AM, Balasubramaniam V, Markham NE, Seedorf G, Gien J, Abman SH. Recombinant human VEGF treatment transiently increases lung edema but enhances lung structure after neonatal hyperoxia. Am J Physiol Lung Cell Mol Physiol. 2006;291(5):L1068–78.
163. Bhandari V, Elias JA. Cytokines in tolerance to hyperoxia-induced injury in the developing and adult lung. Free Radic Biol Med. 2006;41(1):4–18.
164. D'Angio CT, Maniscalco WM. The role of vascular growth factors in hyperoxia-induced injury to the developing lung. Front Biosci. 2002;7:d1609–23.
165. Thebaud B, Ladha F, Michelakis ED, Sawicka M, Thurston G, Eaton F, et al. Vascular endothelial growth factor gene therapy increases survival, promotes lung angiogenesis, and prevents alveolar damage in hyperoxia-induced lung injury: evidence that angiogenesis participates in alveolarization. Circulation. 2005;112(16):2477–86.
166. Thomas W, Seidenspinner S, Kawczynska-Leda N, Kramer BW, Chmielnicka-Kopaczyk M, Marx A, et al. Systemic fetal inflammation and reduced concentrations of macrophage migration inhibitory factor in tracheobronchial aspirate fluid of extremely premature infants. Am J Obstet Gynecol. 2008;198(1):64.e1–6.
167. Kunzmann S, Seher A, Kramer BW, Schenk R, Schutze N, Jakob F, et al. Connective tissue growth factor does not affect transforming growth factor-beta 1-induced Smad3 phosphorylation and T lymphocyte proliferation inhibition. Int Arch Allergy Immunol. 2008;147(2):152–60.
168. Danan C, Franco ML, Jarreau PH, Dassieu G, Chailley-Heu B, Bourbon J, et al. High concentrations of keratinocyte growth factor in airways of premature infants predicted absence of bronchopulmonary dysplasia. Am J Respir Crit Care Med. 2002;165(10):1384–7.
169. Lassus P, Heikkila P, Andersson LC, von Boguslawski K, Andersson S. Lower concentration of pulmonary hepatocyte growth factor is associated with more severe lung disease in preterm infants. J Pediatr. 2003;143(2):199–202.
170. Huusko JM, Karjalainen MK, Mahlman M, Haataja R, Kari MA, Andersson S, et al. A study of genes encoding cytokines (IL6, IL10, TNF), cytokine receptors (IL6R, IL6ST), and glucocorticoid receptor (NR3C1) and susceptibility to bronchopulmonary dysplasia. BMC Med Genet. 2014;15:120.
171. Genc MR, Onderdonk A. Endogenous bacterial flora in pregnant women and the influence of maternal genetic variation. BJOG. 2011;118(2):154–63.
172. Strassberg SS, Cristea IA, Qian D, Parton LA. Single nucleotide polymorphisms of tumor necrosis factor-alpha and the susceptibility to bronchopulmonary dysplasia. Pediatr Pulmonol. 2007;42(1):29–36.
173. Miller TL, Shashikant BN, Pilon AL, Pierce RA, Shaffer TH, Wolfson MR. Effects of an intratracheally delivered anti-inflammatory protein (rhCC10) on physiological and lung structural indices in a juvenile model of acute lung injury. Biol Neonate. 2006;89(3): 159–70.
174. Chang YS, Ahn SY, Yoo HS, Sung SI, Choi SJ, Oh WI, et al. Mesenchymal stem cells for bronchopulmonary dysplasia: phase 1 dose-escalation clinical trial. J Pediatr. 2014;164(5): 966–72.e6.
175. O'Reilly M, Thebaud B. Stem cells for the prevention of neonatal lung disease. Neonatology. 2015;107(4):360–4.
176. Pawelec K, Gladysz D, Demkow U, Boruczkowski D. Stem cell experiments moves into clinic: new hope for children with bronchopulmonary dysplasia. Adv Exp Med Biol. 2015;839:47–53.

Chapter 4
Mycoplasma in Bronchopulmonary Dysplasia

Rose M. Viscardi

Introduction

The mycoplasma species *Ureaplasma parvum*, *U. urealyticum*, and *Mycoplasma hominis* are genitourinary tract commensals in adults but are associated with adverse pregnancy outcomes [1] and neonatal morbidities of prematurity including bronchopulmonary dysplasia (BPD) [2], necrotizing enterocolitis [3], and severe intraventricular hemorrhage [4]. These organisms are the most commonly isolated organisms from infected placentas and amniotic fluid [1, 5]. They have been detected in respiratory secretions [2, 6], gastric aspirates [7], cord blood [4, 8, 9], cerebrospinal fluid [4], and brain [10] and lung tissue [11] of preterm infants. *Ureaplasma* spp. are detected in respiratory samples from 28 to 33 % of infants <1501 g birthweight [2] and the colonization rate is inversely proportional to gestational age [6]. In a recent study at our institution, 65 % of infants <26 weeks gestation were *Ureaplasma* spp. culture or polymerase chain reaction (PCR)-positive one or more times during the first month of life compared with 31 % infants ≥26 weeks gestational age. Colonized infants are more likely to be born extremely preterm by vaginal delivery to women with pregnancies complicated by chorioamnionitis and preterm labor or preterm premature rupture of membranes [12–15] with increasing vertical transmission with longer duration of membrane rupture [16]. *M. hominis* is detected in respiratory samples from preterm infants less frequently than the *Ureaplasma* species and is commonly a co-colonizer with *Ureaplasma* species in vaginal, placental, and neonatal respiratory samples [7, 17, 18]. Despite changes in clinical care over the past 25 years, three meta-analyses that include data from over 4000 infants and more than 40 individual studies during this period have demonstrated persistence of

R.M. Viscardi, MD (✉)
Department of Pediatrics, University of Maryland School of Medicine,
110 S. Paca Street, 8th floor, Baltimore, MD 21201, USA
e-mail: rviscard@peds.umaryland.edu

V. Bhandari (ed.), *Bronchopulmonary Dysplasia*, Respiratory Medicine,
DOI 10.1007/978-3-319-28486-6_4

the *Ureaplasma*–BPD association over time and no significant effect of differences in gestational ages between colonized and non-colonized infants on the strength of the association [2, 19, 20].

Microbiology

Mycoplasmas are members of the class *Mollicutes* characterized by their lack of a rigid cell wall that are the smallest self-replicating organisms both in cellular and genome size capable of cell-free existence [21]. There are 14 serovars among the two *Ureaplasma* species with *U. parvum* serovars 1, 3, 6, and 14 more commonly detected in clinical isolates than *U. urealyticum* serovars [2, 4, 7–13]. All have limited biosynthetic functions, have the capacity to adhere to human mucosal surfaces, and hydrolyze urea to generate adenosine triphosphate (ATP) and ammonia (NH_3) [22]. In contrast, *M. hominis* hydrolyzes arginine to generate ATP with CO_2 and NH_3 as end products [21]. Most *Ureaplasma* spp. laboratory reference strains and clinical respiratory isolates from preterm infants have the capacity to form biofilms in vitro [23]. If confirmed in vivo, biofilm formation may protect the organisms from host defenses and antibiotics.

Virulence Factors

The proposed major ureaplasmal virulence factor is the multiple-banded antigen (MBA), a surface lipoprotein that is the predominant pathogen-associated molecular pattern (PAMP) detected by the host immune system [24]. The MBA consists of a N-terminal conserved domain containing a signal peptide, lipoprotein attachment site, and one transmembrane domain and a C-terminal variable domain consisting of tandem repeating units. Phase variants (loss of MBA expression) have been generated in vitro [25–27] but have not been demonstrated in vivo. However, ureaplasmal MBA size variation has been demonstrated in vitro [24] and in vivo [27–29], suggesting that it may be the major mechanism through which these organisms colonize the host by evading immune defenses.

In addition, functional and enzymatic assays identified potential ureaplasmal virulence factors including IgA protease and phospholipase A1, A2, and C, but gene sequences for these proteins have not been identified in any reference or clinical ureaplasmal strain [30–33]. Ammonia generated by urea hydrolysis by *Ureaplasma* spp. urease enzyme and arginine hydrolysis by *M. hominis* may react with water in tissues to form ammonium hydroxide that may contribute to mucosal injury and inflammation [29]. The *U. parvum* serovar 3 clinical strain SV3F4 genome contains a putative new virulence factor serine/threonine kinase and protein phosphatase (STK/STP) [34] that may contribute to host cell cytotoxicity since mutant genitalium strains lacking the STP gene produce less hydrogen peroxide than wild-type strains [35]. Xiao et al. [36] demonstrated that *Ureaplasma* spp. suppress expression of antimicrobial peptide genes *DEFB1*, *DEFA5*, *DEFA6*, and *CAMP* in vitro as a potential mechanism to avoid the host immune response. Recently, a "gene of interest" was identified in the sequences of two *M. hominis* amniotic fluid isolates that was significantly associated with upper genital tract colonization and preterm birth [37]. Further characterization of this gene and its protein product may identify a previously unknown mycoplasmal virulence factor.

Host Immune Response

Mammalian Toll-like receptor (TLR) proteins are "pattern recognition receptors" that are key components of the innate immune response to microbial products. Engagement of TLRs activates the conserved TLR domain and leads to recruitment of the cytoplasmic signaling molecules such as MyD88, TRIF, and IRAK4 and activation of NF-κB and downstream inflammatory cytokine production and microbial killing. In vitro studies of murine macrophages [38] and human amniotic epithelial cells and transfected HEK cells [39] have confirmed that the ureaplasmal cell surface MBA protein is a ligand for TLR2 with the heterodimer partner TLR6 and the whole bacterium activates intracellular TLR9 with subsequent increases in tumor necrosis factor alpha (TNFα), interleukin-1beta (IL-1ß), IL-6, and IL-8. Recently, we identified four single nucleotide polymorphisms (SNPs) in *TLR2* and *TLR6* that were significantly associated with *Ureaplasma* respiratory tract colonization [40]. Interestingly, a *TLR6* SNP (rs5743827) was associated with both a decreased risk for *Ureaplasma* respiratory tract colonization and decreased risk for BPD, suggesting that this variant may alter susceptibility to *Ureaplasma* infection and the severity of the inflammatory response that contributes to the development of BPD.

Ureaplasma infection-induced stimulation of inflammatory cytokines may be the causative link between intrauterine infection and lung injury. *Ureaplasma* spp. stimulates release of TNFα, IL-1ß, IL-8, monocyte chemoattractant-1 (MCP-1), transforming growth factor beta 1 ($TGFß_1$), and other mediators by various cell types in vitro, and *Ureaplasma* spp. colonization is associated with increased concentrations of these cytokines in tracheal aspirates during the first week of life in infants who develop BPD [22]. Upregulation of these cytokine networks leads to inflammatory cell recruitment and activation, local tissue injury, and alterations in normal developmental pathways during critical periods of lung development [22] (See Chap. 3). Since *Ureaplasma* has been detected as early as mid-trimester, the fetal lung may be exposed to this infection as early as the canalicular stage of development (Table 4.1). Animal models described in the subsequent sections have provided the critical evidence that the mycoplasmas are pathogens, which contribute to preterm birth, altered immune responses, and fetal lung development.

Table 4.1 Embryonic stages of lung development in different species

Lung stages	Human (weeks)	Rhesus (days)	Sheep (days)	Mouse (days)
Embryonic (E)	3–6	21–55	10–35	E9–9.5
Pseudo-glandular	5–17	59–80	35–80	E9.5–16.6
Canalicular	16–26	82–130	80–120	E16.6–17.4
Saccular	24–38	141–168	120–140	E17.4–P5
Alveolar	36 weeks–7 years	155-postnatal	135-postnatal	P5–30
Term	40	155–172	145	21

Animal Models

Human BPD is characterized by an impairment of alveolar and vascular development. Multiple animal models that mimic the BPD phenotype have been developed by exposing newborn wild-type and genetically modified animals to hyperoxia and/or mechanical ventilation [41], and perinatal exposures to lipopolysaccharide (LPS) as an inflammatory stimulus [42]. These models, primarily in rodents, sheep, and nonhuman primates, have provided mechanistic insights into the pathogenesis of BPD and identified the saccular stage as the critical window of vulnerability for inflammation-mediated alterations in alveolar and vascular lung development (reviewed in [43, 44] and Chap. 3).

As summarized in Table 4.2, experimental mycoplasma in vivo models have been developed that have demonstrated that these organisms can elicit an inflammatory response in the lung [45], establish a chronic intrauterine infection [54, 61], and contribute to a BPD phenotype alone or when combined with another inflammatory stimulus such as hyperoxia or mechanical ventilation [59, 60]. There are a number of limitations of these models. Rodents and sheep differ in important aspects in placental anatomy and mechanisms of parturition compared to humans [53, 62]. In addition, since humans are the specific host for *U. parvum* and *U. urealyticum*, these organisms need to be adapted to another species by serial passage in the new host, but may elicit less intense inflammatory responses than in the natural human host [45, 46, 49]. Despite these limitations, important lessons have been learned from these models as summarized in Table 4.2 and the following sections. Taken together, the studies suggest that *Ureasplasma* infection initiated in utero and augmented postnatally by exposure to hyperoxia and volutrauma elicits a sustained dysregulated inflammatory response in the immature lung that impairs alveolarization and stimulates myofibroblast proliferation and excessive collagen and elastin deposition (Fig. 4.1).

Pneumonia Models

Mice and nonhuman primate *Ureasplasma* pneumonia models demonstrate that an infection established in the pulmonary compartment leads to inflammation and lung injury. Intratracheal ureasplasmal inoculation in 140 days preterm baboons caused an

Table 4.2 Animal models for the study of Mycoplasma infections

Species	Advantages	Disadvantages	Major observations
Mice	• Cost-effective • Short gestation (20–22 days) • Well-characterized lung and immune system development (see Table 4.1) • Can be combined with other BPD models (e.g., hyperoxia) • Genetic manipulations	• Not a natural host for *U. parvum*, *U. urealyticum*, *M. hominis* • Need to "adapt" mycoplasma isolates to mouse host [45, 46] • Strain differences in susceptibility to mycoplasmas [47, 48]	• Postnatal age-dependent susceptibility to UP1[a] and UU10 nasal inoculation in newborn mice [46] • Hyperoxia exposure augmented UU10-mediated lung inflammation, delayed clearance, and increased mortality in newborn mice [49] • Juvenile *U. urealyticum* mouse pneumonia model [45] • SP-A-deficient mice exhibited delayed clearance and exaggerated lung inflammatory response to intratracheal *U. parvum* inoculation [50] • Antenatal UP1 inoculation at E13.4 combined with postnatal O_2 exposure resulted in increase inflammatory cytokines in fetal lung and augmented O_2 lung injury [51]
Sheep	• Due to long gestation (147 days), excellent for studies of chronic *U. parvum* intrauterine infection • Fetal lamb size allows instrumentation and postnatal ventilation	• Not a natural host for human mycoplasmas • Intrauterine inflammation does not trigger preterm labor [52] • Layered epithelial–chordial cotyledonary placenta limits transplacental transfer of antibiotics and antibodies [53]	• Establish chronic intrauterine infection from 1 to 10 weeks with variable inflammatory response (histologic chorioamnionitis) and fetal lung infection [28, 54] • Intra-amniotic UP3 induced lung maturation, surfactant production, but abnormal elastin and collagen deposition altering lung structure [54, 55] • Antenatal UP intra-amniotic infection did not affect subsequent lung injury from short-term high tidal volume ventilation [56]

(continued)

Table 4.2 (continued)

Species	Advantages	Disadvantages	Major observations
Nonhuman primates	• Most similar to human pregnancies • Long gestations (~160 day) • Similar hemomonochordial villous, discoid placenta as humans • Intrauterine infection stimulates preterm labor • Established preterm baboon BPD model [41] • Potential for survival of offspring for long-term studies	• Most expensive model • Small sample sizes	• Postnatal intratracheal inoculation baboons delivered at 140 days gestation (term 180 days) resulted in lung infection and acute bronchiolitis [57] • Demonstrated vertical transmission to fetus following second and third trimester maternal IV *Ureaplasma* clinical isolate inoculation in pigtail macaques [58] • Antenatal UP1 inoculation at 122 days gestation baboon delivered at 125 days variable duration of postnatal lung colonization and lung injury and lung fibrosis [59, 60] • Intramniotic UP1 or *M hominis* inoculation elicits an inflammatory response in intrauterine compartment and fetal lung that contributes to preterm labor and fetal lung injury [61]

[a]Abbreviations: *BPD* bronchopulmonary dysplasia, *SP-A* surfactant protein-A, *UP U. parvum*, *UU U. urealyticum*

acute pneumonitis with alveolar septal thickening [57] and an acute interstitial pneumonia in newborn, but not 14-day-old newborn mice [46]. In support of the hypothesis that *Ureasplasma* respiratory tract colonization augments the inflammatory response to a second stimulus, addition of hyperoxia exposure in the newborn mouse pneumonia model increased lung inflammation and mortality and delayed pathogen clearance in the *Ureasplasma*-infected animals [49]. In 6-week-old mice, *U. urealyticum* intratracheal inoculation caused an acute pneumonitis and sustained inflammation up to 28 days postinoculation despite apparent clearance of the organism [45]. Studies of the pneumonia model in knockout mice have provided additional insights. Compared to *U. parvum* intratracheally inoculated wild-type mice, infected surfactant protein-A (SP-A)-deficient mice had delayed ureasplasmal clearance from the lungs and increased inflammatory cells and pro-inflammatory cytokine expression [50]. This observation may be relevant to preterm fetuses and neonates who will have low levels of SP-A and other innate host defense factors in the lungs. Although vertical transmission of ureaplasmas and colonization of the preterm infant respiratory tract may occur at the time of delivery, these pneumonia models lack the prolonged exposure of the early lung developmental stages to an intrauterine infection.

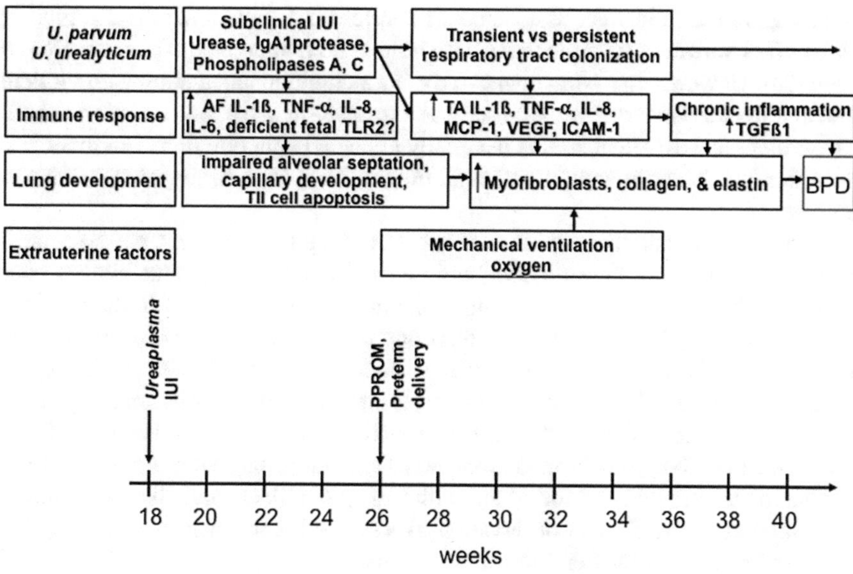

Fig. 4.1 Proposed model for role of Ureaplasma infection in BPD pathogenesis. In this schematic, prolonged intra-amniotic exposure of the fetal lung to Ureaplasma infection and maternal and fetal derived cytokines recruits inflammatory cells and alters TGFß1 signaling in the lung. Postnatal exposure to hyperoxia and ventilation augments this proinflammatory response, leading to impaired alveolarization, disordered myofibroblast proliferation, and excessive collagen and elastin deposition [22]. *IUI* intrauterine infection, *AF* amniotic fluid, *IL-1β* interleukin-1beta, *TNFα* tumor necrosis factor alpha, *TLR* toll-like receptor, *MCP* monocyte chemoattractant protein, *VEGF* vascular endothelial growth factor, *ICAM* intercellular adhesion molecule, *TGF* transforming growth factor, *TII* Type II, *BPD* bronchopulmonary dysplasia, *PPROM* preterm premature rupture of membranes

Intrauterine Infection Models

To address the effects of ureaplasmal infection on the fetal lung, intrauterine infection models have been developed in mice [51], sheep [27, 29, 52, 54–56, 63] and nonhuman primates [58, 59, 61, 64, 65] (Table 4.2). Intra-amniotic *U. parvum* serovar 1 inoculation at E13.4 (pseudo-glandular stage) combined with postnatal hyperoxia exposure resulted in increased inflammatory cytokines in fetal lung and augmented hyperoxia lung injury [51]. In the sheep model, intra-amniotic injection of *Ureaplasma* in early gestation resulted in efficient colonization with persistent infection for 3 months to term [54]. The severity of *Ureasplasma*-mediated chorioamnionitis was variable with 10 % of sheep not demonstrating any chorioamnionitis despite efficient colonization [28]. This may be explained by *Ureasplasma* evading immune detection by the host. MBA size variation was observed in the sheep model with the differences in the number of MBA size variants associated with differences in histologic chorioamniontis severity. Five or fewer MBA size variants detected within amniotic fluid were associated with severe inflammation, whereas nine or more MBA variants were associated with little or no inflammation in the chorioamnion [28]. However, in a subsequent study, intra-amniotic inoculation with virulent and avirulent strains of *U. parvum* serovar 6 resulted in MBA size variation in both the virulent and avirulent strains in serially collected amniotic fluid, but there was no difference in chorioamnion and fetal lung inflammation in response to the two strains [27].

Long-term intrauterine exposure of the fetal sheep to *U. parvum* was associated with improvement in lung function and increased surfactant production but poor fetal growth, fetal acidemia, and lung inflammation [52, 54, 56]. Although effects on lung physiology suggest "lung maturation," they probably represent "dysmaturation" since the improved lung physiology was accompanied by evidence of impaired lung development [55]. Fourteen days after intra-amniotic *Ureaplasma* injection, preterm fetal sheep delivered at 80 % gestation had decreased elastic foci and increased smooth muscle around bronchioles and pulmonary artery/arterioles [55], similar to changes reported for infants with BPD [66–68]. Overall, the sheep studies lend support to the clinical observation of less respiratory distress syndrome but increased risk for BPD after *Ureaplasma* exposure.

Although *Ureaplasma* effectively establishes a chronic infection in the intrauterine compartment in the sheep, it does not stimulate preterm labor due to differences in parturition between sheep and humans [54] and sheep are not natural hosts for *U. parvum* or *U. urealyticum*. In Rhesus monkeys, intra-amniotic *U. parvum* serovar 1 inoculation at 130 days gestation (term 167 days, see Table 4.1) was associated with increased amniotic fluid TNFα, IL-1ß, IL-6, and IL-8, histologic chorioamnionitis, and increased uterine contractility (see Fig. 4.1) [64, 65]. Additional studies in the Rhesus monkey infection model demonstrated that intra-amniotic *U. parvum* serovar 1 or *M. hominis* inoculation elicited an inflammatory response in the intrauterine compartment and fetal lung that contributed to preterm labor and fetal lung injury [61]. Similar findings were observed in the 125 days baboon model infected with *U. parvum* serovar 1 in utero and postnatal exposure to mechanical ventilation and oxygen [59]. Intra-amniotic inoculation of ureaplasmal organisms 2 days before delivery at 125 days in the baboon resulted in an inflammatory response in the intrauterine and fetal lung compartments and vertical transmission to the fetal lung that persisted up to 14 days postnatally in half of the antenatal-exposed animals. Compared with lungs from noninfected animals and gestational controls, *Ureasplasma*-infected lungs demonstrated an imbalance of pro- and anti-fibrotic signaling factors with (1) increased lung lavage IL-1ß and active $TGFß_1$, but no difference in IL-10; (2) more extensive fibrosis, increased myofibroblasts phenotype, and $TGFß_1$ immunostaining; and (3) trend toward greater activation of pro-fibrotic transcription factors Smad-2 and-3 relative to anti-fibrotic Smad-7 in lung homogenates [60]. Although these studies involved direct inoculation of the amniotic cavity, intravenous inoculation of pregnant pigtail macaques (*Macaca nemstrina*) at either late second trimester or early third trimester resulted in infection of the amniotic fluid and multiple fetal tissues including lymph nodes, joints, lungs, and gastrointestinal tract, demonstrating that *Ureasplasma* can cross the placenta and result in hematogenous dissemination in the fetus [58). Taken together, these data provide compelling evidence that antenatal ureaplasmal infection alters lung development and augments a prolonged, proinflammatory, profibrotic response in the preterm lung exposed postnatally to ventilation and hyperoxia [22].

Anti-infective Agents

Since there is increasing recognition that *Ureaplasma* species are pathogens in the preterm lung, therapeutic strategies have been investigated in the animal models (Table 4.3). In the Rhesus macque intrauterine *U. parvum* infection model, azithromycin alone or in combination with anti-inflammatory agents dexamethasone and indomethacin delayed onset of labor, eradicated the infection, and prevented fetal lung injury [70–72]. In contrast, following mid-gestation intra-amniotic *U. parvum* inoculation, maternal intravenous azithromycin or solithromycin for 5 days ± single intra-amniotic dose of the same antibiotic prior to delivery at 125 days gestation effectively cleared infection, but had no effect on fetal lung or chorioamnion histologic inflammation scores [69]. These data suggest that fetal lung injury that occurs

Table 4.3 Efficacy of antibiotics and anti-inflammatory drugs to ameliorate adverse effects of ureaplasmal infection

Drug	Species	Infection model	Outcome
Maternal IV AZI[a] or solithromycin (SOLI) × 5 days ± single intra-amniotic dose same antibiotic	Sheep	Intra-amniotic UP inoculation midgestation, antibiotic therapy 5 days prior to delivery at 125 days	All antibiotic regimens (IV ± intra-amniotic dose) effectively cleared infection, but no effect on fetal lung or chorioamnion histologic inflammation scores [69]
Maternal IV AZI	Rhesus monkeys	Intra-amniotic UP infection	Maternal IV AZI prevents fetal lung lesions [70]
Maternal IV AZI +dexamethasone +indomethacin	Rhesus monkeys	Intra-amniotic UP infection	Maternal IV AZI ± dex + indomethacin clears infection, delays preterm delivery, and reduced fetal lung injury [71]
Maternal IV AZI + intra-amniotic AZI	Rhesus monkeys	Intra-amniotic UP infection	Intra-amniotic AZI + IV AZI × 10 days resulted in UP eradication and intra-amniotic accumulation of AZI [72]
Postnatal IP AZI versus erythromycin	FVB albino mice	Postnatal IM UP14 inoculation d1–3 ± 0.8 FiO_2 exposure × 14days	IP AZI d1-3, but not IP erythromycin improved survival and growth in hyperoxia + IM-infected newborn animals [73]

[a]Abbreviations: *IV* intravenous, *AZI* azithromycin, *SOLI* solithromycin, *UP U. parvum*, *IM* intramuscular, *FiO_2* fraction of inspired oxygen, *IP* intraperitoneal

with prolonged antenatal exposure to *Ureaplasma* infection may not be altered by late eradication of the organisms by either maternal or postnatal antibiotic treatment. In a mouse model, simultaneous treatment of *U. parvum* infected, hyperoxia-exposed newborn pups with intraperitoneal azithromycin, but not erythromycin, improved survival and growth compared to no antibiotic treatment [73]. These studies suggest that early detection of intrauterine infection will be essential for optimal timing of therapeutic interventions and antibiotic therapy alone may be insufficient to prevent BPD in *Ureaplasma*-infected preterm infants.

Conclusions

There is a strong association of *Ureaplasma* colonization and BPD in human neonates. Various animal models have provided evidence of the pathogenic nature of mycoplasma infections, their contribution to preterm birth, and impact on fetal lung development. A combination of intrauterine infection with postnatal factors (hyperoxia, ventilation) has been shown in some of these animal models to mimic the pulmonary phenotype of human BPD. Further studies to optimize therapeutic strategies for the prevention of BPD in premature infants infected with *Ureaplasma* are needed.

References

1. Murtha AP, Edwards JM. The role of mycoplasma and ureaplasma in adverse pregnancy outcomes. Obstet Gynecol Clin North Am. 2014;41(4):615–27.
2. Lowe J, Watkins WJ, Edwards MO, Spiller OB, Jacqz-Aigrain E, Kotecha SJ, et al. Association between pulmonary ureaplasma colonization and bronchopulmonary dysplasia in preterm infants: updated systematic review and meta-analysis. Pediatr Infect Dis J. 2014;33(7):697–702.
3. Okogbule-Wonodi AC, Gross GW, Sun CC, Agthe AG, Xiao L, Waites KB, et al. Necrotizing enterocolitis is associated with ureaplasma colonization in preterm infants. Pediatr Res. 2011;69(5 Pt 1):442–7.
4. Viscardi RM, Hashmi N, Gross GW, Sun CC, Rodriguez A, Fairchild KD. Incidence of invasive ureaplasma in VLBW infants: relationship to severe intraventricular hemorrhage. J Perinatol. 2008;28(11):759–65.
5. Romero R, Miranda J, Chaemsaithong P, Chaiworapongsa T, Kusanovic JP, Dong Z, et al. Sterile and microbial-associated intra-amniotic inflammation in preterm prelabor rupture of membranes. J Matern Fetal Neonatal Med. 2015;12:1394–409.
6. Sung TJ, Xiao L, Duffy L, Waites KB, Chesko KL, Viscardi RM. Frequency of ureaplasma serovars in respiratory secretions of preterm infants at risk for bronchopulmonary dysplasia. Pediatr Infect Dis J. 2011;30(5):379–83.
7. Payne MS, Goss KC, Connett GJ, Kollamparambil T, Legg JP, Thwaites R, et al. Molecular microbiological characterization of preterm neonates at risk of bronchopulmonary dysplasia. Pediatr Res. 2010;67(4):412–8.
8. Goldenberg RL, Andrews WW, Goepfert AR, Faye-Petersen O, Cliver SP, Carlo WA, et al. The Alabama Preterm Birth Study: umbilical cord blood *Ureaplasma urealyticum* and *Mycoplasma hominis* cultures in very preterm newborn infants. Am J Obstet Gynecol. 2008;198(1):43.e1–5.

9. Kacerovsky M, Pliskova L, Menon R, Kutova R, Musilova I, Maly J, et al. Microbial load of umbilical cord blood Ureaplasma species and *Mycoplasma hominis* in preterm prelabor rupture of membranes. J Matern Fetal Neonatal Med. 2014;27(16):1627–32.
10. Rao RP, Ghanayem NS, Kaufman BA, Kehl KS, Gregg DC, Chusid MJ. *Mycoplasma hominis* and Ureaplasma species brain abscess in a neonate. Pediatr Infect Dis J. 2002;21(11):1083–5.
11. Madan E, Meyer MP, Amortegui AJ. Isolation of genital mycoplasmas and *Chlamydia trachomatis* in stillborn and neonatal autopsy material. Arch Pathol Lab Med. 1988;112(7):749–51.
12. Theilen U, Lyon AJ, Fitzgerald T, Hendry GM, Keeling JW. Infection with *Ureaplasma urealyticum*: is there a specific clinical and radiological course in the preterm infant? Arch Dis Child Fetal Neonatal Ed. 2004;89(2):F163–7.
13. Olomu IN, Hecht JL, Onderdonk AO, Allred EN, Leviton A. Perinatal correlates of *Ureaplasma urealyticum* in placenta parenchyma of singleton pregnancies that end before 28 weeks of gestation. Pediatrics. 2009;123(5):1329–36.
14. Namba F, Hasegawa T, Nakayama M, Hamanaka T, Yamashita T, Nakahira K, et al. Placental features of chorioamnionitis colonized with Ureaplasma species in preterm delivery. Pediatr Res. 2010;67(2):166–72.
15. Doyle RM, Alber DG, Jones HE, Harris K, Fitzgerald F, Peebles D, et al. Term and preterm labour are associated with distinct microbial community structures in placental membranes which are independent of mode of delivery. Placenta. 2014;35(12):1099–101.
16. Grattard F, Soleihac B, De Barbeyrac B, Bebear C, Seffert P, Pozzetto B. Epidemiologic and molecular investigations of genital mycoplasmas from women and neonates at delivery. Pediatr Infect Dis J. 1995;14:853–8.
17. Leli C, Meucci M, Vento S, D'Alo F, Farinelli S, Perito S, et al. Microbial and vaginal determinants influencing *Mycoplasma hominis* and *Ureaplasma urealyticum* genital colonization in a population of female patients. Infez Med. 2013;21(3):201–6.
18. Kwak DW, Hwang HS, Kwon JY, Park YW, Kim YH. Co-infection with vaginal *Ureaplasma urealyticum* and *Mycoplasma hominis* increases adverse pregnancy outcomes in patients with preterm labor or preterm premature rupture of membranes. J Matern Fetal Neonatal Med. 2014;27(4):333–7.
19. Wang EE, Cassell GH, Sanchez PJ, Regan JA, Payne NR, Liu PP. *Ureaplasma urealyticum* and chronic lung disease of prematurity: critical appraisal of the literature on causation. Clin Infect Dis. 1993;17 Suppl 1:S112–6.
20. Schelonka RL, Katz B, Waites KB, Benjamin Jr DK. Critical appraisal of the role of Ureaplasma in the development of bronchopulmonary dysplasia with metaanalytic techniques. Pediatr Infect Dis J. 2005;24(12):1033–9.
21. Waites KB, Xiao L, Paralanov V, Viscardi RM, Glass JI. Molecular methods for the detection of Mycoplasma and ureaplasma infections in humans: a paper from the 2011 William Beaumont Hospital Symposium on molecular pathology. J Mol Diagn. 2012;14(5):437–50.
22. Viscardi RM, Hasday JD. Role of Ureaplasma species in neonatal chronic lung disease: epidemiologic and experimental evidence. Pediatr Res. 2009;65(5 Pt 2):84R–90.
23. Pandelidis K, McCarthy A, Chesko KL, Viscardi RM. Role of biofilm formation in Ureaplasma antibiotic susceptibility and development of bronchopulmonary dysplasia in preterm neonates. Pediatr Infect Dis J. 2013;32(4):394–8.
24. Zheng X, Teng L-J, Watson HL, Glass JI, Blanchard A, Cassell GH. Small repeating units within the *Ureaplasma urealyticum* MB antigen gene encode serovar specificity and are associated with antigen size variation. Infect Immun. 1995;63:891–8.
25. Monecke S, Helbig JH, Jacobs E. Phase variation of the multiple banded protein in *Ureaplasma urealyticum* and *Ureaplasma parvum*. Int J Med Microbiol. 2003;293(2–3):203–11.
26. Zimmerman CU, Stiedl T, Rosengarten R, Spergser J. Alternate phase variation in expression of two major surface membrane proteins (MBA and UU376) of *Ureaplasma parvum* serovar 3. FEMS Microbiol Lett. 2009;292(2):187–93.
27. Dando SJ, Nitsos I, Kallapur SG, Newnham JP, Polglase GR, Pillow JJ, et al. The role of the multiple banded antigen of *Ureaplasma parvum* in intra-amniotic infection: major virulence factor or decoy? PLoS One. 2012;7(1):e29856.

28. Knox CL, Dando SJ, Nitsos I, Kallapur SG, Jobe AH, Payton D, et al. The severity of chorioamnionitis in pregnant sheep is associated with in vivo variation of the surface-exposed multiple-banded antigen/gene of *Ureaplasma parvum*. Biol Reprod. 2010;83(3):415–26.
29. Robinson JW, Dando SJ, Nitsos I, Newnham J, Polglase GR, Kallapur SG, et al. *Ureaplasma parvum* serovar 3 multiple banded antigen size variation after chronic intra-amniotic infection/colonization. PLoS One. 2013;8(4):e62746.
30. Kilian M, Brown MB, Brown TA, Freundt EA, Cassell GH. Immunoglobulin A1 protease activity in strains of *Ureaplasma urealyticum*. Acta Pathol Microbiol Immunol Scand B. 1984;92(1):61–4.
31. DeSilva NS, Quinn PA. Characterization of phospholipase A_1, A_2, C activity in *Ureaplasma urealyticum* membranes. Mol Cell Biochem. 1999;201:159–67.
32. Glass JI, Lefkowitz EJ, Glass JS, Heiner CR, Chen EY, Cassell GH. The complete sequence of the mucosal pathogen *Ureaplasma urealyticum*. Nature. 2000;407(6805):757–62.
33. Paralanov V, Lu J, Duffy LB, Crabb DM, Shrivastava S, Methe BA, et al. Comparative genome analysis of 19 *Ureaplasma urealyticum* and *Ureaplasma parvum* strains. BMC Microbiol. 2012;12(1):88.
34. Wu HN, Nakura Y, Motooka D, Nakamura S, Nishiumi F, Ishino S, et al. Complete genome sequence of *Ureaplasma parvum* Serovar 3 strain SV3F4, isolated in Japan. Genome Announc. 2014; 2(3):e00256–14.
35. Martinez MA, Das K, Saikolappan S, Materon LA, Dhandayuthapani S. A serine/threonine phosphatase encoded by MG_207 of *Mycoplasma genitalium* is critical for its virulence. BMC Microbiol. 2013;13:44.
36. Xiao L, Crabb DM, Dai Y, Chen Y, Waites KB, Atkinson TP. Suppression of antimicrobial peptide expression by ureaplasma species. Infect Immun. 2014;82(4):1657–65.
37. Allen-Daniels MJ, Serrano MG, Pflugner LP, Fettweis JM, Prestosa MA, Koparde VN, et al. Identification of a gene in *Mycoplasma hominis* associated with preterm birth and microbial burden in intraamniotic infection. Am J Obstet Gynecol. 2015;212(6):779.e1–e13.
38. Shimizu T, Kida Y, Kuwano K. *Ureaplasma parvum* lipoproteins, including MB antigen, activate NF-{kappa}B through TLR1, TLR2 and TLR6. Microbiology. 2008;154(Pt 5): 1318–25.
39. Triantafilou M, De Glanville B, Aboklaish AF, Spiller OB, Kotecha S, Triantafilou K. Synergic activation of toll-like receptor (TLR) 2/6 and 9 in response to *ureaplasma parvum* & urealyticum in human amniotic epithelial cells. PLoS One. 2013;8(4):e61199.
40. Winters AH, Levan TD, Vogel SN, Chesko KL, Pollin TI, Viscardi RM. Single nucleotide polymorphism in toll-like receptor 6 is associated with a decreased risk for ureaplasma respiratory tract colonization and bronchopulmonary dysplasia in preterm infants. Pediatr Infect Dis J. 2013;32(8):898–904.
41. Coalson JJ, Winter VT, Siler-Khodr T, Yoder BA. Neonatal chronic lung disease in extremely immature baboons. Am J Respir Crit Care Med. 1999;160(4):1333–46.
42. Moss TJ, Newnham JP, Willett KE, Kramer BW, Jobe AH, Ikegami M. Early gestational intra-amniotic endotoxin: lung function, surfactant, and morphometry. Am J Respir Crit Care Med. 2002;165(6):805–11.
43. Yoder BA, Coalson JJ. Animal models of bronchopulmonary dysplasia. The preterm baboon models. Am J Physiol Lung Cell Mol Physiol. 2014;307(12):L970–7.
44. Hilgendorff A, Reiss I, Ehrhardt H, Eickelberg O, Alvira CM. Chronic lung disease in the preterm infant. Lessons learned from animal models. Am J Respir Cell Mol Biol. 2014;50(2):233–45.
45. Viscardi RM, Kaplan J, Lovchik JC, He JR, Hester L, Rao S, et al. Characterization of a murine model of *Ureaplasma urealyticum* pneumonia. Infect Immun. 2002;70:5721–9.
46. Rudd PT, Cassell GH, Waites KB, Davis JK, Duffy LB. *Ureaplasma urealyticum* pneumonia: experimental production and demonstration of age-related susceptibility. Infect Immun. 1989;57:918–25.
47. von Chamier M, Allam A, Brown MB, Reinhard MK, Reyes L. Host genetic background impacts disease outcome during intrauterine infection with *Ureaplasma parvum*. PLoS One. 2012;7(8):e44047.

48. Allam AB, von Chamier M, Brown MB, Reyes L. Immune profiling of BALB/C and C57BL/6 mice reveals a correlation between *Ureaplasma parvum*-Induced fetal inflammatory response syndrome-like pathology and increased placental expression of TLR2 and CD14. Am J Reprod Immunol. 2014;71(3):241–51.
49. Crouse DT, Cassell GH, Waites KB, Foster JM, Cassady G. Hyeroxia potentiates *Ureaplasma urealyticum* pneumonia in newborn mice. Infect Immun. 1990;58:3487–93.
50. Famuyide ME, Hasday JD, Carter HC, Chesko KL, He JR, Viscardi RM. Surfactant protein-A limits Ureaplasma-mediated lung inflammation in a murine pneumonia model. Pediatr Res. 2009;66(2):162–7.
51. Normann E, Lacaze-Masmonteil T, Eaton F, Schwendimann L, Gressens P, Thebaud B. A novel mouse model of Ureaplasma-induced perinatal inflammation: effects on lung and brain injury. Pediatr Res. 2009;65(4):430–6.
52. Moss TJ, Knox CL, Kallapur SG, Nitsos I, Theodoropoulos C, Newnham JP, et al. Experimental amniotic fluid infection in sheep: effects of *Ureaplasma parvum* serovars 3 and 6 on preterm or term fetal sheep. Am J Obstet Gynecol. 2008;198(1):122.e1–8.
53. Enders AC, Carter AM. What can comparative studies of placental structure tell us?—a review. Placenta. 2004;25(Suppl A):S3–9.
54. Moss TJ, Nitsos I, Ikegami M, Jobe AH, Newnham JP. Experimental intrauterine *Ureaplasma* infection in sheep. Am J Obstet Gynecol. 2005;192(4):1179–86.
55. Collins JJ, Kallapur SG, Knox CL, Nitsos I, Polglase GR, Pillow JJ, et al. Inflammation in fetal sheep from intra-amniotic injection of *Ureaplasma parvum*. Am J Physiol Lung Cell Mol Physiol. 2010;299(6):L852–60.
56. Polglase GR, Hillman NH, Pillow JJ, Nitsos I, Newnham JP, Knox CL, et al. Ventilation-mediated injury after preterm delivery of *Ureaplasma parvum* colonized fetal lambs. Pediatr Res. 2010;67(6):630–5.
57. Walsh WF, Butler J, Coalson J, Hensley D, Cassell GH, de Lemos RA. A primate model of *Ureaplasma urealyticum* infection in the premature infant with hyaline membrane disease. Clin Infect Dis. 1993;17 Suppl 1:S158–62.
58. Dohm ED, Richards DS, Robertson JA, Theele DP, Schoeb TR, Davis JK, et al. Vertical transmision of *Ureaplasma uralyticum* in pregnant pigtail macaques (*Macaca nemestrina*). Infect Dis Rev. 1999;1:208–13.
59. Yoder BA, Coalson JJ, Winter VT, Siler-Khodr T, Duffy LB, Cassell GH. Effects of antenatal colonization with *Ureaplasma urealyticum* on pulmonary disease in the immature baboon. Pediatr Res. 2003;54:797–807.
60. Viscardi RM, Atamas SP, Luzina IG, Hasday JD, He JR, Sime PJ, et al. Antenatal *Ureaplasma urealyticum* respiratory tract infection stimulates proinflammatory, profibrotic responses in the preterm baboon lung. Pediatr Res. 2006;60(2):141–6.
61. Novy MJ, Duffy L, Axthelm MK, Sadowsky DW, Witkin SS, Gravett MG, et al. *Ureaplasma parvum* or *Mycoplasma hominis* as sole pathogens cause chorioamnionitis, preterm delivery, and fetal pneumonia in rhesus macaques. Reprod Sci. 2009;16(1):56–70.
62. Mitchell BF, Taggart MJ. Are animal models relevant to key aspects of human parturition? Am J Physiol Regul Integr Comp Physiol. 2009;297(3):R525–45.
63. Dando SJ, Nitsos I, Polglase GR, Newnham JP, Jobe AH, Knox CL. *Ureaplasma parvum* undergoes selection in utero resulting in genetically diverse isolates colonizing the chorioamnion of fetal sheep. Biol Reprod. 2014;90(2):27.
64. Gravett MG, Novy MJ, Rosenfeld RG, Reddy AP, Jacob T, Turner M, et al. Diagnosis of intra-amniotic infection by proteomic profiling and identification of novel biomarkers. JAMA. 2004;292(4):462–9.
65. Gravett MG, Thomas A, Schneider KA, Reddy AP, Dasari S, Jacob T, et al. Proteomic analysis of cervical-vaginal fluid: identification of novel biomarkers for detection of intra-amniotic infection. J Proteome Res. 2007;6(1):89–96.
66. Husain AN, Siddiqui NH, Stocker JT. Pathology of arrested acinar development in postsurfactant bronchopulmonary dysplasia. Hum Pathol. 1998;29:710–7.
67. Viscardi RM, Manimtim WM, Sun CCJ, Duffy L, Cassell GH. Lung pathology in premature infants with *Ureaplasma urealyticum* infection. Pediatr Dev Pathol. 2002;5:141–50.

68. Viscardi R, Manimtim W, He JR, Hasday JD, Sun CC, Joyce B, et al. Disordered pulmonary myofibroblast distribution and elastin expression in preterm infants with *Ureaplasma urealyticum* pneumonitis. Pediatr Dev Pathol. 2006;9(2):143–51.
69. Miura Y, Payne MS, Keelan JA, Noe A, Carter S, Watts R, et al. Maternal intravenous treatment with either azithromycin or solithromycin clears *Ureaplasma parvum* from the amniotic fluid in an ovine model of intrauterine infection. Antimicrob Agents Chemother. 2014;58(9):5413–20.
70. Novy MJ, Sadowsky DW, Grigsby PL, Duffy LB, Waites KB. Maternal azithromcyin (AZI) therapy in ureaplasma intramniotic infection (IAI) prevents advanced fetal lung lesions in rhesus monkeys. Reprod Sci. 2008;15(Suppl):184A.
71. Grigsby PL, Novy MJ, Sadowsky DW, Morgan TK, Long M, Acosta E, et al. Maternal azithromycin therapy for Ureaplasma intraamniotic infection delays preterm delivery and reduces fetal lung injury in a primate model. Am J Obstet Gynecol. 2012;207(6):475.e1–e14.
72. Acosta EP, Grigsby PL, Larson KB, James AM, Long MC, Duffy LB, et al. Transplacental transfer of Azithromycin and its use for eradicating intra-amniotic ureaplasma infection in a primate model. J Infect Dis. 2014;209(6):898–904.
73. Walls SA, Kong L, Leeming HA, Placencia FX, Popek EJ, Weisman LE. Antibiotic prophylaxis improves Ureaplasma-associated lung disease in suckling mice. Pediatr Res. 2009;66(2):197–202.

Chapter 5
Chronic Obstructive Pulmonary Disease Following Bronchopulmonary Dysplasia

Alice Hadchouel and Christophe Delacourt

Chronic obstructive pulmonary disease (COPD) is characterized by a slowly progressive airflow limitation that is not fully reversible [1] and is considered as a major cause of death and disability worldwide [2]. More than 2.5 million people die of the disease each year, and most of them are in poor countries [2]. About 400,000 deaths occur each year from COPD in industrialized countries [2]. The overall COPD prevalence in adults appears to lie between 4 and 10 % in Europe [3], implying a major economic burden on society. COPD is, therefore, currently one of the leading causes of disease burden in the world, and its contribution is expected to rise in the near future [2], unless urgent action is taken to implement new prevention policies or to develop novel therapies.

No single mechanism can account for the complex pathology in COPD. There are clearly individual susceptibility factors and sex differences of major importance in the pathogenesis and progression of COPD [4, 5], making COPD as the result of interactions between host and environmental factors. Although the majority of COPD is attributable to smoking or to other environmental exposures, with a consistent exposure–response relationship (see review in [6]), a substantive burden of disease occurs in nonsmokers and nonoccupationally exposed individuals, notably young people and women [6]. Additionally, COPD develops in only a minority of smokers [7]. An increasing number of arguments suggest that the mechanisms

A. Hadchouel, MD, PhD (✉) • C. Delacourt, MD, PhD
Pediatric Pulmonology, Necker-Enfants Malades Hospital,
149 rue de Sèvres, Paris 75015, France

INSERM, U955, IMRB Equipe 04, Créteil 94000, France

Paris-Descartes University, Sorbonne Paris Cité, Paris 75006, France
e-mail: alice.hadchouel-duverge@aphp.fr; christophe.delacourt@nck.aphp.fr

V. Bhandari (ed.), *Bronchopulmonary Dysplasia*, Respiratory Medicine,
DOI 10.1007/978-3-319-28486-6_5

involved in early lung development may contribute as a susceptibility factor for adult COPD (see reviews in [5, 8]). In particular, there are increasing data demonstrating that the quality of lung development is critical to the level of pulmonary function in adults. Normal lung development is characterized by a growth of lung function during the prenatal period, childhood, and adolescence, to reach a peak in young adulthood, followed by a progressive decline in lung function, which is a normal feature of aging. Developmental processes that affect the growth phase, and as a consequence lead to a decreased peak lung function, could lead to COPD [6]. Indeed, it was demonstrated that lung function in young adults predicted airflow obstruction 20 years later [9]. In a longitudinal study, with repeated lung function measurements over a 20-year period in adults who were aged 18–30 years at study entry, the initial forced expiratory volume in 1 s/forced vital capacity (FEV1/FVC) was found highly predictive of airflow obstruction 20 years later [9]. Airflow obstruction in young and middle age adults was cross-sectionally associated with self-reported COPD [9]. Very recently, it was confirmed, from three independent cohorts, that low FEV1 in early adulthood is important in the occurrence of COPD. This study added that accelerated decline in FEV1 was not an obligate feature of COPD, strengthening the role of initial FEV1 [10]. Because premature birth interferes with normal lung development, it may represent a significant risk factor for COPD occurrence.

Altered Lung Development and Lung Functions in Adults

Although most studies demonstrating a relationship between disrupted fetal development and lower FEV1 in adults did not consider COPD as a specific study outcome, they strongly suggest that early developmental processes are key susceptibility factors for COPD. If we assume that the birth weight reflects the overall quality of prenatal development, Barker showed more than 20 years ago that birth weight was directly correlated to FEV1 in adults [11]. This important study suggested that intrauterine influences which interfere with fetal growth may irrecoverably constrain the growth of the airways. In keeping with these results, death rates from COPD in adult life, but not from another disease related to smoking, were associated with lower birth weight and weight at 1 year [11]. Moreover, it has been shown in a birth cohort of term children that diminished airway function present shortly after birth was a risk factor for airflow obstruction in early adult life [12]. Participants who had infant maximal flow at FRC [*V*max(FRC)] in the lowest quartile also had lower values for the FEV1/FVC ratio, forced expiratory flow 25–75 % (FEF25–75), and FEV1 up to age 22 years [12]. This study strongly suggests that fetal determinants of airway function may predispose to adult airflow obstruction and COPD. Noxious prenatal environmental exposures were also demonstrated to be able to induce irreversible airway obstruction. In particular, in utero cigarette smoke exposure was associated with a nonreversible airway obstruction at birth that persisted in adolescence [13] and early adulthood [14]. Experimentally, airway geometry was found to be strongly altered by prenatal nicotine exposure, with increased airway length and decreased diameter [15]. As a result, adult mice exposed to prenatal nicotine exhibit an increased response to methacholine challenge, even in the absence of allergic sensitization [15]. These results are consistent with the findings in human studies, where the increased prevalence of asthma and wheezing in adolescents with maternal smoking during pregnancy was found independent of atopy [13].

In connection with these previous studies, premature birth can be viewed as a disruption of the physiologic prenatal growth, and per se, as a risk factor for alterations in airway growth. A complete chapter (See Chap. 15) of this book is dedicated to long-term functional consequences of bronchopulmonary dysplasia (BPD). A particular issue is the persistent airway obstructive pattern in the post-surfactant generations of so-called "new" BPD [16]. A long-term impairment in FEV1 was extensively described in cohorts from the pre-surfactant era [17] and was interpreted as the result of direct airway injury during the neonatal period. Advances in neonatal care have led to some of historical BPD lesions becoming less frequent: the airway lesions are currently not observed, and septal fibrosis is now found in fewer cases [18]. These pathological findings have been confirmed by imaging investigations in children with less severe BPD: airway lesions are absent as assessed by chest computed tomography (CT) [19]. Despite these changes, premature birth is still associated with a definitive obstructive airflow pattern in children and adults, even in non-ventilated late preterm infants [20–22]. FEV1 values are about 20 % lower for BPD patients than controls [21], a decrease similar to that observed in cohorts from the pre-surfactant era [17]. This persistence of poor FEV1 values, despite rare airway lesions (as noted above in chest CT images), raises the issue of the consequences of prematurity and BPD for airway growth, in addition to those for alveolar growth [16]. Longitudinal measurements in preterm infants, with or without BPD, demonstrate persistently reduced flows and the absence of catch-up growth [23, 24]. This raises the possibility of an increased risk of COPD in this population.

Mechanisms for Reduced Lung Function in BPD

Impaired alveolarization is a characteristic pathophysiological feature of BPD [16]. During lung development, the first distal airspaces are represented by primitive saccules during the saccular stage, once the majority of lung branching has been completed and before extensive alveolarization. Airway morphogenesis and alveolarization are controlled by separate factors, whose expression is tightly regulated in time and spatially. The molecular pathways which are currently considered to significantly contribute to the occurrence of BPD in preterm infants are those whose disruption potentially results in alveolar growth disorders [16]. Since these factors have no known direct regulatory role in airway morphogenesis, it seems difficult to argue that abnormal expression of these factors in BPD would be both responsible for alveolar growth impairment and for long-term structural airway abnormalities.

A first hypothesis to explain airway obstruction in BPD would be that hypoalveolarization contributes to changes in respiratory mechanics, by reducing attachments between bronchioles and alveoli, resulting in an obstructive profile. Experimentally, impaired alveolar growth can be induced by exposing rodents during the alveolar phase to environmental injuries, such as hyperoxia, or to various drugs, such as glucocorticosteroids [25]. In these models, alveolar hypoplasia is attested by reduced lung volume, alveolar number, and surface area. Of interest, peripheral airway walls were also analyzed in the glucocorticosteroid model [26]. Dexamethasone had direct effect on small peripheral airway walls, which were thinner and had fewer alveolar attachment points with greater distance between attachments than controls. These data suggest that mechanisms leading to impaired alveolarization had an impact also on the mechanical properties of the lung parenchyma, by reducing the forces opposing airway narrowing. Such changes have been demonstrated to be related to abnormal airway function. In a model of in utero smoke exposure, the mean distance between alveolar attachment points was increased in animals exposed to cigarette smoke in utero, and as a consequence, airway responsiveness was increased [27]. Similar findings were observed in the hyperoxic model [28]. Exposure of neonatal mice to hyperoxia induces remodeling of the bronchiolar walls and loss of bronchiolar–alveolar attachments in adulthood. The fact that alveolar attachment points are rarefied in BPD infants has not been investigated.

A second hypothesis would be that molecular factors involved in branching morphogenesis have additional roles in later stages of development, or during repair processes after injury, thus contributing to disrupted airway growth (Fig. 5.1). This hypothesis has been poorly investigated in the context of BPD. For the most premature infants, birth occurs at the beginning of saccular phase of lung development, which appears as a critical period for various events to affect distal lung development as well as growth and differentiation of airways. In a mouse model of prenatal exposure to nicotine, the offspring's pulmonary function was affected only when nicotine was given from Gestation Day 14 to Postnatal Day 7, and not when given from Gestation Day 7 to 21, or from Postnatal Day 3 to 15 [15]. Thus, abnormal lung function was observed only when interference with normal lung development encompassed the entirety of the saccular phase of mouse lung development. It is, therefore, urgent to evaluate in BPD the role of candidate molecules that might be involved in the processes of growth and differentiation of the airways that take place after early branching. Impaired expression of these factors may contribute to the occurrence of definite functional obstruction and finally in the susceptibility to adult COPD. A possible contributor is the fibroblast growth factor (FGF) 10 pathway. FGF10 is a mesenchymal growth factor which may act on the epithelium through its receptor FGFR2b to control pulmonary morphogenesis [29]. Its expression has been found to be decreased in the lung of infants with BPD, as compared with age-matched controls [30]. It is known to play a key role in branching morphogenesis [31]. FGF10, as well as other FGFs that bind to the receptor FGFR2, may not be involved in the emergence of secondary septa. The FGFR2 pathway has been blocked during the alveolar stage, but no structural alterations were observed [32].

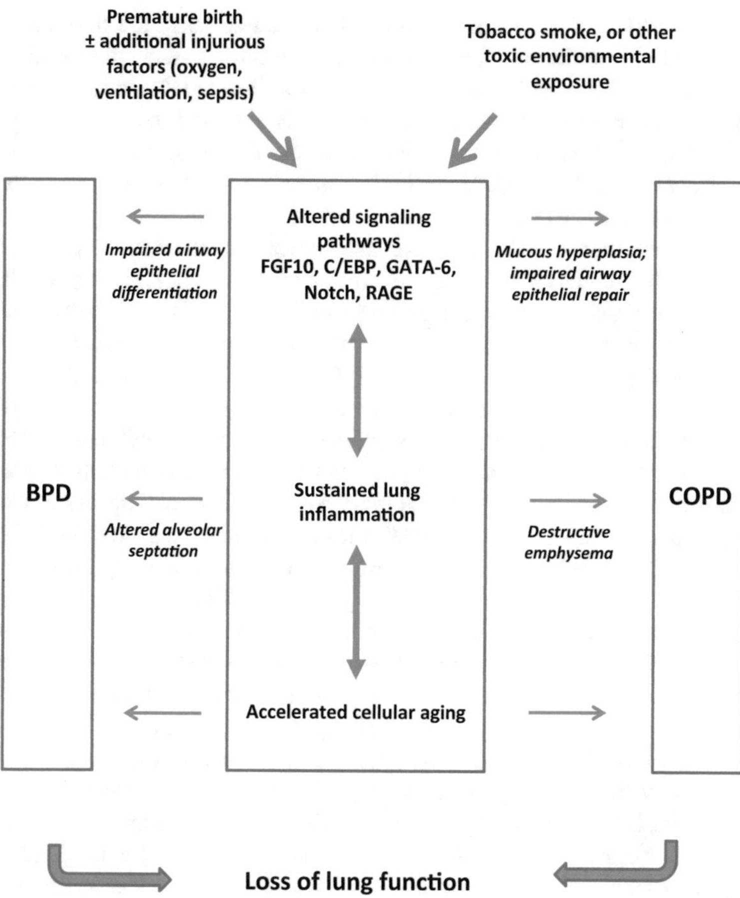

Fig. 5.1 Common pathogenic pathways to BPD and COPD. *BPD* bronchopulmonary dysplasia, *FGF* fibroblast growth factor, *C/EBP* CCAAT/enhancer-binding protein, *RAGE* receptor for advanced glycation end products, *COPD* chronic obstructive pulmonary disease

The role of FGF10 in the postnatal lung has been recently suggested. A strong postnatal lung expression was recently reported [33]. It was demonstrated that FGF10-positive lung cells represent a progenitor cell population [33], which may contribute to injury and repair processes. In a FGF10 hypomorphic mouse model, it has been demonstrated that FGF10 plays a pivotal role in maintaining epithelial progenitor cell proliferation, as well as coordinating alveolar smooth muscle cell formation and vascular development [34]. It was also demonstrated recently in adult mice that FGF10 expression was induced in parabronchial smooth muscle cells after airway epithelial injury, and this in turn initiated epithelial repair [35]. FGF10 may therefore be an important factor for airway homeostasis, both in baseline conditions and during injury. Of interest, constitutive FGF10 insufficiency could also be observed in humans and was demonstrated to be associated with reduced pulmonary function providing a model for a dosage sensitive effect of FGF10 in the development of adult COPD [36]. Furthermore, independent genome-wide association studies have recently identified the hedgehog interacting protein (HHIP), which is a critical regulator of the FGF10 pathway, as a susceptibility gene for COPD and airflow obstruction [37–41]. HHIP is also involved in the fetal lung response to adverse antenatal events, as for example, in utero smoke exposure, which are associated with subsequent airway obstruction [42].

Factors other than FGF10 influence lung development through the control of airway epithelial maturation, and as such may be involved in pathological changes associated with COPD [43]. Their effective roles in both BPD and COPD need to be confirmed. Most relevant candidates are the transcriptional regulators CCAAT/enhancer-binding protein (C/EBP)α and C/EBPβ, the GATA-binding protein (GATA)-6, the Notch signaling pathway, and the receptor for advanced glycation end products (RAGE). Mice with a lung epithelial-specific disruption of the C/EBPα gene exhibit impaired lung development and epithelial differentiation [44, 45]. More specifically for their potential implication in COPD pathogenesis, C/EBPα and C/EBPβ were shown to play pivotal roles in determining airway epithelial differentiation. Compared to wild-type littermates, mice with lung epithelial-specific deletion of both C/EBPα and C/EBPβ displayed undifferentiated Clara cells and ectopic mucus-producing cells in the conducting airways [46]. Additionally, C/EBPα was shown to regulate the expression of serine protease inhibitors that are required for the normal increase of fibronectin and the restoration of ciliated cells after ablation of bronchiolar epithelial cells by naphthalene in mice [47]. The role for C/EBPs in COPD pathogenesis is suggested by the demonstration of a decreased C/EBP activity in airway epithelial cells of COPD patients compared to healthy smokers, with C/EBPβ being the dominant C/EBP in the airway epithelium in all groups [48]. Furthermore, C/EBPα-deficient mice that survive until adulthood develop a majority of the histopathological and inflammatory characteristics of COPD [45]. These lesions develop spontaneously, without tobacco smoke exposure, reinforcing the hypothesis that developmental factors can lead to the onset of COPD, even regardless of environmental exposure. GATA-6 is known to be expressed in the epithelial cells of the developing airway epithelium and is especially involved in the maturation of terminal airways and alveoli [49]. GATA-6-induced air space enlargement persisted into adulthood [50], suggesting a potential role in emphysema. Notch signaling was demonstrated crucial to control the balance of differentiated cell profiles both in developing airways [51] and in postnatal airways [52]. During development, disruption of Notch signaling dramatically expands the population of distal progenitors, altering morphogenetic boundaries and preventing formation of proximal structures [53]. During postnatal life, Notch is required to prevent Clara cells from differentiating into goblet cells [52]. Altered Notch signaling may therefore contribute to the metaplastic changes in the respiratory epithelium that occur in pathological conditions, such as COPD. Indeed, several Notch ligands, receptors, and downstream effector genes were found downregulated in the small airway epithelium of smokers, with more genes downregulated in smokers with COPD than in healthy smokers [54]. Furthermore, Notch is known to interact with Sox family transcription factors [51]. Pharmacological inhibition of Notch in the early lung interferes with the establishment of proximal cell fate, resulting in a substantial reduction in the *Sox2* expression domain in the forming airways [51]. Besides its role during development, Sox2 also has a role in the adult airway epithelium. Sox2 was demonstrated to control the capacity of adult epithelial tracheal cells to proliferate in culture and to repair after injury in vivo, functions that might be crucial in COPD occurrence [55]. The cell surface protein RAGE serves as a receptor for nonenzymatically glycated adducts, including proinflammatory cytokine-like mediators of the S100/calgranulin family [56]. In particular, S100A12 protein was recently shown to induce MUC5AC mRNA and the protein in human bronchial epithelial cells via RAGE signaling [57]. RAGE may be involved in both control of lung development and adult lung diseases, but available data linking the two processes are controversial. Experimentally, overexpression of RAGE resulted in BPD-like histological changes in the neonatal lung, and in emphysema with persistent inflammatory status in the adult lung [58]. In human pathology, however, emphysema severity in COPD is associated with lower circulating sRAGE levels [59, 60]. Interaction between environmental factors and lung RAGE expression may contribute to these discrepancies. Recently, it was shown that RAGE-deficient mice exposed to chronic cigarette smoke demonstrated an impaired early recruitment of neutrophils and were significantly protected from smoke-induced emphysema [61].

Finally, recent data suggest that accelerated cellular aging would also contribute to the long-term respiratory consequences of premature birth. Lung function decline over age is known to partially reflect biological aging due to intrinsic processes [62]. Telomere length, which is considered to be a robust biomarker of cellular senescence, is positively associated with the pre-bronchodilator values of FEV1, independent of any pathological respiratory status [62]. The association between preterm birth, cellular senescence, and risk of diseases later in life was recently demonstrated for cardiovascular-related diseases. Preterm birth was found to promote endothelial colony-forming cell dysfunction by triggering a stress-induced premature senescence [63]. We recently reported an association between telomere length and distal airway obstruction in a population of adolescents born extremely preterm, independent of perinatal events [64]. This provides evidence that prematurity per se may be an independent risk factor for a persistent biological stress throughout life that may lead to both continuing airway disease and inflammation and also to an accelerated shortening of telomeres. A previous study reported higher levels of 8-isoprostane in exhaled breath condensates of ex-premature adolescents, regardless of BPD status, compared to healthy controls born at term [65]. More recently, using a metabolomic approach, altered biochemical–metabolic patterns were still identifiable in the lung of adolescents with BPD as compared with control subjects [66]. These studies strengthen the hypothesis of the existence of an ongoing disease in the airways of prematurely born children, because of persistently deregulated metabolic processes, and especially of a persistent oxidative stress [65]. Long-term airway obstruction in prematurely born children may not be just the functional expression of structural airway abnormalities that occurred during the first months of life, but may at least be partly related to persistent deregulated metabolic processes in the lung. Of interest, several studies found that telomere length was also associated with COPD [67, 68], suggesting an accelerated aging process in the development of the disease and establishing new links between post-BPD airway obstruction and susceptibility to COPD (Fig. 5.1).

Such a process could also contribute to the worsening of COPD lesions, and especially to the development of emphysema lesions. Although BPD leads to impaired alveolar development and COPD's emphysema to alveolar destruction, there are striking similarities in the pathophysiology of these two processes, which have been reviewed in detail [69]. In particular, both diseases include oxidative stress phenomena, sustained inflammation, and alteration of the extracellular matrix. The confirmation that these common pathological processes may not need to be reactivated in adulthood, but persist abnormally since the neonatal period, would represent a major risk factor for a rapid development of COPD lesions in adults born prematurely.

Synergistic Effect of Reduced Lung Function and Environmental Exposure

A large fraction of COPD is attributable to environmental exposures, and especially to active smoking. In response to noxious particles or gases, an accelerated decline in lung function was observed, associated with an abnormal inflammatory response of the lungs [5]. The rate with which the respiratory function declines and reaches the threshold for a COPD diagnosis depends on several factors, including the maximum lung function attained after childhood lung growth [5]. Disorders that compromise lung growth, including premature birth and BPD, would therefore increase the risk of early COPD occurrence following environmental exposures. As an aggravating factor, it is possible that the rate of decline in lung function is all the higher as that airway caliber is smaller to begin with (Fig. 5.2). There are several studies providing arguments for a synergistic deleterious effect between active smoking in adolescence and impaired growth of the airways. In particular, it was suggested that prenatal exposure to cigarette smoke and active smoking act synergistically to affect early lung function deficits in young adulthood. Upton and coworkers showed that maternal and paternal smoking were associated with significantly lower levels of the FEV1/FVC ratio among active smokers but not among nonsmokers [70]. Using the data from the Tucson cohort, Guerra et al. found that at the age of 26, participants with exposure to parental and active smoking had significantly lower FEV1/FVC levels than those who were not exposed to parental or active smoking [71]. Interestingly, young adults who were only exposed to active smoking or only exposed to parental smoking did not differ from those who were not exposed to either. Further, participants with exposure to parental and active smoking had the steepest decline in FEV1/ FVC between year 11 and year 26. The combination of early impaired airway development and active smoking also probably has a deleterious effect on the occurrence of respiratory symptoms. It was shown that active smoking during

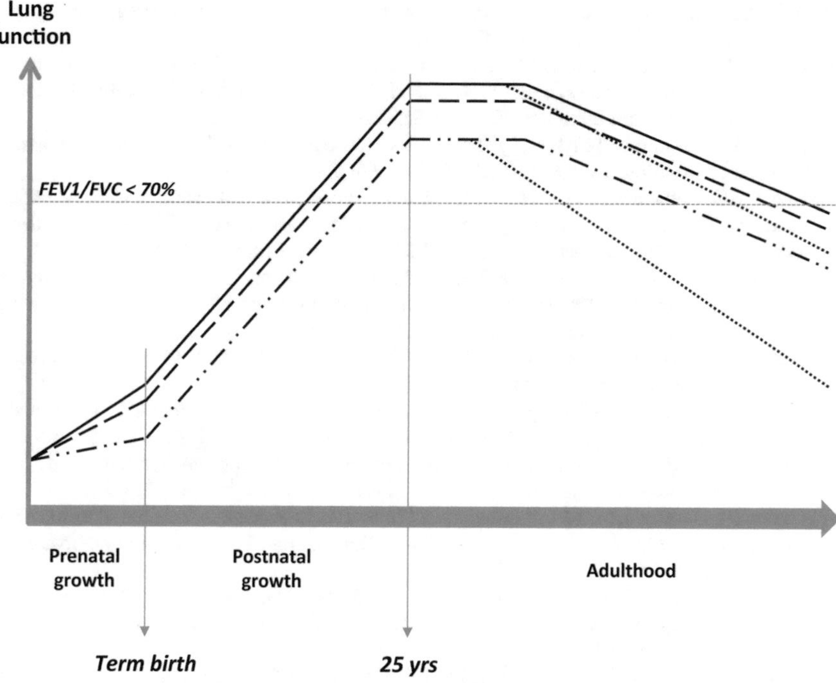

Fig. 5.2 Schematic representation of lung function growth and decline through life. The threshold for COPD diagnosis is mentioned. *Plain line*: healthy individuals; *dashed line*: individuals born prematurely, without BPD; *dashed* and *dotted line*: individuals born prematurely, with BPD; *dotted lines* during adulthood: changes in lung function decline related to early active smoking, in healthy individuals and in BPD individuals. *FEV1/FVC* forced expiratory volume in 1 s/forced vital capacity

adolescence was associated with wheeze at age 18 years, only among those with reduced lung function in infancy [72]. Finally, in a longitudinal study, including 2496 adults who were 18–30 years of age at entry, the effect of cigarette smoking on lung function decline with age was most evident in young adults with pre-existing airflow obstruction [9].

Taken together, these data support a high risk of progression to early COPD for young adults who are born prematurely and who have the most important functional alterations, that is, those with BPD. In these subjects, active smoking should be strongly discouraged, as this most likely results in a faster deleterious effect than in subjects who are born at term and have normal lung function.

References

1. Celli BR, MacNee W. Standards for the diagnosis and treatment of patients with COPD: a summary of the ATS/ERS position paper. Eur Respir J. 2004;23(6):932–46.
2. Lopez AD, Shibuya K, Rao C, Mathers CD, Hansell AL, Held LS, et al. Chronic obstructive pulmonary disease: current burden and future projections. Eur Respir J. 2006;27(2):397–412.

3. Halbert RJ, Isonaka S, George D, Iqbal A. Interpreting COPD prevalence estimates: what is the true burden of disease? Chest. 2003;123(5):1684–92.
4. Kohler M, Sandberg A, Kjellqvist S, Thomas A, Karimi R, Nyren S, et al. Gender differences in the bronchoalveolar lavage cell proteome of patients with chronic obstructive pulmonary disease. J Allergy Clin Immunol. 2013;131(3):743–51.
5. Rennard SI, Drummond MB. Early chronic obstructive pulmonary disease: definition, assessment, and prevention. Lancet. 2015;385(9979):1778–88.
6. Eisner MD, Anthonisen N, Coultas D, Kuenzli N, Perez-Padilla R, Postma D, et al. An official American Thoracic Society public policy statement: novel risk factors and the global burden of chronic obstructive pulmonary disease. Am J Respir Crit Care Med. 2010;182(5):693–718.
7. Lamprecht B, McBurnie MA, Vollmer WM, Gudmundsson G, Welte T, Nizankowska-Mogilnicka E, et al. COPD in never smokers: results from the population-based burden of obstructive lung disease study. Chest. 2011;139(4):752–63.
8. Postma DS, Bush A, van den Berge M. Risk factors and early origins of chronic obstructive pulmonary disease. Lancet. 2015;385(9971):899–909.
9. Kalhan R, Arynchyn A, Colangelo LA, Dransfield MT, Gerald LB, Smith LJ. Lung function in young adults predicts airflow obstruction 20 years later. Am J Med. 2010;123(5):468.e1–7.
10. Lange P, Celli B, Agustí A, Jensen G, Divo M, Faner R, et al. Lung-function trajectories leading to chronic obstructive pulmonary disease. N Engl J Med. 2015;373(2):111–22.
11. Barker DJ, Godfrey KM, Fall C, Osmond C, Winter PD, Shaheen SO. Relation of birth weight and childhood respiratory infection to adult lung function and death from chronic obstructive airways disease. BMJ. 1991;303(6804):671–5.
12. Stern DA, Morgan WJ, Wright AL, Guerra S, Martinez FD. Poor airway function in early infancy and lung function by age 22 years: a non-selective longitudinal cohort study. Lancet. 2007;370(9589):758–64.
13. Hollams EM, de Klerk NH, Holt PG, Sly PD. Persistent effects of maternal smoking during pregnancy on lung function and asthma in adolescents. Am J Respir Crit Care Med. 2014;189(4):401–7.
14. Hayatbakhsh MR, Sadasivam S, Mamun AA, Najman JM, Williams GM, O'Callaghan MJ. Maternal smoking during and after pregnancy and lung function in early adulthood: a prospective study. Thorax. 2009;64(9):810–4.
15. Wongtrakool C, Wang N, Hyde DM, Roman J, Spindel ER. Prenatal nicotine exposure alters lung function and airway geometry through alpha7 nicotinic receptors. Am J Respir Cell Mol Biol. 2012;46(5):695–702.
16. Hadchouel A, Franco-Montoya ML, Delacourt C. Altered lung development in bronchopulmonary dysplasia. Birth Defects Res A Clin Mol Teratol. 2014;100(3):158–67.
17. Baraldi E, Filippone M. Chronic lung disease after premature birth. N Engl J Med. 2007;357(19):1946–55.
18. Husain AN, Siddiqui NH, Stocker JT. Pathology of arrested acinar development in postsurfactant bronchopulmonary dysplasia. Hum Pathol. 1998;29:710–7.
19. Mahut B, De Blic J, Emond S, Benoist MR, Jarreau PH, Lacaze-Masmonteil T, et al. Chest computed tomography findings in bronchopulmonary dysplasia and correlation with lung function. Arch Dis Child Fetal Neonatal Ed. 2007;92(6):F459–64.
20. Fawke J, Lum S, Kirkby J, Hennessy E, Marlow N, Rowell V, et al. Lung function and respiratory symptoms at 11 years in children born extremely preterm: the EPICure study. Am J Respir Crit Care Med. 2010;182(2):237–45.
21. Kotecha SJ, Edwards MO, Watkins WJ, Henderson AJ, Paranjothy S, Dunstan FD, et al. Effect of preterm birth on later FEV1: a systematic review and meta-analysis. Thorax. 2013;68(8):760–6.
22. Kotecha SJ, Watkins WJ, Paranjothy S, Dunstan FD, Henderson AJ, Kotecha S. Effect of late preterm birth on longitudinal lung spirometry in school age children and adolescents. Thorax. 2012;67(1):54–61.
23. Fakhoury KF, Sellers C, Smith EO, Rama JA, Fan LL. Serial measurements of lung function in a cohort of young children with bronchopulmonary dysplasia. Pediatrics. 2010;125(6):e1441–7.

24. Friedrich L, Pitrez PM, Stein RT, Goldani M, Tepper R, Jones MH. Growth rate of lung function in healthy preterm infants. Am J Respir Crit Care Med. 2007;176(12):1269–73.
25. Hilgendorff A, Reiss I, Ehrhardt H, Eickelberg O, Alvira CM. Chronic lung disease in the preterm infant: lessons learned from animal models. Am J Respir Cell Mol Biol. 2014;50(2):233–45.
26. Kovar J, Willet KE, Hislop A, Sly PD. Impact of postnatal glucocorticoids on early lung development. J Appl Physiol (1985). 2005;98(3):881–8.
27. Elliot J, Carroll N, Bosco M, McCrohan M, Robinson P. Increased airway responsiveness and decreased alveolar attachment points following in utero smoke exposure in the guinea pig. Am J Respir Crit Care Med. 2001;163(1):140–4.
28. O'Reilly M, Harding R, Sozo F. Altered small airways in aged mice following neonatal exposure to hyperoxic gas. Neonatology. 2014;105(1):39–45.
29. Morrisey E, Hogan B. Preparing for the first breath: genetic and cellular mechanisms in lung development. Dev Cell. 2010;18:8–23.
30. Benjamin JT, Smith RJ, Halloran BA, Day TJ, Kelly DR, Prince LS. FGF-10 is decreased in bronchopulmonary dysplasia and suppressed by Toll-like receptor activation. Am J Physiol Lung Cell Mol Physiol. 2007;292(2):L550–8.
31. El Agha E, Bellusci S. Walking along the fibroblast growth factor 10 route: a key pathway to understand the control and regulation of epithelial and mesenchymal cell-lineage formation during lung development and repair after injury. Scientifica (Cairo). 2014;2014:538379.
32. Hokuto I, Perl AK, Whitsett JA. Prenatal, but not postnatal, inhibition of fibroblast growth factor receptor signaling causes emphysema. J Biol Chem. 2003;278(1):415–21.
33. El Agha E, Herold S, Al Alam D, Quantius J, MacKenzie B, Carraro G, et al. Fgf10-positive cells represent a progenitor cell population during lung development and postnatally. Development. 2014;141(2):296–306.
34. Ramasamy SK, Mailleux AA, Gupte VV, Mata F, Sala FG, Veltmaat JM, et al. Fgf10 dosage is critical for the amplification of epithelial cell progenitors and for the formation of multiple mesenchymal lineages during lung development. Dev Biol. 2007;307(2):237–47.
35. Volckaert T, Campbell A, De Langhe S. c-Myc regulates proliferation and Fgf10 expression in airway smooth muscle after airway epithelial injury in mouse. PLoS One. 2013;8(8):e71426.
36. Klar J, Blomstrand P, Brunmark C, Badhai J, Hakansson HF, Brange CS, et al. Fibroblast growth factor 10 haploinsufficiency causes chronic obstructive pulmonary disease. J Med Genet. 2011;48(10):705–9.
37. Hancock DB, Eijgelsheim M, Wilk JB, Gharib SA, Loehr LR, Marciante KD, et al. Meta-analyses of genome-wide association studies identify multiple loci associated with pulmonary function. Nat Genet. 2010;42(1):45–52.
38. Pillai SG, Ge D, Zhu G, Kong X, Shianna KV, Need AC, et al. A genome-wide association study in chronic obstructive pulmonary disease (COPD): identification of two major susceptibility loci. PLoS Genet. 2009;5(3):e1000421.
39. Repapi E, Sayers I, Wain LV, Burton PR, Johnson T, Obeidat M, et al. Genome-wide association study identifies five loci associated with lung function. Nat Genet. 2010;42(1):36–44.
40. Van Durme YM, Eijgelsheim M, Joos GF, Hofman A, Uitterlinden AG, Brusselle GG, et al. Hedgehog-interacting protein is a COPD susceptibility gene: the Rotterdam study. Eur Respir J. 2010;36(1):89–95.
41. Wilk JB, Chen TH, Gottlieb DJ, Walter RE, Nagle MW, Brandler BJ, et al. A genome-wide association study of pulmonary function measures in the Framingham heart study. PLoS Genet. 2009;5(3):e1000429.
42. Kerkhof M, Boezen HM, Granell R, Wijga AH, Brunekreef B, Smit HA, et al. Transient early wheeze and lung function in early childhood associated with chronic obstructive pulmonary disease genes. J Allergy Clin Immunol. 2014;133(1):68–76.e1–4.
43. Roos AB, Berg T, Nord M. A relationship between epithelial maturation, bronchopulmonary dysplasia, and chronic obstructive pulmonary disease. Pulm Med. 2012;2012:196194.
44. Basseres DS, Levantini E, Ji H, Monti S, Elf S, Dayaram T, et al. Respiratory failure due to differentiation arrest and expansion of alveolar cells following lung-specific loss of the transcription factor C/EBPalpha in mice. Mol Cell Biol. 2006;26(3):1109–23.

45. Didon L, Roos AB, Elmberger GP, Gonzalez FJ, Nord M. Lung-specific inactivation of CCAAT/enhancer binding protein alpha causes a pathological pattern characteristic of COPD. Eur Respir J. 2010;35(1):186–97.
46. Roos AB, Berg T, Barton JL, Didon L, Nord M. Airway epithelial cell differentiation during lung organogenesis requires C/EBPalpha and C/EBPbeta. Dev Dyn. 2012;241(5):911–23.
47. Sato A, Xu Y, Whitsett JA, Ikegami M. CCAAT/enhancer binding protein-alpha regulates the protease/antiprotease balance required for bronchiolar epithelium regeneration. Am J Respir Cell Mol Biol. 2012;47(4):454–63.
48. Didon L, Qvarfordt I, Andersson O, Nord M, Riise GC. Decreased CCAAT/enhancer binding protein transcription factor activity in chronic bronchitis and COPD. Chest. 2005;127(4):1341–6.
49. Liu C, Morrisey EE, Whitsett JA. GATA-6 is required for maturation of the lung in late gestation. Am J Physiol Lung Cell Mol Physiol. 2002;283(2):L468–75.
50. Liu C, Ikegami M, Stahlman MT, Dey CR, Whitsett JA. Inhibition of alveolarization and altered pulmonary mechanics in mice expressing GATA-6. Am J Physiol Lung Cell Mol Physiol. 2003;285(6):L1246–54.
51. Tsao PN, Vasconcelos M, Izvolsky KI, Qian J, Lu J, Cardoso WV. Notch signaling controls the balance of ciliated and secretory cell fates in developing airways. Development. 2009;136(13):2297–307.
52. Tsao PN, Wei SC, Wu MF, Huang MT, Lin HY, Lee MC, et al. Notch signaling prevents mucous metaplasia in mouse conducting airways during postnatal development. Development. 2011;138(16):3533–43.
53. Tsao PN, Chen F, Izvolsky KI, Walker J, Kukuruzinska MA, Lu J, et al. Gamma-secretase activation of notch signaling regulates the balance of proximal and distal fates in progenitor cells of the developing lung. J Biol Chem. 2008;283(43):29532–44.
54. Tilley AE, Harvey BG, Heguy A, Hackett NR, Wang R, O'Connor TP, et al. Down-regulation of the notch pathway in human airway epithelium in association with smoking and chronic obstructive pulmonary disease. Am J Respir Crit Care Med. 2009;179(6):457–66.
55. Que J, Luo X, Schwartz RJ, Hogan BL. Multiple roles for Sox2 in the developing and adult mouse trachea. Development. 2009;136(11):1899–907.
56. Schmidt AM, Yan SD, Yan SF, Stern DM. The multiligand receptor RAGE as a progression factor amplifying immune and inflammatory responses. J Clin Invest. 2001;108(7):949–55.
57. Kang JH, Hwang SM, Chung IY. S100A8, S100A9 and S100A12 activate airway epithelial cells to produce MUC5AC via extracellular signal-regulated kinase and nuclear factor-kappaB pathways. Immunology. 2015;144(1):79–90.
58. Fineschi S, De Cunto G, Facchinetti F, Civelli M, Imbimbo BP, Carnini C, et al. Receptor for advanced glycation end products contributes to postnatal pulmonary development and adult lung maintenance program in mice. Am J Respir Cell Mol Biol. 2013;48(2):164–71.
59. Carolan BJ, Hughes G, Morrow J, Hersh CP, O'Neal WK, Rennard S, et al. The association of plasma biomarkers with computed tomography-assessed emphysema phenotypes. Respir Res. 2014;15:127.
60. Cheng DT, Kim DK, Cockayne DA, Belousov A, Bitter H, Cho MH, et al. Systemic soluble receptor for advanced glycation endproducts is a biomarker of emphysema and associated with AGER genetic variants in patients with chronic obstructive pulmonary disease. Am J Respir Crit Care Med. 2013;188(8):948–57.
61. Sambamurthy N, Leme AS, Oury TD, Shapiro SD. The receptor for advanced glycation end products (RAGE) contributes to the progression of emphysema in mice. PLoS One. 2015;10(3):e0118979.
62. Albrecht E, Sillanpaa E, Karrasch S, Alves AC, Codd V, Hovatta I, et al. Telomere length in circulating leukocytes is associated with lung function and disease. Eur Respir J. 2014;43(4):983–92.
63. Vassallo PF, Simoncini S, Ligi I, Chateau AL, Bachelier R, Robert S, et al. Accelerated senescence of cord blood endothelial progenitor cells in premature neonates is driven by SIRT1 decreased expression. Blood. 2014;123(13):2116–26.

64. Hadchouel A, Marchand-Martin L, Franco-Montoya M, Peaudecerf L, Ancel P, Delacourt C, et al. Salivary telomere length and lung function in adolescents born very preterm. PLoS One. 2015;in press.
65. Filippone M, Bonetto G, Corradi M, Frigo AC, Baraldi E. Evidence of unexpected oxidative stress in airways of adolescents born very pre-term. Eur Respir J. 2012;40(5):1253–9.
66. Carraro S, Giordano G, Pirillo P, Maretti M, Reniero F, Cogo PE, et al. Airway metabolic anomalies in adolescents with bronchopulmonary dysplasia: new insights from the metabolomic approach. J Pediatr. 2015;166(2):234–9.e1.
67. Rode L, Bojesen SE, Weischer M, Vestbo J, Nordestgaard BG. Short telomere length, lung function and chronic obstructive pulmonary disease in 46,396 individuals. Thorax. 2013;68(5):429–35.
68. Savale L, Chaouat A, Bastuji-Garin S, Marcos E, Boyer L, Maitre B, et al. Shortened telomeres in circulating leukocytes of patients with chronic obstructive pulmonary disease. Am J Respir Crit Care Med. 2009;179(7):566–71.
69. Bourbon JR, Boucherat O, Boczkowski J, Crestani B, Delacourt C. Bronchopulmonary dysplasia and emphysema: in search of common therapeutic targets. Trends Mol Med. 2009;15(4):169–79.
70. Upton MN, Smith GD, McConnachie A, Hart CL, Watt GC. Maternal and personal cigarette smoking synergize to increase airflow limitation in adults. Am J Respir Crit Care Med. 2004;169(4):479–87.
71. Guerra S, Stern DA, Zhou M, Sherrill DL, Wright AL, Morgan WJ, et al. Combined effects of parental and active smoking on early lung function deficits: a prospective study from birth to age 26 years. Thorax. 2013;68(11):1021–8.
72. Mullane D, Turner SW, Cox DW, Goldblatt J, Landau LI, le Souef PN. Reduced infant lung function, active smoking, and wheeze in 18-year-old individuals. JAMA Pediatr. 2013;167(4):368–73.

Part II
BPD: Translational Aspects

Chapter 6
Genetics of Bronchopulmonary Dysplasia

Pascal M. Lavoie

Introduction

Bronchopulmonary dysplasia (BPD) is a common and serious complication of prematurity, occurring mainly in infants born below 32 weeks of gestation [1]. Clinically, BPD manifests as a prolonged need for respiratory support and supplemental oxygen during the neonatal period. In the long term, BPD is associated with increased risk of neurodevelopment impairment in very low-birth weight infants and is a precursor to life-long restrictions in pulmonary function [2]. Based on data from epidemiological studies and animal models, inflammation and oxidative stress from repeated exposure to supplemental oxygen, inadequate nutritional support, pulmonary congestion due to blood shunts, baro and volutrauma due to mechanical ventilation, and infections cause the prolonged respiratory dysfunction characteristic of BPD. Microbial colonization, in the face of mucosal barrier disrupting interventions and an immature immune system also contribute to the pathophysiology of BPD [3].

The clinical presentation of the disease has changed considerably over the years. Fifty years ago, BPD was described in more mature, mid-term gestation infants [4]. With advances in neonatal care, together with improved survival of more immature preterm infants, this original form of BPD has virtually disappeared to make place for a new form of BPD [5]. This new BPD now almost exclusively affects very low gestation preterm infants and is characterized by delayed pulmonary development leading to impaired vascular gas exchange and obstructive lung disease throughout

P.M. Lavoie, MDCM, PhD, FRCPC (✉)
Child and Family Research Institute, Vancouver, BC, Canada

Division of Neonatology, Department of Pediatrics, University of British Columbia, Vancouver, BC, Canada

Department of Pediatrics, Division of Neonatology, Children's and Women's Health Centre of British Columbia, room 1R47 – 4480 Oak Street, Vancouver, BC, Canada V6H3V4
e-mail: plavoie@cw.bc.ca

V. Bhandari (ed.), *Bronchopulmonary Dysplasia*, Respiratory Medicine,
DOI 10.1007/978-3-319-28486-6_6

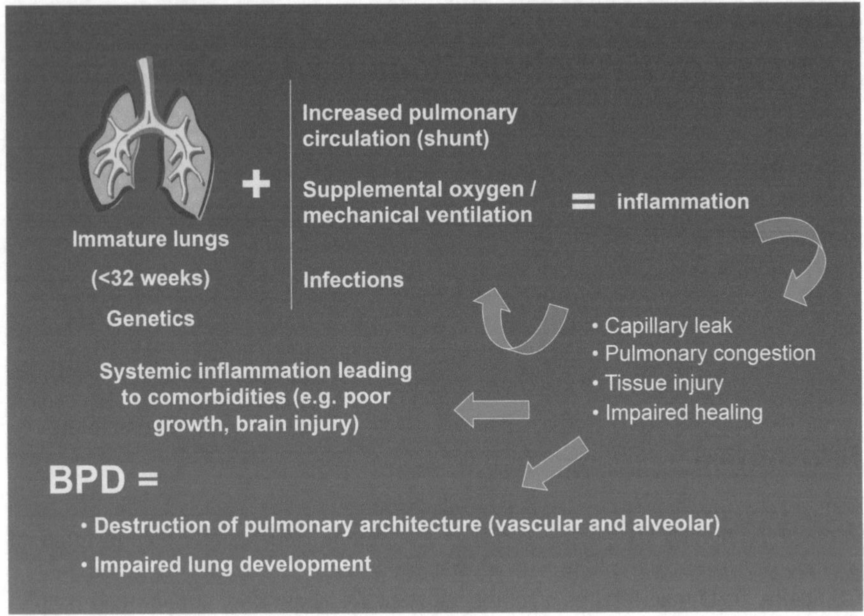

Fig. 6.1 Pathogenesis of bronchopulmonary dysplasia

childhood [5]. This "new" BPD often occurs in infants relatively unexposed to mechanical ventilation and supplemental oxygen, raising the possibility that genetic factors play a major predisposing role. Evidence indicates an important role for delayed mechanisms of pulmonary development, which may explain why some infants develop the disease whereas others do not [6]. See Fig. 6.1. In this chapter, we present the latest evidence supporting a role for genetic factors in determining susceptibility to BPD in at-risk infants.

Bronchopulmonary Dysplasia, a Genetic Disease

The concept that susceptibility to BPD is influenced by genetic factors was proposed nearly 40 years ago. In 1980, Nickerson reported an increased incidence of asthma in siblings affected with BPD compared to relatives of control infants with hyaline membrane disease without BPD. However, this observation was based on a small number of children (i.e., less than 40 index cases) that were also born in the "old" BPD era, and the authors of this study did not take into account major confounders making it impossible to confirm whether familial factors play a role [7]. The role of genetics in BPD was, however, more formally proposed by Parker who found a high concordance in 108 twin pairs of birth weight below 1500 g [8]. Because of a lack of data on the zygosity of these infants, it was not possible to discern a specific role for genetic factors from similar environmental factors. Almost 10 years later, two studies analyzed cohorts of multiple births and estimated heritability using traditional twin study designs incorporating data on the zygosity of these infants. These two studies showed that up to 50–80 % of the susceptibility to BPD may be inherited [9, 10]. These seminal articles fueled a growing interest in neonatology research to identify genetic risk factors to illuminate potential biological pathways linked to BPD susceptibility, but also with a promise that this will help stratify which infants are at highest risk so that specific therapies can be tailored early on [11].

Genetic Approaches to Study BPD

The human genome is an extremely vast source of information that governs the function of hundreds of thousands of protein composing cells in our body. It consists of three billion nucleotide bases duplicated on 22 chromosome pairs plus sex chromosomes X and Y (in boys). Genomic DNA is organized in regulatory and protein-encoding regions, with less than 1–2 % of base pairs encoding for proteins. Humans vary genetically among each other in about 0.1–1 % of their nucleotide base pairs. Single nucleotide polymorphisms (SNPs, pronounced "snips") are the most common and most studied type of genetic polymorphism. They can either represent additions, deletions, or permutations of a single nucleotide. They occur at a frequency of about 1 in 100–1 in 300 base pairs in the human genome. At the time of writing this chapter, over 50 million SNPs have been cataloged in the human genome National Centre for Biotechnology Information (NCBI) SNP database (dbSNP). SNPs are, by definition, found in 1 % or more of the general population and represent a common source of genetic variation, in contrast to rare mutations which are also much less common. SNPs are expected to modulate disease risk to a modest extent in relation to environmental factors. For this reason, identification of a functional impact of SNPs requires large cohorts of infants, and this is a major challenge in neonatology.

Copy-number variations (CNVs) represent another less common source of genomic diversity [12]. CNVs compose less than 10 % of the variability in the human genome and can either be deletions or duplications of either very short (i.e., <1000 base pairs) or larger (e.g., several millions base pairs) nucleotide sequences. The impact of CNVs on the biological diversity of human protein functions has been less studied. So far, the vast majority of genetic association studies in BPD have concentrated on SNPs, except for one study that examined CNVs [13].

Genetic variants are not necessarily transmitted together during cell meiosis due to chromosomal recombination events occurring between genes. However, genetic variants (or alleles) are not randomly passed on from parents to the offspring, a phenomenon referred to as linkage disequilibrium. Rather, alleles may co-segregate during meiosis by virtue of a reduced rate of recombination between two nearby genes on a chromosome.

The structural relationships between alleles and how they co-segregate within ethnic populations are defined in haplotypes, which are sections of the genome that are transmitted together during cell meiosis. The HapMap project is a large-scale project that defined haplotype linkage disequilibrium relationships between genetic variants across several human populations [14]. The knowledge of haplotype structures has considerably facilitated the conduct of genetic association studies by allowing to consider groups of genetic variants co-transmitted in the same haplotype represented by unique "tag-SNPs." In complex diseases like BPD, it is likely that many of the reported association are not causally due to the SNP directly examined, but rather to a SNP that is linked or co-transmitted within the same haplotype. Imputation techniques can be used in data analysis to address this question [15]. This analysis technique has not been sufficiently employed in studies of BPD.

The structural linkage relationships between nearby genetic variants within haplotypes are better understood in humans in contrast to our understanding of the functional interactions between multiple genetic variants which are still poorly understood. Different alleles of a gene can functionally interact in their combined effect on a disease phenotype. These effects are also referred to as epistasis effects [16]. A classic example is the allele determining the color of the hair that can be expressed differently in the presence of another allele resulting in baldness. As a gross simplification, most genetic association studies in BPD have assumed that each gene variant has isolated cumulative (additive) effect on the risk of BPD. However, this is unlikely to be the case and the identification of functional interactions between genetic variants pose considerable challenges in studying complex traits in a population of relatively limited sample sizes such as in preterm infant populations. To circumvent these challenges, studies have combined genetic association studies with genomic approaches looking at downstream expression of these genes as a way to provide information about the net functional impact of genetic variants [17, 18] (see below).

Linkage analyses constitute powerful ways of detecting genetic influences on disease traits. However, for complex diseases like BPD that virtually only affects infants born very preterm, linkage analyses are not practical and genetic association studies have therefore been employed. Two general approaches can be applied in this context: candidate gene and whole-genome approaches. The advantage of the whole-genome approach is that it "casts the net more widely", making no a priori assumptions on the nature of gene variants, whereas the candidate gene approach has the advantage of being more focused and generally less expensive, also necessitating smaller sample size. The latter approach has been used in most studies of BPD [19]. In clinical practice, important variations in the incidence of BPD as well as clinical practices related to major known risk factors for this disease have been reported, and therefore, replication studies are particularly important to confirm that results could be generalized to other populations.

Genetic Variants in BPD

Since the publication of twin studies supporting a strong heritability of BPD [9, 10], over 65 genetic association studies have been published with BPD-related outcomes. Table 6.1 lists genes that have been implicated in candidate gene association studies. The vast majority have been selected within genes implicated in inflammation and antioxidant responses. Most studies were generally of small sample size and did not include a replication cohort, therefore limiting the power of associations. These studies have recently been reviewed [20–23] and will not be detailed again here in this chapter. Nonetheless, a few studies published more recently or more remarkable in the approach used by their authors are discussed below.

Table 6.1 Genetic variants associated with BPD in previous studies

Gene	Protein	Reference(s)
ACE	Angiotensin-converting enzyme isoform 1	[102, 103]
BICC1	BicC family RNA binding protein 1	[34]
COL23A1	Collagen, type XXIII, alpha 1	[34]
DAG1	Dystroglycan 1 (dystrophin-associated glycoprotein 1)	[104]
F7	Coagulation factor VII	[105]
FGFR4	Fibroblast growth factor receptor 4	[106]
GC	Vitamin D-binding protein (Gc globulin)	[42]
GSTM1	Glutathione S-transferase mu 1	[38]
GSTT1	Glutathione S-transferase theta 1	[38]
GSTP1	Glutathione S-transferase Pi 1	[107]
HLA-A	Human leukocyte adhesion molecule class I (type A)	[108]
HLA-B	Human leukocyte adhesion molecule class I (type B)	[108]
HLA-C	Human leukocyte adhesion molecule class I (type C)	[108]
IFNG	Interferon gamma	[109]
IL1RN	Interleukin-1 receptor antagonist	[45]
IL6	Interleukin-6	[44]
IL6ST	Interleukin-6 signal transducer	[31]
IL10	Interleukin-10	[31, 110]
IL12B	Interleukin-12 (p40 subunit)	[109]
IL18R1	Interleukin-18 receptor	[33]
IL18RAP	Interleukin-18 receptor accessory molecule	[33]
KITLG	Kit ligand (Stem cell factor)	[30]
MBL	Mannose-binding lectin	[46]
MBL2	Mannose-binding lectin 2	[45, 105, 111]
MIF	Macrophage migration inhibitory factor	[112]
MMP16	Matrix metallopeptidase 16	[113]
NFE2L2	Nuclear factor, erythroid 2-like 2	[35]
NFKBIA	Nuclear factor of kappa light polypeptide gene enhancer in B-cells inhibitor, alpha	[55]
NFE2L2	Nuclear factor erythroid-2 related factor-2	[35]
NQO1	NAD(P)H dehydrogenase, quinone 1 (also known as quinone oxidoreductase 1)	[35]

(continued)

Table 6.1 (continued)

Gene	Protein	Reference(s)
SELL	L-selectin	[114]
SOD2	Mitochondrial superoxide dismutase	[37, 115]
SOD3	Extracellular superoxide dismutase	[37]
SFTPA	Surfactant protein A	[116]
SFTPB	Surfactant protein B	[80–82, 117]
SFTPD	Surfactant protein D	[103]
SPOCK2	Sparc/Osteonectin, cwcv and kazal-like domains proteoglycan (testican) 2	[24]
TIRAP	Toll-interleukin-1 receptor (TIR) domain containing adaptor protein	[118]
TLR2	Toll-like receptor 2	[47]
TLR4	Toll-like receptor 4	[32]
TLR5	Toll-like receptor 5	[118]
TLR6	Toll-like receptor 6	[47]
TLR10	Toll-like receptor 10	[119]
TNFA	Tumor necrosis factor-alpha	[119–124]
VDR	Vitamin D receptor	[41]
VEGF	Vascular endothelial growth factor	[43, 119, 125]
VEGFR2	Vascular endothelial growth factor receptor 2	[29]

The first study to provide a replication cohort was a French study, which included 418 preterm infants and detected a genetic association with a variant in *SPOCK2*, a gene potentially affecting lung alveolarization [24]. This study is also remarkable as it examined polymorphisms at the genome-wide significance level. However, whereas findings from the French cohort were replicated in a Finnish cohort of infants, they were not reproduced in a Canadian cohort raising a question of whether they can be applied to North American infants of mixed ethnicity (Hadchouel A and Delacourt C, personal communication). Indeed, the incidence of BPD in many parts of Europe is considerably less than North America, and it is possible that environmental factors may differentially modulate the impact of variants in the *SPOCK2* gene [25–28]. This study also illustrated well the challenges in replicating associations across cohorts where the incidence of BPD and clinical practice varies considerably. This was also evidenced in a number of Canadian-Finnish studies from the BPD and Genetics Study Group, where independent replication has proven extremely difficult within an achievable sample size [29–32].

Floros and colleagues found significant associations between BPD, defined as oxygen-dependency at 28 days, and genetic variants in the interleukin-18 receptor 1 (IL18R1) and accessory protein (IL18RAP) genes, among African-American infants. Similar findings were detected in a separate mixed ethnic cohort [33]. The IL-18 receptor and its accessory molecule mediate signals from its corresponding cytokine IL-18. IL-18 is an inflammatory cytokine that triggers potent cell-mediated immunity in tissues. Associations between polymorphisms in the genes encoding for IL-18 receptor components are consistent with an important role for inflammation in BPD. In another relatively large study, authors examined genetic associations in two regional retrospective BPD cohorts of infants ($n = 1726/795$ infants in the discovery/replication cohorts, respectively) including those who required ventilation for at least 3 days. This study identified potential variants, but none remained associated after adjusting for multiple comparisons [34]. While this study used a nontraditional definition of BPD which may have biased the results, it further highlights the difficulty in replicating genetic effects of the low-to-moderate magnitude generally detectable in complex diseases such as BPD. The same authors also examined associations with copy-number variants in this multiethnic cohort predominantly of Mexican-Hispanic origin [13].

In light of a role for oxidative stress, a few studies have tested associations between polymorphisms in antioxidant defense-related genes and the occurrence or severity of BPD [35–39]. Functional loss of antioxidant responses (ARE) has been shown to modulate the severity of lung injury in humans and animal exposed to oxidants [35]. The rare allele for a functional variant in the gene encoding the ARE-related protein NF-E2-related factor 2 (*NFE2L2*) protected against severe BPD in a Caucasian population of very low birth weight (VLBW) infants. Interestingly, promoter variants have been linked to acute lung injury in humans, and expression of the *NFE2L2* gene prevents lung injury and bacterial infection in a hyperoxia mouse model [40]. More studies are required to replicate these findings in neonatal populations.

Vitamin D plays pleiotropic roles in alveolar type cell growth, angiogenesis, and innate immune functions. Genetic variants in the vitamin D-binding protein and vitamin D receptor gene were recently shown to influence the risk of BPD in Turkish preterm infants [41, 42]. Authors from the GEN-BPD Study Group recently systematically reviewed published data on the potential role of common genetic variants in the VEGF pathway in modulating the risk of BPD. Although they found significant associations between BPD and an intronic SNP in the VEGF receptor 2, this association was not replicated in a mixed Canadian/Finnish Caucasian cohort of infants [29]. In another study, a noncoding 5′ untranslated variant in the vascular endothelial growth factor (VEGF) also showed a marginally significant association with BPD in a Japanese cohort of preterm infants [43].

Associations between innate immune and inflammatory genes, and BPD have been frequently examined [44]. The mannose-binding lectin proteins 1 and 2 are plasma proteins involved in antibacterial and antifungal immunity. Common genetic variants in these genes were associated with pulmonary outcomes as well as serum levels of MBL in preterm infants [45, 46]. A recent study showed an association between a noncoding variant in the 3′ untranslated region of the gene encoding the Toll-like receptor protein (*TLR6*) and a decreased risk of BPD and decreased colonization with the BPD-associated microbial pathogen *Ureaplasma*, although this association did not meet a Bonferonni-adjusted significance threshold below 0.05 [47].

Genetic Pathway Analyses

To address a main limitation of sample size in populations of preterm infants, authors have recently employed genome-wide gene expression profiling to examine functional genomic interactions during BPD. This has been facilitated by considerable improvement and reduction in the cost of these technologies over the last few years. The expression of genes can either be measured by quantifying the amount of known transcripts using hybridization techniques, such as arrays, or more directly using next-generation sequencing that also allows the identification of new transcript isoforms. Using these approaches, authors have identified major differences in the gene expression of inflammatory [48] and chromatin remodeling genes in infants with BPD [49], although these studies have been carried out on blood which may not reflect changes occurring in tissues, such as lungs. One study compared gene expression profiles on postmortem lung tissues and identified a novel potential role for mast cells in BPD [50].

In a recent study, Carrera et al. reported preliminary data from a study combining exome sequencing in a candidate approach based on previously associated BPD susceptibility loci [51, 52]. While these data also require confirmation in larger cohorts including controls, they reported several variants in genes involved in immune recognition and responses in infants with severe disease validating the role of inflammation in BPD. Li et al. also performed whole-exome sequencing in a small group of 50 infants affected with BPD, comparing to their unaffected twin [53]. They provide evidence of a dose-dependent effect of haploinsufficiency across 258 candidate gene loci in highly conserved molecular pathways across species. Unexpectedly, another remarkable finding of this study is that pathways covered by these gene variants involved mechanisms of embryonic development and lung remodeling. These include connective tissue structure proteins and the evolutionarily conserved Wnt signaling pathway that have been shown to play an important role in vascular development [54]. Although the implication of these pathways will require a more thorough confirmation in an experimental model as well as in infants with BPD, this study illustrates the power of genetic association studies in illuminating unsuspected pathways in the pathogenesis of BPD. Moreover, based on an increased likelihood of BPD in infants heterozygous at these loci, they postulated that genetic variants in these pathways influence the risk of BPD according to a dominant inheritance [53].

Ali et al. provided strong evidence of a functional effect of common variants in the *NFKBIA* gene encoding a principal inhibitor of the master inflammatory transcription factor NF-κB, using an allele-specific gene expression reporter strategy. Functional haplotype variants were reproducibly implicated as main transcriptional response hubs in three pediatric lung disease cohorts of infants with respiratory syncytial virus infection, asthma, and BPD [55]. In another study, authors further illustrate the power of systems-based genomic approaches combining data from over eight million SNPs, including 1.2 million genotyped SNPs and an additional seven million imputed SNPs (i.e., associated through the knowledge of their haplotype segregation within the human genome), to whole-genome gene expression profiling [56]. Using a molecular pathway analysis, they identified functionally interacting groups of molecules associated with BPD using a false-discovery rate method of adjusting for multiple statistical comparisons (FDR<0.1). Variants nearby the *ADARB2*, *CD44* genes, and the miR-29 pathway were implicated in their genome-wide association analysis. Expression of two of candidate genes, miR-219 and CD44, was shown to be increased in human lungs of infants with BPD. MiR-219 belongs to a group of small inhibitor microribonucleic acids (miRNAs). miRNAs are small molecules that regulate the translation of specific proteins by activating or silencing messenger RNAs through binding of nucleotide-specific sequences. Another group has reported changes in expression of miRNA in the blood of infants at risk of BPD [57]. The role of miRNA in regulating cell function and organ development has gained considerable interest over the last few years and offers new perspectives in our understanding of the molecular mechanisms of BPD [58].

Summary of Genetic Association Studies

Over the last few decades, considerable technological progress has been made, which greatly improves the feasibility of genetic studies by reducing costs. However, the integration of the extraordinary amount of data generated from these studies, in ways that inform clinical outcomes, remains a major unachieved challenge. Clearly, there is a need to re-examine genetic associations in other populations of infants with BPD, using robust outcome measures incorporating systems-based genomic approaches [22]. In the future, strict efforts should be invested to ensure that findings from genetic association and genomic studies are replicated and published even in situations where the outcome of a well-designed study is a negative study, in order to avoid a publication bias. In order to address the impact of clinical heterogeneity modulating genetic influences on BPD, efforts should also concentrate on replication analyses in large independent cohorts enrolled within the same center as well as between centers, combining gene–environment analyses.

Rare Mutations in Neonatal-Onset Respiratory Disease

The above-mentioned studies have largely focused on common variants having relatively modest effects on the risk of BPD. In addition, rare genetic mutations may have more profound effects on the course of neonatal lung diseases. Most studies which examined disease-causing mutations in neonatal lung disease have focused on term infants. However, it is likely that the same mutations may affect the course of BPD in preterm infants. Indeed an atypical, more severe, or early-onset clinical presentation for BPD in a preterm infant should prompt the search for some of these gene defects after more common causes have been excluded (e.g., large atrial or ventricular septal defect) [59, 60]. Defects in the surfactant proteins B and C, as well as the ATP-binding cassette subfamily A member 3 (ABCA3) protein, have been reported in infants with severe neonatal lung disease. In some cases, a lung biopsy with an electron microscopy examination may also aid the specific molecular diagnosis [61–65].

ABCA3 Gene Mutations in the *ABCA3* gene are the most common cause of genetic cases of neonatal-onset respiratory disease [66–70]. The *ABCA3* gene is located on the 16p13 chromosome locus and encodes a membrane lipid transporter that plays an important role in the formation of lamellar bodies and in the synthesis of surfactant by mediating the transport of phospholipids in type II alveolar cells [71, 72]. A systematic review of phenotype–genotype relationships in 185 infants with *ABCA3* gene mutations showed that a majority of infants with severe neonatal lung disease and poor outcome had homozygous frameshift or nonsense mutations (i.e., resulting in truncated proteins) [73, 74]. In the case of compound heterozygous or missense mutations, infants can present with varying disease severity and age of onset [73]. In another study involving a cohort of 228 late preterm Caucasian infants with severe respiratory distress syndrome *ABCA3* gene mutations were identified in up to 5 % of them [75]. In a Finnish cohort of 267 preterm infants born between 25 and 35 weeks of gestation, common haplotypes were associated with varying severity of lung disease [76]. In some cases, mutations in the *ABCA3* gene have also been associated with delayed cerebral and cerebellar neuronal migration, an entity referred to as cerebropulmonary dysgenetic syndrome [77]. In a large cohort of 3177 VLBW infants, no discernable clinical features could be identified in babies carrying a missense E292V mutation suspected to cause later-onset pediatric interstitial lung disease [78]. More studies are needed to understand how common mutations in the *ABCA3* gene affect the course of BPD and to assess their functional impact specifically in preterm age groups.

SFTPB Gene The *SFTPB* gene is about 10 kb and located on the 2p12 chromosome locus. Mutations in surfactant protein B (*SFTPB* gene) is the second most common genetic defect linked to surfactant deficiency. Deleterious mutations in the *SFTPB* gene are most often inherited as an autosomal recessive manner [79]. Neonatal respiratory insufficiency due to surfactant deficiency usually presents in more severe, early-onset intractable respiratory failure [66]. Other than a lung transplant, limited treatment options exist for infants with complete loss-of-function in this gene [60]. The hypothesis that common genetic variants in the general population that may also affect the synthesis surfactant protein B alter the course of neonatal lung diseases was assessed in a few studies. In these studies, common intronic deletion [80–82], missense mutations in exon 4 [83], and other mutations affecting protein glycosylation [84–87] in the *SFTPB* gene have been linked to the neonatal lung outcomes.

SFTPC Gene Mutations in the surfactant protein C (*SFTPC* gene) follow more of an autosomal dominant inheritance pattern and are therefore often sporadic [88]. The *SFTPC* gene spans a short 3.5 kb area located at the 8p21 chromosome locus.

It encodes a small hydrophobic component of surfactant. Mutations in the *SFTPC* gene result in interstitial lung disease of variable severity and age of onset from the neonatal to adult age period [89]. These mutations are relatively uncommon even in neonatal-onset lung diseases. The vast majority of cases have been reported in term-born infants with clinical features ranging from severe neonatal respiratory distress syndrome to later onset acute exacerbations from respiratory viral infections [89]. Recently, an infant born at 23 weeks of gestation with a mutation at position 176 in the surfactant C protein causing a change in aminoacid from an arginine to a glutamine (termed R167Q mutation) required prolonged mechanical ventilation, suggesting that this variant may have contributed to this infant's clinical course [90]. The potential availability of treatments for defects in surfactant protein C synthesis makes screening for this condition particularly more interesting in the clinical setting. Indeed, two groups have claimed successful treatment of infants using hydroxychloroquine, a drug that may prevent misfolding of the surfactant C protein. However, the exact mechanism of action of the drug in this situation remains unclear [91, 92]. In addition to these rare disease-causing mutations, common genetic variants in the *SFTPC* gene may also influence the course of neonatal lung disease in preterm infants to a more modest extent [88].

Other Genes Missense mutations in the *FLNA* gene, encoding the filamin A, alpha protein, associated with diffuse lung disease have been linked with features of cerebral periventricular nodular heterotopia [93]. The thyroid transcription factor-1 (TTF1) induces surfactant expression [94]. Mutations in the regulator TTF1 have been linked to neonatal-onset respiratory insufficiency in association with other neurological deficits and/or hypopituitarism [94–97]. Other gene defects in the *SCL34A2* gene encoding a pH-sensitive sodium-dependent phosphate transporter [98] and in the telomerase reverse transcriptase gene *TERT* have been linked to worse neonatal respiratory outcomes [99], although more in-depth phenotypic evaluation in cases involving these mutations is lacking.

Concluding Remarks

Despite improvements in survival and outcomes in very preterm infants, BPD continues to represent a major health burden. Few interventions are available to clinicians to prevent this disease. Early postnatal corticosteroids may reduce the risk of BPD, but the high occurrence of unacceptable side-effects due to these medications seriously restricts their use in medical practice [100]. Given the ethical challenges in conducting mechanistic studies in populations of preterm infants, the identification of genetic risk factors is important not only to improve our understanding of the pathology of BPD, but also to help orient treatments in high-risk groups. The conduct of genetic association studies in human preterm populations is complicated by practical challenges, issues of clinical heterogeneity, as well as differences in clinical practices and incidence of BPD between neonatal centers. The combinations of genomic approaches involving molecular pathway analyses, with well-powered genetic association studies, may provide better means to obtain information about the molecular factors underlying susceptibility to BPD in some infants. Clearly, other major questions concerning the genetics of BPD need to be addressed in the future. First, we currently have little knowledge of how clinical practices modulate genetic influences on BPD across populations. It is likely that differences in clinical practice or even ethnicity across populations may affect reproducibility of data between studies. Second, the biological impact of genetic variants needs to be experimentally confirmed in human cells, mimicking conditions that are relevant to the pathogenesis of BPD in human preterm infants. The development of lung humanoid models on-a-chip, coupled with targeted mutagenesis technologies, opens tremendous possibilities to tackle these questions [101]. Third, we do not understand well the role of common mutations, for example, in surfactant protein genes and in the etiology of severe neonatal lung diseases in very preterm infants, and clarifying this question through more detailed phenotype–genotype studies will improve diagnostic possibilities.

Acknowledgement I am thankful to Mikko Hallmann and Vineet Bhandari for critical comments on this manuscript.

References

1. Kinsella JP, Greenough A, Abman SH. Bronchopulmonary dysplasia. Lancet. 2006;367(9520):1421–31. PubMed.
2. El Mazloum D, Moschino L, Bozzetto S, Baraldi E. Chronic lung disease of prematurity: long-term respiratory outcome. Neonatology. 2014;105(4):352–6. PubMed Epub 2014/06/17. eng.
3. Bhandari V. Postnatal inflammation in the pathogenesis of bronchopulmonary dysplasia. Birth Defects Res A Clin Mol Teratol. 2014;100(3):189–201. PubMed Epub 2014/03/01. eng.
4. Northway Jr WH, Rosan RC, Porter DY. Pulmonary disease following respirator therapy of hyaline-membrane disease. Bronchopulmonary dysplasia. N Engl J Med. 1967;276(7): 357–68. PubMed.
5. Jobe AH. The new bronchopulmonary dysplasia. Curr Opin Pediatr. 2010;23(2):167–72. PubMed Epub 2010/12/21. eng.
6. Hadchouel A, Franco-Montoya ML, Delacourt C. Altered lung development in bronchopulmonary dysplasia. Birth Defects Res A Clin Mol Teratol. 2014;100(3):158–67. PubMed Epub 2014/03/19. eng.
7. Nickerson BG, Taussig LM. Family history of asthma in infants with bronchopulmonary dysplasia. Pediatrics. 1980;65(6):1140–4. PubMed.
8. Parker RA, Lindstrom DP, Cotton RB. Evidence from twin study implies possible genetic susceptibility to bronchopulmonary dysplasia. Semin Perinatol. 1996;20(3):206–9. PubMed.
9. Bhandari V, Bizzarro MJ, Shetty A, Zhong X, Page GP, Zhang H, et al. Familial and genetic susceptibility to major neonatal morbidities in preterm twins. Pediatrics. 2006;117(6):1901–6. PubMed.
10. Lavoie PM, Pham C, Jang KL. Heritability of bronchopulmonary dysplasia, defined according to the consensus statement of the national institutes of health. Pediatrics. 2008;122(3):479–85. PubMed.

11. Walsh MC, Szefler S, Davis J, Allen M, Van Marter L, Abman S, et al. Summary proceedings from the bronchopulmonary dysplasia group. Pediatrics. 2006;117(3 Pt 2):S52–6. PubMed.
12. Wain LV, Armour JA, Tobin MD. Genomic copy number variation, human health, and disease. Lancet. 2009;374(9686):340–50. PubMed.
13. Hoffmann TJ, Shaw GM, Stevenson DK, Wang H, Quaintance CC, Oehlert J, et al. Copy number variation in bronchopulmonary dysplasia. Am J Med Genet A. 2014;164A(10):2672–5. PubMed Central PMCID: 4167221.
14. International HapMap C, Altshuler DM, Gibbs RA, Peltonen L, Altshuler DM, Gibbs RA, et al. Integrating common and rare genetic variation in diverse human populations. Nature. 2010;467(7311):52–8. PubMed Central PMCID: 3173859.
15. Li Y, Willer C, Sanna S, Abecasis G. Genotype imputation. Annu Rev Genomics Hum Genet. 2009;10:387–406. PubMed Epub 2009/09/01. eng.
16. Wei WH, Hemani G, Haley CS. Detecting epistasis in human complex traits. Nat Rev Genet. 2014;15(11):722–33. PubMed Epub 2014/09/10. eng.
17. Stranger BE, Raj T. Genetics of human gene expression. Curr Opin Genet Dev. 2013;23(6):627–34. PubMed.
18. Atias N, Istrail S, Sharan R. Pathway-based analysis of genomic variation data. Curr Opin Genet Dev. 2013;23(6):622–6. PubMed.
19. Patnala R, Clements J, Batra J. Candidate gene association studies: a comprehensive guide to useful in silico tools. BMC Genet. 2013;14:39. PubMed Central PMCID: 3655892.
20. Shaw GM, O'Brodovich HM. Progress in understanding the genetics of bronchopulmonary dysplasia. Semin Perinatol. 2013;37(2):85–93. PubMed Central PMCID: 3628629.
21. Hallman M, Marttila R, Pertile R, Ojaniemi M, Haataja R. Genes and environment in common neonatal lung disease. Neonatology. 2007;91(4):298–302. PubMed.
22. Lavoie PM, Dubé MP. Genetics of bronchopulmonary dysplasia in the age of genomics. Curr Opin Pediatr. 2010;22(2):134–8. PubMed.
23. Prosnitz A, Gruen JR, Bhandari V. The genetics of disorders affecting the premature newborn. In: Rimoin DL, Connor JM, Pyeritz RE, Korf BR, editors. Emery and Rimoin's principles and pactice of medical genetics. 6th ed. Philadelphia: Elsevier; 2013. p. 1–22.
24. Hadchouel A, Durrmeyer X, Bouzigon E, Incitti R, Huusko J, Jarreau PH, et al. Identification of SPOCK2 as a susceptibility gene for bronchopulmonary dysplasia. Am J Respir Crit Care Med. 2011;184(10):1164–70. PubMed.
25. Ruegger C, Hegglin M, Adams M, Bucher HU, Swiss Neonatal Network. Population based trends in mortality, morbidity and treatment for very preterm- and very low birth weight infants over 12 years. BMC Pediatr. 2012;12:17. PubMed Central PMCID: 3311070.
26. Costeloe KL, Hennessy EM, Haider S, Stacey F, Marlow N, Draper ES. Short term outcomes after extreme preterm birth in England: comparison of two birth cohorts in 1995 and 2006 (the EPICure studies). BMJ. 2012;345:e7976. PubMed Central PMCID: 3514472.
27. Gortner L, Misselwitz B, Milligan D, Zeitlin J, Kollee L, Boerch K, et al. Rates of bronchopulmonary dysplasia in very preterm neonates in Europe: results from the MOSAIC cohort. Neonatology. 2011;99(2):112–7. PubMed.
28. Lundqvist P, Kallen K, Hallstrom I, Westas LH. Trends in outcomes for very preterm infants in the southern region of Sweden over a 10-year period. Acta Paediatr. 2009;98(4):648–53. PubMed.
29. Mahlman M, Huusko JM, Karjalainen MK, Kaukola T, Marttila R, Ojaniemi M, et al. Genes encoding vascular endothelial growth factor A (VEGFA) and VEGF receptor 2 (VEGFR2) and risk for bronchopulmonary dysplasia. Neonatology. 2015;108(1):53–9.
30. Huusko JM, Mahlman M, Karjalainen MK, Kaukola T, Haataja R, Marttila R, et al. Polymorphisms of the gene encoding kit ligand are associated with bronchopulmonary dysplasia. Pediatr Pulmonol. 2015;50:260–70. (Epub ahead of print). PubMed Epub 2014/03/13. eng.
31. Huusko JM, Karjalainen MK, Mahlman M, Haataja R, Kari MA, Andersson S, et al. A study of genes encoding cytokines (IL6, IL10, TNF), cytokine receptors (IL6R, IL6ST), and glucocorticoid receptor (NR3C1) and susceptibility to bronchopulmonary dysplasia. BMC Med Genet. 2014;15:120. PubMed Epub 2014/11/21. eng.

32. Lavoie PM, Ladd M, Hirschfeld AF, Huusko J, Mahlman M, Speert DP, et al. Influence of common non-synonymous Toll-like receptor 4 polymorphisms on bronchopulmonary dysplasia and prematurity in human infants. PLoS One. 2012;7(2):e31351. PubMed Central PMCID: 3279371.
33. Floros J, Londono D, Gordon D, Silveyra P, Diangelo SL, Viscardi RM, et al. IL-18R1 and IL-18RAP SNPs may be associated with bronchopulmonary dysplasia in African-American infants. Pediatr Res. 2012;71(1):107–14. PubMed Epub 2012/02/01. eng.
34. Wang H, St Julien KR, Stevenson DK, Hoffmann TJ, Witte JS, Lazzeroni LC, et al. A genome-wide association study (GWAS) for bronchopulmonary dysplasia. Pediatrics. 2013;132(2):290–7. PubMed Pubmed Central PMCID: 3727675.
35. Sampath V, Garland JS, Helbling D, Dimmock D, Mulrooney NP, Simpson PM, et al. Antioxidant response genes sequence variants and BPD susceptibility in VLBW infants. Pediatr Res. 2015;77(3):477–83. PubMed Epub 2014/12/18. eng.
36. Askenazi DJ, Halloran B, Patil N, Keeling S, Saeidi B, Koralkar R, et al. Genetic polymorphisms of heme-oxygenase 1 (HO-1) may impact on acute kidney injury, bronchopulmonary dysplasia, and mortality in premature infants. Pediatr Res. 2015;77(6):793–8. PubMed Central PMCID: 4439308.
37. Poggi C, Giusti B, Vestri A, Pasquini E, Abbate R, Dani C. Genetic polymorphisms of antioxidant enzymes in preterm infants. J Matern Fetal Neonatal Med. 2012;25 Suppl 4:131–4. PubMed Epub 2012/09/14. eng.
38. Wang X, Li W, Liu W, Cai B, Cheng T, Gao C, et al. GSTM1 and GSTT1 gene polymorphisms as major risk factors for bronchopulmonary dysplasia in a Chinese Han population. Gene. 2013;533(1):48–51. PubMed Epub 2013/10/15. eng.
39. Karagianni P, Rallis D, Fidani L, Porpodi M, Kalinderi K, Tsakalidis C, et al. Glutathion-S-Transferase P1 polymorphisms association with broncopulmonary dysplasia in preterm infants. Hippokratia. 2013;17(4):363–7. PubMed Central PMCID: 4097420.
40. Cho HY, Kleeberger SR. Noblesse oblige: NRF2 functions in the airways. Am J Respir Cell Mol Biol. 2014;50(5):844–7. PubMed Central PMCID: 4068955.
41. Koroglu OA, Onay H, Cakmak B, Bilgin B, Yalaz M, Tunc S, et al. Association of vitamin D receptor gene polymorphisms and bronchopulmonary dysplasia. Pediatr Res. 2014;76(2):171–6. PubMed Epub 2014/05/07. eng.
42. Serce Pehlevan O, Karatekin G, Koksal V, Benzer D, Gursoy T, Yavuz T, et al. Association of vitamin D binding protein polymorphisms with bronchopulmonary dysplasia: a case-control study of gc globulin and bronchopulmonary dysplasia. J Perinatol. 2015;35(9):763–7. PubMed Epub 2015/06/13. eng.
43. Fujioka K, Shibata A, Yokota T, Koda T, Nagasaka M, Yagi M, et al. Association of a vascular endothelial growth factor polymorphism with the development of bronchopulmonary dysplasia in Japanese premature newborns. Sci Rep. 2014;4:4459. PubMed Epub 2014/03/26. eng.
44. Usuda T, Kobayashi T, Sakakibara S, Kobayashi A, Kaneko T, Wada M, et al. Interleukin-6 polymorphism and bronchopulmonary dysplasia risk in very low-birthweight infants. Pediatr Int. 2012;54(4):471–5. PubMed Epub 2012/03/28. eng.
45. Cakmak BC, Calkavur S, Ozkinay F, Koroglu OA, Onay H, Itirli G, et al. Association between bronchopulmonary dysplasia and MBL2 and IL1-RN polymorphisms. Pediatr Int. 2012;54(6):863–8. PubMed Epub 2012/08/14. eng.
46. Ozkan H, Koksal N, Cetinkaya M, Kilic S, Celebi S, Oral B, et al. Serum mannose-binding lectin (MBL) gene polymorphism and low MBL levels are associated with neonatal sepsis and pneumonia. J Perinatol. 2012;32(3):210–7. PubMed Epub 2011/06/18. eng.
47. Winters AH, Levan TD, Vogel SN, Chesko KL, Pollin TI, Viscardi RM. Single nucleotide polymorphism in toll-like receptor 6 is associated with a decreased risk for ureaplasma respiratory tract colonization and bronchopulmonary dysplasia in preterm infants. Pediatr Infect Dis J. 2013;32(8):898–904. PubMed Epub 2013/03/23. eng.
48. Pietrzyk JJ, Kwinta P, Wollen EJ, Bik-Multanowski M, Madetko-Talowska A, Gunther CC, et al. Gene expression profiling in preterm infants: new aspects of bronchopulmonary dysplasia development. PLoS One. 2013;8(10):e78585. PubMed Epub 2013/11/07. eng.

49. Cohen J, Van Marter LJ, Sun Y, Allred E, Leviton A, Kohane IS. Perturbation of gene expression of the chromatin remodeling pathway in premature newborns at risk for bronchopulmonary dysplasia. Genome Biol. 2007;8(10):R210. PubMed Epub 2007/10/06. eng.
50. Bhattacharya S, Go D, Krenitsky DL, Huyck HL, Solleti SK, Lunger VA, et al. Genome-wide transcriptional profiling reveals connective tissue mast cell accumulation in bronchopulmonary dysplasia. Am J Respir Crit Care Med. 2012;186(4):349–58. PubMed Epub 2012/06/23. eng.
51. Carrera P, Di Resta C, Volonteri C, Castiglioni E, Bonfiglio S, Lazarevic D, et al. Exome sequencing and pathway analysis for identification of genetic variability relevant for bronchopulmonary dysplasia (BPD) in preterm newborns: a pilot study. Clin Chim Acta. 2015;451:39–45. PubMed Epub 2015/01/13. eng.
52. Somaschini M, Castiglioni E, Volonteri C, Cursi M, Ferrari M, Carrera P. Genetic predisposing factors to bronchopulmonary dysplasia: preliminary data from a multicentre study. J Matern Fetal Neonatal Med. 2012;25 Suppl 4:127–30. PubMed Epub 2012/09/14. eng.
53. Li J, Yu KH, Oehlert J, Jeliffe-Pawlowski LL, Gould JB, Stevenson DK, et al. Exome sequencing of neonatal blood spots identifies genes implicated in bronchopulmonary dysplasia. Am J Respir Crit Care Med. 2015;192(5):589–98. PubMed Epub 2015/06/02. eng.
54. Cohen ED, Ihida-Stansbury K, Lu MM, Panettieri RA, Jones PL, Morrisey EE. Wnt signaling regulates smooth muscle precursor development in the mouse lung via a tenascin C/PDGFR pathway. J Clin Invest. 2009;119(9):2538–49. PubMed Epub 2009/08/20. eng.
55. Ali S, Hirschfeld AF, Mayer ML, Fortuno 3rd ES, Corbett N, Kaplan M, et al. Functional genetic variation in NFKBIA and susceptibility to childhood asthma, bronchiolitis, and bronchopulmonary dysplasia. J Immunol. 2013;190(8):3949–58. PubMed.
56. Ambalavanan N, Cotten CM, Page GP, Carlo WA, Murray JC, Bhattacharya S, et al. Integrated genomic analyses in bronchopulmonary dysplasia. J Pediatr. 2015;166(3):531–7.e13. PubMed Epub 2014/12/03. eng.
57. Wu YT, Chen WJ, Hsieh WS, Tsao PN, Yu SL, Lai CY, et al. MicroRNA expression aberration associated with bronchopulmonary dysplasia in preterm infants: a preliminary study. Respir Care. 2013;58(9):1527–35. PubMed Epub 2013/03/14. eng.
58. Yang Y, Qiu J, Kan Q, Zhou XG, Zhou XY. MicroRNA expression profiling studies on bronchopulmonary dysplasia: a systematic review and meta-analysis. Genet Mol Res. 2013;12(4):5195–206. PubMed Epub 2013/12/05. eng.
59. Wert SE, Whitsett JA, Nogee LM. Genetic disorders of surfactant dysfunction. Pediatr Dev Pathol. 2009;12(4):253–74. PubMed Epub 2009/02/18. eng.
60. Turcu S, Ashton E, Jenkins L, Gupta A, Mok Q. Genetic testing in children with surfactant dysfunction. Arch Dis Child. 2013;98(7):490–5. PubMed Epub 2013/04/30. eng.
61. Edwards V, Cutz E, Viero S, Moore AM, Nogee L. Ultrastructure of lamellar bodies in congenital surfactant deficiency. Ultrastruct Pathol. 2005;29(6):503–9. PubMed Epub 2005/12/01. eng.
62. Bruder E, Hofmeister J, Aslanidis C, Hammer J, Bubendorf L, Schmitz G, et al. Ultrastructural and molecular analysis in fatal neonatal interstitial pneumonia caused by a novel ABCA3 mutation. Mod Pathol. 2007;20(10):1009–18. PubMed Epub 2007/07/31. eng.
63. Flamein F, Riffault L, Muselet-Charlier C, Pernelle J, Feldmann D, Jonard L, et al. Molecular and cellular characteristics of ABCA3 mutations associated with diffuse parenchymal lung diseases in children. Hum Mol Genet. 2011;21(4):765–75. PubMed Epub 2011/11/10. eng.
64. Carrera P, Ferrari M, Presi S, Ventura L, Vergani B, Lucchini V, et al. Null ABCA3 in humans: large homozygous ABCA3 deletion, correlation to clinical-pathological findings. Pediatr Pulmonol. 2014;49(3):E116–20. PubMed Epub 2014/01/15. eng.
65. Citti A, Peca D, Petrini S, Cutrera R, Biban P, Haass C, et al. Ultrastructural characterization of genetic diffuse lung diseases in infants and children: a cohort study and review. Ultrastruct Pathol. 2013;37(5):356–65. PubMed Epub 2013/09/21. eng.
66. Somaschini M, Nogee LM, Sassi I, Danhaive O, Presi S, Boldrini R, et al. Unexplained neonatal respiratory distress due to congenital surfactant deficiency. J Pediatr. 2007;150(6):649–53, 53.e1. PubMed Epub 2007/05/23. eng.

67. Wambach JA, Wegner DJ, Depass K, Heins H, Druley TE, Mitra RD, et al. Single ABCA3 mutations increase risk for neonatal respiratory distress syndrome. Pediatrics. 2012;130(6):e1575–82. PubMed Epub 2012/11/21. eng.
68. Bullard JE, Wert SE, Whitsett JA, Dean M, Nogee LM. ABCA3 mutations associated with pediatric interstitial lung disease. Am J Respir Crit Care Med. 2005;172(8):1026–31. PubMed Epub 2005/06/25. eng.
69. Saugstad OD, Hansen TW, Ronnestad A, Nakstad B, Tollofsrud PA, Reinholt F, et al. Novel mutations in the gene encoding ATP binding cassette protein member A3 (ABCA3) resulting in fatal neonatal lung disease. Acta Paediatr. 2007;96(2):185–90. PubMed Epub 2007/04/13. eng.
70. Goncalves JP, Pinheiro L, Costa M, Silva A, Goncalves A, Pereira A. Novel ABCA3 mutations as a cause of respiratory distress in a term newborn. Gene. 2014;534(2):417–20. PubMed Epub 2013/11/26. eng.
71. Fitzgerald ML, Xavier R, Haley KJ, Welti R, Goss JL, Brown CE, et al. ABCA3 inactivation in mice causes respiratory failure, loss of pulmonary surfactant, and depletion of lung phosphatidylglycerol. J Lipid Res. 2007;48(3):621–32. PubMed Epub 2006/12/05. eng.
72. Besnard V, Matsuzaki Y, Clark J, Xu Y, Wert SE, Ikegami M, et al. Conditional deletion of Abca3 in alveolar type II cells alters surfactant homeostasis in newborn and adult mice. Am J Physiol Lung Cell Mol Physiol. 2010;298(5):L646–59. PubMed Epub 2010/03/02. eng.
73. Wambach JA, Casey AM, Fishman MP, Wegner DJ, Wert SE, Cole FS, et al. Genotype-phenotype correlations for infants and children with ABCA3 deficiency. Am J Respir Crit Care Med. 2014;189(12):1538–43. PubMed Epub 2014/05/30. eng.
74. Shulenin S, Nogee LM, Annilo T, Wert SE, Whitsett JA, Dean M. ABCA3 gene mutations in newborns with fatal surfactant deficiency. N Engl J Med. 2004;350(13):1296–303. PubMed.
75. Naderi HM, Murray JC, Dagle JM. Single mutations in ABCA3 increase the risk for neonatal respiratory distress syndrome in late preterm infants (gestational age 34–36 weeks). Am J Med Genet A. 2014;164A(10):2676–8. PubMed Epub 2014/07/31. eng.
76. Karjalainen MK, Haataja R, Hallman M. Haplotype analysis of ABCA3: association with respiratory distress in very premature infants. Ann Med. 2008;40(1):56–65. PubMed.
77. Shanklin DR, Mullins AC, Baldwin HS. Cerebropulmonary dysgenetic syndrome. Exp Mol Pathol. 2008;85(2):112–6. PubMed Epub 2008/07/08. eng.
78. Hartel C, Felderhoff-Muser U, Gebauer C, Hoehn T, Kribs A, Laux R, et al. ATP-binding cassette member A3 (E292V) gene mutation and pulmonary morbidity in very-low-birth-weight infants. Acta Paediatr. 2011;101(4):380–3. PubMed Epub 2011/12/08. eng.
79. Nogee LM. Genetic mechanisms of surfactant deficiency. Biol Neonate. 2004;85(4):314–8. PubMed Epub 2004/06/26. eng.
80. Makri V, Hospes B, Stoll-Becker S, Borkhardt A, Gortner L. Polymorphisms of surfactant protein B encoding gene: modifiers of the course of neonatal respiratory distress syndrome? Eur J Pediatr. 2002;161(11):604–8. PubMed.
81. Rova M, Haataja R, Marttila R, Ollikainen V, Tammela O, Hallman M. Data mining and multiparameter analysis of lung surfactant protein genes in bronchopulmonary dysplasia. Hum Mol Genet. 2004;13(11):1095–104. PubMed.
82. Cai BH, Chang LW, Li WB, Liu W, Wang XJ, Mo LX, et al. Association of surfactant protein B gene polymorphisms (C/A-18, C/T1580, intron 4 and A/G9306) and haplotypes with bronchopulmonary dysplasia in chinese han population. J Huazhong Univ Sci Technol Med Sci. 2013;33(3):323–8. PubMed Epub 2013/06/19. eng.
83. Yin X, Meng F, Wang Y, Xie L, Kong X, Feng Z. Surfactant protein B deficiency and gene mutations for neonatal respiratory distress syndrome in China Han ethnic population. Int J Clin Exp Pathol. 2013;6(2):267–72. PubMed Epub 2013/01/19. eng.
84. Taponen S, Huusko JM, Petaja-Repo UE, Paananen R, Guttentag SH, Hallman M, et al. Allele-specific N-glycosylation delays human surfactant protein B secretion in vitro and associates with decreased protein levels in vivo. Pediatr Res. 2013;74(6):646–51. PubMed Epub 2013/09/05. eng.
85. Marttila R, Haataja R, Guttentag S, Hallman M. Surfactant protein A and B genetic variants in respiratory distress syndrome in singletons and twins. Am J Respir Crit Care Med. 2003;168(10):1216–22. PubMed.

86. Marttila R, Haataja R, Ramet M, Lofgren J, Hallman M. Surfactant protein B polymorphism and respiratory distress syndrome in premature twins. Hum Genet. 2003;112(1):18–23. PubMed.
87. Hamvas A, Heins HB, Guttentag SH, Wegner DJ, Trusgnich MA, Bennet KW, et al. Developmental and genetic regulation of human surfactant protein B in vivo. Neonatology. 2009;95(2):117–24. PubMed Epub 2008/09/09. eng.
88. Wambach JA, Yang P, Wegner DJ, An P, Hackett BP, Cole FS, et al. Surfactant protein-C promoter variants associated with neonatal respiratory distress syndrome reduce transcription. Pediatr Res. 2010;68(3):216–20. PubMed Epub 2010/06/12. eng.
89. Peca D, Boldrini R, Johannson J, Shieh JT, Citti A, Petrini S, et al. Clinical and ultrastructural spectrum of diffuse lung disease associated with surfactant protein C mutations. Eur J Hum Genet. 2015;23(8):1033–41. PubMed Epub 2015/03/19. eng.
90. Jon C, Nolan PK, Ekong M, Mosquera RA, Stark JM. SFTPC gene mutation p.R167Q in a premature infant. Pediatr Pulmonol. 2013;49(3):E66–8. PubMed Epub 2013/06/19. eng.
91. Rosen DM, Waltz DA. Hydroxychloroquine and surfactant protein C deficiency. N Engl J Med. 2005;352(2):207–8. PubMed Epub 2005/01/14. eng.
92. Hepping N, Griese M, Lohse P, Garbe W, Lange L. Successful treatment of neonatal respiratory failure caused by a novel surfactant protein C p.Cys121Gly mutation with hydroxychloroquine. J Perinatol. 2013;33(6):492–4. PubMed Epub 2013/05/31. eng.
93. Lord A, Shapiro AJ, Saint-Martin C, Claveau M, Melancon S, Wintermark P. Filamin A mutation may be associated with diffuse lung disease mimicking bronchopulmonary dysplasia in premature newborns. Respir Care. 2014;59(11):e171–7. PubMed Epub 2014/07/24. eng.
94. Peca D, Petrini S, Tzialla C, Boldrini R, Morini F, Stronati M, et al. Altered surfactant homeostasis and recurrent respiratory failure secondary to TTF-1 nuclear targeting defect. Respir Res. 2011;12:115. PubMed Epub 2011/08/27. eng.
95. Pohlenz J, Dumitrescu A, Zundel D, Martine U, Schonberger W, Koo E, et al. Partial deficiency of thyroid transcription factor 1 produces predominantly neurological defects in humans and mice. J Clin Invest. 2002;109(4):469–73. PubMed Epub 2002/02/21. eng.
96. Salerno T, Peca D, Menchini L, Schiavino A, Petreschi F, Occasi F, et al. Respiratory insufficiency in a newborn with congenital hypothyroidism due to a new mutation of TTF-1/NKX2.1 gene. Pediatr Pulmonol. 2014;49(3):E42–4. PubMed Epub 2013/09/03. eng.
97. Kleinlein B, Griese M, Liebisch G, Krude H, Lohse P, Aslanidis C, et al. Fatal neonatal respiratory failure in an infant with congenital hypothyroidism due to haploinsufficiency of the NKX2-1 gene: alteration of pulmonary surfactant homeostasis. Arch Dis Child Fetal Neonatal Ed. 2010;96(6):F453–6. PubMed Epub 2010/06/30. eng.
98. Yin X, Wang H, Wu D, Zhao G, Shao J, Dai Y. SLC34A2 Gene mutation of pulmonary alveolar microlithiasis: report of four cases and review of literatures. Respir Med. 2012;107(2):217–22. PubMed Epub 2012/11/21. eng.
99. Whitsett JA, Wert SE, Weaver TE. Alveolar surfactant homeostasis and the pathogenesis of pulmonary disease. Annu Rev Med. 2009;61:105–19. PubMed Epub 2009/10/15. eng.
100. Committee on Fetus and Newborn. Postnatal corticosteroids to treat or prevent chronic lung disease in preterm infants. Pediatrics. 2002;109(2):330–8. PubMed.
101. Huh DD. A human breathing lung-on-a-chip. Ann Am Thorac Soc. 2015;12 Suppl 1:S42–4. PubMed Epub 2015/04/02. eng.
102. Kazzi SN, Quasney MW. Deletion allele of angiotensin-converting enzyme is associated with increased risk and severity of bronchopulmonary dysplasia. J Pediatr. 2005;147(6):818–22. PubMed.
103. Ryckman KK, Dagle JM, Kelsey K, Momany AM, Murray JC. Genetic associations of surfactant protein D and angiotensin-converting enzyme with lung disease in preterm neonates. J Perinatol. 2011;32(5):349–55. PubMed Epub 2011/10/01. eng.
104. Concolino P, Capoluongo E, Santonocito C, Vento G, Tana M, Romagnoli C, et al. Genetic analysis of the dystroglycan gene in bronchopulmonary dysplasia affected premature newborns. Clin Chim Acta. 2007;378(1–2):164–7. PubMed Epub 2007/01/02. eng.

105. Hartel C, Konig I, Koster S, Kattner E, Kuhls E, Kuster H, et al. Genetic polymorphisms of hemostasis genes and primary outcome of very low birth weight infants. Pediatrics. 2006;118(2):683–9. PubMed.
106. Rezvani M, Wilde J, Vitt P, Mailaparambil B, Grychtol R, Krueger M, et al. Association of a FGFR-4 gene polymorphism with bronchopulmonary dysplasia and neonatal respiratory distress. Dis Markers. 2013;35(6):633–40. PubMed Epub 2013/11/30. eng.
107. Manar MH, Brown MR, Gauthier TW, Brown LA. Association of glutathione-S-transferase-P1 (GST-P1) polymorphisms with bronchopulmonary dysplasia. J Perinatol. 2004; 24(1):30–5. PubMed.
108. Rocha G, Proenca E, Areias A, Freitas F, Lima B, Rodrigues T, et al. HLA and bronchopulmonary dysplasia susceptibility: a pilot study. Dis Markers. 2011;31(4):199–203. PubMed Epub 2011/11/03. eng.
109. Bokodi G, Derzbach L, Banyasz I, Tulassay T, Vasarhelyi B. Association of interferon gamma T+874A and interleukin 12 p40 promoter CTCTAA/GC polymorphism with the need for respiratory support and perinatal complications in low birthweight neonates. Arch Dis Child Fetal Neonatal Ed. 2007;92(1):F25–9. PubMed.
110. Yanamandra K, Boggs P, Loggins J, Baier RJ. Interleukin-10 -1082 G/A polymorphism and risk of death or bronchopulmonary dysplasia in ventilated very low birth weight infants. Pediatr Pulmonol. 2005;39(5):426–32. PubMed.
111. Hilgendorff A, Heidinger K, Pfeiffer A, Bohnert A, Konig IR, Ziegler A, et al. Association of polymorphisms in the mannose-binding lectin gene and pulmonary morbidity in preterm infants. Genes Immun. 2007;8(8):671–7. PubMed Epub 2007/09/28. eng.
112. Prencipe G, Auriti C, Inglese R, Devito R, Ronchetti MP, Seganti G, et al. A polymorphism in the macrophage migration inhibitory factor promoter is associated with bronchopulmonary dysplasia. Pediatr Res. 2010;69(2):142–7. PubMed Epub 2010/11/04. eng.
113. Hadchouel A, Decobert F, Franco-Montoya ML, Halphen I, Jarreau PH, Boucherat O, et al. Matrix metalloproteinase gene polymorphisms and bronchopulmonary dysplasia: identification of MMP16 as a new player in lung development. PLoS One. 2008;3(9):e3188. PubMed.
114. Derzbach L, Bokodi G, Treszl A, Vasarhelyi B, Nobilis A, Rigo Jr J. Selectin polymorphisms and perinatal morbidity in low-birthweight infants. Acta Paediatr. 2006;95(10):1213–7. PubMed.
115. Giusti B, Vestrini A, Poggi C, Magi A, Pasquini E, Abbate R, et al. Genetic polymorphisms of antioxidant enzymes as risk factors for oxidative stress-associated complications in preterm infants. Free Radic Res. 2012;46(9):1130–9. PubMed Epub 2012/05/12. eng.
116. Weber B, Borkhardt A, Stoll-Becker S, Reiss I, Gortner L. Polymorphisms of surfactant protein A genes and the risk of bronchopulmonary dysplasia in preterm infants. Turk J Pediatr. 2000;42(3):181–5. PubMed.
117. Pavlovic J, Papagaroufalis C, Xanthou M, Liu W, Fan R, Thomas NJ, et al. Genetic variants of surfactant proteins A, B, C, and D in bronchopulmonary dysplasia. Dis Markers. 2006;22(5–6):277–91. PubMed.
118. Sampath V, Garland JS, Le M, Patel AL, Konduri GG, Cohen JD, et al. A TLR5 (g.1174C > T) variant that encodes a stop codon (R392X) is associated with bronchopulmonary dysplasia. Pediatr Pulmonol. 2011;47(5):460–8. PubMed Epub 2011/11/08. eng.
119. Mailaparambil B, Krueger M, Heizmann U, Schlegel K, Heinze J, Heinzmann A. Genetic and epidemiological risk factors in the development of bronchopulmonary dysplasia. Dis Markers. 2010;29(1):1–9. PubMed Epub 2010/09/10. eng.
120. Elhawary NA, Tayeb MT, Abdel-Ghafar S, Rashad M, Alkhotani AA. TNF-238 polymorphism may predict bronchopulmonary dysplasia among preterm infants in the Egyptian population. Pediatr Pulmonol. 2013;48(7):699–706. PubMed Epub 2013/01/30. eng.
121. Kazzi SN, Kim UO, Quasney MW, Buhimschi I. Polymorphism of tumor necrosis factor-alpha and risk and severity of bronchopulmonary dysplasia among very low birth weight infants. Pediatrics. 2004;114(2):e243–8. PubMed.
122. Kazzi SN, Jacques SM, Qureshi F, Quasney MW, Kim UO, Buhimschi IA. Tumor necrosis factor-alpha allele lymphotoxin-alpha+250 is associated with the presence and severity of placental inflammation among preterm births. Pediatr Res. 2004;56(1):94–8. PubMed.

123. Strassberg SS, Cristea IA, Qian D, Parton LA. Single nucleotide polymorphisms of tumor necrosis factor-alpha and the susceptibility to bronchopulmonary dysplasia. Pediatr Pulmonol. 2007;42(1):29–36. PubMed.
124. Chauhan M, Bombell S, McGuire W. Tumour necrosis factor (−308A) polymorphism in very preterm infants with bronchopulmonary dysplasia: a meta-analysis. Arch Dis Child Fetal Neonatal Ed. 2009;94(4):F257–9. PubMed Epub 2008/12/11. eng.
125. Kwinta P, Bik-Multanowski M, Mitkowska Z, Tomasik T, Legutko M, Pietrzyk JJ. Genetic risk factors of bronchopulmonary dysplasia. Pediatr Res. 2008;64(6):682–8. PubMed Epub 2008/07/11. eng.

Chapter 7
Biomarkers of Bronchopulmonary Dysplasia

Wesley Jackson and Matthew M. Laughon

Introduction

The pathophysiology of bronchopulmonary dysplasia (BPD) includes two processes which are closely linked: inflammation and growth impairment of the preterm lung. The role of inflammation in the development of BPD was first proposed following the observation that tracheal aspirate samples of infants with BPD had elevated neutrophil counts [1]. Current models of the pathophysiology of BPD suggest a preceding inflammatory state occurring in the prenatal environment and often initiated in response to a bacterial infection in utero. This leads to further impaired alveolarization of the preterm lung if the inflammatory process is not well controlled in the first weeks after birth. There are a number of early sources of inflammation which preterm infants are exposed to, such as in utero infection (e.g., chorioamnionitis), relative hyperoxia, and high tidal volumes used in the delivery room, which may act as an initiator for BPD by promoting the influx of inflammatory cells into the neonatal lung and eventually leading to decreased number of alveoli and reduced alveolar septation. This process can be augmented and sustained by important postnatal events such as neonatal sepsis, ventilator-associated pneumonia/lung injury, and necrotizing enterocolitis, which may result in a prolonged inflammatory state, further contributing to lung injury and eventually, though much less pronounced than "old" BPD, lung fibrosis.

Given the important role that inflammation plays in the pathophysiology of BPD, a considerable amount of research has been conducted to identify important proteins, hormones, and growth factors which are involved in the initiation and mediation of the inflammatory cascade in an attempt to develop strategies to prevent and/or mitigate the effects of lung injury and to identify infants who are most at risk of developing

W. Jackson, MD (✉) • M.M. Laughon, MD, MPH
Division of Neonatal-Perinatal Medicine, University of North Carolina at Chapel Hill, UNC Hospitals, CB#7596, 101 Manning Dr, Chapel Hill, NC 27599-7596, USA
e-mail: Wesley.Jackson@unchealth.unc.edu; matt_laughon@med.unc.edu

V. Bhandari (ed.), *Bronchopulmonary Dysplasia*, Respiratory Medicine,
DOI 10.1007/978-3-319-28486-6_7

BPD. The inflammatory process occurs via complex interactions between certain proteins which attract inflammatory cells to the lungs (i.e., chemokines), proteins which allow the inflammatory cells to attach to the endothelium of blood vessels and migrate into the pulmonary interstitium and alveoli (i.e., adhesion molecules), proteins which are involved in the destruction of tissue in the lungs via the inflammatory process (i.e., proinflammatory cytokines and proteases), and proteins which are important in the regulation of the inflammatory cascade (anti-inflammatory cytokines, binding proteins, and receptor antagonists). There are additional hormones, growth factors, and other molecules which regulate lung homeostasis and may influence lung injury and recovery (see Fig. 7.1). These biomarkers have been collected and studied from a variety of in vivo sources, including amniotic fluid, cord blood, maternal and neonatal serum, tracheal aspirates from bronchoalveolar lavage (BAL), and urine samples. In addition to collecting samples from living infants who are at the highest risk of developing BPD, additional research on biomarkers has come from studying autopsies of infants who have succumbed to BPD or other causes of prematurity-related death and animal research studies.

Studies using human preterm infants as subjects have limitations. For instance, serum levels of biomarkers do not necessarily correlate with the presence or concentrations of these markers in the developing lung of the neonate. Samples of the epithelial lining fluid of the lung may be obtained using either tracheal aspirate (TA), which consists of infusing a small amount of saline into the trachea and recovering the fluid, or by BAL [2, 3]. While BAL allows sampling of distal airways where inflammation is more likely to be occurring, it tends to be more invasive and carries a higher risk of inducing bleeding into the fluid which may prevent obtaining an accurate measurement of biomarkers in the epithelial lining fluid (ELF) [3]. As a result, most studies rely on the use of TA. TA and BAL samples provide a more accurate reflection of the environment of the epithelial lining of the lung, in contrast to the alveoli and pulmonary interstitium, which are the compartments where more active inflammation may be occurring. Sampling biases are inherent in many studies using human subjects as lung tissue can typically only be obtained from autopsies, and TA samples must be taken from infants who are intubated. Without the availability of samples from healthy, age-matched control subjects, these studies often select for the most severe cases of BPD. Technological advances in multiplex assays have allowed for the simultaneous detection and quantification of multiple biomarkers in a small sample, and the development of automated gene chip array assays allow measurement of the activity of certain genes involved in the inflammatory process by detecting mRNA.

The primary purpose of studying the biomarkers associated with BPD is to develop potential therapeutic agents and management strategies which may either prevent or mitigate the lung inflammation and impairment in development which is characteristic of BPD, as well as to provide an objective process to identify the neonates who are at highest risk of developing BPD and prognosticate their long-term outcomes. Biomarkers are most likely to be useful when combined with available clinical data in predicting an individual infant's risk of developing BPD and appropriate management. In this chapter, we will review the major categories of inflammatory biomarkers and provide a general overview of each (see Table 7.1).

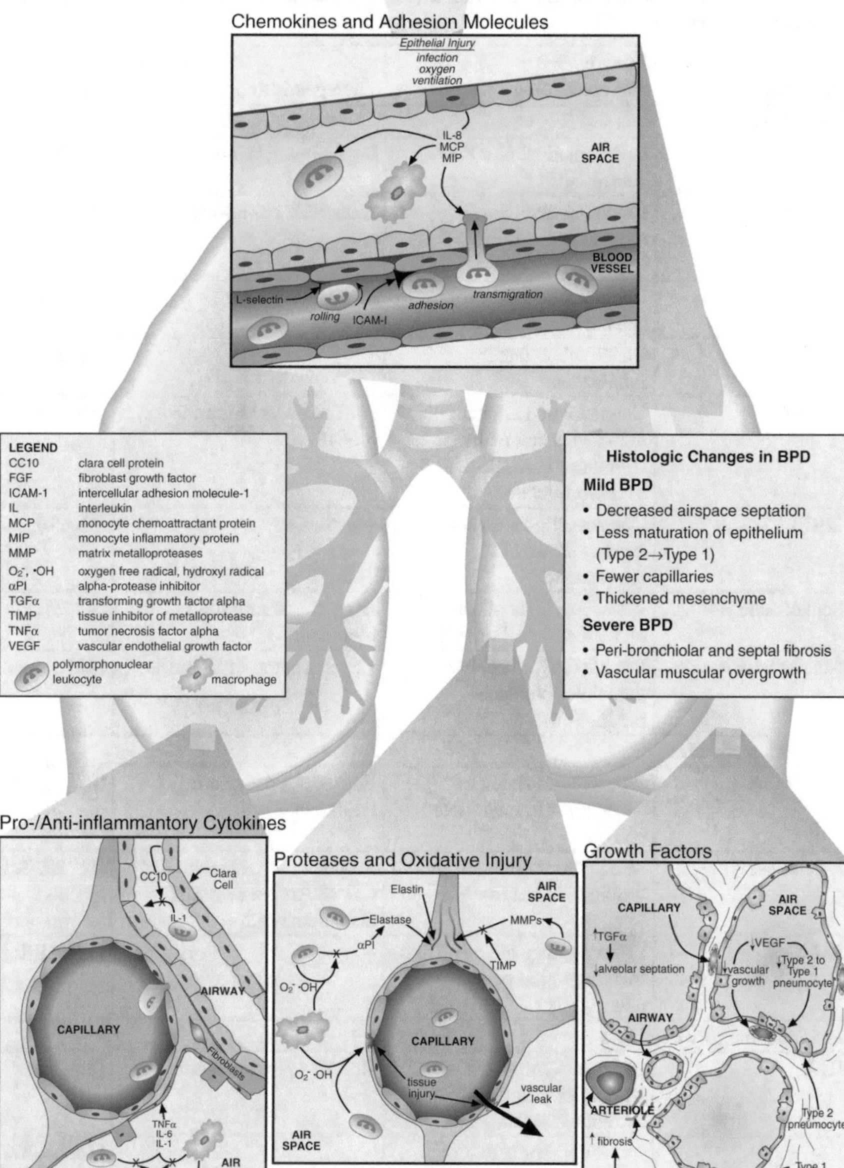

Fig. 7.1 Diagram of important mediators of inflammation, lung injury, and remodeling involved in the pathogenesis of BPD. Reproduced from "Bronchopulmonary dysplasia and inflammatory biomarkers in the premature neonate" CL Bose, CEL Dammann, MM Laughon, *Arch Dis Child Fetal Neonatal Ed*, Vol 93: F457, 2008 with permission from BMJ Publishing Group Ltd.

Table 7.1 Common markers of inflammation involved in the development of BPD and potential therapeutic approaches

Biomarker	Role in BPD pathophysiology	Therapeutic approach	References
Chemokines			
IL-8	Chemotactic factor for neutrophils	Inhaled or systemic steroids	[7–15, 26]
MCP-1	Chemotactic factor for monocytes and lymphocytes	Anti-MCP1 antibody	[16–20, 25]
MCP-2	Chemotactic factor for mast cells, monocytes, NK cells	–	[19, 20]
MCP-3	Chemotactic factor for monocytes	–	[19, 20]
MIP-1α	Chemotactic factor for monocytes and neutrophils; stimulates IL-8, IL-6, and TNFα production	Anti-MIP-1α in murine models	[18, 20]
MIP-1β	Chemotactic factor for monocytes and T lymphocytes	–	[18, 20]
Leukotriene B4	Attracts neutrophils and increases formation of ROS	Early dexamethasone treatment	[22, 23]
Anaphylatoxin C5a	Recruits myofibroblasts and stimulates collagen production	C5a Receptor Antagonists	[24]
Adhesion molecules			
E-selectins	Promotes adhesion of neutrophils to endothelial cell	Early dexamethasone treatment	[27, 28, 31]
L-selectins	Mediates margination or "rolling" of neutrophils	Monoclonal L-selectin and CD 18 Antibodies; early dexamethasone	[28, 29, 32]
ICAM-1	Promotes firm adhesion and transmigration of neutrophils	–	[13, 30, 31]
Pro-inflammatory cytokines			
IL-1	Activates lymphocytes; stimulates proinflammatory cytokine cascade	IL-1 receptor antagonists	[35–38, 43]
IL-6	Increases production of cytokines, supports growth of B lymphocytes	–	[34, 35, 37, 77]
TNFα	Activates macrophages and T lymphocytes	Polyclonal anti-TNFα antibodies	[34, 35, 39, 42]
IFN-γ	Stimulates phagocytic activity	–	[40]

(continued)

Table 7.1 (continued)

Biomarker	Role in BPD pathophysiology	Therapeutic approach	References
Proteases and Inhibitors			
MMPs	Breakdown of collagen in extracellular matrix	IV α1-antitrypsin, secretory leukocyte protease inhibitors	[45–50, 54]
TIMPs	Inhibits activity of matrix metalloproteases	–	[47, 48]
Anti-inflammatory cytokines			
IL-10	Inhibits production of proinflammatory cytokines and upegulates IL-1 receptor antagonist	–	[6, 69–72]
CC10	Inhibits activity of phospholipase A2, supports endogenous production of surfactant	Intratracheal recombinant human CC10	[73, 74, 76, 77]
Growth factors and other			
VEGF	Supports lung alveolarization and angiogenesis	–	[76, 79–81]
TGFα	Regulates lung remodeling following injury	–	[87, 88]
TGFβ	Stimulates fibroblasts and enhances fibrosis	Phosphodiesterase inhibitors (e.g., caffeine, theophylline, rolipram)	[82–86]
Bombesin-like peptide	Growth factor in normal lung development	–	[64–66]
GM-CSF	Stimulates production of granulocytes and macrophages	–	[80]
PTHrP	Regulates surfactant production	Rosiglitazone stimulates myofibroblast differentiation	[89, 90]
Angiopoietin-2	Growth factor involved in angiogenesis and vascular endothelial cell integrity	Dexamethasone treatment	[61, 93, 94]

Please see text for the expanded names of the abbreviations used in the table.

Chemokines

The acute phase of inflammation is initiated and mediated by certain regulatory proteins called chemokines which are categorized into four subtypes (CC, CSC, CX3C, and XC) [4]. Chemokines promote an influx of neutrophils followed by macrophages and other inflammatory cells [5, 6]. The presence of chemokines in samples collected from TA of preterm infants who develop BPD has led to investigations into the possible role they may have in the pathogenesis of BPD. However, attempts to develop predictive models of incidence and severity of disease based on quantitative levels and their timing in the postnatal period have remained elusive.

The chemokine studied most extensively in association with BPD is interleukin-8 (IL-8; also known as CXCL8), a chemotactic cytokine which is released by fibroblasts, endothelial cells, and alveolar epithelial cells and is associated with the early stages of inflammation marked by the influx of neutrophils and their degranulation [7–9]. Experimental models in animals have shown that blockade of IL-8 or its receptor by anti-CXCL8 antibodies in the setting of lipopolysaccharide-induced inflammation reduces the influx of neutrophils and thereby attenuates lung injury [10]. Various studies have demonstrated an elevation in IL-8 in TA samples obtained from preterm infants in the first 10 days of life who develop BPD or early death compared to those who do not develop BPD [11, 12]. A multicenter, prospective cohort study of extremely low birth weight infants found that elevated serum IL-8 levels in the first 3 days of life were associated with a higher incidence of BPD [13]. This association with the development of BPD was preserved even when evaluating only those infants who had survived to the postmenstrual age (PMA) of 36 weeks. In contrast, one study demonstrated that concentrations of IL-8 in TA samples from ventilated preterm infants predicted the combined outcome of BPD and death but not BPD alone [12]. High tidal volumes have also been associated with elevations in IL-8 [14]. The influx of neutrophils and subsequent pulmonary edema associated with the early elevation of IL-8 in TA and serum samples of those preterm infants who develop BPD may reflect a causal role of IL-8 in the pathophysiology of BPD; however it remains unclear whether elevated IL-8 levels are a marker of critical illness in the neonate or if it is specific for BPD [15].

Other groups of chemokines associated with the development of BPD are monocyte chemoattractant proteins, MCP-1 (CCL2), MCP-2 (CCL8), and MCP-3 (CCL7), which are chemotactic cytokines attracting monocytes and lymphocytes, and macrophage inflammatory proteins, MIP-1α (CCL3) and MIP-1β (CCL4). These chemokines are important mediators of the influx of macrophages and lymphocytes associated with the subacute phase of airway inflammation, as evidenced by animal studies using hyperoxia-induced models of inflammation which found that peak MCP-1 expression preceded the influx of macrophages [16]. One study using postmortem lung samples from preterm newborns ventilated in the first 3 days of life found increased mRNA expression of MCP-1 compared to age-matched control samples, which is consistent with early monocyte infiltration of lungs in newborns with respiratory distress syndrome (RDS) who may go on to develop BPD [17]. The activation of alveolar macrophages by CCL2, CCL3, CCL4, CCL7, and CCL8 prolongs lung injury by producing toxic oxygen metabolites such as superoxide anion and hydrogen peroxide.

Macrophages also release chemoattractant proteins which result in further influx of neutrophils to the lung and prolong the inflammatory process. TA samples of preterm infants colonized with *Ureaplasma urealyticum*, a proposed risk factor for the development of BPD, and histologic chorioamnionitis have shown increased levels of MCP-1, MIP-1α, and MIP-1β [18]. There is also a close association between pulmonary hemorrhage and the presence of MCP-1, MCP-2, and MCP-3 in TA samples [19]. TA samples from 56 ventilated infants born at <1500 g found increased levels of MCP-1, MCP-2, MCP-3, and MIP-1β in the first week of life in those infants with RDS. The increased levels of these chemokines and their maximal TA concentrations were greater in those infants who went on to develop an oxygen requirement at 28 days of life, compared to those who did not. In addition, higher TA concentrations of MCP-1, MCP-2, and MCP-3, but not MIP-1α and MIP-1β, were predictive of BPD when defined as oxygen dependence at 36 weeks PMA [20].

Additional chemokines include leukotriene B4 (LTB4), complement component C5-derived anaphylatoxin (C5a), and regulated on activation, normal T cell expressed and secreted (RANTES), all of which have been found to be elevated in TA samples in the first 2 weeks of life in infants who develop BPD [15, 21]. LTB4 is an oxidative product of arachidonic acid, which acts as a chemoattractant for neutrophils and leads to lung injury by the formation of reactive oxygen species (ROS). It is also an important mediator of smooth muscle airway constriction which characterizes the airway hyperreactivity seen in BPD. Dexamethasone inhibits the production of LTB4 by enhancing the activity of antiphospholipase A2. Several studies have shown decreased levels of LTB4 in TA samples from ventilated preterm infants who were administered early dexamethasone treatment, with one study revealing a significant decrease in LTB4 levels in TA samples if dexamethasone was given on day 10 of life but no decrease if treated later (i.e., day of life 16) [22, 23]. In addition to its role as a chemoattractant of phagocytic cells and complement in the presence of inflammation, anaphylatoxin C5a has been recently shown using in vitro human models to promote myofibroblast migration to the alveolar microenvironment, leading to pulmonary fibrosis due to collagen production via the extrinsic coagulation cascade [24]. Ambalavanan et al. also found that a lower serum concentration of RANTES, an important chemokine for T lymphocytes, in the first 3 days of life was associated with the development of BPD. These findings suggest that unregulated neutrophil activity in the absence of effector T cell activity may play a role in the pathogenesis of BPD [15].

Due to the important role that chemokines play in the inflammatory process preceding BPD, attempts have been made to develop potential treatment modalities which may attenuate the oxidative damage and influx of neutrophils caused by these cells. Vozzelli et al. found that in newborn rats exposed to a hyperoxia environment, the injection of anti-MCP-1 on day of life 3–5 resulted in reduced levels of polymorphonuclear neutrophils (PMN) and macrophages in BAL samples taken at 1 week of life compared to immunoglobulin-G (IgG)-treated controls. It was also found that the anti-MCP-1-treated pups had decreased levels of cytokine-induced neutrophil chemoattractant-1 (CINC-1), the analog of IL-8 in rats, which prevented the influx of neutrophils and reduced the level of lung injury due to oxidative stress [25]. A randomized, placebo-controlled trial of 161 ventilated preterm infants found that, in those infants with elevated baseline IL-8 levels, the early use of inhaled beclomethasone decreased the need for subsequent systemic glucocorticoid therapy and resulted in a lower incidence of BPD [26].

Adhesion Molecules

Adhesion molecules are proteins on the surface of cells which mediate transmigration, a process whereby inflammatory cells move from the peripheral blood to their site of action. It is clear that the cell–cell interactions between inflammatory cells and the endothelium play an important role in the inflammatory-mediated lung injury, characteristic of BPD. The process begins with leukocytes slowly rolling along the surface of the endothelium. The leukocytes at first transiently, then firmly, adhere to the endothelium and transmigrate from the capillary into the airspace. The adhesion molecules most commonly studied in the context of BPD are selectins, which are responsible for rolling and transient adhesion, including E-selectins (expressed on endothelial cells), L-selectins (expressed on leukocytes), P-selectins (expressed on endothelial cells and platelets), and intercellular adhesion molecule-1 (ICAM-1).

Concentrations of soluble E-selectin in cord blood obtained at birth have been found to be higher in preterm infants who develop BPD [27]. One study found that decreased soluble L-selectin level in the serum was associated with an increased risk of developing BPD, which was theorized to be secondary to decreased shedding of soluble L-selectin from the surface of the neutrophil, leading to increased neutrophil–endothelial interaction and subsequent transmigration into the lung, while increased serum soluble E-selectin levels were found in those preterm infants who developed BPD [28]. The same study found that administration of dexamethasone was shown to modulate the activity of adhesion molecules by increasing the serum concentration of soluble L-selectin (possibly by inducing shedding of the molecule from the surface of leukocytes) and decreasing the concentration of soluble E-selectin, providing additional support for the use of early administration of postnatal steroids in the management of ventilated infants at risk for BPD. In TA samples, concentrations of soluble L-selectin were similar in all infants on the first day of life, while levels of soluble L-selectin were elevated at 1 week of life in infants who developed BPD compared with infants who were healthy and infants who had RDS at birth but did not develop BPD [29].

ICAM-1 is a molecule which promotes firm leukocyte adhesion and transmigration and binds to membrane immunoglobulin-M (IgM) for intracellular signaling. Animal models using newborn mice and adult rats have shown upregulation of ICAM-1, P-selectin, and E-selectin in the lungs of animals exposed to prolonged supplemental oxygen, suggesting the influence of a hyperoxia-induced environment in the regulation of adhesion molecules [30, 31]. Elevated concentrations of ICAM-1 in TA samples have been observed at day of life 10 in infants who develop BPD [13].

Preliminary research into agents such as humanized CD 18 monoclonal antibodies and monoclonal antibodies to L-selectin, which block selectin-mediated interactions between leukocytes and endothelial cells in the context of systemic inflammatory response syndrome in patients with sepsis, may prove useful in the future as a potential strategy for preventing BPD [32].

Proinflammatory Cytokines

Extensive studies in neonates and animal models indicate that the amount of inflammation present in the lung is largely determined by the balance between proinflammatory and anti-inflammatory cytokines such that a predominance of proinflammatory cytokines and a deficiency in the production/release of anti-inflammatory cytokines increases the risk of developing BPD [33]. Cytokines are regulatory peptides which are produced and released by neutrophils and other inflammatory cells in the airway, as well as alveolar epithelial cells, fibroblasts, and endothelial cells in the lung parenchyma and mediate the tissue injury associated with inflammation via the regulation of humoral and cell-mediated immune responses. By interacting with cell-surface receptors, cytokines initiate intracellular signaling mechanisms which lead to upregulation or downregulation of certain genes and transcription factors in the nucleus important to the cellular response to inflammatory stress.

The proinflammatory cytokines which have been studied most extensively and have been consistently shown to be associated with the development of chronic lung disease in neonates are IL-1, IL-6, IL-8 (which is also a chemokine, see above), and tumor necrosis factor alpha (TNFα) [34–36]. While the majority of studies have focused on identifying individual cytokines which may offer predictive value in the development of BPD, one study examined TA samples obtained from 27 very low birth weight (VLBW) infants at 24 h of life and classified the infants into two outcome groups (±BPD) by simultaneously measuring 12 proinflammatory mediators [37]. Using a linear discriminant analysis model, the study found that measuring the levels of 12 mediators [IL-1receptor antagonist or IL-1ra, IL-1β, IL-6, IL-8, IL-10, granulocyte macrophage colony-stimulating factor (GM-CSF), vascular endothelial growth factor (VEGF), MCP-1, MIP-1a, MIP-1b, and TNFα] provided a useful predictive model which correctly classified 96 % of the cases in the study. A higher incidence of the combined outcome of BPD and death has been associated with lower infant serum levels of IL-17 [13].

IL-1β represents a prototypical proinflammatory cytokine which is released by alveolar macrophages and plays an important role in the amplification of the inflammatory cascade by recruiting inflammatory cells, inducing the production of other proinflammatory cytokines and adhesion molecules in addition to stimulating the activity of fibroblasts, thereby contributing to the process of fibrosis. An increased level of IL-1β in TA samples from preterm infants has been shown to be correlated with adverse pulmonary outcomes likely due to its association with maternal chorioamnionitis [36, 38].

IL-6 has both pro- and anti-inflammatory properties and may serve a compensatory role in protecting the lung against the harmful effects of the inflammatory process. Elevated concentrations of IL-1β and an increased ratio of IL-1β to IL-6 in TA samples of VLBW infants have been associated with airway colonization of *U. urealyticum*, a pathogen which has been implicated as a risk factor for BPD [35].

TNFα, a potent activator of macrophages, plays an integral role in the host defense against pathogenic bacteria; however, overproduction of the cytokine leads to parenchymal lung damage by promoting capillary leak. Elevated levels of TNFα in BAL samples from ventilated preterm infants were associated with increased mortality [39].

Additional proinflammatory cytokines which have been investigated in the context of RDS and BPD include interferon-gamma (IFN-γ) and macrophage migration inhibitory factor (MIF). IFN-γ is a T helper cell cytokine which if overexpressed can lead to pulmonary edema and alveolar damage. Elevated concentration of IFN-γ in serum and TA samples have been associated with the combined outcomes of death or development of BPD in preterm infants, supporting its role in lung injury in animal models using a hyperoxia-induced environment [40]. MIF is expressed by alveolar macrophages, endothelial cells, and bronchial epithelial cells and is thought to be protective to the lung by promoting angiogenesis and stimulating type 2 alveolar cells to produce surfactant. Reduced intrapulmonary levels of MIF were observed in preterm infants with RDS who developed BPD [41]. The release of intracellular stores of MIF by the administration of corticosteroids provides a potential role for its use in the early stages of BPD.

The use of pharmacological agents to block the activation of proinflammatory cytokines, such as polyclonal anti-TNFα antibodies and IL-1 receptor antagonists, has been studied in adult models of severe sepsis [42, 43]. These strategies may eventually provide insight into the development of treatment modalities for decreasing the cytokine cascade involved in BPD [44].

Proteases and Their Inhibitors

Inflammatory cells contribute to the pathogenesis of BPD by releasing proteinases which promote the breakdown of collagen in the alveolar/capillary interface and extracellular matrix leading to decreased alveolar septation and impairment in lung development. Matrix metalloproteases (MMPs) are a tightly regulated family of proteinases which contribute to lung remodeling by breaking down proteins in the extracellular matrix. MMPs have a role in normal lung development and are important in the process of lung tissue repair [45]. However, an imbalance in factors which promote proteinase activity relative to specific proteinase inhibitors which decrease their activity, which often occurs in preterm infants, can lead to lung damage [46]. MMP-8 and MMP-9, in addition to the tissue inhibitor of metalloproteases (TIMPs), have been studied in TA samples from preterm infants and support the theory that an imbalance in proteinase activity increases the risk of BPD. This has been demonstrated by the association of an increased incidence of BPD with low concentrations of TIMPs and high concentrations of MMPs [47, 48].

While antenatal steroids had no effect on MMP-8 or MMP-9 levels in BAL fluid obtained from preterm infants, higher concentrations of MMP-8 and-9 were found in infants exposed to environments in utero in which histologic chorioamnionitis was present [49, 50]. The destruction of cross-linked elastin fibers in the presence of infection and/or hyperoxia environment, supported by the increase in urinary excretion of desmosine, an elastolytic degradation product of elastin, in preterm infants with BPD suggests an important role in the pathogenesis of chronic lung disease [51, 52]. Increased levels of trypsin-2 were found in TA samples taken in the early postnatal period in preterm infants who developed BPD [53]. Trypsin-2 acts as a potent matrix-degrading proteinase in addition to activating the G-protein-coupled receptor proteinase-activated receptor 2 (PAR2) found in the bronchial epithelium, leading to the release of proinflammatory cytokines, chemokines, and MMPs [54].

Several studies have taken advantage of the inhibitory activity of α1-antitrypsin on elastase activity as well as the use of secretory leukocyte protease inhibitors (SLPIs) to investigate potential therapeutic agents to prevent BPD. A randomized, controlled trial using intravenous α1-antitrypsin supplementation in preterm infants found a decrease in the incidence of pulmonary hemorrhage in the treated group but no statistically significant difference in the incidence of BPD [55]. The administration of recombinant SLPIs has been shown to reduce elastase-induced injury in animal models; however, its use in the newborn population has remained limited [56].

Reactive Oxygen Species and Oxidative Injury

The oxidative stress leading to cellular damage caused by exposure of the preterm infant to high fractions of inspired oxygen has been shown to be strongly linked to inflammation in the lungs and is mediated by the production of free oxygen radicals resulting from lipid peroxidation [57]. Increased levels of ethane and pentane, two products of the peroxidation of lipids, were found in expired air from VLBW infants with RDS who developed BPD or death compared to those infants with RDS who survived without BPD [58]. These ROS lead to degradation of the basement membrane and extracellular matrix of the lung by promoting microvascular permeability with subsequent pulmonary edema [24] in addition to inhibiting antiproteases, which regulate elastase activity. ROS such as superoxide anions, hydrogen peroxide, and hydroxyl anions are produced by neutrophils and macrophages in the lung, and their production has been found to be increased in BAL samples taken from infants who developed BPD compared to those without lung disease [59].

Enzymes and products associated with oxidative stress have been used as biomarkers in attempts to identify which infants are at the highest risk for the development of BPD. TA samples from preterm infants in the first week of life found increases in myeloperoxidase and elastase activity in addition to increased xanthine oxidase in infants who developed BPD compared to those infants who did not [60]. 3-Chlorotyrosine, a product of myeloperoxidase activity in neutrophils, and malondialdehyde have also been found to be correlated with the development of BPD [61]. The relative deficiency of antioxidant enzymes such as superoxide dismutase, catalase, and glutathione peroxidase and lower levels of anti-proteases in preterm infants places them at an increased risk of lung damage due to oxidative stress [62, 63].

Exposure to a hyperoxia environment contributes to the development of BPD by inducing oxidative stress which can overwhelm the preterm infant's antioxidant capacity. In addition, hyperoxia potentiates lung injury due to secondary effects such as enhancing the production of bombesine-like peptides (BLPs), growth factors produced by pulmonary neuroendocrine cells which are important to normal fetal development but can lead to lung injury due to proinflammatory effects of mast cell stimulation [64]. Elevated concentrations of urinary BLPs have been associated with increased risk of developing BPD [65, 66].

There is some evidence to support a role for antioxidant therapy in the prevention of BPD. A multicenter, randomized control trial involving 302 preterm infants found that while multiple doses of intratracheal recombinant human CuZn superoxide dismutase did not decrease the incidence of BPD or death, the treatment was associated with improved pulmonary outcome in survivors at 1 year corrected age [67]. *N*-acetylcysteine (NAC) has been investigated for its antioxidant properties, which occurs via repletion of intracellular glutathione stores; however, a randomized, controlled trial using a 6-day course of intravenous NAC in ELBW infants failed to show an effect on death or incidence of BPD [68].

Anti-inflammatory Cytokines

It is clear that while inflammation plays a significant role in the development of BPD, those infants who are able to recover from the initial stages of inflammation are less likely to develop the pulmonary sequelae associated with prematurity. The ability to regulate the inflammatory cascade and recover from the initial injury to the lung has been shown to be highly dependent on the activity of anti-inflammatory cytokines, the most important of which is IL-10. The decreased expression of IL-10 in preterm infants is associated with the development of BPD.

IL-10 has been studied extensively due to its counter-regulatory role in the inflammatory cascade by inhibiting the production of TNFα, IL-1β, IL-6, and IL-8 and upregulating IL-1ra, thereby promoting lung protection [6, 69]. The absence of IL-10 in airway secretions from preterm infants compared to detectable levels in term infants may in part be due to the decreased ability of alveolar macrophages to produce IL-10 in preterm infants [70, 71]. While IL-10 levels rise earlier and are preceded by an increase in IL-8 in BAL samples from ventilated preterm infants who develop BPD, IL-10 concentrations also fall more quickly within the first 5 days compared with infants who do not develop BPD, supporting the concept of BPD as attributable to a cytokine imbalance [72].

Clara cell secretory protein 10 (CC10), produced in non-ciliated pulmonary epithelial cells, has also been identified for its important anti-inflammatory properties due to the inhibition of chemotaxis of inflammatory cells and fibronectin binding. CC10 may also offer lung protection in the setting of inflammation by preventing the degradation of phospholipid components of surfactant by phospholipase A2. Preterm infants have a decreased level of CC10 in TA samples compared to adults [73]. Decreased expression of CC10 in TA samples of preterm infants who developed BPD compared to those who did not suggests that a deficiency in CC10 may predispose preterm infants to BPD [74]. While one study found lower levels of CC16, an additional protein secreted by pulmonary mucosal cells, in the cord blood of preterm infants who developed BPD, the transient nature of plasma levels of CC16 have led to conflicting results and prevent the use of CC16 as a reliable biomarker for BPD [75].

Intratracheal administration of recombinant human CC10 (rhCC10) has shown promising results in reducing pulmonary inflammation and upregulating surfactant and VEGF production [76]. One study found decreased levels of neutrophil and IL-6 from TA samples in preterm infants treated with rhCC10, however, the study was not sufficiently powered to demonstrate a difference in incidence of BPD [77]. Further studies using a randomized, control trial design with larger sample sizes are required to determine the effectiveness and optimal dosing of rhCC10 prior to its widespread use as a therapeutic approach to preventing BPD.

Growth Factors and Other Important Mediators of Inflammation

Fetal lung development occurs in a highly regulated manner and is dependent on a variety of growth factors and hormones, the disruption of which secondary to lung injury and inflammation may lead to impaired growth and function [78]. Since the shift in our understanding of the pathophysiology of "new" BPD in the post-surfactant age, there has been an increased interest in studying growth factors due to their role in the regulation of pulmonary vasculature formation. VEGF, produced in endothelial and bronchial epithelial cells, is of particular interest in BPD research given its role in the stimulation of lung alveolarization and angiogenesis [79]. One study involving the measurement of several growth factors in the BAL samples from ventilated preterm infants in the first week of life found that, of the growth factors studied, low levels of VEGF as early as the first 24 h of life were associated with an increased risk of BPD [80]. While the precise temporal course of VEGF levels in preterm infants has not yet been determined, one study has proposed a bimodal distribution in which VEGF levels are relatively increased in the first 12 h after birth and by 3–4 weeks postnatal [81]. The correlation of VEGF with gestational age and phospholipid concentration in BAL fluid also suggests a role in surfactant synthesis and supports its use as a general biomarker of lung development.

The role of transforming growth factor (TGF) β provides an example of the fine balance that certain growth factors have in the role of lung development. While TGFβ has been shown in animal models to promote lung repair after hyperoxia and reduces the production of proinflammatory cytokines [82, 83], its overexpression has also been implicated in the process of fibrosis and decreased alveolarization and may represent a useful marker of severe BPD [84, 85]. Investigations using phosphodiesterase (PDE) inhibitors, such as caffeine, theophylline, and rolipram (a PDE-4 selective inhibitor) to block downstream targets of TGFβ, such as connective tissue growth factor have shown promising results and may represent a novel therapeutic approach to preventing abnormal lung tissue remodeling [86].

TGFα also requires strict regulation of its expression in order to provide benefits for lung maturation as murine models have shown disruptions in lung development with both overexpression and knockout of the growth factor [87, 88], while decreased levels of TGFα in BAL fluid of preterm infants have been associated with increased BPD [40]. Additional growth factors which have been studied for their role in lung protection include fibroblast growth factors, keratinocyte and pulmonary hepatocyte growth factors, placental growth factor, epithelial growth factor, platelet-derived growth factor, and insulin-like growth factor; however, their utility as biomarkers for BPD has not been well established [81].

Other factors which have been studied as potential markers of BPD include parathyroid hormone-related protein (PTHrP) which is an important paracrine factor regulating the production of surfactant. Lower levels of PTHrP in TA samples of preterm infants were found to correlate with increased duration of mechanical ventilation [89]. The administration of certain drugs which activate pathways involved in PTHrP signaling, such as rosiglitazone, has been proposed as novel therapeutic approaches to preventing BPD by stimulating myofibroblast differentiation [90]. Krebs von den Lungen-6 (KL-6) has been found to be a useful indicator of lung injury in the peripheral blood with serum levels of KL-6 correlating well with severity of BPD [91]. Hyperoxia models in newborn rats confirm the correlation of circulating levels of KL-6 with increased expression in pulmonary tissue consistent with impaired alveolarization [92]. Angiopoietin-2 is a growth factor which has been studied extensively in the context of BPD due to its role in disrupting the formation of blood vessels and promoting pulmonary vascular leak and endothelial cell necrosis in conditions of hyperoxia [93]. Increased TA levels of angiopoietin-2 have been observed in preterm infants who developed BPD and/or died compared to those infants who developed RDS and recovered [61]. The early administration of dexamethasone to preterm infants significantly reduced TA levels of angiopoietin-2, presumably due to the anti-inflammatory properties of steroids, and may provide evidence to support the potentially beneficial effects of developing anti-angiopoietin-2 agents [94].

GM-CSF is a growth factor which stimulates the production of granulocytes and macrophages and elevated levels of GM-CSF in BAL fluids obtained from ventilated infants in the first week of life correlates temporally with the influx of inflammatory cells into the airways [80].

Additional biomarkers obtained from a variety of biological sources which have been studied for their potential link to the development of BPD have been reviewed elsewhere and are included here for the sake of completion: maternal serum alpha-fetoprotein, human chorionic gonadotropin and unconjugated estriol, endostatin, endothelial colony-forming cells, type IV collagen, CD9, C-terminal fragment of type I collagen, eosinophilic cationic protein, 8-isoprostanes, N-terminal pro-B-type natriuretic peptide, granulocyte-specific S100A12, urinary levels of 8-iso-prostaglandin F2 alpha and 8-hydroxydeoxyguanosine, cathepsin K, chitinase-like proteins, endothelin-1, endoglin (a TGFβ co-receptor), inducible nitric oxide synthase, nuclear factor-kappa B, fibronectin, plasminogen activator inhibitor-1, lysozyme, polyunsaturated fatty acids, dimethylacetals, neutrophil-gelatinase-associated lipocalin, pepsin, Sirtuin1, connective tissue mast cell, breath condensate end-tidal carbon monoxide, and exhaled nitric oxide [81].

Limitations of the Utility of Biomarkers and Future Research

It remains unclear whether the biomarkers discussed in this chapter represent causal agents in the process of lung injury characteristic of BPD or whether their presence is merely a reflection of an environment which has already caused lung inflammation and injury. Of the various molecules reviewed in this chapter which have been studied for their potential link to BPD, the biomarkers which have shown the strongest evidence as reliable markers of BPD include: IL-1β, IL-6, MCP-1, TGFβ1, VEGF, KGF, bombesin-like peptide, MMP-9, PTHrP, MIF, and IFN-γ. Despite promising results in numerous studies suggesting their role in the early identification of infants at risk for BPD, biomarkers are not currently used in the routine care of neonates given a general lack of understanding of how these markers interact with one another in the clinical setting. Much of the existing research involves the measurement of biomarkers in response to a single environmental factor, making it difficult to apply to clinical contexts in which multiple conditions may be occurring simultaneously. As demonstrated in this chapter, the regulation of the body's immune response is complex and multifactorial; while a cytokine may offer protection from lung injury in certain instances, an alteration in its regulation or expression by a variety of other factors can lead to a cascading inflammatory response which disrupts normal lung development. A better understanding of how these factors interact with one another at multiple time points will be essential in developing individual infant risk profiles and determining clinical applicability.

References

1. Merritt TA, Cochrane CG, Holcomb K, Bohl B, Hallman M, Strayer D, et al. Elastase and alpha 1-proteinase inhibitor activity in tracheal aspirates during respiratory distress syndrome. Role of inflammation in the pathogenesis of bronchopulmonary dysplasia. J Clin Invest. 1983;72(2):656–66.
2. Dargaville PA, South M, Vervaart P, McDougall PN. Validity of markers of dilution in small volume lung lavage. Am J Respir Crit Care Med. 1999;160:778–84.
3. Dargaville PA, South M, McDougall PN. Comparison of two methods of diagnostic lung lavage in ventilated infants with lung disease. Am J Respir Crit Care Med. 1999;160:771–7.
4. Charo IF, Ransohoff RM. The many roles of chemokines and chemokine receptors in inflammation. N Engl J Med. 2006;354:610–21.
5. Whicher JT, Evans SW. Cytokines in disease. Clin Chem. 1990;36:1269–81.
6. Ozdemir A, Brown MA, Morgan WJ. Markers and mediators of inflammation in neonatal lung disease. Pediatr Pulmonol. 1997;23:292–306.
7. Truog WE, Ballard PL, Norberg M, et al. Inflammatory markers and mediators in tracheal fluid of premature infants treated with inhaled nitric oxide. Pediatrics. 2007;119:670–8.
8. Takasaki J, Ogawa Y. Interleukin 8 and granulocyte elastase alpha 1 proteinase inhibitor complex in the tracheobronchial aspirate of infants with chronic lung disease following interuterine infection. Acta Paediatr Jpn. 1996;38:132–6.

9. Groneck P, Speer CP. Interleukin-8 in pulmonary effluent fluid of preterm infants. J Pediatr. 1993;123:839–40.
10. D'Angio CT, Finkelstein JN, Lomonaco MB, Paxhia A, Wright SA, Baggs RB, et al. Changes in surfactant protein gene expression in a neonatal rabbit model of hyperoxia-induced fibrosis. Am J Physiol Lung Cell Mol Physiol. 1997;272:720–30.
11. De Dooy J, Ieven M, Stevens W, et al. High levels of CXCL8 in tracheal aspirate samples taken at birth are associated with adverse respiratory outcome only in preterm infants younger than 28 weeks gestation. Pediatr Pulmonol. 2007;42:193–203.
12. Kotecha S, Chan B, Azam N, et al. Increase in interleukin-8 and soluble intercellular adhesion molecule-1 in bronchoalveolar lavage fluid from premature infants who develop chronic lung disease. Arch Dis Child Fetal Neonatal Ed. 1995;72:F90–6.
13. Ambalavanan N, Carlo WA, D'Angio CT, McDonald SA, Das A, Schendel D, Thorsen P, Higgins RD, Eunice Kennedy Shriver National Institute of Child Health and Human Development Neonatal Research Network. Cytokines associated with bronchopulmonary dysplasia or death in extremely low birth weight infants. Pediatrics. 2009;123(4):1132–41.
14. Lista G, Castoldi F, Fontana P, et al. Lung inflammation in preterm infants with respiratory distress syndrome: effects of ventilation with different tidal volumes. Pediatr Pulmonol. 2006;41:357–63.
15. Munshi UK, Niu JO, Siddiq MM, et al. Elevation of interleukin-8 and interleukin-6 precedes the influx of neutrophils in tracheal aspirates from preterm infants who develop bronchopulmonary dysplasia. Pediatr Pulmonol. 1997;24:331–6.
16. D'Angio CT, LoMonaco MB, Chaudhry SA, Paxhia A, Ryan RM. Discordant pulmonary proinflammatory cytokine expression during acute hyperoxia in the newborn rabbit. Exp Lung Res. 1999;25(5):443–65.
17. De Paepe ME, Greco D, Mao Q. Angiogenesis-related gene expression profiling in ventilated preterm human lungs. Exp Lung Res. 2010;36(7):399–410.
18. Baier RJ, Loggins J, Kruger TE. Monocyte chemoattractant protein-1 and interleukin-8 are increased in bronchopulmonary dysplasia: relation to isolation of *Ureaplasma urealyticum*. J Investig Med. 2001;49:362–9.
19. Baier RJ, Loggins J, Kruger TE. Increased interleukin-8 and monocyte chemoattractant protein-1 concentrations in mechanically ventilated preterm infants with pulmonary hemorrhage. Pediatr Pulmonol. 2002;34:131–7.
20. Baier RJ, Majid A, Parupia H, Loggins J, Kruger TE. CC chemokine concentrations increase in respiratory distress syndrome and correlate with development of bronchopulmonary dysplasia. Pediatr Pulmonol. 2004;37:137–48.
21. Groneck P, Gotze-Speer B, Oppermann M, et al. Association of pulmonary inflammation and increased microvascular permeability during the development of bronchopulmonary dysplasia: a sequential analysis of inflammatory mediators in respiratory fluids of high-risk preterm neonates. Pediatrics. 1994;93:712–8.
22. Wang JY, Yeh TF, Lin YJ, Chen WY, Lin CH. Early postnatal dexamethasone therapy may lessen lung inflammation in premature infants with respiratory distress syndrome on mechanical ventilation. Pediatr Pulmonol. 1997;23(3):193–7.
23. Groneck P, Reuss D, Götze-Speer B, Speer CP. Effects of dexamethasone on chemotactic activity and inflammatory mediators in tracheobronchial aspirates of preterm infants at risk for chronic lung disease. J Pediatr. 1993;122(6):938–44.
24. Kambas K, Chrysanthopoulou A, Kourtzelis I, Skordala M, Mitroulis I, Rafail S, Vradelis S, Sigalas I, Wu YQ, Speletas M, Kolios G, Ritis K. Endothelin-1 signaling promotes fibrosis in vitro in a bronchopulmonary dysplasia model by activating the extrinsic coagulation cascade. J Immunol. 2011;186(11):6568–75.
25. Vozzelli MA, Mason SN, Whorton MH, Auten RL. Antimacrophage chemokine treatment prevents neutrophil and macrophage influx in hyperoxia-exposed newborn rat lung. Am J Physiol Lung Cell Mol Physiol. 2004;286(3):L488–93.

26. Gupta GK, Cole CH, Abbasi S, Demissie S, Njinimbam C, Nielsen HC, Colton T, Frantz 3rd ID. Effects of early inhaled beclomethasone therapy on tracheal aspirate inflammatory mediators IL-8 and IL-1ra in ventilated preterm infants at risk for bronchopulmonary dysplasia. Pediatr Pulmonol. 2000;30(4):275–81.
27. Kim BI, Lee HE, Choi CW, Jo HS, Choi EH, Koh YY, Choi JH. Increase in cord blood soluble E-selectin and tracheal aspirate neutrophils at birth and the development of new bronchopulmonary dysplasia. J Perinat Med. 2004;32(3):282–7.
28. Ballabh P, Kumari J, Krauss AN, Shin JJ, Jain A, Auld PA, Lesser ML, Cunningham-Rundles S. Soluble E-selectin, soluble L-selectin and soluble ICAM-1 in bronchopulmonary dysplasia, and changes with dexamethasone. Pediatrics. 2003;111(3):461–8.
29. Kotecha S, Silverman M, Shaw RJ, Klein N. Soluble L-selectin concentration in bronchoalveolar lavage fluid obtained from infants who develop chronic lung disease of prematurity. Arch Dis Child Fetal Neonatal Ed. 1998;78:F143–7.
30. Zeb T, Piedboeuf B, Gamache M, Langston C, Welty SE. P-selectin is upregulated early in the course of hyperoxic lung injury in mice. Free Radic Biol Med. 1996;21(4):567–74.
31. Ramsay PL, Geske RS, Montgomery CA, Welty SE. Increased soluble E-Selectin is associated with lung inflammation, and lung injury in hyperoxia-exposed rats. Toxicol Lett. 1996;87(2–3):157–65.
32. Chandra A, Enkhbaatar P, Nakano Y, Traber LD, Traber DL. Sepsis: emerging role of nitric oxide and selectins. Clinics (Sao Paulo). 2006;61(1):71–6.
33. Speer CP. Inflammation and bronchopulmonary dysplasia: a continuing story. Semin Fetal Neonatal Med. 2006;11(5):354–62.
34. Jonsson B, Tullus K, Brauner A, et al. Early increase of TNF alpha and IL-6 in tracheobronchial aspirate fluid indicator of subsequent chronic lung disease in preterm infants. Arch Dis Child Fetal Neonatal Ed. 1997;77:F198–201.
35. Patterson AM, Taciak V, Lovchik J, et al. *Ureaplasma urealyticum* respiratory tract colonization is associated with an increase in interleukin 1-beta and tumor necrosis factor alpha relative to interleukin 6 in tracheal aspirates of preterm infants. Pediatr Infect Dis J. 1998;17:321–8.
36. Cayabyab RG, Jones CA, Kwong KY, et al. Interleukin-1beta in the bronchoalveolar lavage fluid of premature neonates: a marker for maternal chorioamnionitis and predictor of adverse neonatal outcome. J Matern Fetal Neonatal Med. 2003;14:205–11.
37. Schneibel KR, Fitzpatrick AM, Ping XD, Brown LA, Gauthier TW. Inflammatory mediator patterns in tracheal aspirate and their association with bronchopulmonary dysplasia in very low birth weight neonates. J Perinatol. 2013;33(5):383–7.
38. Kotecha S, Wilson L, Wangoo A, et al. Increase in interleukin (IL)-1 beta and IL-6 in bronchoalveolar lavage fluid obtained from infants with chronic lung disease of prematurity. Pediatr Res. 1996;40:250–6.
39. Mahieu LM, De Dooy JJ, Ieven MM, et al. Increased levels of tumor necrosis factor-alpha and decreased levels of interleukin-12 p 70 in tracheal aspirates, within 2 hrs after birth, are associated with mortality among ventilated preterm infants. Pediatr Crit Care Med. 2005;6:682–9.
40. Aghai ZH, Saslow JG, Mody K, Eydelman R, Bhat V, Stahl G, Pyon K, Bhandari V. IFN-γ and IP-10 in tracheal aspirates from premature infants: relationship with bronchopulmonary dysplasia. Pediatr Pulmonol. 2013;48(1):8–13.
41. Kevill KA, Bhandari V, Kettunen M, Leng L, Fan J, Mizue Y, et al. A role for macrophage migration inhibitory factor in the neonatal respiratory distress syndrome. J Immunol. 2008;180:601–8.
42. Rice TW, Wheeler AP, Morris PE, et al. Safety and efficacy of affinity-purified, anti-tumor necrosis factor-alpha, ovine Fab for injection (CytoFab) in severe sepsis. Crit Care Med. 2006;34(9):2271–81.
43. Eichacker PQ, Parent C, Kalil A, et al. Risk and the efficacy of antiinflammatory agents: retrospective and confirmatory studies of sepsis. Am J Respir Crit Care Med. 2002;166(9):1197–205.
44. Nold MF, Mangan NE, Rudloff I, Cho SX, Shariatian N, Samarasinghe TD, et al. Interleukin-1 receptor antagonist prevents murine bronchopulmonary dysplasia induced by perinatal inflammation and hyperoxia. Proc Natl Acad Sci USA. 2013;110(35):14384–9.

45. Greenlee KJ, Werb Z, Kheradmand F. Matrix metalloproteinases in lung: multiple, multifarious, and multifaceted. Physiol Rev. 2007;87:69–98.
46. Sweet DG, Curley AE, Chesshyre E, et al. The role of matrix metalloproteinases -9 and -2 in development of neonatal chronic lung disease. Acta Paediatr. 2004;93:791–6.
47. Ekekezie II, Thibeault DW, Simon SD, et al. Low levels of tissue inhibitors of metalloproteinases with a high matrix metalloproteinase-9/tissue inhibitor of metalloproteinase-1 ratio are present in tracheal aspirate fluids of infants who develop chronic lung disease. Pediatrics. 2004;113:1709–14.
48. Cederqvist K, Sorsa T, Tervahartiala T, et al. Matrix metalloproteinases-2, -8, and -9 and TIMP-2 in tracheal aspirates from preterm infants with respiratory distress. Pediatrics. 2001;108:686–92.
49. Curley AE, Sweet DG, Thornton CM, O'Hara MD, Chesshyre E, Pizzotti J, et al. Chorioamnionitis and increased neonatal lung lavage fluid matrix metalloproteinase-9 levels: implications forantenatal origins of chronic lung disease. Am J Obstet Gynecol. 2003;188(4):871–5.
50. Curley AE, Sweet DG, MacMahon KJ, O'Connor CM, Halliday HL. Chorioamnionitis increases matrix metalloproteinase-8 concentrations in bronchoalveolar lavage fluid from preterm babies. Arch Dis Child Fetal Neonatal Ed. 2004;89(1):F61–4.
51. Bruce MC, Schuyler M, Martin RJ, et al. Risk factors for the degradation of lung elastic fibers in the ventilated neonate. Implications for impaired lung development in bronchopulmonary dysplasia. Am Rev Respir Dis. 1992;146:204–12.
52. Thibeault DW, Mabry SM, Ekekezie II, Truog WE. Lung elastic tissue maturation and perturbations during the evolution of chronic lung disease. Pediatrics. 2000;106:1452–9.
53. Cederqvist K, Haglund C, Heikkila P, et al. Pulmonary trypsin-2 in the development of bronchopulmonary dysplasia in preterm infants. Pediatrics. 2003;112:570–7.
54. Cederqvist K, Haglund C, Heikkilä P, Hollenberg MD, Karikoski R, Andersson S. High expression of pulmonary proteinase-activated receptor 2 in acute and chronic lung injury in preterm infants. Pediatr Res. 2005;57(6):831–6.
55. Stiskal JA, Dunn MS, Shennan AT, O'Brien KK, Kelly EN, Koppel RI, et al. alpha1-Proteinase inhibitor therapy for the prevention of chronic lung disease of prematurity: a randomized, controlled trial. Pediatrics. 1998;101(1 Pt 1):89–94.
56. Watterberg KL, Carmichael DF, Gerdes JS, Werner S, Backstrom C, Murphy S. Secretory leukocyte protease inhibitor and lung inflammation in developing bronchopulmonary dysplasia. J Pediatr. 1994;125(2):264–9.
57. Saugstad OD. Oxidative stress in the newborn—a 30-year perspective. Biol Neonate. 2005;88:228–36.
58. Pitkänen OM, Hallman M, Andersson SM. Correlation of free oxygen radical-induced lipid peroxidation with outcome in very low birth weight infants. J Pediatr. 1990;116(5):760–4.
59. Clement A, Chadelat K, Sardet A, Grimfeld A, Tournier G. Alveolar macrophage status in bronchopulmonary dysplasia. Pediatr Res. 1988;23(5):470–3.
60. Contreras M, Hariharan N, Lewandoski JR, et al. Bronchoalveolar oxyradical inflammatory elements herald bronchopulmonary dysplasia. Crit Care Med. 1996;24:29–37.
61. Thompson A, Bhandari V. Pulmonary biomarkers of bronchopulmonary dysplasia. Biomarker Insights. 2008;3:361–73.
62. Frank L, Sosenko IR. Development of lung antioxidant enzyme system in late gestation: possible implications for the prematurely born infant. J Pediatr. 1987;110:9–14.
63. Autor AP, Frank L, Roberts RJ. Developmental characteristics of pulmonary superoxide dismutase: relationship to idiopathic respiratory distress syndrome. Pediatr Res. 1976;10:154–8.
64. Sunday ME, Yoder BA, Cuttitta F, et al. Bombesin-like peptide mediates lung injury in a baboon model of bronchopulmonary dysplasia. J Clin Invest. 1998;102:584–94.
65. Cullen A, Van Marter LJ, Allred EN, et al. Urine bombesin-like peptide elevation precedes clinical evidence of bronchopulmonary dysplasia. Am J Respir Crit Care Med. 2002;165:1093–7.
66. Subramaniam M, Sugiyama K, Coy DH, et al. Bombesin-like peptides and mast cell responses: relevance to bronchopulmonary dysplasia? Am J Respir Crit Care Med. 2003;168:601–11.

67. Davis JM, Parad RB, Michele T, Allred E, Price A, Rosenfeld W, North American Recombinant Human CuZnSOD Study Group. Pulmonary outcome at 1 year corrected age in premature infants treated at birth with recombinant human CuZn superoxide dismutase. Pediatrics. 2003;111(3):469–76.
68. Ahola T, Lapatto R, Raivio KO, Selander B, Stigson L, Jonsson B, et al. N-acetylcysteine does not prevent bronchopulmonary dysplasia in immature infants: a randomized controlled trial. J Pediatr. 2003;143:713–9.
69. Spits H, de Waal Malefyt R. Functional characterization of human IL-10. Int Arch Allergy Immunol. 1992;99:8–15.
70. Jones CA, Cayabyab RG, Kwong KY, et al. Undetectable interleukin (IL)-10 and persistent IL-8 expression early in hyaline membrane disease: a possible developmental basis for the predisposition to chronic lung inflammation in preterm newborns. Pediatr Res. 1996;39:966–75.
71. Blahnik MJ, Ramanathan R, Riley CR, Minoo P. Lipopolysaccharide-induced tumor necrosis factor-alpha and IL-10 production by lung macrophages from preterm and term neonates. Pediatr Res. 2001;50:726–31.
72. Beresford MW, Shaw NJ. Detectable IL-8 and IL-10 in bronchoalveolar lavage fluid from preterm infants ventilated for respiratory distress syndrome. Pediatr Res. 2002;52:973–8.
73. Bernard A, Roels H, Lauwerys R, et al. Human urinary protein 1: evidence for identity with the Clara cell protein and occurrence in respiratory tract and urogenital secretions. Clin Chim Acta. 1992;207:239–49.
74. Ramsay PL, DeMayo FJ, Hegemier SE, et al. Clara cell secretory protein oxidation and expression in premature infants who develop bronchopulmonary dysplasia. Am J Respir Crit Care Med. 2001;164:155–61.
75. Zhang ZQ, Huang XM, Lu H. Early biomarkers as predictors for bronchopulmonary dysplasia in preterm infants: a systematic review. Eur J Pediatr. 2014;173(1):15–23.
76. Wolfson MR, Funanage VL, Kirwin SM, Pilon AL, Shashikant BN, Miller TL, Shaffer TH. Recombinant human Clara cell secretory protein treatment increases lung mRNA expression of surfactant proteins and vascular endothelial growth factor in a premature lamb model of respiratory distress syndrome. Am J Perinatol. 2008;25(10):637–45.
77. Levine CR, Gewolb IH, Allen K, Welch RW, Melby JM, Pollack S, et al. The safety, pharmacokinetics, and anti-inflammatory effects of intratracheal recombinant human Clara cell protein in premature infants with respiratory distress syndrome. Pediatr Res. 2005;58:15–21.
78. Gross I, Wilson CM, Ingleson LD, et al. The influence of hormones on the biochemical development of fetal rat lung in organ culture. I Estrogen. Biochim Biophys Acta. 1979;575:375–83.
79. Thebaud B. Angiogenesis in lung development, injury and repair: implications for chronic lung disease of prematurity. Neonatology. 2007;91:291–7.
80. Been JV, Debeer A, van Iwaarden JF, Kloosterboer N, Passos VL, Naulaers G, Zimmermann LJ. Early alterations of growth factor patterns in bronchoalveolar lavage fluid from preterm infants developing bronchopulmonary dysplasia. Pediatr Res. 2010;67(1):83–9.
81. Bhandari A, Bhandari V. Biomarkers in bronchopulmonary dysplasia. Paediatr Respir Rev. 2013;14(3):173–9.
82. Buckley S, Shi W, Barsky L, Warburton D. TGF-beta signaling promotes survival and repair in rat alveolar epithelial type 2 cells during recovery after hyperoxic injury. Am J Physiol Lung Cell Mol Physiol. 2008;294:L739–48.
83. Sime PJ, Xing Z, Graham FL, et al. Adenovector-mediated gene transfer of active transforming growth factor-beta1 induces prolonged severe fibrosis in rat lung. J Clin Invest. 1997;100:768–76.
84. Gauldie J, Galt T, Bonniaud P, Robbins C, Kelly M, Warburton D. Transfer of the active form of transforming growth factor-beta 1 gene to newborn rat lung induces changes consistent with bronchopulmonary dysplasia. Am J Pathol. 2003;163:2575–84.
85. Lecart C, Cayabyab R, Buckley S, et al. Bioactive transforming growth factor-beta in the lungs of extremely low birthweight neonates predicts the need for home oxygen supplementation. Biol Neonate. 2000;77:217–23.

86. Fehrholz M, Speer CP, Kunzmann S. Caffeine and rolipram affect Smad signalling and TGF-β1 stimulated CTGF and transgelin expression in lung epithelial cells. PLoS One. 2014;9(5):e97357.
87. Kramer EL, Deutsch GH, Sartor MA, Hardie WD, Ikegami M, Korfhagen TR, Le Cras TD. Perinatal increases in TGF-{alpha} disrupt the saccular phase of lung morphogenesis and cause remodeling: microarray analysis. Am J Physiol Lung Cell Mol Physiol. 2007;293:L314–27.
88. Minami S, Iwamoto R, Mekada E. HB-EGF decelerates cell proliferation synergistically with TGFalpha in perinatal distal lung development. Dev Dyn. 2008;237:247–58.
89. Rehan VK, Torday JS. Lower parathyroid hormone-related protein content of tracheal aspirates in very low birth weight infants who develop bronchopulmonary dysplasia. Pediatr Res. 2006;60(2):216–20.
90. Cerny L, Torday JS, Rehan VK. Prevention and treatment of bronchopulmonary dysplasia: contemporary status and future outlook. Lung. 2008;186(2):75–89.
91. Wang K, Huang X, Lu H, Zhang Z. A comparison of KL-6 and Clara cell protein as markers for predicting bronchopulmonary dysplasia in preterm infants. Dis Markers. 2014;2014:736536.
92. Zhu Y, Fu J, You K, Jin L, Wang M, Lu D, Xue X. Changes in pulmonary tissue structure and KL-6/MUC1 expression in a newborn rat model of hyperoxia-induced bronchopulmonary dysplasia. Exp Lung Res. 2013;39(10):417–26.
93. Bhandari V, Choo-Wing R, Lee CG, et al. Hyperoxia causes angiopoietin 2-mediated acute lung injury and necrotic cell death. Nat Med. 2006;12(11):1286–93.
94. Aghai Z, Faqiri S, Saslow J, Nakhla T, Farhath S, Kumar A, et al. Angiopoietin 2 concentrations in infants developing bronchopulmonary dysplasia: attenuation with dexamethasone. J Perinatol. 2008;28:148–55.

Chapter 8
Pathology of Bronchopulmonary Dysplasia

Monique E. De Paepe

Introduction

The pulmonary pathology of surviving premature infants over the past half century faithfully reflects contemporaneous neonatal management practices. The introduction of mechanical ventilation for newborns in the 1960s allowed survival of relatively preterm infants (saccular stage of lung development), but led to a fulminant fibroproliferative and inflammatory injury response, as described by Northway [1]. Introduction of exogenous surfactant and antenatal steroid administration in the 1990s associated with improved ventilation strategies and better nutrition, allowed survival at very young age (late canalicular/early saccular stage of development). This modified the pulmonary phenotype to a less fibroproliferative condition with as the main characteristic a disruption of alveolar and microvascular remodeling [2].

In this chapter, the major features of lung morphogenesis are reviewed, with emphasis on the postglandular stages of development. We then describe the main histologic patterns of lung disease in preterm infants over the past six decades. From a clinicopathological viewpoint, this time period can be divided into the pre-ventilation (and pre-surfactant) era (prior to 1960); the pre-surfactant era (from 1960 to 1990); and the current "surfactant" era (from 1990 on). Each of these time periods is associated with a more or less typical pulmonary phenotype, namely, Wilson–Mikity syndrome, "old" or "classical" bronchopulmonary dysplasia (BPD), and "new" BPD, respectively (Table 8.1). Finally, we review what is known presently about the lung pathology of long-term (adolescent and adult) BPD survivors. The focus of this chapter is on the human disease, even though important insights into the human condition have been gained from studies in animal models of BPD [3–6].

M.E. De Paepe, MD (✉)
Department of Pathology, Women and Infants Hospital of Rhode Island,
101 Dudley Street, Providence, RI 02806, USA
e-mail: mdepaepe@wihri.org

V. Bhandari (ed.), *Bronchopulmonary Dysplasia*, Respiratory Medicine,
DOI 10.1007/978-3-319-28486-6_8

Table 8.1 Pathology of chronic lung disease in preterm infants—historical perspective

Time period	Lung disease	Clinical context	Pathology
<1960	Wilson–Mikity syndrome [20]	• No ventilation, no surfactant	• Alveolar growth abnormalities • Minimal fibrosis
1960–1990	"Old" or "classical" BPD [1, 24]	• Ventilation, no surfactant	• Severe fibroinflammatory process • Four stages: exudative, early reparative, subacute, and chronic fibroproliferative • Emphysema/atelectasis • Severe airway injury • Alveolar growth abnormalities
>1990	'New' BPD [2]	• Surfactant, glucocorticoids, improved ventilation, and nutrition • Survival at 23–28 weeks' gestation	• Alveolar growth abnormalities • Dysmorphic microvasculature • Minimal airway injury and fibrosis

Descriptions of earlier forms of prematurity-associated lung pathology provide important insights into the plasticity of the immature lungs, in particular the gestational age- and/or insult-dependent reaction patterns to injury. Furthermore, such historical reports remain highly relevant as selected features of "classical" BPD may still be encountered in preterm infants today, at least at autopsy. Finally, a thorough understanding of the wide spectrum of alveolar, bronchial, and vascular pathology associated with prematurity may contribute to optimal care of the expanding cohort of former preterm individuals who survived the classical or new forms of BPD and have now reached adulthood.

Lung Development

A basic understanding of the stages of normal lung development, and in particular of the *postglandular* stages of lung development, is essential to comprehend the adverse effects of preterm birth on the developing organ. Using morphologic criteria, lung development is traditionally classified into five stages [7] that conform to the classical stages of organogenesis, namely induction, morphogenesis, and differentiation [8] (Table 8.2). While the division of lung development into five histologic stages is somewhat arbitrary and artificial in view of the continuity of lung organogenesis, it emphasizes the concepts of progressive phases of fetal lung development.

The *embryonic stage* is initiated by the formation of the lung bud. This epithelial diverticulum protrudes from the ventral aspect of the foregut into the adjacent mesenchyme and branches into left and right primary bronchial buds, which eventually develop into the left and right bronchial trees. By the fifth week, elongation, branching,

Table 8.2 Structural stages of fetal lung development

Stage	Postconceptional age	Major events
Embryonal	21 days to 8 weeks	Development of trachea, major and segmental bronchi
Pseudoglandular	8–16 weeks	Development of bronchial tree up to the level of terminal bronchioles; differentiation of respiratory epithelial cells; development of preacinar vasculature
Canalicular	16 to 26–28 weeks	Development of framework of acinus and corresponding vascular bed: flattening of epithelium; differentiation of type I and type II alveolar epithelial cells; development of distal pulmonary circulation; formation of air–blood barrier; appearance of surfactant
Saccular	26–28 to 32–36 weeks	Increased complexity of terminal saccules by secondary crest formation; interstitial thinning; doubling of capillary layer
Alveolar	≥32–36 weeks to 2–8 years of age	Completion of alveolarization by septation; microvascular maturation; fusion of capillaries

and budding of the two bronchial buds give rise to three bronchial stems on the right and two on the left—the basis for the lobar organization of the mature lung. At the end of the embryonic period, the primitive pulmonary arteries start to form from the sixth aortic arch [9, 10]. The pulmonary veins form as evaginations from the left atrium during the fourth week of gestation and fuse with the mesenchymal capillary plexus in week 5 [11, 12].

During the subsequent *pseudoglandular stage* (Fig. 8.1a), the bronchial buds undergo 12–23 rapid cycles of centrifugal dichotomous branching via complex epithelial–mesenchymal interactions, resulting in the formation of the conductive airway tree down to the level of the terminal bronchioles. At the end of this stage, the branching pattern is essentially that of the adult lung [13]. The term *pseudoglandular* reflects the histologic appearance of the lungs, which on cross-section display hollow gland-like epithelial structures surrounded by a dense cuff of mesenchymal cells. The pulmonary arteries develop in parallel with the conducting portion of the lungs and follow the same branching pattern. The arteries are originally connected to systemic veins that drain the trachea and foregut, but subsequently anastomose with the pulmonary veins derived from the cardiac atrium. At the end of the pseudoglandular stage, all major elements of the conducting system are formed, but gas exchange is not yet possible.

The pseudoglandular sequence is followed by the *canalicular stage* (Fig. 8.1b), characterized by further expansion of the airway tree and brisk organ growth along with cytodifferentiation of the airway epithelium. In this stage, acinar development begins with the formation of primitive airspaces and the apposition of capillaries to their wall, resulting in the formation of a primitive potential air–blood barrier. The terminal bronchioles divide into respiratory bronchioles, which in turn branch to form primitive alveolar ducts ending in terminal sacs. The canalicular stage is

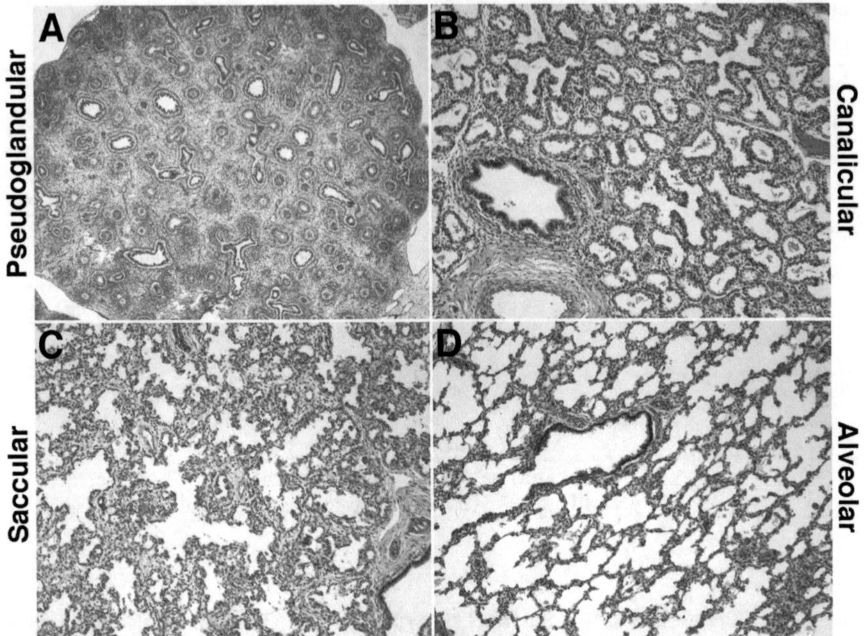

Fig. 8.1 Postembryonic stages of lung development. (**a**) Human fetal lung at pseudoglandular stage (12 weeks' gestation) showing simple tubular structures branching out in a primitive mesenchymal matrix. (**b**) Fetal lung at canalicular stage (20 weeks' gestation). The primitive airspaces are wavy, irregularly shaped, and separated by thinning interstitium containing a dense, often subepithelially placed capillary network. (**c**) Saccular stage (28 weeks' gestation) characterized by protrusion of vascularized secondary crests from the previously smooth air space walls. Efficient gas exchange is made possible by thinning of the interstitium, epithelial differentiation, and formation of an extensive, complex double-walled capillary system. (**d**) Term fetal lung at early alveolar stage (37 weeks' gestation) showing focal formation of thin-walled polygonal structures (alveoli) supported by a single-layered capillary network. [(**a**–**d**) Hematoxylin–eosin, original magnification: ×100]

also characterized by extensive angiogenesis within the peripheral respiratory mesenchyme, leading to vascularization of the developing respiratory structures by formation of a dense capillary network. The potential airspaces are thus "canalized" and approximated by a vast network of capillaries [14]. Through this period, the mesenchyme continues to thin, and the epithelial lining in the lung periphery starts to attenuate with initial differentiation of type I and type II cells. By the end of the canalicular stage, a potentially functional albeit rudimentary blood–gas barrier has formed, sufficiently thin to support gas exchange. Because cranial segments of the lung mature faster than caudal segments, this stage partially overlaps with the subsequent saccular stage.

At the onset of the *saccular (terminal sac) stage* (Fig. 8.1c), vascularized ridges called secondary crests protrude into the terminal saccules, pulling a capillary network with them (or propelled outward by a capillary network) and causing branching of the previously smooth-walled saccules, which eventually differentiate into alveolar complexes. The secondary crests contain a double-walled capillary system. Division of the saccules into smaller units by the secondary crests, associated with a marked decrease in interstitial tissue and a further expansion of the capillary bed, results in the development of a complex capillary network in the saccular wall. This ensures efficient gas exchange as alveoli begin to form at the end of this stage. As vascularized septa form within growing terminal sacs, type I cells continue to flatten and spread, increasing the surface area available for gas exchange. Type II cells, as well, continue to expand and differentiate with the accumulation of surfactant lipids. The end result of the saccular stage is a marked increase in the gas-exchange surface of the lung and a robust thinning of the interstitium.

The final maturation of the respiratory system takes place during the *alveolar stage* (Fig. 8.1d). Alveoli develop as flask-shaped, polygonal structures with thin walls supported by a single-layered capillary bed. Alveolar formation is closely linked to the deposition of elastin in the saccular lung [15]. Alveolar structures can be recognized in some fetuses at as early as 32 weeks of gestation and are present uniformly by 36 weeks [15]. The majority of alveoli form during the first 2 years of life; after 2–5 years, the lung continues to grow in proportion to body growth mainly by an increase in alveolar size and volume rather than further increase in alveolar number. Septal maturation continues beyond the alveolar stage during what is sometimes called the (sixth) stage of *microvascular maturation*. This phase extends until 2–5 (or 8) years of age [16] and is associated with rapid growth of the arterial bed [17].

Wilson–Mikity Syndrome

Before mechanical ventilation methods were successfully adapted to the specific dimensions and physiology of the premature newborn in the 1960s, prolonged survival at gestational ages younger than 28 weeks was exceptional [18]. In the 1950s and early 1960s, many preterm infants died with respiratory failure soon after birth and showed hyaline membrane disease at autopsy. In 1960, Wilson and Mikity [19] reported a chronic pulmonary syndrome in a small cohort of surviving very small premature infants. This early report was followed by a larger series of infants with this condition, by this time formally designated “Wilson–Mikity syndrome” [20], as well as smaller case reports worldwide [18]. Wilson–Mikity syndrome was observed around two weeks after birth in very premature infants (average birth weight of 1280 g) [19, 20]. These infants usually had little or no oxygen requirements initially, but later required increasing supplemental oxygen concentrations to prevent cyanosis. Some infants recovered spontaneously over the course of weeks or months; those who died demonstrated hyperaeration and reduced alveolar septa at autopsy. Biopsies during the early stage (20 weeks) showed an immature pattern with wide, cellular alveolar septa. Later specimens showed hyperexpansion with reduced alveolar septa. In the series reported by Hodgman et al. [20], histopathologic evidence of inflammation was minimal and only 1 of 23 cases had interstitial fibrosis.

"Old" or "Classical" Bronchopulmonary Dysplasia

The introduction of mechanical ventilation for management of respiratory distress syndrome (RDS) in the mid-1960s was followed by reports of pathologic abnormalities that were attributed to ventilation-associated exposure to high oxygen concentrations, barotrauma, and volutrauma. The first description of BPD is generally attributed to Northway et al. [1] in 1967, even though Hawker et al. [21] described almost identical findings in the same year.

This pre-surfactant BPD, now known as "classical" or "old" BPD, had an evolution of injury and repair that started with an exudative and early reparative stage and progressed through a subacute fibroproliferative stage to a chronic fibroproliferative stage [1, 22–24]. The exudative stage was marked by hyaline membranes and bronchial epithelial necrosis with bronchiolar plugging and early fibroblast activation in the septal interstitium (Fig. 8.2a). The subacute stage showed a progression of these processes with variable bronchiolar obliteration and dilation, bronchiolar squamous metaplasia, peribronchiolar fibrosis, hyperplasia of airway smooth muscle with extension into adjacent lobular parenchyma, alveolar epithelial cell hyperplasia, and increasing interstitial fibrosis (Fig. 8.2b). Chronic or late-stage BPD (beyond 1 month) showed changes that varied from lobule to lobule, with alternation of severely affected lobules with less affected areas (Fig. 8.2c–d). Changes of late-stage BPD included interstitial fibrosis, lobular remodeling, occasionally marked extension of airway smooth muscle into the lobular parenchyma, arterial smooth muscle hyperplasia, and the development of pseudofissures caused by compression of collapsed lobules between regions with overexpansion and fibrosis. All stages might further be complicated by pulmonary interstitial emphysema.

Long-term damage persisted several months after birth. In 1986, Stocker [24] reported on the histopathology of long-standing healed BPD in 3- to 40-month-old infants who had moderate or severe BPD in the neonatal period. In his experience, alveolar septal fibrosis was the most constant residual feature in the healed stage of BPD. The degree of alveolar septal fibrosis was strikingly variable within individual infants, with moderate to severe fibrosis in one lobe or lobule and normally inflated or hyperinflated lung in the adjacent lobe or lobule [24] (Fig. 8.2e–f). This remarkable variability was attributed to the presence of obstructive bronchiolar lesions, such as the necrotizing bronchiolitis commonly observed in the acute stages of BPD. Occlusion of the bronchioles was speculated to protect the more distal lung parenchyma from the injurious effects of high oxygen tension and ventilatory pressures used to treat the preceding hyaline membrane disease [24].

In addition to the typical variable degrees of alveolar septal fibrosis and alternating areas of hyperexpansion and atelectasis, other long-term findings were described in "classical" BPD, involving virtually all lung compartments. In addition to epithelial injury, bronchi and bronchioles displayed submucosal fibrosis, smooth muscle hyperplasia, and increased numbers of mucus-secreting goblet cells [22, 25]. Elastic fiber architecture was abnormal [24, 26, 27]. Morphometric studies revealed a marked reduction in the total alveolar number [26, 28, 29], with deficient new alve-

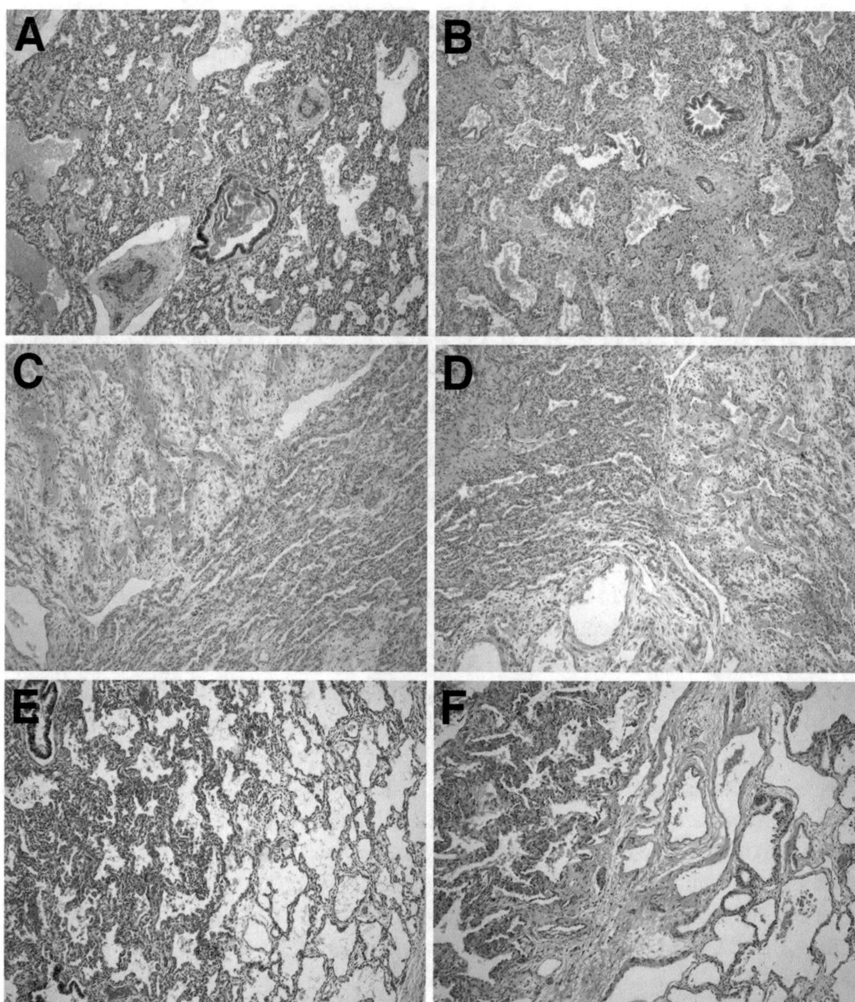

Fig. 8.2 Pathology of "classical," pre-surfactant bronchopulmonary dysplasia. (**a**) Exudative stage. Airspaces are lined by densely eosinophilic hyaline membranes; a centrally placed bronchiole shows epithelial necrosis and plugging of the lumen by necrotic debris. A pulmonary arteriole is affected by pulmonary interstitial emphysema (infant born at 29 weeks, lived 28 h). (**b**) Subacute fibroproliferative stage. There is marked septal widening due to prominent interstitial and peribronchiolar fibrosis (infant born at 23 weeks, lived 15 days). (**c**–**d**) Transition to chronic disease. There is abrupt juxtaposition of areas of fibrosis, atelectasis, and overexpansion (infant born at 25 weeks, lived 24 days). (**e**) Late-stage, healed old BPD. A region with moderate septal fibrosis (*left*) is noted adjacent to a region with alveolar enlargement and simplification, indicative of alveolar growth abnormalities (*right*) (infant born at 25 weeks, lived 57 days). (**f**) Late-stage, healed old BPD. A lobule with marked septal fibrosis (*left*) is separated by a prominent interlobular septum from a lobule with marked emphysematous changes (*right*). The fibrotic and overexpanded regions both exhibit severe alveolar growth abnormalities (infant born at 25 weeks, lived 22 weeks). [(**a**–**f**) Hematoxylin–eosin, original magnification: ×100]

olar growth at the periphery of the lobules [26]. Pulmonary arteries and intra-acinar arterioles showed increased muscularization, consistent with pulmonary hypertensive vascular disease [30–32].

"New" Bronchopulmonary Dysplasia

In 1980, Fujiwara et al. [33] reported the first successful treatment of RDS with exogenous surfactant. By the early 1990s, exogenous surfactant replacement had become universally incorporated in the management of the preterm infant, soon to be followed by the widespread use of antenatal corticosteroid therapy. These new treatment strategies, combined with improved ventilation techniques and better nutrition, allowed survival of extremely preterm infants (23–28 weeks gestation, <1000 g birth weight) with lungs in the late canalicular/early saccular stage of development at birth, and substantially modified the clinical as well as histopathologic presentation of BPD. In 1999, Jobe [2] coined the term "new BPD" to refer to the chronic lung disease of preterm infants at that time.

Largely attributable to the improved survival of preterm infants in the surfactant era, histologic descriptions of "new BPD" are limited and primarily based on an autopsy series by Husain et al. [34] and a surgical biopsy series by Coalson et al. [35], both reported more than a decade ago. Husain et al. [34] described the lungs of 14 surfactant-treated infants and children born prematurely between 1988 and 1994 at gestational ages ranging from 24 to 32 weeks. In contrast to the often severe fibroproliferative response seen in "old BPD," alveolar septal fibrosis was completely absent in 65 % of the surfactant-treated infants and only mild to moderate in the others. The more striking and constant finding in this series was a partial or complete impairment in acinar development, as determined morphometrically by a significantly lower radial alveolar count compared with age-matched controls without BPD. Lungs of surfactant-treated infants showed limited or no airway damage [34].

Autopsy findings likely reflect the most severe end of the spectrum in BPD and may not be representative of the appearance of new BPD in survivors. To determine the histopathologic findings in infants with severe, but not necessarily lethal, disease, Coalson [35] reviewed a small series of open lung biopsies in low-birth weight infants on ventilatory support at a postnatal age between 2 weeks and 7 months [35]. The gestational ages at birth ranged from 24 to 28 weeks and the birth weights ranged from 570 to 1100 g. Simplification of the distal lung acinus with lack of significant alveolar septation ("alveolar hypoplasia") was the principal finding in all biopsy specimens [35]. In this series, the degree of cellularity and fibrosis in the simplified alveolar structures was highly variable: some cases studied between 1 and 2.5 months showed only thin alveolar walls, whereas others showed interspersed or diffuse septal thickening [35]. As in the autopsy series by Husain et al. [34], airway epithelial changes, typical of pre-surfactant BPD, were negligible at all stages of disease [35].

Based mainly on these two landmark studies, alveolar simplification is recognized as the dominant histopathologic feature of the current BPD. In this context, alveolar simplification refers to the enlargement and decreased septation of the airspaces, which, at least morphologically, resembles emphysematous changes in adult lungs (Fig. 8.3). The alveolar pathology of new BPD is included in the most recent classification of diffuse lung disease in infants and children prepared by the Children's Interstitial Lung Disease (ChILD) Research Network [36]. In this proposed classification scheme for pediatric diffuse lung disease, prematurity-related chronic lung disease (BPD) is listed under a general pathologic category of "growth abnormalities" reflecting deficient alveolarization [36].

In view of the tight correlation and developmental interdependence between microvasculature, epithelium, and interstitial matrix during lung morphogenesis [37–41], disruption of microvascular development in premature lungs has been implicated in the dysregulation of alveolar development that is characteristic of new BPD, leading to the "vascular hypothesis" of BPD [42, 43]. Most, if not all, studies describing the distal lung vasculature in new BPD have found the pulmonary microvasculature to be structurally abnormal, variably described as dysmorphic, decreased in extent, abnormally distributed, abnormally centrally positioned within septa, or immature and non-sprouting, reminiscent of the microvasculature during the saccular stage of development [34, 35, 44–46]. While there is uniform agreement that the pulmonary microvasculature in new BPD is structurally abnormal (i.e., dysmorphic) (Fig. 8.4), it remains unsettled whether the underlying mechanism is arrested or aberrant, dysregulated angiogenesis ('dysangiogenesis') [44–47]. This may be explained, in part, by differences in use or interpretation of morphometric and biochemical techniques [45].

Alveolar simplification and dysmorphic microvasculature are the hallmark histologic features of new BPD. Additional reported findings include bronchial and bronchiolar smooth muscle hyperplasia [48, 49], which has been implicated, in part, in the pathophysiology of airflow limitation and bronchial hyperreactivity observed in some ex-BPD patients. Others have described an apparent increase in alveolar lymphatics [50], expansion of bronchial circulation-derived peribronchial vessels [51], and persistence or expansion of precapillary arteriovenous anastomoses [52] in BPD. New BPD further has been linked to altered numbers of pulmonary neuroendocrine cells [53, 54] and increased distal acinar arterial muscularization in severe cases [47].

Long Term Pathology of 'New BPD'

As the first cohort of surfactant-treated former BPD patients has reached adulthood, it has become increasingly more relevant to identify the life-long pulmonary consequences of extreme prematurity and associated disruption of normal postcanalicular lung remodeling. Assessment of the long-term (>10 years) pulmonary outcome of very preterm infants with a history of BPD is mainly based on clinical grounds, as

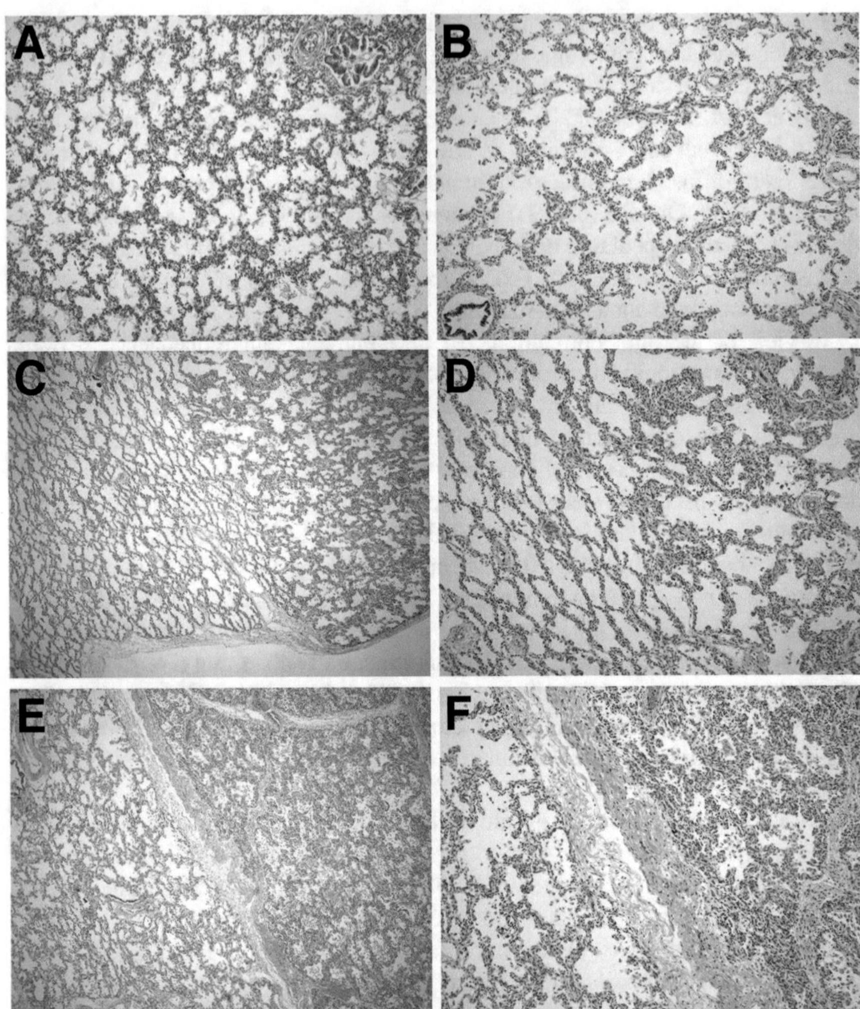

Fig. 8.3 Pathology of "new" bronchopulmonary dysplasia. (**a**) Control, non-BPD lung in early alveolar stage of development showing relative small and complex airspaces, abundant secondary crest formation, and thin alveolar septa (infant born at 38 weeks, lived 6 h). (**b**) Representative "new" BPD lung showing large, simplified airspaces, consistent with diffuse alveolar growth abnormalities (infant born at 25 weeks, treated with surfactant and antenatal steroids, lived 15 weeks, corrected post-conceptional age 40 weeks). (**c–d**) "New" BPD lung showing a region with severe emphysematous changes (*left*) adjacent to a region with less prominent alveolar growth abnormalities (*right*). Depression and thickening of the pleura overlying the emphysematous region correlated with macroscopically observed fissure formation (infant born at 27 weeks, lived 14 weeks). (**e–f**) Left upper and lower lung lobes of infant with "new" BPD. Moderate interstitial fibrosis is noted in one lobe (*right*); both lobes display alveolar growth abnormalities (infant born at 27 weeks, lived 14 weeks). [(**a–f**) Hematoxylin–eosin, original magnification: ×40 (**c**, **e**) and ×100 (**a**, **b**, **d**, **f**)]

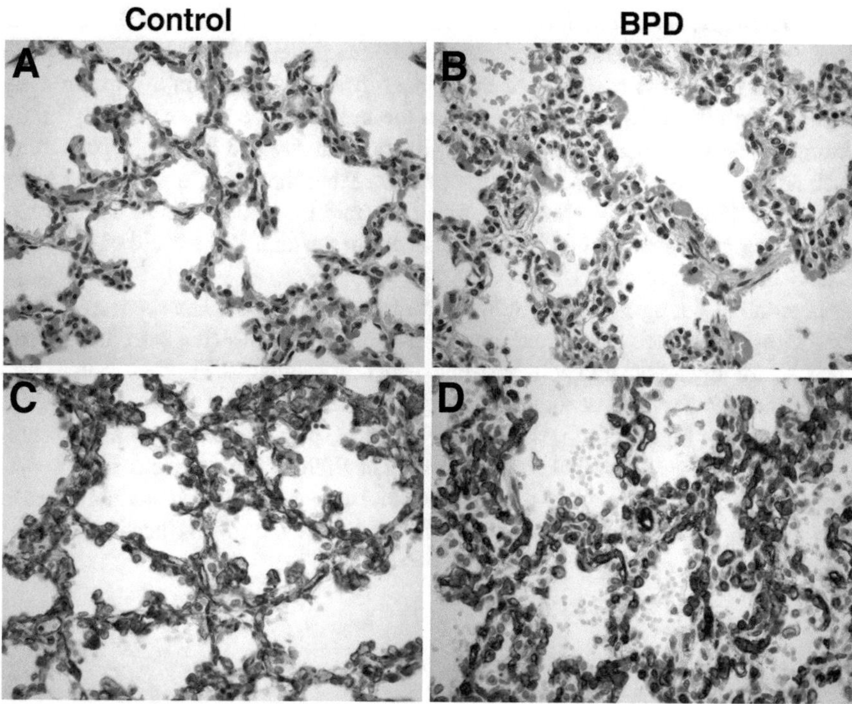

Fig. 8.4 Microvascular pathology of "new" bronchopulmonary dysplasia. (**a**) Control non-BPD lung in early alveolar stage of development showing complex distal lung parenchyma with numerous secondary crests and thin alveolar septa (stillborn at 38 weeks). (**b**) Lung of infant with "new" BPD showing simple, large-sized airspaces separated by relatively thick and hypercellular septa (infant born at 27 weeks, lived 12 weeks, treated with antenatal steroids and exogenous surfactant). (**c**) Anti-CD31 immunostaining of control lung highlighting a complex, variably single and double capillary network with abundant outsproutings toward secondary crests in thin alveolar septa (same infant as **a**). (**d**) Anti-CD31 immunostaining of lung with "new" BPD demonstrates the typical dysmorphic capillary network within the wide septa: the capillaries are tortuous and dilated and mostly arranged in a double-track parallel pattern. Secondary crests are sparse (same infant as B). [(**a**–**b**) Hematoxylin-eosin, (**c**–**d**) anti-CD31 (platelet endothelial cell adhesion molecule (PECAM)-1) immunohistochemistry); all: original magnification: ×400]

pathology data are sparse. Most available histology data do not extend beyond infancy, i.e., the early stages of the disease, with the exception of an 8-year-old child included in the series reported by Husain et al. [34].

The persistence of abnormalities in lung function tests in former preterm infants is suggestive of a failure of catch-up lung (alveolar) growth [55–57]. In support of these lung function studies, occasional case reports have illustrated the persistence of enlarged airspaces with reduced alveolar septation, replicating the alveolar growth abnormalities seen in the earlier stages of BPD [58], although a recent study by Narayanan et al. [59] suggests that there may be some degree of catch-up in alveolarization during childhood.

Interestingly, lung function studies in the generation of "new BPD" survivors have demonstrated a persistent airway obstructive pattern [60, 61] that tracks into adulthood [62]. This evidence of significant airway obstruction after extremely preterm birth needs to be reconciled with the near-absence of overt airway injury during the neonatal period and suggests that prematurity and BPD may have long-term adverse consequences for airway growth. Parenthetically, the case report by Cutz et al. [58] also described changes of chronic bronchial asthma with airway remodeling and peribronchial inflammatory infiltrates in a 12-year-old child with a history of prematurity and BPD.

In summary, lung function studies and rare pathologic studies seem to suggest long-term persistence of alveolar growth abnormalities following extreme preterm birth, seemingly associated with obstructive airway anomalies. However, interpretation of these few reports is complicated by the small number of cases, variability in clinical factors (age at birth, duration of survival, postnatal course, and management) and uneven selection of control tissue. The lifelong impact of extreme prematurity on the morphology of the various lung compartments, including alveoli, interstitium, conducting airways, vascular bed, and blood–gas barrier, remains undetermined at present.

Conclusions

The pulmonary histopathology of preterm infants has undergone remarkable changes over the past half century, as it transitioned from the Wilson–Mikity syndrome prior to the 1960s, through three decades of variable fibroproliferative lung injury ("classical BPD") in ventilated preterm infants during the pre-surfactant era, to the current alveolar simplification seen in extremely preterm infants with "new BPD.".

While reasonable from a clinicopathologic perspective, categorization of preterm lung disease according to these three distinct patterns is inevitably overly simplistic. The transition from "classical" to "new" BPD, in particular, is not abrupt, but rather represents a continuum with a heterogeneous spectrum of pulmonary abnormalities. Cases of "classical" acute BPD with necrotizing bronchiolitis, alveolar cell hyperplasia, and/or peribronchial and alveolar septal fibrosis may still be seen today, albeit very rarely. Similarly, older infants may still exhibit focal or diffuse alveolar septal fibrosis at autopsy, which is generally considered to be more typical of healing "classical" BPD. The mechanisms underlying the variability of these structural abnormalities and the impact of clinical factors, such as gestational age at time of birth, types of antenatal and postnatal injuries, and host responses, remain poorly understood.

Alveolar growth abnormalities arise as the common thread among the three historical patterns of lung pathology in preterm infants. Alveolar enlargement was the most characteristic feature of preterm infants surviving prior to the introduction of assisted mechanical ventilation (Wilson–Mikity). During the pre-surfactant era, alveolar growth abnormalities were a constant feature of healed "old BPD," as documented by detailed morphometric studies [26, 28, 29], even though they may have been obscured by the more dramatic interstitial fibrosis and airway injury. In fact, the alveolar morphology of healed "old BPD" illustrated in some of the presurfactant studies [26, 63] is virtually indistinguishable from the alveolar growth abnormalities regarded as typical of "new" BPD. It thus appears alveolar growth abnormalities have been present in preterm lungs at all time points and likely reflect a nonspecific reaction of postcanalicular lungs to any insult.

Finally, from a pathologist's point of view, it is important to recognize that the diagnosis of "new BPD" is primarily based on clinical, not pathological, grounds. In the pre-surfactant era, the striking fibroproliferation and ubiquitous airway lesions allowed a confident pathologic diagnosis of BPD, even followed by histopathologic staging of the disease according to well-described criteria [24]. In the absence of overt bronchial lesions or alveolar septal fibrosis, the pathologist's contribution to the diagnosis of current-day BPD is usually limited to confirmation of the presence of—often subtle—alveolar simplification. Definitive diagnosis of alveolar enlargement and diminished alveolar septation may require morphometric studies (e.g., radial alveolar count and/or mean linear intercept) [8, 34], which, in turn, require standardized lung preparation and availability of appropriate, age-matched, and similarly prepared lungs. In accordance with the recent classification by the ChILD network [36], it seems appropriate to describe the observed alveolar findings (usually at autopsy) as "alveolar growth abnormalities, consistent with BPD in the appropriate clinical context." It needs to be understood that such alveolar growth abnormalities are not unique to "new" BPD, but represent a nonspecific reaction pattern of developing lungs that may be seen in a wide range of perinatal and neonatal conditions [8].

References

1. Northway Jr WH, Rosan RC, Porter DY. Pulmonary disease following respirator therapy of hyaline-membrane disease. Bronchopulmonary dysplasia. N Engl J Med. 1967;276(7): 357–68.
2. Jobe AJ. The new BPD: an arrest of lung development. Pediatr Res. 1999;46(6):641–3.
3. Berger J, Bhandari V. Animal models of bronchopulmonary dysplasia. I: The term mouse models. Am J Physiol Lung Cell Mol Physiol. 2014. doi:10.1152/ajplung.00159.2014. Epub 2014/10/12.
4. D'Angio CT, Ryan RM. Animal models of bronchopulmonary dysplasia. Iii: The preterm and term rabbit models. Am J Physiol Lung Cell Mol Physiol. 2014. doi:10.1152/ajplung.00228.2014. Epub 2014/10/19.
5. O'Reilly M, Thebaud B. Animal models of bronchopulmonary dysplasia. II: The term rat models. Am J Physiol Lung Cell Mol Physiol. 2014. doi:10.1152/ajplung.00160.2014. Epub 2014/10/12.
6. Yoder BA, Coalson JJ. Animal models of bronchopulmonary dysplasia. V: The preterm baboon models. Am J Physiol Lung Cell Mol Physiol. 2014. doi:10.1152/ajplung.00171.2014. Epub 2014/10/05.
7. Burri PH. Structural aspects of prenatal and postnatal development and growth of the lung. In: McDonald JA, editor. Lung growth and development. New York: Marcel Dekker; 1997. p. 1–36.

8. De Paepe ME. Lung growth and development. In: Churg AM, Myers JL, Tazelaar HD, Wright JL, editors. Thurlbeck's pathology of the lung. 3rd ed. New York: Thieme Medical; 2005.
9. Hislop A, Reid L. Intra-pulmonary arterial development during fetal life-branching pattern and structure. J Anat. 1972;113(1):35–48.
10. Hall SM, Hislop AA, Pierce CM, Haworth SG. Prenatal origins of human intrapulmonary arteries: formation and smooth muscle maturation. Am J Respir Cell Mol Biol. 2000;23(2): 194–203.
11. Hislop A, Reid L. Fetal and childhood development of the intrapulmonary veins in man—branching pattern and structure. Thorax. 1973;28(3):313–9.
12. Hall SM, Hislop AA, Haworth SG. Origin, differentiation, and maturation of human pulmonary veins. Am J Respir Cell Mol Biol. 2002;26(3):333–40.
13. Bucher U, Reid LM. Development of intrasegmental bronchial tree: the pattern of branching and development of cartilage at various stages of intra-uterine life. Thorax. 1961; 16:207–18.
14. Boyden EA. The programming of canalization in fetal lungs of man and monkey. Am J Anat. 1976;145(1):125–7.
15. Langston C, Kida K, Reed M, Thurlbeck WM. Human lung growth in late gestation and in the neonate. Am Rev Respir Dis. 1984;129(4):607–13.
16. Zeltner TB, Burri PH. The postnatal development and growth of the human lung. II Morphology. Respir Physiol. 1987;67(3):269–82.
17. Davies G, Reid L. Growth of the alveoli and pulmonary arteries in childhood. Thorax. 1970;25(6):669–81.
18. Philip AG. Chronic lung disease of prematurity: a short history. Semin Fetal Neonatal Med. 2009;14(6):333–8. Epub 2009/08/25.
19. Wilson MG, Mikity VG. A new form of respiratory disease in premature infants. AMA J Dis Child. 1960;99:489–99. Epub 1960/04/01.
20. Hodgman JE, Mikity VG, Tatter D, Cleland RS. Chronic respiratory distress in the premature infant. Wilson-Mikity syndrome. Pediatrics. 1969;44(2):179–95. Epub 1969/08/01.
21. Hawker JM, Reynolds EO, Taghizadeh A. Pulmonary surface tension and pathological changes in infants dying after respirator treatment for severe hyaline membrane disease. Lancet. 1967;2(7506):75–7. Epub 1967/07/08.
22. Bonikos DS, Bensch KG, Northway Jr WH, Edwards DK. Bronchopulmonary dysplasia: the pulmonary pathologic sequel of necrotizing bronchiolitis and pulmonary fibrosis. Hum Pathol. 1976;7(6):643–66.
23. Anderson WR, Engel RR. Cardiopulmonary sequelae of reparative stages of bronchopulmonary dysplasia. Arch Pathol Lab Med. 1983;107(11):603–8. Epub 1983/11/01.
24. Stocker JT. Pathologic features of long-standing "healed" bronchopulmonary dysplasia: a study of 28 3- to 40-month-old infants. Hum Pathol. 1986;17(9):943–61. Epub 1986/09/01.
25. Lee RM, O'Brodovich H. Airway epithelial damage in premature infants with respiratory failure. Am Rev Respir Dis. 1988;137(2):450–7. Epub 1988/02/01.
26. Margraf LR, Tomashefski Jr JF, Bruce MC, Dahms BB. Morphometric analysis of the lung in bronchopulmonary dysplasia. Am Rev Respir Dis. 1991;143(2):391–400.
27. Takemura T, Akamatsu H. Ultrastructural study on the pulmonary parenchyma of the neonates following prolonged mechanical ventilation. Acta Pathol Jpn. 1987;37(7):1115–26. Epub 1987/07/01.
28. Hislop AA, Wigglesworth JS, Desai R, Aber V. The effects of preterm delivery and mechanical ventilation on human lung growth. Early Hum Dev. 1987;15(3):147–64. Epub 1987/05/01.
29. Sobonya RE, Logvinoff MM, Taussig LM, Theriault A. Morphometric analysis of the lung in prolonged bronchopulmonary dysplasia. Pediatr Res. 1982;16(11):969–72. Epub 1982/11/01.
30. Bush A, Busst CM, Knight WB, Hislop AA, Haworth SG, Shinebourne EA. Changes in pulmonary circulation in severe bronchopulmonary dysplasia. Arch Dis Child. 1990;65(7):739–45. Epub 1990/07/01.
31. Reid L. Bronchopulmonary dysplasia—pathology. J Pediatr. 1979;95(5 Pt 2):836–41. Epub 1979/11/01.

32. Tomashefski Jr JF, Oppermann HC, Vawter GF, Reid LM. Bronchopulmonary dysplasia: a morphometric study with emphasis on the pulmonary vasculature. Pediatr Pathol. 1984;2(4):469–87.
33. Fujiwara T, Maeta H, Chida S, Morita T, Watabe Y, Abe T. Artificial surfactant therapy in hyaline-membrane disease. Lancet. 1980;1(8159):55–9. Epub 1980/01/12.
34. Husain AN, Siddiqui NH, Stocker JT. Pathology of arrested acinar development in postsurfactant bronchopulmonary dysplasia. Hum Pathol. 1998;29(7):710–7.
35. Coalson JJ. Pathology of new bronchopulmonary dysplasia. Semin Neonatol. 2003;8(1):73–81. Epub 2003/04/02.
36. Kurland G, Deterding RR, Hagood JS, Young LR, Brody AS, Castile RG, et al. An official American Thoracic Society clinical practice guideline: classification, evaluation, and management of childhood interstitial lung disease in infancy. Am J Respir Crit Care Med. 2013;188(3):376–94. Epub 2013/08/03.
37. Jakkula M, Le Cras TD, Gebb S, Hirth KP, Tuder RM, Voelkel NF, et al. Inhibition of angiogenesis decreases alveolarization in the developing rat lung. Am J Physiol Lung Cell Mol Physiol. 2000;279(3):L600–7.
38. Le Cras TD, Markham NE, Tuder RM, Voelkel NF, Abman SH. Treatment of newborn rats with a VEGF receptor inhibitor causes pulmonary hypertension and abnormal lung structure. Am J Physiol Lung Cell Mol Physiol. 2002;283(3):L555–62.
39. Gerber HP, Hillan KJ, Ryan AM, Kowalski J, Keller GA, Rangell L, et al. VEGF is required for growth and survival in neonatal mice. Development. 1999;126(6):1149–59.
40. Galambos C, Ng YS, Ali A, Noguchi A, Lovejoy S, D'Amore PA, et al. Defective pulmonary development in the absence of heparin-binding vascular endothelial growth factor isoforms. Am J Respir Cell Mol Biol. 2002;27(2):194–203.
41. Thebaud B. Angiogenesis in lung development, injury and repair: implications for chronic lung disease of prematurity. Neonatology. 2007;91(4):291–7. Epub 2007/06/19.
42. Abman SH. Bronchopulmonary dysplasia: "a vascular hypothesis". Am J Respir Crit Care Med. 2001;164(10 Pt 1):1755–6.
43. Thebaud B, Abman SH. Bronchopulmonary dysplasia: where have all the vessels gone? Roles of angiogenic growth factors in chronic lung disease. Am J Respir Crit Care Med. 2007;175(10):978–85.
44. Bhatt AJ, Pryhuber GS, Huyck H, Watkins RH, Metlay LA, Maniscalco WM. Disrupted pulmonary vasculature and decreased vascular endothelial growth factor, Flt-1, and TIE-2 in human infants dying with bronchopulmonary dysplasia. Am J Respir Crit Care Med. 2001;164(10 Pt 1):1971–80.
45. De Paepe ME, Mao Q, Powell J, Rubin SE, DeKoninck P, Appel N, et al. Growth of pulmonary microvasculature in ventilated preterm infants. Am J Respir Crit Care Med. 2006;173(2):204–11.
46. Thibeault DW, Mabry SM, Norberg M, Truog WE, Ekekezie II. Lung microvascular adaptation in infants with chronic lung disease. Biol Neonate. 2004;85(4):273–82. Epub 2004/01/24.
47. Thibeault DW, Truog WE, Ekekezie II. Acinar arterial changes with chronic lung disease of prematurity in the surfactant era. Pediatr Pulmonol. 2003;36(6):482–9. Epub 2003/11/18.
48. Sward-Comunelli SL, Mabry SM, Truog WE, Thibeault DW. Airway muscle in preterm infants: changes during development. J Pediatr. 1997;130(4):570–6. Epub 1997/04/01.
49. Tiddens HA, Hofhuis W, Casotti V, Hop WC, Hulsmann AR, de Jongste JC. Airway dimensions in bronchopulmonary dysplasia: implications for airflow obstruction. Pediatr Pulmonol. 2008;43(12):1206–13. Epub 2008/11/11.
50. McNellis EM, Mabry SM, Taboada E. Ekekezie. II Altered pulmonary lymphatic development in infants with chronic lung disease. BioMed Res Int. 2014;2014:109891. Epub 2014/02/15.
51. Ghelfi E, Karaaslan C, Berkelhamer S, Akar S, Kozakewich H, Cataltepe S. Fatty acid-binding proteins and peribronchial angiogenesis in bronchopulmonary dysplasia. Am J Respir Cell Mol Biol. 2011;45(3):550–6. Epub 2010/12/24.
52. Galambos C, Sims-Lucas S, Abman SH. Histologic evidence of intrapulmonary anastomoses by three-dimensional reconstruction in severe bronchopulmonary dysplasia. Ann Am Thorac Soc. 2013;10(5):474–81. Epub 2013/08/31.

53. Cutz E, Yeger H, Pan J. Pulmonary neuroendocrine cell system in pediatric lung disease-recent advances. Pediatr Dev Pathol. 2007;10(6):419–35. Epub 2007/11/16.
54. Johnson DE, Anderson WR, Burke BA. Pulmonary neuroendocrine cells in pediatric lung disease: alterations in airway structure in infants with bronchopulmonary dysplasia. Anat Rec. 1993;236(1):115–9. 72–3; discussion 20–1. Epub 1993/05/01.
55. Balinotti JE, Chakr VC, Tiller C, Kimmel R, Coates C, Kisling J, et al. Growth of lung parenchyma in infants and toddlers with chronic lung disease of infancy. Am J Respir Crit Care Med. 2010;181(10):1093–7. Epub 2010/02/06.
56. Welsh L, Kirkby J, Lum S, Odendaal D, Marlow N, Derrick G, et al. The EPICure study: maximal exercise and physical activity in school children born extremely preterm. Thorax. 2010;65(2):165–72. Epub 2009/12/10.
57. Fakhoury KF, Sellers C, Smith EO, Rama JA, Fan LL. Serial measurements of lung function in a cohort of young children with bronchopulmonary dysplasia. Pediatrics. 2010;125(6):e1441–7. Epub 2010/05/05.
58. Cutz E, Chiasson D. Chronic lung disease after premature birth. N Engl J Med. 2008;358(7):743–5. author reply 5–6. Epub 2008/02/15.
59. Narayanan M, Beardsmore CS, Owers-Bradley J, Dogaru CM, Mada M, Ball I, et al. Catch-up alveolarization in ex-preterm children: evidence from (3)He magnetic resonance. Am J Respir Crit Care Med. 2013;187(10):1104–9. Epub 2013/03/16.
60. Fawke J, Lum S, Kirkby J, Hennessy E, Marlow N, Rowell V, et al. Lung function and respiratory symptoms at 11 years in children born extremely preterm: the EPICure study. Am J Respir Crit Care Med. 2010;182(2):237–45. Epub 2010/04/10.
61. Kotecha SJ, Edwards MO, Watkins WJ, Henderson AJ, Paranjothy S, Dunstan FD, et al. Effect of preterm birth on later FEV1: a systematic review and meta-analysis. Thorax. 2013;68(8):760–6. Epub 2013/04/23.
62. Vollsaeter M, Roksund OD, Eide GE, Markestad T, Halvorsen T. Lung function after preterm birth: development from mid-childhood to adulthood. Thorax. 2013;68(8):767–76. Epub 2013/06/12.
63. Erickson AM, de la Monte SM, Moore GW, Hutchins GM. The progression of morphologic changes in bronchopulmonary dysplasia. Am J Pathol. 1987;127(3):474–84.

Part III
BPD: Clinical Aspects

Chapter 9
Bronchopulmonary Dysplasia: Definitions and Epidemiology

Eduardo Bancalari and Nelson Claure

Chronic respiratory sequelae are a major health problem in surviving premature infants. Bronchopulmonary dysplasia (BPD) is the pathological condition resulting from abnormal lung development following premature birth and respiratory support. Alterations in lung function in infants with BPD are manifested throughout their hospital course as the initial respiratory failure evolves into the more chronic forms of lung disease. The impairment in lung function associated with BPD can persist through childhood and into adulthood [1–7]. Therefore, it is important to have diagnostic criteria that clearly defines the severity of the pulmonary abnormalities following premature birth and provides a prognostic indication on the respiratory impairment beyond hospital discharge. One of the important aspects of using a diagnostic definition of BPD is to identify infants who have different severities of lung disease. The BPD definitions are also used to compare outcomes between groups of infants exposed to different interventions in clinical trials, for epidemiological identification of risk factors and to compare outcomes between centers or within centers over time for quality control and improvement progress.

The following sections provide an update on the epidemiology of BPD, describe the different diagnostic definitions of BPD and their rationale, and discuss their advantages and limitations in face of the changing epidemiology of BPD.

E. Bancalari, MD (✉) • N. Claure, MSc, PhD
Division of Neonatology, Department of Pediatrics, University of Miami School of Medicine, 1611 NW 12 Avenue, Central Building #740, Miami, FL 33136, USA
e-mail: ebancalari@miami.edu; nclaure@miami.edu

V. Bhandari (ed.), *Bronchopulmonary Dysplasia*, Respiratory Medicine,
DOI 10.1007/978-3-319-28486-6_9

Epidemiology of BPD

Premature infants with respiratory failure are at risk of lung damage because of structural and functional immaturity of their respiratory system that makes them more susceptible to mechanical, oxidant, and inflammatory injury.

The term BPD was introduced by Northway and collaborators to define a clinical, radiographic, and pathological entity occurring in preterm infants with severe respiratory distress syndrome (RDS) who survived after aggressive mechanical ventilation and exposure to high concentrations of inspired oxygen [8]. These infants evolved with severe respiratory failure from the time of birth and required mechanical ventilation and supplemental oxygen for long periods of time. The severity of the respiratory failure and the radiographic images in these infants provided clear evidence of their serious lung derangement and poor short and long-term prognoses.

The epidemiology of BPD has changed over the years following the introduction of prenatal steroid therapy and postnatal exogenous surfactant, better understanding of the mechanisms leading to lung injury, and advances in respiratory support. The severe forms of BPD described earlier are less frequent now and have been replaced by less severe forms that occur more frequently as the survival of extreme premature infants has markedly increased.

The underlying abnormality in the developing lungs of the premature infant is an alteration in the normal process of alveolar and capillary formation. The more severe cases are frequently associated with airway and vascular remodeling leading to airway obstruction and pulmonary hypertension that can be accompanied by interstitial edema and fibrous tissue proliferation.

Although the classic forms of BPD are less common today, there are still some infants who have a severe course and prolonged need for respiratory support who end up with significant respiratory failure, pulmonary hypertension, and marked alterations in their chest radiographs. These infants offer minimal diagnostic or prognostic difficulty.

The difficulty with the diagnosis occurs with the less severe forms of BPD when the infants have a milder initial respiratory failure and require lower levels of respiratory support and for shorter lengths of time. The clinical and radiographic evidence in these infants is in general less conclusive than that from the severe BPD described earlier [8]. The radiographs frequently show mainly haziness reflecting diffuse loss of volume or fluid accumulation. Dense areas of segmental or lobar atelectasis or pneumonic infiltrates are occasionally observed, but they do not present with the areas of severe over inflation typical of the severe BPD.

Severe BPD cases were characterized by morphologic alterations, including emphysema, atelectasis and fibrosis and marked epithelial squamous metaplasia and smooth muscle hypertrophy in the airways and in the pulmonary vasculature. These alterations were associated with airway obstruction, pulmonary hypertension, and cor pulmonale that resulted from prolonged respiratory failure.

There are some striking differences between the populations of preterm infants developing BPD at present time compared to those infants who developed severe

BPD in earlier years. Infants developing BPD today are considerably more premature than the earlier cases of severe BPD. In fact, the incidence of BPD, even in milder forms, among infants weighing more than 1000 or 1500 g at birth or among infants born after 32 weeks gestation has become negligible in modern neonatal centers. This is in line with the decline in the number of infants in those birth weight or gestational age ranges that present with severe RDS.

Today, the most important determinant of the incidence of BPD is the degree of prematurity, with BPD predominantly occurring in infants of less than 29 weeks of gestation age (GA) or birth weight (BW) below 1000 g. The incidence of BPD in infants of less than 29 weeks GA in the centers of the Eunice Kennedy Shriver National Institute of Child Health and Human Development (NICHD)-Neonatal Research Network was 42 % during years 2003–2007 [9]. According to a recent report from stratified samples of nearly one-fifth of US hospitals, the incidence of BPD among surviving infants of BW below 1500 g has declined from 50 to 60 % in the 1990s to nearly 40 % in the years 2000–2006 years [10].

The initial presentation of the infants who develop BPD, even when more premature, is more heterogeneous than in earlier years. Most infants who had BPD in earlier years had severe RDS and it is likely that the incidence of BPD would have been even higher if it was not for the relatively high early mortality rate due to severe respiratory failure in those years. At present, not every extreme premature infant who develops BPD presents with severe early RDS. Instead, many infants have only a mild initial respiratory failure that requires relatively low levels of respiratory support and for shorter lengths of time.

The BPD cases today are mainly characterized by accumulation of fluid in the lung, diffuse areas of inflammation, and a striking reduction in alveolar septation and vascular development [11–16]. These changes suggest that the underlying lung immaturity plays a dominant role in the pathogenesis and the clinical presentation of BPD. These changes are compatible with an impairment in lung development but it is not clear to what extent they are secondary to the exposure of the immature lung to gas breathing versus the effects of mechanical trauma and oxygen toxicity. Additional factors including inflammatory processes due to ante or postnatal infections, increased pulmonary blood flow due to a patent ductus arteriosus (PDA), and hormonal and nutritional factors are also associated with the pathogenesis of BPD [17–27].

BPD Diagnostic Definitions

The severe forms of BPD described in earlier years did not offer a major diagnostic ambiguity because those infants presented with a severe and persistent initial respiratory failure, required high mechanical ventilatory support and oxygen supplementation for prolonged periods of time, and had typical radiographic changes. All these characteristics noted within a few weeks after preterm birth provided clear evidence of the chronic lung damage and conveyed a poor long-term prognosis.

In contrast, premature infants who develop BPD today frequently have only mild or transient initial respiratory distress [28–30] and are not exposed to high levels of mechanical ventilatory support or supplemental oxygen. Their cumulative need for mechanical ventilation and oxygen supplementation is often prolonged but not necessarily continuous. This new presentation has created some inconsistencies in the definition and in the diagnostic criteria of BPD [31].

The need for supplemental oxygen has been used as a surrogate for alteration in gas exchange and as a marker of the severity of lung damage. The duration of the supplemental oxygen requirement and the fraction of inspired oxygen needed to keep adequate arterial oxygen levels have been used to define BPD and its severity as well as to predict later respiratory impairment.

Although the need for oxygen supplementation can be a reliable marker of lung dysfunction with obvious practical advantages, there are some important caveats with its use. There is a striking lack of uniformity in the diagnostic definition of BPD among clinical centers and as an endpoint in clinical trials or observational studies. This explains, in part, the wide variation in the reported incidence of BPD among different centers. The indications for supplemental oxygen vary from center to center because there is no conclusive evidence on what is the optimal arterial oxygen level for these infants. Moreover, the need for supplemental oxygen can be influenced by drugs such as steroids, diuretics, and respiratory stimulants and by the use of the alternate methods of respiratory support.

An important issue when defining BPD by the need for supplemental oxygen is that oxygen administration is also implicated in oxidant lung damage that contributes to the pathogenesis of BPD. Unless carefully managed, supplemental oxygen can induce more lung injury and further worsen the underlying lung disease and perpetuate the need for oxygen.

BPD Definitions Based on the Duration of Oxygen Supplementation

Continuous Oxygen Requirement During the First 4 Weeks

In 1979, a workshop sponsored by the National Institutes of Health (NIH) proposed a criteria to define BPD based on a continued need for supplemental oxygen during the first 28 days plus clinical and radiographic findings compatible with lung disease [32]. This definition essentially classified as BPD cases those infants with the most severe and persistent respiratory failure.

This definition was largely adequate to classify the presentation of severe BPD at the time it was first described, but it may not be suitable to the preterm infants who develop chronic lung disease at the present time. Today, except for the most severe cases of respiratory failure, the majority of premature infants do not require supplemental oxygen continuously during the first weeks after birth. Many of these infants have periods of time when they are able to maintain good arterial oxygen levels

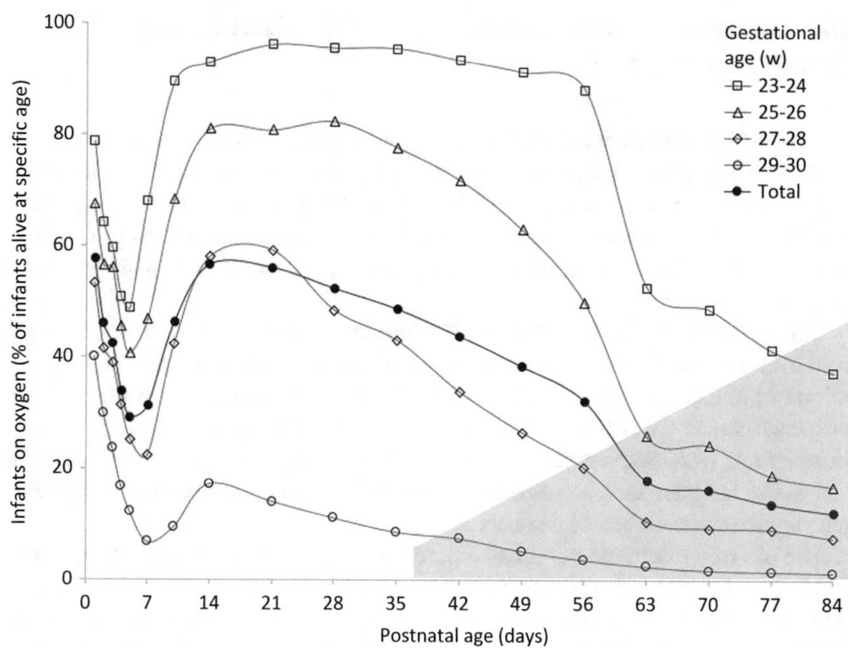

Fig. 9.1 Proportion of infants on supplemental oxygen during first 12 weeks after birth. The figure shows the proportion of infants who require supplemental oxygen at different postnatal days during the first 12 weeks after birth. Varying proportions of infants require oxygen supplementation at different time points during the first 4 weeks after birth with a decreasing proportion in the higher gestational age stratum. While most preterm infants have an initial decline in the need for supplemental oxygen, the need for oxygen surges after the first week or two and remains elevated for several weeks. This is more evident in infants of lower gestational age. The *shaded area* shows the proportion of infants who would be classified as BPD based on their need for oxygen at or beyond 36 weeks PMA across different strata of gestational age. Data from 1554 infants of 23–30 weeks gestational age admitted to the neonatal ICU of Holtz Children's Hospital of the Jackson Health System/University of Miami during years 2005–2014. The proportion of infants are calculated from the infants alive at each postnatal day

without supplemental oxygen. This is illustrated in Fig. 9.1 showing how the proportion of premature infants who require supplemental oxygen decreases at different time points during the first 4 weeks. This is particularly evident among infants of more advanced gestational age.

Although a prolonged duration of oxygen supplementation during the first 4 weeks is associated with a greater cumulative duration of oxygen supplementation during the hospital stay, a brief initial oxygen need is not always associated with a short cumulative total duration of oxygen supplementation. Many infants who initially require oxygen for only a few days end up with a prolonged oxygen dependency during the rest of their hospital stay. The respiratory course of these infants presents a diagnostic and terminology dilemma because they show a relatively mild but persistent respiratory insufficiency that cannot be clearly attributed as a remnant of their initial RDS or to chronic lung changes [33].

Cumulative Oxygen Requirement for More Than 28 Days During Hospital Stay

The use of the cumulative duration of oxygen supplementation for more than 28 days over the entire hospitalization was proposed as an alternative to define BPD. This definition classifies BPD based on the persistency of the respiratory insufficiency and different from assessing BPD at specific time points or over specific periods of time; it classifies as BPD cases only those infants with prolonged oxygen dependency.

This definition differs from that using a minimum duration of continuous oxygen need over the first 4 weeks and can reflect the chronicity of lung disease in the population of premature infants seen today who have varying degrees of milder pulmonary insufficiency over time. This definition is more likely to classify as BPD cases those infants who have a relatively brief duration of oxygen dependency during the first weeks but later have a protracted course and accumulate several weeks of oxygen supplementation before discharge.

The use of a minimum cumulative duration of 28 days of oxygen supplementation before discharge is arbitrary. Although it is a reasonable estimate of the oxygen dependency for most premature infants and may provide some indication of the severity of the clinical course, it does not necessarily describe the respiratory status at discharge. This is because many premature infants that require oxygen for more than 4 weeks are eventually weaned off oxygen and have a relatively mild residual lung disease. This is particularly common among infants of less than 28 weeks of gestation. While a longer threshold of cumulative oxygen supplementation could be used to classify the more chronic infants, it may not be sufficiently sensitive to classify more mature infants of 30 weeks gestational age or higher who may be discharged before censoring time.

BPD Definitions Based on Oxygen Requirement at Specific Postnatal Ages

Oxygen Requirement at Day 28

The 1979 NIH workshop definition has been simplified and many clinicians and investigators classify as BPD infants who require supplemental oxygen *at* day 28. The intent of this simpler approach was to classify as cases of BPD those infants who remain oxygen dependent continuously after the initial respiratory failure. This approach simplified the definition of BPD by eliminating the time consuming task of counting days of oxygen supplementation.

Although more practical and easier to use, defining BPD as the need for oxygen *at* day 28 has important limitations. When applied to the current population of extreme premature infants, this liberal definition is highly sensitive for classifying as BPD cases all infants who would remain oxygen dependent for a long time, but it lacks sufficient specificity. As mentioned before, many infants with mild initial respiratory failure have a relatively brief oxygen need during the first few days and later present with an increased need for oxygen after week 1 or 2. In most infants this increase in the need for oxygen persists for a few days or weeks, and only in some of them the dependency for supplemental oxygen becomes protracted. Figure 9.1 shows an increasing proportion of infants who require oxygen after weeks 1 or 2 of whom only a fraction remain on oxygen some weeks later. Some infants who do not have significant lung disease may require supplemental oxygen just around day 28 due to a transient deterioration.

These shortcomings are in part due to the changes in the baseline population of premature infants with respect to earlier years when these classifications were implemented. The population of infants developing BPD today are born at a considerable earlier gestational age and the 4 week postnatal age assessment time may be too early to be a reliable indicator of chronic lung disease.

Oxygen Requirement at 36 Weeks Postmenstrual Age

The criterion based on the need for supplemental oxygen at 36 weeks postmenstrual age (PMA) has become the most accepted definition for BPD [3]. It classifies premature infants afflicted by a more chronic lung disease that persists to near term corrected age, a point when their lungs are expected to have reached a more complete development. Because this is a stricter criterion, this definition better reflects long-term pulmonary health than other less stringent criteria.

The introduction of this criterion was also based on the assumption that smaller infants require longer periods of supplemental oxygen because of their immaturity, and therefore selecting a given corrected age would adjust for the gestation-dependent oxygen need. The criteria of oxygen dependency at 36 weeks PMA requires for an infant born at 24 weeks of gestation to remain on oxygen 12 weeks after birth while an infant born at 30 weeks of gestation is labeled as having BPD if he or she remains on oxygen 6 weeks after birth. The shaded area in Fig. 9.1 shows the proportion of infants who are still oxygen dependent at or beyond 36 weeks PMA across different gestational age groups.

These are the important limitations resulting from defining BPD only by the need for oxygen at a specific point in time and ignoring the rest of the clinical evolution. Although it is true that more premature infants require longer periods of time on supplemental oxygen, the relationship between gestational age and oxygen dependency is highly variable. Many infants remain oxygen dependent for many weeks and are weaned from oxygen shortly before they reach 36 weeks PMA. Many of these infants still have significant lung disease reflected by the prolonged need for supplemental oxygen and other signs of chronic lung involvement but are classified as non-BPD cases. The opposite can also occur; an infant with a relatively mild respiratory course develops an acute deterioration around 36 weeks PMA and ends up being classified as BPD when the long-term respiratory outcome of this infant may not be consistent with this diagnosis.

BPD Definition Based on Duration of Oxygen Dependency and Need at a Specific Postnatal Age.

Oxygen Requirement for More Than 28 Days and at 36 Weeks PMA

In order to address some of the limitations described above, the NIH organized a workshop in the year 2000 [34]. The diagnostic classification of BPD recommended by this workshop addressed some of the limitations of using oxygen requirement at a single time point or the duration of oxygen dependency as single indicators of BPD. The recommendation from this group of experts included the use of a cumulative duration of oxygen supplementation of at least 28 days to indicate the chronicity of the problem plus it considered the concentration of oxygen required at 36 weeks PMA to define the severity of the chronic lung damage. The definitions of mild, moderate, and severe BPD as per the NIH workshop consensus are presented in Table 9.1.

The striking differences between the definitions of BPD when applied to the same population of infants are illustrated in Fig. 9.2. This figure shows that the proportion of infants who continuously require supplemental oxygen for the first 28

Table 9.1 NIH Consensus definition of BPD (adapted from Jobe and Bancalari)

Gestational age	<32 weeks	≥32 weeks
Time point of assessment	36 weeks PMA or discharge to home, whichever comes first	>28 days but <56 days postnatal age or discharge to home, whichever comes first
Treatment with oxygen >21 % for at least 28 days plus		
Mild BPD	Breathing room air at 36 weeks PMA or discharge, whichever comes first	Breathing room air by 56 days postnatal age or discharge, whichever comes first
Moderate BPD	Need[a] for <30 % at 36 weeks PMA or discharge, whichever comes first	Need[a] for <30 % at 56 days postnatal age or discharge, whichever comes first
Severe BPD	Need[a] for ≥30 % oxygen and/or positive pressure (PPV or NCPAP) at 36 weeks PMA or discharge, whichever comes first	Need[a] for ≥30 % oxygen and/or positive pressure (PPV or NCPAP) at 56 days postnatal age or discharge, whichever comes first

BPD bronchopulmonary dysplasia, *NCPAP* nasal continuous positive airway pressure, *PMA* postmenstrual age, *PPV* positive-pressure ventilation

[a]A physiologic test confirming that the oxygen requirement at the assessment time point remains to be defined. This assessment may include a pulse oximetry saturation range. BPD usually develops in neonates being treated with oxygen and positive pressure ventilation for respiratory failure, most commonly respiratory distress syndrome. Persistence of clinical features of respiratory disease (tachypnea, retractions, rales) are considered common to the broad description of BPD and have not been included in the diagnostic criteria describing the severity of BPD. Infants treated with oxygen >21 % and/or positive pressure for non-respiratory disease (e.g., central apnea or diaphragmatic paralysis) do not have BPD unless they also develop parenchymal lung disease and exhibit clinical features of respiratory distress. A day of treatment with oxygen >21 % means that the infant received oxygen >21 % for more than 12 h on that day. Treatment with oxygen >21 % and/or positive pressure at 36 weeks PMA, or at 56 days postnatal age or discharge, should not reflect an "acute" event, but should rather reflect the infant's usual daily therapy for several days preceding and following 36 weeks PMA, 56 days postnatal age, or discharge

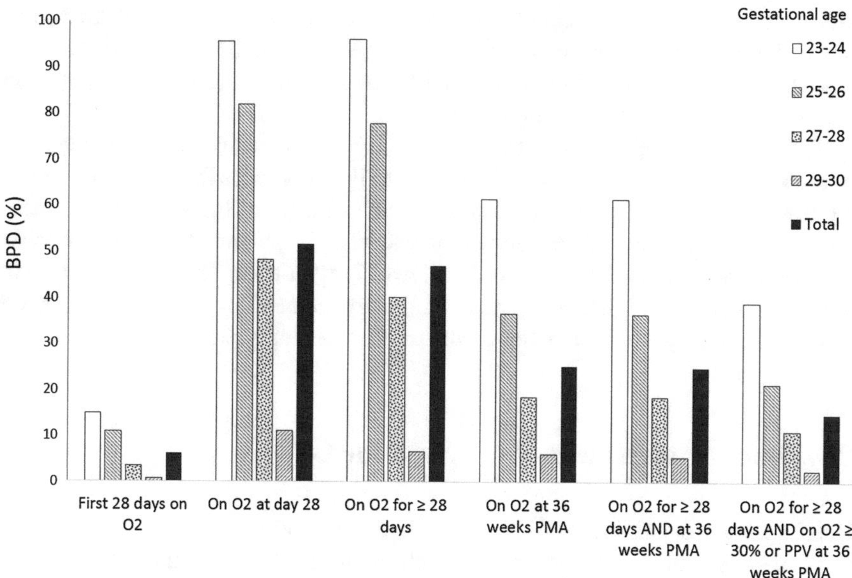

Fig. 9.2 Incidence of BPD by diagnostic criteria across gestational age. The figure shows the incidence of BPD for each diagnostic definition of BPD across gestational age groups. A small proportion of infants require oxygen continuously during the first 4 weeks. A considerable higher proportion of infants require oxygen at day 28 or longer than 28 days. This is particularly evident in the lower gestational age brackets. Nearly two thirds of those infants remain oxygen dependent at 36 weeks PMA and about a third of them need 30 % oxygen or higher at that age. Data from 1376 infants of 23–30 weeks gestational age admitted to the neonatal ICU of Holtz Children's Hospital of the Jackson Health System/University of Miami during years 2005–2014 who were discharged alive

days is much smaller than the proportion of infants requiring oxygen at 36 weeks PMA. Although small in number, most infants who require oxygen continuously during the first 28 days remain oxygen dependent at 36 weeks PMA. These infants account only for a small fraction of the infants who develop BPD, but they often present with the more severe forms of chronic lung disease.

It is also evident in Fig. 9.2 that the proportion of infants who require oxygen at 36 weeks PMA is nearly half of those who are on oxygen at day 28 or those with a cumulative duration of at least 28 days. This reflects the relatively low specificity of using the need for oxygen at an early age or even the cumulative duration to determine the need for oxygen at a later age or at discharge.

Classification of BPD Severity

The NIH consensus definition recommended classifying as severe BPD infants who require supplemental oxygen at 30 % or higher or need of any form of positive pressure respiratory support at 36 weeks PMA. As shown in Fig. 9.2, nearly half of the infants who need supplemental oxygen at 36 weeks PMA meet this definition of severe BPD. In our center, most infants meet these criteria based on their need for oxygen and very few because of the need for positive pressure respiratory support but this may vary between institutions.

The main advantage of using the need for higher concentrations of supplemental oxygen for the classification of BPD severity is that it reduces the ambiguity resulting from using low supplemental oxygen as an indicator of lung disease. As mentioned before, some infants may require low levels of supplemental oxygen because of unstable respiratory drive and not because of lung disease. This is not the case in infants who require higher concentrations of supplemental oxygen reflecting more severe lung damage and is a better predictor of worse long-term outcome.

Physiologic Assessment of the Need for Oxygen

One important determinant of the need for oxygen supplementation is the target range of oxygenation that is selected by each neonatal center. Centers aiming to keep higher levels of arterial oxygen saturation are bound to keep infants longer on supplemental oxygen. In order to minimize the influence of different strategies for oxygen supplementation on the reported incidence of BPD [35], Walsh et al. developed a test to standardize the need for oxygen at 36 weeks PMA when BPD is assessed [36]. In this test, infants with moderate oxygen dependency at the time of assessment, i.e., on less than 30 % oxygen, are challenged by decreasing the inspired oxygen to 21 % and infants who are unable to maintain arterial oxygen saturation at or above 90 % are classified as BPD cases. When this test was applied to a cohort of premature infants from the NICHD Neonatal Research Network, the incidence of BPD changed from 35 % based on the clinically prescribed oxygen to 25 % with the test. This occurred in spite of applying the test to only 14 % of the cohort who qualified for the test. While the overall reduction in BPD incidence was 10 %, it ranged from 0 to 44 % in different centers and was mainly attributed to differences in oxygen saturation targeting. The individual center reduction in BPD incidence not only demonstrated the wide variation in the use of supplemental oxygen but also brought to light the use of supplemental oxygen for nonpulmonary purposes. More than 40 % of the infants tested passed the challenge test and did not require the clinically prescribed oxygen.

Competing Outcomes

Assessment of BPD at any specific postnatal age, e.g., 36 weeks PMA, in any cohort or clinical trial must adjust for the occurrence of other outcomes or interventions that may change the risk of the cohort prior to the assessment of BPD. For example, differences in mortality before the 36 weeks PMA assessment time can change the incidence of BPD in the surviving population. The use of a composite variable such as "BPD or death before 36 weeks PMA" is a statistical technique to adjust for the competing outcome in a clinical trial or in epidemiologic studies [37]. This approach assigns the negative event, i.e., BPD, to those infants who died before they can be classified as BPD cases and therefore, assumes that if they had survived they would have developed BPD. Although this is a valid statistical approach, it is essential that the rates of the individual components, death, and BPD are also reported separately because of the obvious difference in importance. Any change in death rate should take precedence over any effect of a given intervention on BPD.

Consideration to competing outcomes should also be given when interpreting the results of interventions that could affect other major outcomes, such as neurologic development in the preterm infant. One example of this is the use of postnatal steroids that while improving the short-term respiratory outcome can increase the risk of cerebral palsy [38].

Defining the Populations at Risk

An important aspect to consider when interpreting data using a BPD diagnostic classification for benchmarking purposes or in clinical trials is the baseline characteristic of the cohort or population from which the incidence of BPD is being reported.

Benchmarking comparisons should also account for differences in mortality between populations. The reported incidence per total admissions is likely to be lower than the incidence among premature infant surviving the neonatal period, at 36 weeks PMA or at discharge.

Because BPD is largely influenced by the degree of prematurity, the stratification by GA or BW is very important for comparative interpretations between trials or cohorts. Also important is the approach used to define the range of BW or GA for inclusion in a trial or a cohort. For instance, a cohort that includes only infants born within a specific range of BW, e.g., below 1000 g, may inadvertently include a high proportion of infants of more advanced GA that meet the BW cut off for inclusion because these are small for GA. The risk for BPD in these more mature infants differ from that of other infants in the same weight strata born at lower GA. A more adequate approach would be to use a given range of GA for eligibility regardless of BW.

When interpreting the findings of clinical trials or epidemiologic cohorts, other entry criteria that could change the basal risk for BPD should be considered. For example, studies that include only ventilated preterm infants would have higher BPD rates than studies that include all infants. This is also true for studies that deliberately enroll infants at higher risk of BPD based on their initial respiratory course. The findings obtained in those studies may not be directly applicable to infants of lesser risk or comparable to other studies with different entry criteria.

Application of any BPD diagnostic criteria and interpretation of the results should also consider the use of oxygen or other forms of respiratory support for conditions other than parenchymal lung disease. Transient conditions such as abnormal control of breathing, concomitant respiratory illness, and the use of medications such as caffeine, diuretics or steroids can acutely influence the need for oxygen and thereby the classification of BPD. Center-specific characteristics such as the target range of arterial oxygen saturation and the center's altitude above sea level can also influence the need for supplemental oxygen. More importantly, there may be interactions between these cofactors that further increase the need for oxygen supplementation. A recent study showed that nearly half of the infants who failed an oxygen weaning challenge test developed periodic breathing that led to decreases in arterial oxygen saturation [39]. This suggests that some premature infants may need to be maintained at oxygen saturation levels above 90 % in order to stabilize their respiratory control function.

The use of positive pressure respiratory support in infants with respiratory control issues or airway problems, but with minimal parenchymal involvement, should also be accounted for when defining BPD. This is particularly important in view of the definition of severity of BPD recommended by the NIH workshop. Based on that definition, infants who do not need or need low supplemental oxygen levels would be classified as severe BPD if they receive positive pressure support at 36 weeks PMA. If the control of breathing problems eventually subside, these infants may have normal long-term pulmonary outcomes.

This has become a particularly important issue due to the increased use of nasal cannula (NC) flow. When used at higher flows than those required for oxygen supplementation alone, flow can generate positive airway pressure that can stabilize lung volume. On the other hand, when the NC flow is insufficient to meet the infant's inspiratory demand, the presence of the cannula itself can produce an obstructive effect and increase the need for inspired oxygen. Also, with NC there is uncertainty of the actual fraction of inspired oxygen, and classification of BPD severity becomes difficult to assess.

Prognosis for Long-Term Impairment

One of the purposes of defining BPD is to provide a prognosis for long-term respiratory outcome. The sensitivity and specificity of the different definitions of BPD based on the cumulative duration of oxygen for at least 28 days, need for oxygen at 36 weeks PMA, and the NIH consensus definition were recently evaluated in a cohort of infants from the NICHD Neonatal Research Network at 18–22 months corrected age [40]. As shown in Fig. 9.3, the criteria using oxygen supplementation for at least 28 days is more sensitive in detecting post-discharge respiratory complications than oxygen dependency at 36 weeks PMA, but its specificity is considerably lower. Both definitions using oxygen dependency at 36 weeks PMA are more specific but at a cost of not classifying as BPD infants that may later need additional respiratory care. This is in agreement with a report showing discontinuation of supplemental oxygen after day 28 is a more sensitive test (although less specific) than after 36 weeks PMA in predicting poor long-term pulmonary outcome [41].

The higher specificity of the severe BPD classification ($O_2 \geq 30$ % at 36 weeks PMA) on long-term respiratory prognosis clearly shows how this indicator of severity can avoid some of the limitations of the milder classifications of BPD.

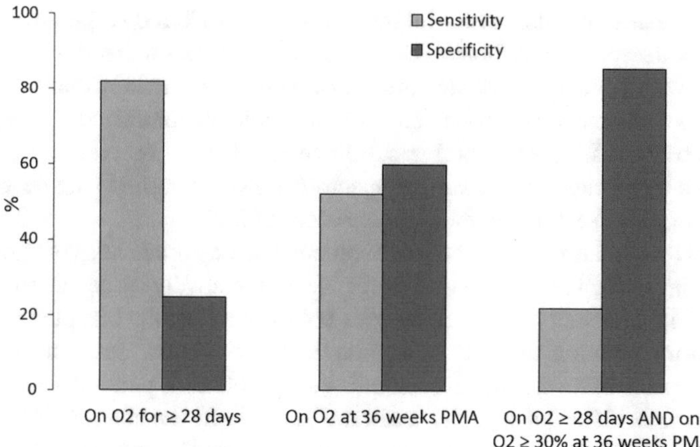

Fig. 9.3 Sensitivity and specificity of BPD definitions for hospitalization for respiratory illness between discharge and 18–22 months corrected age. The figure shows the calculated sensitivity and specificity for hospitalization for respiratory illness within 2 years of discharge for the different diagnostic definitions of BPD. The duration of oxygen is shown as a more sensitive but poorly specific marker of long-term respiratory illness. The need for oxygen at 36 weeks provides a more specific indication of long-term respiratory illness and most particularly when the need for oxygen is high. Data from 3848 infants of birth weight <1000 g, gestational age <32 weeks admitted to centers of the NICHD Neonatal Research Network during years 1995–1999, who were followed until 18–22 months corrected age

This underscores the importance of analyzing not only for the incidence of BPD but also for its severity when doing clinical trials or epidemiologic studies. In spite of this, very few studies report the incidence of severe BPD.

Data from the cohort of the NICHD Neonatal Research Network indicate that the BPD definition of oxygen at 36 weeks PMA is a better predictor of mental and psychomotor developmental impairment [40]. However, it must be noted that the association between poor neurologic outcome and BPD can be confounded by many coexisting morbidities.

The intended use of these diagnostic definitions of BPD has been to characterize the severity of the chronic lung disease and predict respiratory course later in life. However, it is important to consider that these diagnostic definitions of BPD do not indicate that infants who do not meet these criteria have normal lung development and function.

Multiple investigators have shown that long-term lung function in former premature infants is often abnormal when compared to term infants. These alterations are found in many preterm infants but are more common and severe among infants with BPD. Therefore, it is apparent that these working definitions of BPD can identify cases with more severe lung damage from those less affected but its absence cannot assure normal lung function. Most preterm infants can maintain adequate arterial oxygen levels without supplemental oxygen at 36 weeks PMA, but this does not rule out underlying alterations in lung structure and function that could manifest later in life or when exposed to challenges.

The fact that many premature infants present with altered respiratory function later in life, irrespective of their BPD classification, suggests that the lung damage associated with premature birth and the impact of the many factors that can interfere with lung development cannot be defined as a simple dichotomized outcome, presence, or absence. Like most biological processes, it may be more appropriately represented by a continuum across the spectrum between normal lung development and the alterations seen in the more severe cases of BPD.

Arterial oxygenation or the need for supplemental oxygen to keep oxygen saturation in the prescribed range provides a practical but relatively crude measure of lung function. Supplemental oxygen alone does not fully reflect the complex alterations in respiratory function that can be at play in these infants. Tests measuring the different aspects of lung function, including lung volumes, pulmonary mechanics, gas distribution, diffusion capacity, and ventilation/perfusion abnormalities that can be used individually or as a battery, could lead to more specific and sensitive ways to predict lung function later in life. Unfortunately, most of these tests are too complex for clinical use, and their interpretation is not simple. Until more practical and simpler tests to evaluate lung structure and function become available, the only tools available are basic indicators of gas exchange to classify BPD in these infants and to predict their long-term lung function.

In summary, use of standard diagnostic classifications of BPD and its severity is important in order to clearly define end points in clinical trials evaluating therapeutic strategies and for monitoring clinical outcomes between centers and within centers over time. Most definitions of BPD are based on the need for supplemental oxygen to define the chronic lung dysfunction. Although the need for supplemental oxygen largely reflects the severity of the lung damage, it does not provide a precise enough prediction for long-term respiratory outcome. There is a clear need for better markers of lung injury and function that may also provide a reliable prediction of long-term lung health in this population.

References

1. Tepper RS, Morgan WJ, Cota K, Taussig LM. Expiratory flow limitation in infants with bronchopulmonary dysplasia. J Pediatr. 1986;109:1040–6. PMID: 3783328.
2. Gerhardt T, Hehre D, Feller R, Reifenberg L, Bancalari E. Serial determination of pulmonary function in infants with chronic lung disease. J Pediatr. 1987;110:448–56. PMID: 3819948.
3. Shennan AT, Dunn MS, Ohlsson A, Lennox K, Hoskins EM. Abnormal pulmonary outcomes in premature infants: prediction from oxygen requirement in the neonatal period. Pediatrics. 1988;82:527–32. PMID: 3174313.
4. Palta M, Sadek-Badawi M, Evans M, Weinstein MR, McGuinnes G. Functional assessment of a multicenter very low-birth-weight cohort at age 5 years: newborn lung project. Arch Pediatr Adolesc Med. 2000;154:23–30. PMID: 10632246.
5. Baraldi E, Filippone M, Trevisanuto D, Zanardo V, Zacchello F. Pulmonary function until two years of life in infants with bronchopulmonary dysplasia. Am J Respir Crit Care Med. 1997;155:149–55. PMID: 9001304.
6. Korhonen P, Laitinen J, Hyodynmaa E, Tammela O. Respiratory outcome in school-aged, very-low-birth-weight children in the surfactant era. Acta Paediatr. 2004;93:316–21. PMID: 15124832.

7. Doyle LW, The Victorian Infant Collaborative Study Group. Respiratory function at age 8–9 years in extremely low birthweight/very preterm children born in Victoria in 1991–92. Pediatr Pulmonol. 2006;41:570–6. PMID: 22826206.
8. Northway Jr WH, Rosen RC, Porter DY. Pulmonary disease following respirator therapy of hyaline membrane disease: bronchopulmonary dysplasia. N Engl J Med. 1967;276: 357–68.
9. Stoll BJ, Hansen NI, Bell EF, Shankaran S, Laptook AR, Walsh MC, Hale EC, Newman NS, Schibler K, Carlo WA, Kennedy KA, Poindexter BB, Finer NN, Ehrenkranz RA, Duara S, Sánchez PJ, O'Shea TM, Goldberg RN, Van Meurs KP, Faix RG, Phelps DL, Frantz 3rd ID, Watterberg KL, Saha S, Das A, Higgins RD, Eunice Kennedy Shriver National Institute of Child Health and Human Development Neonatal Research Network. Neonatal outcomes of extremely preterm infants from the NICHD neonatal research network. Pediatrics. 2010;126:443–56.
10. Stroustrup A, Trasande L. Epidemiological characteristics and resource use in neonates with bronchopulmonary dysplasia: 1993–2006. Pediatrics. 2010;126:291–7.
11. Margraf LR, Tomashefski Jr JF, Bruce MC, Dahms BB. Morphometric analysis of the lung in bronchopulmonary dysplasia. Am Rev Respir Dis. 1991;143:391–400.
12. Husain AN, Siddiqui NH, Stocker JT. Pathology of arrested acinar development in postsurfactant bronchopulmonary dysplasia. Hum Pathol. 1998;29:710–7.
13. Thibeault DW, Mabry SM, Ekekezie II, Zhang X, Truog WE. Collagen scaffolding during development and its deformation with chronic lung disease. Pediatrics. 2003;111:766–76.
14. Coalson JJ, Winter V, deLemos RA. Decreased alveolarization in baboon survivors with bronchopulmonary dysplasia. Am J Respir Crit Care Med. 1995;152:640–6.
15. Jobe AJ. The new BPD: an arrest of lung development. Pediatr Res. 1999;46:641–3.
16. Abman SH. Pulmonary hypertension in chronic lung disease of infancy. Pathogenesis, pathophysiology and treatment. In: Bland RD, Coalson JJ, editors. Chronic lung disease of infancy. New York: Dekker; 2000.
17. Watterberg KL, Demers LM, Scott SM, et al. Chorioamnionitis and early lung inflammation in infants in whom bronchopulmonary dysplasia develops. Pediatrics. 1996;97:210–5.
18. Yoon BH, Romero R, Jun JK, et al. Amniotic fluid cytokines (interleukin-6, tumor necrosis factor-α, interleukin-1β, and interleukin-8) and the risk for the development of bronchopulmonary dysplasia. Am J Obstet Gynecol. 1997;177:825–30.
19. Groneck P, Gotze-Speer B, Oppermann M, et al. Association of pulmonary inflammation and increased microvascular permeability during the development of bronchopulmonary dysplasia: a sequential analysis of inflammatory mediators in respiratory fluids of high-risk preterm neonates. Pediatrics. 1994;93:712–8.
20. Pierce MR, Bancalari E. The role of inflammation in the pathogenesis of bronchopulmonary dysplasia. Pediatr Pulmonol. 1995;19:371–8.
21. Groneck P, Speer CP. Inflammatory mediators and bronchopulmonary dysplasia. Arch Dis Child. 1995;73:F1–3.
22. Hannaford K, Todd DA, Jeffery H, John E, Blyth K, Gilbert GL. Role of ureaplasma urealyticum in lung disease of prematurity. Arch Dis Child. 1999;81:F162–7.
23. Gonzalez A, Sosenko IRS, Chandar J, Hummler H, Claure N, Bancalari E. Influence of infection on patent ductus arteriosus and chronic lung disease in premature infants weighing 1000 grams or less. J Pediatr. 1996;128:470–8.
24. Marshall DD, Kotelchuck M, Young TE, et al. Risk factors for chronic lung disease in the surfactant era: a North Carolina population-based study of very low birth weight infants. Pediatrics. 1998;104:1345–50.
25. Watterberg KL, Scott SM. Evidence of early adrenal insufficiency in babies who develop bronchopulmonary dysplasia. Pediatrics. 1995;95:120–5.
26. Watterberg KL, Gerdes JS, Gifford KL, et al. Prophylaxis against early adrenal insufficiency to prevent chronic lung disease in premature infants. Pediatrics. 1999;104:1258–63.
27. Watterberg KL, Scott SM, Backstrom C, et al. Links between early adrenal function and respiratory outcome in preterm infants: airway inflammation and patent ductus arteriosus. Pediatrics. 2000;150:320–4.

28. Parker RA, Pagano M, Allred EN. Improved survival accounts for most, but not all, of the increase in bronchopulmonary dysplasia. Pediatrics. 1992;90:663–8.
29. Rojas MA, Gonzalez A, Bancalari E, et al. Changing trends in the epidemiology and pathogenesis of neonatal chronic lung disease. J Pediatr. 1995;126:605–10.
30. Charafeddine L, D'Angio CT, Phelps DL. Atypical chronic lung disease patterns in neonates. Pediatrics. 1999;103:759–65.
31. Bancalari E, Claure N, Sosenko IRS. Bronchopulmonary dysplasia: changes in pathogenesis, epidemiology and definition. Semin Neonatol. 2003;8:63–71.
32. Bancalari E, Abdenour GE, Feller R, et al. Bronchopulmonary dysplasia: clinical presentation. J Pediatr. 1979;95:819–23.
33. Bancalari EH, Jobe AH. The respiratory course of extremely preterm infants: a dilemma for diagnosis and terminology. J Pediatr. 2012;161:585–8.
34. Jobe AH, Bancalari E. Bronchopulmonary dysplasia. NICHD-NHLBI-ORD workshop. Am J Resp Crit Care Med. 2001;163:1723–9.
35. Ellsbury DL, Acarregui MJ, McGuinness GA, Klein JM. Variability in the use of supplemental oxygen for bronchopulmonary dysplasia. J Pediatr. 2002;140:247–9.
36. Walsh MC, Yao Q, Gettner P, et al. Impact of a physiologic definition of bronchopulmonary dysplasia rates. Pediatrics. 2004;114:1305–11.
37. Parekh SA, Field DJ, Johnson S, Juszczak E. Accounting for deaths in neonatal trials: is there a correct approach? Arch Dis Child Fetal Neonatal Ed. 2015;100:F193–7.
38. Doyle LW, Ehrenkranz RA, Halliday HL. Dexamethasone treatment in the first week of life for preventing bronchopulmonary dysplasia in preterm infants: a systematic review. Neonatology. 2010;98:217–24.
39. Coste F, Ferkol T, Hamvas A, Cleveland C, Linneman L, Hoffman J, Kemp J. Ventilatory control and supplemental oxygen in premature infants with apparent chronic lung disease. Arch Dis Child Fetal Neonatal Ed. 2015;100(3):F233–7.
40. Ehrenkranz RA, Walsh MC, Vohr BR, et al. Validation of the national institutes of health consensus definition of bronchopulmonary dysplasia. Pediatrics. 2005;116:1353–60.
41. Davis PG, Thorpe K, Roberts R, et al. Evaluating "old" definitions for the "new" bronchopulmonary dysplasia. J Pediatr. 2002;140:555–60.

Chapter 10
Oxygen Modulation and Bronchopulmonary Dysplasia: Delivery Room and Beyond

Isabel Torres-Cuevas, María Cernada, Antonio Nuñez, and Maximo Vento

Introduction

In the last decades, improvement of regionalization and of perinatal care has substantially increased the survival of extremely preterm infants of ≤28 weeks' gestational age (GA) [1]. Two important consequences of extreme prematurity are: (1) lung's incapability of sustaining aerobic respiration, and as a consequence (2) the need for mechanical ventilation (MV) and oxygen (O_2) supplementation. In a recent epidemiologic study, it was acknowledged that 91.6 % of preterm infants between 22 and 26 weeks GA needed MV, 88.1 % needed O_2 in the delivery room, and 91.3 % in the neonatal intensive care unit (NICU). Moreover, as shown in Fig. 10.1, the overall survival without bronchopulmonary dysplasia (BPD) for this GA represented 32.1 % of the survivors. Of note, the percentage of survivors with a GA <24 weeks without BPD was almost non-existent. Thus, we can conclude that BPD is still the leading cause of chronic disability in survivors of extremely low GA and that BPD is inherent to the condition of being born extremely low birth weight (ELBW) [2].

The lung's capacity to sustain aerobic respiration is not completed until late in gestation. Thus, the lung development of infants born prematurely, especially between 24 and 28 weeks gestation, is in the late canalicular and early saccular stage.

I. Torres-Cuevas, PharmD, MSc • M. Cernada, MD • A. Nuñez, MD
Health Research Institute La Fe, Neonatal Research Group,
Avenida Fernando Abril Martorell 106, Valencia 46026, Spain
e-mail: maria.i.torres@uv.es; mariacernada@gmail.com; aguilllermo9nr@hotmail.com

M. Vento, MD, PhD (✉)
Health Research Institute La Fe, Neonatal Research Group,
Avenida Fernando Abril Martorell 106, Valencia 46026, Spain

Division of Neonatology, University and Polytechnic Hospital La Fe,
Avenida Fernando Abril Martorell 106, Valencia 46026, Spain
e-mail: maximo.vento@uv.es

V. Bhandari (ed.), *Bronchopulmonary Dysplasia*, Respiratory Medicine,
DOI 10.1007/978-3-319-28486-6_10

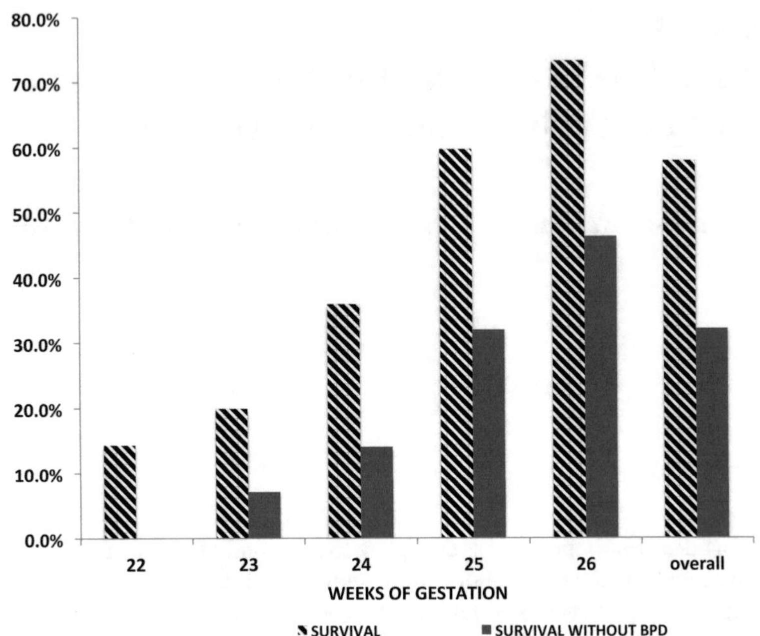

Fig. 10.1 Survival and survival without BPD of extremely low gestational age neonates (22–26 weeks' gestation) retrieved from the database SEN 1500 (Spanish Neonatal Society; Sociedad Española de Neonatología) (Ref. [2])

The anatomic and physiologic characteristics of these primitive structures pose great difficulties in adequately establishing gas exchange. Characteristically, primitive pseudoalveolar structures at this stage have a reduced number of type I pneumocytes and secondary septation and therefore a reduced gas exchange surface. In addition, there is an increased surface tension due to a very limited production of surfactant by type II neumocytes that leads to alveolar collapse during expiration. Moreover, the pulmonary vascularization bed is scarcely developed, and there is a considerable distance between capillaries and alveoli rendering gas exchange extremely difficult. After birth, preterm babies initiate aerial respiration rich in O_2. O_2 availability triggers ubiquitination of hypoxia-inducible factor-1α (HIF-1α), which promotes its degradation. HIF-1α is an essential transcription factor that promotes the expression of a great number of molecules necessary for vascular growth, especially vascular endothelial growth factors (VEGF 1 and 2) and its receptors. The consequence of a decrease in HIF-1α and its downstream-regulated molecules is a slowdown of the alveolar capillary bed development and alveolar secondary septation. The confluence of both these circumstances will cause lung underdevelopment with simplified saccules and diminished vascularization. Under these circumstances, respiratory insufficiency and respiratory distress will ensue. The need for O_2 supplementation and invasive MV, among other factors, will favor the development of chronic respiratory insufficiency and especially BPD, defined as the need for O_2 supplementation at 36 weeks of postmenstrual age [3–7].

In this scenario, different prenatal and postnatal approaches such as antenatal steroids, postnatal surfactant, noninvasive ventilation, postnatal steroids, and caffeine have been pursued to reduce the incidence, or at least the severity of BPD [1]. The association between O_2 therapy and BPD has been clearly established; however, trying to adequately oxygenate preterm infants without causing damage by hypo-or-hyperoxia represents still a challenge for modern neonatology [8, 9].

O_2, Free Radicals, Oxidative Stress, and Antioxidant Defenses

O_2 is probably the most widely employed drug during the neonatal period. O_2 is necessary to provide multicellular organisms with sufficient energy for growth and development. Metabolization of nutritional components such as glucose, fatty acids, or amino acids in the presence of O_2 during the mitochondrial process of oxidative phosphorylation is extremely efficient. Hence, 1 mol of glucose generates a positive balance of two adenosine triphosphates (ATPs) under anaerobic conditions, while in the presence of O_2 it will generate 30–32 ATP molecules. This high efficiency of aerobic metabolism has allowed the development of complex multicellular organisms upon the earth surface [10].

O_2 is present in nature generally as di-oxygen. Dioxygen has four unpaired electrons in the outer orbital that spin in the same direction. This peculiarity confers O_2 paramagnetic properties. Dioxygen needs to be reduced by four electrons to achieve chemical stability. However, this special electronic configuration confers O_2 with a low reactivity rendering it difficult for O_2 to establish chemical bonds with other compounds. Characteristically, O_2 will undergo a step-by-step reduction to complete its outer orbital (tetravalent reduction). Of note, reduction of O_2 with just one electron at a time will lead to the formation of reactive oxygen species (ROS) such as anion superoxide (O_2^-), hydrogen peroxide (H_2O_2), or hydroxyl radical ($OH^•$). Some of these compounds are highly reactive species known as free radicals (e.g., anion superoxide, hydroxyl radical). In the presence of nitric oxide ($NO^•$), O_2 free radicals will react forming highly reactive nitrogen species (RNS) such as peroxynitrite ($ONOO^-$). ROS and RNS are potent oxidizing and reducing agents with an extremely short half-life that will react with any nearby standing molecules altering their structure and function. Free radicals are atomic or molecular species capable of independent existence that contain one or more unpaired electrons in their molecular orbitals. They are able, therefore, to oxidize cellular membranes, structural and functional proteins, and nucleic acids (Fig. 10.2) [11]. Moreover, in recent years the concept of redox code has been put forward. The redox code consists of four principles by which biological systems are organized, and O_2 is central in all of them. These are electron donating and accepting properties of nicotinamide adenine dinucleotide (NAD) and NAD phosphate (NADP) linked to ATP production and catabolism, protein tertiary structure conformation through kinetically controlled redox switches that regulate interactions, trafficking, activity, etc., the role of hydrogen peroxide in redox sensing mechanisms, and finally the ability of redox networks to conform to an adaptive system that responds to the environment. Interestingly, the response to

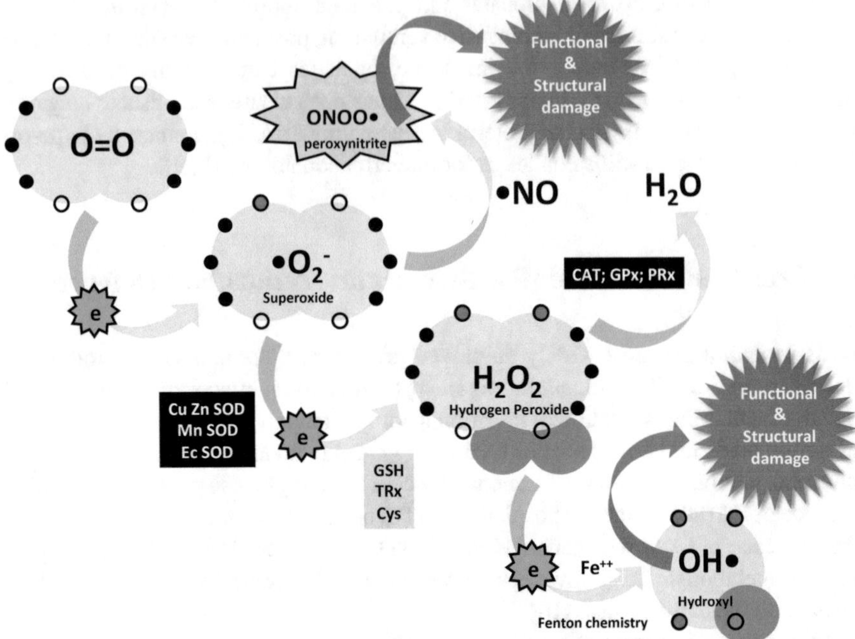

Fig. 10.2 Stepwise monovalent reduction of oxygen leads successively to the formation of anion superoxide ($O_2^{-\bullet}$), hydrogen peroxide (H_2O_2), and hydroxyl radical ($OH^{\bullet}$) known as reactive oxygen species (ROS). Moreover, the combination of nitric oxide ($NO^{\bullet}$) with superoxide will lead to the formation of peroxynitrite ($ONOO^{\bullet}$), a very aggressive reactive nitrogen species (RNS). ROS and RNS can cause functional and structural damage to proteins, lipids, carbohydrates, DNA, and RNA. However, tissues are endowed with an ample array of enzymatic and nonenzymatic antioxidants that prevent or diminish oxidative damage. The most relevant enzymatic antioxidants are the superoxidases family (Cu Zn SOD; Mn SOD; Ec SOD), catalases (CAT), glutathione peroxidases (GPx), and periredoxins (PRx). The most relevant nonenzymatic antioxidants are reduced glutathione (GSH), thioredoxin (TRx), cysteine (Cys), transition metal quenchers such as transferrin, ferritin, or ceruloplasmin, uric acid, bilirubin, etc.

the environment is performed through subcellular systems from microcompartments (cytoplasm, endoplasmic reticulum, nucleus, extracellular space) that have an individual and characteristic redox potential that can be altered individually without a concomitant alteration of the other tissue territories. As a consequence, the older concept of oxidative stress as a global situation affecting the entire economy is under review [11–13].

To overcome the deleterious actions of oxygen free radicals, complex antioxidant (AO) defense systems have evolved. AO defenses can be enzymatic and nonenzymatic in nature. The families of superoxide dismutases (SOD), catalases (CAT), glutathione peroxidases (GPX), and glucose 6-phosphate dehydrogenase (G6PD) represent, from a clinical perspective, the most relevant AO enzymes. In addition, there are a series of compounds capable of neutralizing ROS and free radicals. The most abundant cytoplasmic nonenzymatic AO is glutathione (GSH), a ubiquitous tripeptide formed by γ-glutamine, L-cysteine, and glycine. GSH easily combines with another GSH resulting in GSSG (oxidized glutathione), thus providing electrons needed to neutralize free radicals. GSSG is reduced again to GSH by glutathione reductase (GSH-reductase) with the electrons coming from the Krebs cycle and provided by NADPH (reduced form of NADP). Other relevant nonenzymatic AO are proteins that bind transition metals such as transferrin and ceruloplasmin, or molecules that quench free radicals such as uric acid and bilirubin, and certain vitamins such as A, E, and C [14–16].

Oxidative stress refers to the disequilibrium that ensues in an organism when the formation of free radicals overrides the ability of biologic system to completely neutralize them. Oxidative stress can be physiologic in nature (oxidative eu-stress) and necessary to activate specific metabolic pathways or pathologic (oxidative distress) which causes damage to structures and alters the function of biological systems. Oxidative stress can result from diminished AO levels or AO enzymes' response capacity or defects in the genes that regulate the AO machinery. In addition, oxidative stress may also be the consequence of an increased production of O_2 free radicals, toxic substances, radiation, etc. Preterm infants, especially those who are very preterm (≤28 weeks GA), are endowed with an immature AO defense system characterized by a diminished response of the enzymatic AO defense system to a pro-oxidant aggression [17] and depletion of nonenzymatic AO such as vitamins (E, D, C, flavonoids, carotenoids) or micronutrients (selenium, copper, zinc, etc.) that accumulate in the fetus at the end of gestation [18]. Biomarkers employed to evaluate oxidative stress may directly reflect a pro- or anti-oxidant status (redox status) such as GSH/GSSG ratio. Other biomarkers inform on damage to the cell components such as lipids (malondialdehyde or *n*-aldehydes), nucleic acids (8-oxo-deyhydroguanosine or 8-oxodG) or proteins (oxidized tyrosines, carbonyl compounds). In recent years, isoprostanes and isofurans have evolved as one of the most reliable markers of oxidative stress assessing peroxidation of polyunsaturated fatty acids (PUFA) [19, 20].

ROS and RNS also trigger proinflammatory responses in the cells promoting the activation of nuclear factor-kappaB (NF-κB), a transcription factor for multiple inflammation-related genes and tumor necrosis factor alpha (TNFα), crucial in the inflammatory response as well as in the activation of apoptosis [15]. ROS act upon redox mechanisms, which control gene expression, cell proliferation, and apoptosis. Diffusible H_2O_2 especially, but also other ROS, act reversibly oxidizing and reducing signaling proteins providing a means for control of protein activity, protein–protein interaction, protein trafficking and protein–DNA interaction [13].

Conspicuously, preterm babies are endowed with an immature respiratory and AO defense system. Under these circumstances, theses babies will need O_2 supplementation to overcome respiratory insufficiency but simultaneously are going to be submitted to an intense pro-oxidant status, which undoubtedly will harm especially sensitive organs such as retina, brain, lung, or intestine leading to severe conditions such as retinopathy of prematurity (ROP), periventricular leukomalacia (PVL), BPD, or necrotizing enterocolitis (NEC) [21].

O_2 and the Pathogenesis of BPD

Toxicity of hyperoxia has been widely employed to cause experimental lung injury in animal (especially murine) models of BPD. Hyperoxia causes impairment of late lung development associated with BPD and has allowed exploration of the molecular pathways that become altered during alveolar septation and vascular development and to evaluate possible treatments for these abnormalities. Hyperoxia has been associated with perturbations of growth factor signaling, inadequate assembling of the extracellular matrix, and alterations of lung cell proliferation, differentiation, and apoptosis together with a dysregulation in pulmonary vascular development [22].

The master regulator for the cell's adaptive responses to oxygen is HIF-1, a heterodimeric transcription factor that comprises two subunits HIF-1α and HIF-1β. HIF-1α is posttranscriptionally regulated by the prolyl-hydroxylase enzymes (PHD1–3). PHD's activities directly depend on the O_2 concentration in tissues. Under normoxic conditions, PHDs will cause ubiquitination and proteasomal degradation of HIF-1α. On the contrary, under low O_2 concentrations, HIF-1α is stabilized and accumulates in the hypoxic cell. HIF-1β is constitutively present in the cell nucleus. Under low O_2 conditions, it dimerizes with HIF-1α and binds to the hypoxia response elements (HREs) in the regulatory region of a number of genes, activating their transcription. Activated genes, and especially VEGF and erythropoietin (EPO), enhance O_2 delivery to tissue and promote vascular growth. Interestingly, when babies are born prematurely there is a switch from a relative hypoxic environment in utero to a normoxic or even hyperoxic environment. If the baby needs O_2 supplementation to establish an adequate adaptation, O_2 will promote PHDs ubiquitinization of HIF-1α causing vascular and secondary alveolar development to slow down or even cease (Fig. 10.3). In addition, the enhanced generation of O_2 and nitrogen-free radicals will cause direct damage to the lung structures favoring the development of BPD [23]. The effects exerted by hyperoxia upon the lung structure are extremely varied. Hyperoxia apparently increases the stiffness of lung extracellular matrix increasing the susceptibility of alveolar epithelial cells to mechanical stress secondary to invasive MV or even noninvasive positive pressure ventilation [24]. In addition, prematurity has been related to the relative deficiency of nuclear factor (erythroid derived 2)-like 2 (Nrf2), an essential transcription factor that affords protection against oxidant damage, increased lung injury, and impairment of alveolarization caused by hyperoxia through the activation of the AO responsive elements of nuclear DNA. Moreover, peroxynitrite resulting from the combination of anion superoxide and nitric oxide also play a key role in hyperoxia-induced effects on alveolarization and in vascular reactivity [25–27]. High O_2 concentrations may also alter physiologic apoptosis, which undoubtedly regulates lung remodeling. Apoptosis decisively contributes to the thinning of the alveolocapillary barrier and removes excess of alveolar type II cells and fibroblasts, thus facilitating alveolocapillary gas exchange. Lung exposure to high O_2 concentrations provokes an inhibition of apoptosis in neonatal rodents that leads to an aberrant lung structure with increased number of interstitial cells and septal thickness [28] and even alteration of the smooth muscle development [29].

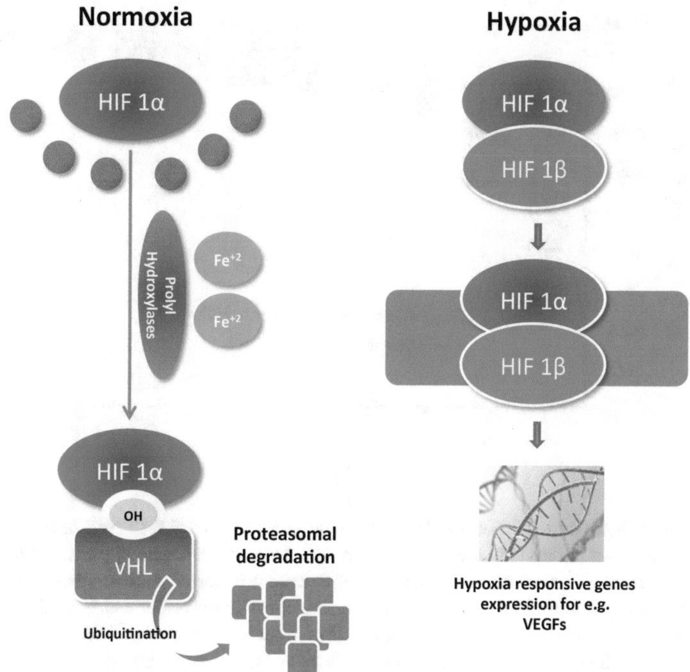

Fig. 10.3 The master regulator responsible for the cell's adaptive mechanisms during hypoxia is hypoxia-inducible factor-1 (HIF-1),)a heterodimeric transcription factor comprising HIF-1α and HIF-1β subunits. HIF-1 α protein is predominantly regulated posttranscriptionally by the oxygen dependent hydroxylation of two proline residues by the prolyl-hydroxylase enzymes and von-Hippel-Lindau (vHL)-ubiquitin ligase complexes. In the presence of elevated oxygen concentrations, activation of these enzymes lead to ubiquitination and proteasomal degradation of HIF-1α. However, under hypoxic conditions when the concentrations of oxygen are below the specific critical oxygen threshold, HIF-1 α is stabilized, thus accumulating in the hypoxic cell and promoting the expression of genes related to vascular development such as vascular endothelial growth factors (VEGFs)

Changes in Oxygenation in Fetal-to-Neonatal Transition

The arterial partial pressure of O_2 (p_aO_2) in utero ranges between 25 and 50 mmHg (3.3–6.6 kPa). The fetus is permanently under a physiologic oxidative and nitrosative stress necessary for morphogenesis and activation of specific metabolic pathways [23]. Of note, arterial O_2 saturation measured with preductal pulse oximetry (SpO_2) in healthy term or near-term newborn infants do not reach values ≥90 % until several minutes after birth. In this regard, it should be underscored that there is a great individual variability and while some babies only need 2–3 min, others will need ≥10 min to achieve $SpO_2 \geq 90$ %. This is clearly reflected in the O_2 saturation nomogram derived from merging preductal SpO_2 values collected for 10 min in healthy term infants' not needing resuscitation [30]. Following this nomogram, international resuscitation guidelines have targeted SpO_2 between 60–65 % at 1 min, 65–70 % at

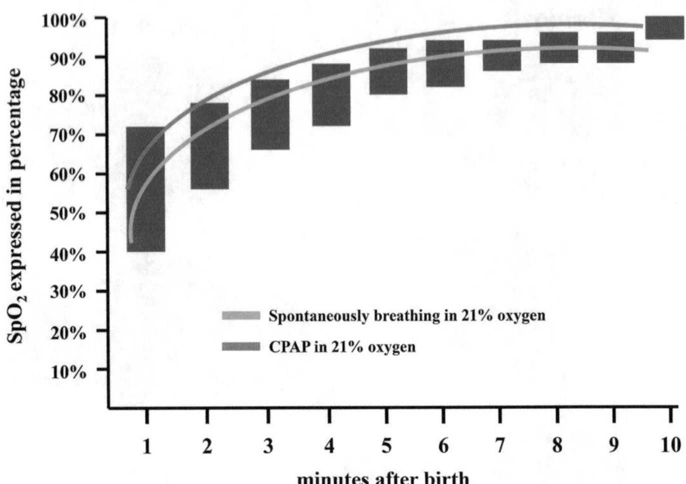

Fig. 10.4 Oxygen saturation measured by preductal pulse oximetry retrieved in the first 10 min after birth in preterm babies <32 weeks gestation who received continuous positive pressure ventilation with face mask and room air. These patients were not treated with supplementary oxygen (>21 %) or require profound resuscitation (intubation, chest compressions, drugs). *Dark bars* represent the range of normality for SpO_2 retrieved from Dawson's nomogram (Ref. [30]). The *blue line* represents the median for preductal SpO_2 in Dawson's nomogram, and the *red line* the median for preterm babies on continuous positive airway pressure (CPAP) and room air. Differences were significant in the first minutes after birth (Ref. [32])

2 min, 70–75 % at 3 min, 75–80 % at 4 min, 80–85 % at 5 min, and 85–95 % at 10 min [31]. The nomogram was constructed with a relatively small representation of preterm infants ≤36 weeks' gestation (31.8 %). Out of these only 75 (16 %) were below 32 weeks' gestation. In addition, SpO_2 below 50–60 % as detected in the first minutes after birth are of relative value since the pulse oximeters used to build up the nomogram have an algorithm that is not fully reliable in these range of saturations. Therefore, reliable values of preductal SpO_2 may not be achieved until 3–4 min after birth have elapsed [9]. In addition, in a recent study it was shown that spontaneously breathing preterm babies aided in the delivery room with positive pressure ventilation of 4-6 cmH_2O in room air achieved targeted SpO_2 in the first minutes after birth faster than babies in the nomogram (Fig. 10.4). Intriguingly, female newborn infants were significantly faster at achieving stable saturations ≥90 % than paired males of the same GA. Therefore, gender, type of ventilation, and the initial fraction of inspired O_2 (FiO_2) should be considered relevant in the delivery room [32].

Cord clamping also influences postnatal SpO_2. Experimental studies in sheep have shown that the initiation of ventilation while cord blood flow was patent increased cardiac preload and improved left ventricular output thus facilitating cardiopulmonary circulation after birth [33]. It could be speculated that under adverse perinatal circumstances increasing the circulating blood volume simultaneously to expanding the lung and reducing the pulmonary vascular resistance could be an effective approach to resuscitation of depressed newborn infants.

However, although allowing newly born infants to start crying while the cord is patent is becoming more and more common in many delivery wards, no randomized controlled clinical studies have confirmed these experimental findings. In addition, it has been shown that blood gases of healthy newborn infants are different if immediate or delayed cord clamping is performed. Hence, p_aO_2 in cord blood shows significant increases in the first 90 s after birth, while no changes in venous cord blood were detected after delayed cord clamping [34]. Moreover, delayed cord clamping also increased cerebral oxygenation in brain oxygenation as measured by near-infrared spectroscopy in preterm babies at 4 and 24 h after birth [34]. For all these reasons, the elaboration of a nomogram in term and preterm infants with delayed clamping of the umbilical cord would provide interesting information to optimize caregiver interventions in the delivery room.

Influence of the O_2 Load in the Delivery Room and the Development of BPD

Postnatal adaptation of very preterm infants is hampered by the immaturity of both the respiratory and AO system [17]. To overcome these difficulties, positive pressure ventilation and O_2 are often needed even in spontaneously breathing babies. However, given the fragility of the lung and the lack of AO response, recent guidelines have advocated a gentle management of the respiratory airways avoiding baro-, volu-, and atelecto-trauma and oxidative damage [35]. In this regard, supplementation of O_2 should be guided by preductal pulse oximetry and titrated as to keep SpO_2 within the recommended ranges [30, 31].

Identification of the appropriate initial FiO_2 ($iFiO_2$) is still a matter of debate. The $iFiO_2$ greatly correlates with the O_2 load received by the patient upon stabilization because titration of the O_2 supplementation cannot be done quickly to avoid alterations in the pulmonary vascular reactivity. O_2 load refers to the amount of pure O_2 per body weight and influences the AO response and the final redox balance upon resuscitation. Hence, in the first blinded studies that were performed in term infants in the delivery room, oxidative stress biomarkers greatly correlated with the O_2 load. Moreover, a highly significant correlation was established between O_2 load, oxidized glutathione (GSSG), and biomarkers of damage to myocardium and kidney [36–38]. The first pilot studies in preterm infants were designed to assess if postnatal stabilization was feasible with $iFiO_2$ lower than 1.0 O_2, thus trying to avoid oxidative stress. In the absence of a nomogram, target saturations were established at specific time points after birth based on clinical experience. The use of room air as $iFiO_2$ in very preterm infants (<32 weeks' gestation) was frequently associated with persistent bradycardia and the need to abruptly increase FiO_2 [39, 40]. However, in a feasibility pilot study by Escrig R. et al., researchers compared an $iFiO_2$ of 0.3 versus 0.9 in ELBW infants and showed that it was not only feasible, but the low O_2 group achieved targeted saturations at pre-established timings, and kept heart rate within normal ranges during the procedure [41]. In a second trial by the same group, biomarkers of oxidative stress and clinical outcomes were assessed and compared between the low O_2 group ($iFiO_2$: 0.3) and the high O_2 group ($iFiO_2$: 0.9). Babies in the low O_2 group had significantly lower values for oxidative stress biomarkers and developed significantly less BPD. There was a correlation between specific markers of arachidonic acid oxidation under hyperoxic conditions (Isofurans) and damage to DNA (8-oxodG) and later development of BPD [42]. Ezaki et al. also showed increased oxidative stress in preterm babies initially ventilated with 100 % O_2 as compared to those who were initially ventilated with 100 % O_2 but FiO_2 was titrated according to pulse oximeter readings [43]. Stola et al. compared the use of progressively lower FiO_2's in the delivery room in three different periods in very low BW (VLBW) infants. Initial FiO_2 was progressively reduced from 1.0 (historical approach) to 0.42 and finally to 0.28. Some well-adapted babies required only room air. No increase in the rate for intubation or positive pressure ventilation in the delivery room was noted. Moreover, there was a significant reduction in the p_aO_2 upon arrival to the NICU and less need for O_2 at 24 h after birth [44]. In a recent study, Kapadia et al. ventilated preterm babies in the delivery room using two different strategies. The low oxygen group received room air initially, and thereafter FiO_2 was titrated according to SpO_2 readings. The high O_2 group started with 100 % and had FiO_2 reduced based on the readings of the pulse oximeter. Babies in the high O_2 group had significantly higher values for oxidative stress biomarkers upon arrival to the NICU, and importantly, they developed significantly more BPD and needed more days of mechanical ventilation [45]. From these pilot studies, it could be deduced that initial FiO_2 around 0.3 seems to be adequate for the majority of ELBW babies, while values of 0.9–1.0, even if O_2 supplementation is titrated according to pulse oximetry readings, promote oxidative stress and in some studies, an increase in the incidence of BPD. Trying to overcome this clinical conundrum, Brown et al. published in 2012 an updated review and meta-analysis of randomized or quasi-randomized controlled studies comparing high (>0.5) versus low (<0.5) $iFiO_2$ in preterm infants <32 weeks gestation and analyzed differences regarding mortality and/or morbidity (BPD, NEC, severe intraventricular hemorrhage or IVH, ROP). There were no differences relative to the main outcomes related to use of a high or low $iFiO_2$. Of note, when trials without an allocation concealment were lumped together with studies with allocation concealment, there was a significant reduction ($p<0.04$) in the risk of death pooled risk ratio for the high O_2 group. However, when only truly randomized trials were included the difference for mortality was rendered nonsignificant [46]. Saugstad et al. published in 2014 a systematic review and meta-analysis which included 10 randomized studies, some of which had not been included in Brown's meta-analysis [47]. The study included a total of 321 preterm infants ≤32 weeks' gestation that were stabilized with a low (0.21–0.30) and 356 with a high (0.60–1.0) $iFiO_2$. Babies with a high $iFiO_2$ had a significantly higher mortality while no differences were found for BPD and IVH [47]. However, in the 2015 Pediatric Academic Societies (PAS) annual meeting, the results from the Targeted Oxygenation in the Resuscitation of Premature Infants and their Developmental Outcome (Torpido trial; ACTRN12610001059055) were presented [48]. This study randomized preterm infants <31 weeks' gestation to initial room air versus 100 % oxygen and titration thereafter according to SpO_2. Babies in the room air group had higher mortality. No significant differences in the other outcomes were present [48]. If results from the Torpido trial were added to Saugstad's meta-analysis, there would be a slight increase in mortality in the low oxygen group given the considerable weight of the Torpido in which a substantial greater number of babies were recruited as compared to the rest of the trials. The authors concluded that very preterm infants should be initially ventilated with a FiO_2 of 0.21–0.3. Thereafter, FiO_2 should be titrated according to the babies' response and recommended guidelines [48].

The Use of O_2 After Delivery Room Stabilization in the NICU

The safety range for SpO_2 in preterm infants needing O_2 supplementation has not yet been clearly established. Moreover, no reliable system to keep SpO_2 within desired ranges is yet available. Fluctuation in the O_2 concentration seems to cause oxidative stress and prompts the activation of specific transduction factors that lead to inflammatory, autophagic, and/or apoptotic responses that cause alterations in the lung, retina, or brain structure and function [49]. Moreover, experimental studies in individuals exposed to similar O_2 concentrations have shown a great variability; while some are highly resistant to O_2, others are highly susceptible [50]. In a review performed by Askie et al., it was shown that preterm babies kept within lower O_2 saturations ranges in the first weeks after birth (<90 %) had increased probability of death, cerebral palsy (CP), patent ductus arteriosus (PDA), persistent pulmonary hypertension (PPHN), or apnea, whilst those targeted to higher SpO_2 (>90 %) had increased risk for ROP or chronic lung disease (CLD) [51]. To establish a safety range for preterm infants in the NICU, five different groups constituted the NeOProM collaborative group (Neonatal Oxygenation Prospective Meta-analysis Collaboration study). Five prospective randomized controlled blinded trials with the primary objective of establishing safe O_2 saturation ranges until 36 completed postmenstrual weeks in very preterm infants (23^{+0} or 24^{+0}–27^{+6} weeks gestation) have been completed. Babies were randomized to low (85–89 %) versus high (91–95 %) SpO_2 ranges when O_2 supplementation was needed in the NICU. Blinding was achieved using electronically altered pulse oximeters (Masimo Radical; Irvine; Ca; USA) [52–54]. Saugstad and Dagfinn have extensively analyzed the results of these studies in a recent publication [55]. The relative risks (RR > 1 favors high O_2 saturation group) when comparing low versus a high O_2 saturation target (low: 85–89 %; high: 91–95 %) were: (1) for mortality at discharge 1.41 (1.14–1.74); (2) for follow-up evaluation using Bayley III scales, 0.74 (0.59–0.92); (3) for severe ROP, 0.95 (0.86–1.04), (4) for physiologic BPD, 1.25 (1.05–1.49); (5) for NEC, 1.02 (0.88–1.19); (6) for brain injury, and (7) for PDA 1.01 (0.95–1.08). Summarizing these results it could be stated that in ELBW infants, low O_2 saturation targeting reduced mortality and NEC and increased severe ROP. No significant effect was found in relation to physiologic BPD. However, the COT trial [54] was the only one in which no differences in mortality between groups was found. In the COT trial, the proportion of babies managed with the old, and the revised version of the pulse oximeter software was lower in the COT trial. Moreover, babies in the COT trial were kept within the established SpO_2 margins more effectively [54]. Di Fiore et al., analyzing the SUPPORT data [52] found that the low O_2 saturation targeted group was associated with an increased risk of hypoxemic events along the entire monitoring period, and increasingly frequent at the end of it [56]. In addition, the BOOST II trial [53] found increasing difference of deaths between the low and high saturation groups up to 70 days after birth indicating that the consequences of intermittent periods of hypoxemia are translated into clinical vulnerability. It could be that duration of hypoxemic periods was longer than detected because the pulse oximeter that was employed overestimated oxygenation [57], there was a reduced O_2 carrying capacity resulting from anemia, and/or remodeling of the pulmonary vascular endothelium that is extremely sensitive to O_2 led to pulmonary hypertension and right cardiac insufficiency [58].

Other investigators who have conducted an independent meta-analysis of the studies to answer the same question have questioned the quality of evidence for the estimate of the effect on mortality and reported no significant differences in death or disability at 24 months, BPD, ROP, neurodevelopmental outcomes, or hearing loss at 24 months [59]. Some recent work has suggested that targeting O_2 saturation between 87 and 93 % improved the outcomes of ROP and BPD, without affecting mortality in the NICU [60]. It is important to mention that setting of alarm limits to avoid hypoxemia (SpO_2<85 %) and hyperoxia (SpO_2>95 %) are important to keeping the SpO_2 between the suggested target range of 88–92 %, with alarm limits of 86–94 % [60–62].

The AVIOX study showed that unstable preterm infants spend a considerable amount of time outside the intended SpO_2 range. Moreover, delayed or insufficient adjustment or conversely, excessive increments of FiO_2 resulted in prolonged periods of hypoxemia, hyperoxemia, or SpO_2 fluctuations [63]. Clucas et al. also showed that recommended ranges for SpO_2 are commonly exceeded especially in the upper limits with a greater tendency towards keeping babies in hyperoxia [64]. Furthermore, Laptook et al. also showed a similar incapacity to keep babies within established limits for more than 60 % of the time even when expanding the limits of the saturation range [65].

In order to avoid oxygen fluctuations out of established limits Claure and collaborators have developed a "closed-loop FiO_2 control system" (CLiO) [66]. Such systems have been developed to achieve a more precise control of FiO_2 for keeping babies within established SpO_2 ranges than with the use of routine manual control by the nursing staff and thus reducing the length and intensity of intermittent periods of hypoxia or hyperoxia in preterm infants needing O_2 supplementation. The CLiO system basically consists of a device to monitor oxygenation (pulse oximeter), gas delivery device (ventilator), and the algorithm that determines the timing and size of the FiO_2 adjustments. The system senses the SpO_2 of the baby and increases or decreases FiO_2 accordingly to recover the pre-established range. Of note, the user previously decides the magnitude or the frequency of the adjustment. The CLiO system has been compared to a manual control by a nurse fully dedicated to adjusting oxygenation targets in a preterm population and has shown to be far more effective especially for affecting periods of hyperoxemia which were drastically reduced [62]. In a multicenter randomized controlled cross-over clinical trial in 34 preterm infants receiving invasive MV or nasal continuous positive airway pressure (nCPAP) and supplemental O_2, 24 h of manual control were compared to 24 h of manual control plus closed loop O_2 control system. The automatic control system was successful in keeping the babies 71.2 % of the time within the established range versus 61.4 % of the manual control. In addition, there was a substantial reduction in the number of manual changes needed when the automatic system was used, thus reducing the workload for the nursing staff [67]. More prospective randomized controlled trials with sufficient statistical power to prove the effectiveness of CLiO to better control targeted saturations in unstable preterm infants needing O_2 are required to not only assess the effectiveness of automatic systems to control limits of saturation prescribed, but also to evaluate if there is a benefit such as a reduction in BPD and/or ROP [66].

Conclusions

BPD is inherent to extreme preterm birth and is characterized by impairment in lung development. The switch from a low to a high O_2 environment and the oxidative and inflammatory aggression to the developing lung are essential to the pathogenesis of BPD. Avoiding O_2 in excess during postnatal stabilization, titration of O_2 supplementation to keep O_2 saturation within the reference range, delaying cord clamping or milking the cord, and using noninvasive ventilation whenever possible have been shown to reduce the incidence and severity of BPD. In preterm babies requiring O_2 in the NICU, O_2 saturation within established ranges should be kept, if possible, at all times. In this regard, the use of close loop automatic oxygen control offers a new and exciting possibility to all clinicians. There is, therefore, a need for randomized controlled trials to confirm if this new technology is effective not only in keeping babies within established SpO_2 margins but also if its use lowers the incidence and/or severity of BPD and ROP.

References

1. Vento M, Cheung PY, Aguar M. The first golden minutes of the extremely-low-gestational-age neonate: a gentle approach. Neonatology. 2009;95:286–98.
2. García-Muñoz Rodrigo F, Díez Recinos A, García-Alix Pérez A, et al. Changes in perinatal care and outcomes in newborns at the limit of viability in Spain: the EPI-SEN study. Neonatology. 2015;107:120–9.
3. Bhandari A, Bhandari V. Pathogenesis and pathophysiology of pulmonary sequelae of bronchopulmonary dysplasia in premature infants. Front Biosci. 2003;8:e370–80.
4. Thebaud B, Abman SH. Bronchopulmonary dysplasia: where have all the vessels gone? Role of angiogenic growth factors in chronic lung disease. Am J Respir Crit Care Med. 2007;175: 978–85.
5. Abman SH, Conway SJ. Developmental determinants and changing patterns of respiratory outcomes after preterm birth. Birth Defects Res A Clin Mol Teratol. 2014;100:811.

6. Baker CD, Abman SH. Impaired pulmonary vascular development in bronchopulmonary dysplasia. Neonatology. 2015;107:344–51.
7. Vento M, Lista GL. Managing preterm in the first minutes of life. Paediatr Respir Rev. 2015 Mar 11. doi:10.1016/j.prrv.2015.02.004. (Epub ahead of print).
8. Buczynski BW, Maduerkwe ET, O'Reilly MA. The role of hyperoxia in the pathogenesis of experimental BPD. Semin Perinatol. 2013;37:69–78.
9. Vento M. Oxygen supplementation in the neonatal period: changing the paradigm. Neonatology. 2014;105:323–31.
10. Kalyanaraman B. Teaching the basics of redox biology to medical and graduate students: oxidants, antioxidants and disease mechanisms. Redox Biol. 2013;1:244–57.
11. Jones DP, Go YM, Anderson CL, et al. Cysteine/cystine couple is a newly recognized node in the circuitry for biologic redox signaling and control. FASEB J. 2004;18:1246–8.
12. Jones DP. Redox sensing: orthogonal control in cell cycle and apoptosis signalling. J Intern Med. 2010;268:432–48.
13. Jones DP, Sies H. The redox code. Antioxid Redox Signal. 2015;23:734–46.
14. Maltepe E, Saugstad OD. Oxygen in health and disease: regulation of oxygen homeostasis-clinical implications. Pediatr Res. 2009;65:261–8.
15. Davis JM, Auten RL. Maturation of the antioxidant system and the effects on preterm birth. Semin Fetal Neonatal Med. 2010;15:191–5.
16. Lu SC. Regulation of glutathione synthesis. Mol Aspects Med. 2009;30:42–59.
17. Vento M, Aguar M, Escobar J, Arduini A, Escrig R, Brugada M, Izquierdo I, Asensi MA, Sastre J, Saenz P, Gimeno A. Antenatal steroids and antioxidant enzyme activity in preterm infants: influence of gender and timing. Antioxid Redox Signal. 2009;11:2945–55.
18. Dömeloff M. Nutritional care of premature infants: microminerals. World Rev Nutr Diet. 2014;110:121–39.
19. Belik J, Gonzalez-Luis GE, Perez-Vizcaino F, Villamor E. Isoprostanes in fetal and neonatal health and disease. Free Radic Biol Med. 2010;48:177–88.
20. Milne GL, Dai Q, Roberts 2nd LJ. The isoprostanes-25 years later. Biochim Biophys Acta. 1851;2015:433–45.
21. Saugstad OD, Sejersted Y, Solberg R, Wollen EJ, Bjørås M. Oxygenation of the newborn: a molecular approach. Neonatology. 2012;101(4):315–25.
22. Madurga A, Mizikova I, Ruiz-Camp J, Morty RE. Recent advances in late lung development and the pathogenesis of bronchopulmonary dysplasia. Am J Physiol Lung Cell Mol Physiol. 2013;305:L893–905.
23. Vento M, Teramo K. Evaluating the fetus at risk for cardiopulmonary compromise. Semin Fetal Neonatal Med. 2013;18:324–9.
24. Roan E, Wilhelm K, Bada A, Makena PS, Gorantla VK, Sinclair SE, Waters CM. Hyperoxia alters the mechanical properties of alveolar epithelial cells. Am J Physiol Lung Cell Mol Physiol. 2012;302:L1235–41.
25. Cho HY, van Houten B, Wang X, Miller-DeGraff L, Fostel J, Gladwell W, Perrow L, Panduri V, Kobzik L, Yamamoto M, Bell DA, Kleeberger SR. Targeted deletion of nrf2 impairs lung development and oxidant injury in neonatal mice. Antioxid Redox Signal. 2012;17:1066–82.
26. Masood A, Belcastro R, Li J, Kantores C, Jankov RP, Tanswell AK. A peroxynitrite decomposition catalyst prevents 60% O2-mediated rat chronic neonatal lung injury. Free Radic Biol Med. 2010;49:1182–91.
27. Wedgwood S, Lakshminrusimha S, Czech L, Schumacker PT, Steinhorn RH. Increased p22(phox)/Nox4 expression is involved in remodeling through hydrogen peroxide signaling in experimental persistent pulmonary hypertension of the newborn. Antioxid Redox Signal. 2013;18:1765–76.
28. Yi M, Masood A, Ziino A, Johnson BH, Belcastro R, Li J, Shek S, Kantores C, Jankov RP, Tanswell AK. Inhibition of apoptosis by 60% oxygen: a novel pathway contributing to lung injury in neonatal rats. Am J Physiol Lung Cell Mol Physiol. 2011;300:L319–29.
29. Hartman WR, Smelter DF, Sathish V, Karass M, Kim S, Aravamudan B, Thompson MA, Amrani Y, Pandya HC, Martin RJ, Prakash YS, Pabelick CM. Oxygen dose responsiveness of human fetal airway smooth muscle cells. Am J Physiol Lung Cell Mol Physiol. 2012;303:L711–9.

30. Dawson JA, Kamlin CO, Vento M, Wong C, Cole TJ, Donath SM, Davis PG, Morley CJ. Defining the reference range for oxygen saturation for infants after birth. Pediatrics. 2010;125:e1340–7.
31. Perlman JM, Wyllie J, Kattwinkel J, et al. Part 11: Neonatal resuscitation: 2010 international consensus on cardiopulmonary resuscitation and emergency cardiovascular care science with treatment recommendations. Circulation. 2010;122:S516–38.
32. Vento M, Cubells E, Escobar JJ, Escrig R, Aguar M, Brugada M, Cernada M, Saénz P, Izquierdo I. Oxygen saturation after birth in preterm infants treated with continuous positive airway pressure and air: assessment of gender differences and comparison with a published nomogram. Arch Dis Child Fetal Neonatal Ed. 2013;98:F228–32.
33. Hooper SB, Polglase GR, Roehr CC. Cardiopulmonary changes with aeration of the newborn lung. Paediatr Respir Rev. 2015 Mar 17. pii: S1526-0542(15)00028-7. doi: 10.1016/j.prrv.2015.03.003. (Epub ahead of print).
34. Baenziger O, Stolkin F, Keel M, von Siebenthal K, Fauchere JC, Das Kundu S, Dietz V, Bucher HU, Wolf M. The influence of timing of cord clamping on postnatal cerebral oxygenation in preterm neonates: a randomized controlled trial. Pediatrics. 2007;119:445–59.
35. Sweet DG, Carnielli V, Greisen G, Hallman M, Ozek E, Plavka R, Saugstad OD, Simeoni U, Speer CP, Vento M, Halliday HL. European consensus guidelines on the management of neonatal respiratory distress syndrome in preterm infants – 2013 update. Neonatology. 2013;103:353–68.
36. Vento M, Asensi M, Sastre J, García-Sala F, Pallardó FV, Viña J. Resuscitation with room air instead of 100% oxygen prevents oxidative stress in moderately asphyxiated term neonates. Pediatrics. 2001;107:642–7.
37. Vento M, Asensi M, Sastre J, Lloret A, García-Sala F, Viña J. Oxidative stress in asphyxiated term infants resuscitated with 100% oxygen. J Pediatr. 2003;142:240–6.
38. Vento M, Sastre J, Asensi MA, Viña J. Room-air resuscitation causes less damage to heart and kidney than 100% oxygen. Am J Respir Crit Care Med. 2005;172:1393–8.
39. Wang CL, Anderson C, Leone TA, Rich W, Govindaswami B, Finer NN. Resuscitation of preterm neonates by using room air or 100% oxygen. Pediatrics. 2008;121:1083–9.
40. Dawson JA, Kamlin CO, Wong C, te Pas AB, O'Donnell CP, Donath SM, Davis PG, Morley CJ. Oxygen saturation and heart rate during delivery room resuscitation of infants <30 weeks' gestation with air or 100% oxygen. Arch Dis Child Fetal Neonatal Ed. 2009;94:F87–91.
41. Escrig R, Arruza L, Izquierdo I, Villar G, Sáenz P, Gimeno A, Moro M, Vento M. Achievement of targeted saturation values in extremely low gestational age neonates resuscitated with low or high oxygen concentrations: a prospective, randomized trial. Pediatrics. 2008;121:875–81.
42. Vento M, Moro M, Escrig R, Arruza L, Villar G, Izquierdo I, Roberts 2nd LJ, Arduini A, Escobar JJ, Sastre J, Asensi MA. Preterm resuscitation with low oxygen causes less oxidative stress, inflammation, and chronic lung disease. Pediatrics. 2009;124:e439–49.
43. Ezaki S, Suzuki K, Kurishima C, Miura M, Weilin W, Hoshi R, Tanitsu S, Tomita Y, Takayama C, Wada M, Kondo T, Tamura M. Resuscitation of preterm infants with reduced oxygen results in less oxidative stress than resuscitation with 100% oxygen. J Clin Biochem Nutr. 2009;44:111–8.
44. Stola A, Schulman J, Perlman J. Initiating delivery room stabilization/resuscitation in very low birth weight (VLBW) infants with an FiO2 less than 100% is feasible. J Perinatol. 2009;29:548–52.
45. Kapadia VS, Chalak LF, Sparks JE, Allen JR, Savani RC, Wyckoff MH. Resuscitation of preterm neonates with limited versus high oxygen strategy. Pediatrics. 2013;132:e1488–96.
46. Brown JVE, Moe-Byrne T, Harden M, Mc-Guire W. Lower versus higher oxygen concentration for delivery room stabilisation of preterm neonates: systematic review. PLoS One. 2013;7:e52033.
47. Saugstad OD, Aune D, Aguar M, Kapadia V, Finer N, Vento M. Resuscitation of premature infants with low or high oxygen. A systematic review and meta-analysis. Acta Paediatr. 2014;103:744–51.
48. Oei JL, Lui K, Wright IM, Craven P, Saugstad OD, Coates E, Tarnow-Mordi WO. Targeted oxygen in the resuscitation of preterm infants and their developmental outcomes (To2rpido): a randomised controlled study. EPAS. 2015;751387.

49. Di Fiore JM, Kaffashi F, Loparo K, Sattar A, Luchter M, et al. The relationship between patterns of intermittent hypoxia and retinopathy of prematurity in preterm infants. Pediatr Res. 2012;72:606–12.
50. Zhou D, Haddad GG. Genetic analysis of hypoxia tolerance and susceptibility in *Droshophila* and humans. Annu Rev Gen Hum Gen. 2013;14:25–43.
51. Askie LM, Brocklehurst P, Darlow BA, Finer N, Schmidt B, Tarnow-Mordi W, NeOProM Collaborative Group. NeOProM: neonatal oxygenation prospective meta-analysis collaboration study protocol. BMC Pediatr. 2011;11:6.
52. SUPPORT Study Group of the Eunice Kennedy Shriver NICHD Neonatal Research Network, Carlo WA, Finer NN, Walsh MC, Rich W, Gantz MG, Laptook AR, et al. Target ranges of oxygen saturation in extremely preterm infants. N Engl J Med. 2010;362:1959–69.
53. BOOST II United Kingdom Collaborative Group, BOOST II Australia Collaborative Group, BOOST II New Zealand Collaborative Group, Stenson BJ, Tarnow-Mordi WO, Darlow BA, Simes J, Juszczak E, Askie L, et al. Oxygen saturation and outcomes in preterm infants. N Engl J Med. 2013;368:2094–104.
54. Schmidt R, Whyte RK, Asztalos EV, Modemann D, Poets C, Rabi Y, Solimano A, Roberts RS, Canadian Oxygen Trial (COT) Group. Effects of targeting higher vs. lower arterial oxygen saturations on death or disability in extremely preterm infants: a randomized clinical trial. JAMA. 2013;309:2111–20.
55. Saugstad OD, Dagfinn A. Optimal oxygenation of extremely low birth weight infants: a meta-analysis and systematic review of the oxygen saturation target studies. Neonatology. 2014;105: 55–63.
56. Di Fiore JM, Walsh M, Wrage L, Rich W, Finer N, Carlo WA, Martin RJ, SUPPORT Study Group of Eunice Kennedy-Shriver National Institute of Child Health and Human Development Neonatal Research Network. Low oxygen saturation target range is associated with increased incidence of intermittent hypoxemia. J Pediatr. 2012;161:1047–52.
57. Rosychuk RJ, Hudson-Mason A, Eklund D, Lacaze-Masmonteil T. Discrepancies between arterial oxygen saturation and functional oxygen saturation measured with pulse oximetry in very preterm infants. Neonatology. 2012;101:14–9.
58. Prabhakar NR, Semenza GL. Adaptive and maladaptive cardiorespiratory responses to continuous and intermittent hypoxia mediated by hypoxia-inducible factors 1 and 2. Physiol Rev. 2012;92:967–1003.
59. Manja V, Lakshminrusimha S, Cook DJ. Oxygen saturation target range for extremely preterm infants: a systematic review and meta-analysis. JAMA Pediatr. 2015;169:332–40.
60. Bizzarro MJ, Li FY, Katz K, Shabanova V, Ehrenkranz RA, Bhandari V. Temporal quantification of oxygen saturation ranges: an effort to reduce hyperoxia in the neonatal intensive care unit. J Perinatol. 2014;34:33–8.
61. Sola A, Golombek SG, Montes Bueno MT, Lemus-Varela L, Zuluaga C, Domínguez F, Baquero H, Young Sarmiento AE, Natta D, Rodriguez Perez JM, Deulofeut R, Quiroga A, Flores GL, Morgues M, Pérez AG, Van Overmeire B, van Bel F. Safe oxygen saturation targeting and monitoring in preterm infants: can we avoid hypoxia and hyperoxia? Acta Paediatr. 2014;103:1009–18.
62. Lakshminrusimha S, Manja V, Mathew B, Suresh GK. Oxygen targeting in preterm infants: a physiological interpretation. J Perinatol. 2015;35:8–15.
63. Hagadorn JI, Furey AM, Nghiem TH, et al. Achieved versus intended pulse oximeter saturation in infants born less than 28 weeks' gestation: the AVIOx study. Pediatrics. 2006;118:1574–82.
64. Clucas L, Doyle LW, Dawson J, Donath S, Davis PG. Compliance with alarm limits for pulse oximetry in very preterm infants. Pediatrics. 2007;119:1056–60.
65. Laptook AR, Salhab W, Allen J, Saha S, Walsh M. Pulse oximetry in very low birth weight infants: can oxygen saturation be maintained in the desired range? J Perinatol. 2006;26:337–41.
66. Claure N, Bancalari E. Closed-loop control of inspired oxygen in premature infants. Semin Fetal Neonatal Med. 2015;20:198–204.
67. Hallenberger A, Poets CF, Horn W, Seyfang A, Urschitz MS, CLAC Study Group. Closed-loop automatic oxygen control (CLAC) in preterm infants: a randomized controlled trial. Pediatrics. 2014;133:e379–85.

Chapter 11
Noninvasive Ventilation for the Prevention of Bronchopulmonary Dysplasia

Louise S. Owen, Brett J. Manley, Vineet Bhandari, and Peter G. Davis

Introduction

The search for reliable, effective methods of supporting the breathing of preterm babies marks the beginning of modern neonatal intensive care. Nasal continuous positive airway pressure (CPAP) was developed to avoid the complications associated with endotracheal intubation. Subsequently nasal intermittent positive pressure (NIPPV) was used in an attempt to augment the benefits of CPAP. Most recently, high-flow nasal cannulae have become popular as an alternative to CPAP using a simpler, more comfortable interface. This chapter examines in detail these modes of non-invasive ventilation, examining their usefulness in a variety of clinical settings.

L.S. Owen, MBChB, MRCPCH, FRACP, MD (✉) • B.J. Manley, MBBS (Hons), PhD
P.G. Davis, MD, MBBS
Royal Women's Hospital, Neonatal Services and Newborn Research Centre;
Department of Obstetrics and Gynaecology, University of Melbourne,
Level 7, 20 Flemington Road, Parkville, Melbourne, VIC 3052, Australia
e-mail: louise.owen@thewomens.org.au; brett.manley@thewomens.org.au; pgd@unimelb.edu.au

V. Bhandari, MBBS, MD, DM
Department of Neonatology (Pediatrics), Drexel University College of Medicine,
St. Christopher's Hospital for Children, 160 East Erie Avenue, Philadelphia, PA 19134, USA

Hahnemann University Hospital, Philadelphia, PA, USA

Temple University Hospital, Philadelphia, PA, USA
e-mail: vineet.bhandari@drexelmed.edu

V. Bhandari (ed.), *Bronchopulmonary Dysplasia*, Respiratory Medicine,
DOI 10.1007/978-3-319-28486-6_11

Nasal Continuous Positive Airway Pressure

History of Continuous Positive Airway Pressure

The use of CPAP in neonates was first reported by George Gregory in 1971 [1], around 10 years after the introduction of endotracheal ventilation in this population. Ongoing high mortality and frequent air leaks seen during endotracheal ventilation led to the search for a better alternative. Initially, CPAP was delivered using an endotracheal tube and was shown to improve both oxygenation and survival [1]. Since that first report, nasal CPAP has increased in popularity; for the treatment of respiratory distress syndrome (RDS) and apnea of prematurity, for the prevention of re-intubation, and for many other neonatal respiratory conditions. CPAP has been enthusiastically adopted around the world, with modern, cheap, disposable devices making it a viable therapy in resource-limited settings [2, 3]. It has been hailed as a means of avoiding endotracheal ventilation and of reducing bronchopulmonary dysplasia (BPD) in preterm infants.

Physiological Effects of CPAP

CPAP has been to shown to have numerous physiological benefits. It stabilizes the chest wall and helps splint open the upper airway [4] and pharyngeal walls [5], reducing upper airway collapse, decreasing resistance [6], and increasing the laryngeal opening [7]. These mechanical effects reduce obstructive [8] and mixed apneas [9]. CPAP alters the shape of the diaphragm, leading to decreased lung resistance and increased lung compliance [10]. This in turn results in reduced work of breathing [11] and a smaller phase angle between the thorax and abdomen [4], allowing larger tidal volumes for the same respiratory effort [12, 13] and improved oxygenation [14]. CPAP increases functional residual capacity (FRC) [15, 16], conserves surfactant, reduces ventilation-perfusion mismatch, and decreases left-to-right shunting [17]. Dynamic volume-preserving mechanisms, such as expiratory braking, are seen less often during CPAP, as infants are able to maintain FRC without these maneuvers [18].

CPAP Pressure Generation and Delivery

Several CPAP pressure-generating devices are available. “Bubble” CPAP utilizes circuit pressure generated by placing the distal limb of the circuit under a measured depth of water. This is a simple, cheap technique and is characterized by variations in the pressure generated by gas bubbling under water. Neonatal ventilators may be used to generate CPAP; the expiratory valve controls the CPAP delivered and there are no pressure oscillations. "Variable flow" CPAP devices generate pressures in proportion to the gas flow set by the clinician. There is little high-quality evidence to support one form of CPAP delivery over another [19]. High-frequency ventilation using the nasal CPAP interface has been developed, with encouraging preliminary, short-term animal and bench top studies. One small human study reported beneficial short-term effects [20], but this mode requires further evaluation.

CPAP may be delivered through a variety of nasal interfaces. The original method of using an endotracheal tube is no longer recommended due to high tube resistance leading to increased work of breathing. Modern CPAP interfaces are most commonly short bi-nasal prongs of various shapes and sizes. Alternatives include longer single, and bi-nasal, nasopharyngeal prongs. These have higher resistance than short prongs, and therefore the delivered pressure is attenuated [21]; they are not as effective at preventing re-intubation as short bi-nasal prongs [19]. Triangular-shaped nasal masks are also commonly used, although less data exist to support their efficacy.

Use of CPAP in the Post-extubation Period

As the adverse effects of endotracheal ventilation became apparent, clinicians endeavored to wean support and remove the endotracheal tube as soon as possible. Traditionally, infants were extubated and treated with supplemental oxygen. Later, CPAP was used post-extubation. Systematic review of nine randomized studies of CPAP versus supplemental oxygen following extubation ($n = 726$) clearly demonstrated that provision of CPAP resulted in higher rates of extubation success (number needed to treat, NNT = 6) [22]. However, benefits were only observed when pressures ≥5 cm of water (cmH_2O) were used. There was no significant difference between groups in rates of BPD, defined as the need for supplemental oxygen at 28 days, relative risk (RR) 1.00 [95 % confidence interval (CI) 0.81, 1.24]. No outcomes beyond 28 days were reported [22]. Extubation of premature infants to CPAP is now established as standard practice and is incorporated into international guidelines [23].

Studies Using Primary CPAP from Birth

Studies of the use of CPAP from birth fall into distinct categories:

CPAP Versus Supplemental Oxygen

A 2002 Cochrane review [24], updated in 2008, compared the effects of early continuous distending pressures (including both CPAP and continuous negative pressure), with supplemental oxygen alone, in preterm infants (<37 weeks' gestation). Six small studies were included ($n = 355$), three using CPAP and three using continuous negative pressure. CPAP resulted in a lower rate of failed treatment (death or need for additional respiratory support), RR 0.61 (95 % CI 0.45, 0.81). BPD (supplemental oxygen at 28 days) was only reported as a pooled outcome from two CPAP studies and one negative pressure study; no difference was shown, RR 1.22 (95 % CI 0.44, 3.39). The authors acknowledged that four of the studies were performed prior to the introduction of antenatal steroids and surfactant replacement, and therefore, these results may not currently be applicable in the developed world. However, these findings remain relevant in resource-limited settings which do not have access to steroids and surfactant.

Prophylactic Early CPAP Versus Rescue CPAP

Preterm Infants <37 Weeks' Gestational Age (GA)

A 2002 Cochrane review [25], updated in 2009, compared the effects of early continuous distending pressures (again including both CPAP and continuous negative pressure), with delayed application of distending pressures, in preterm infants (<37 weeks' gestation). Six small studies were included ($n=165$), all carried out prior to 1981, four using CPAP, two using continuous negative pressure. For the four CPAP studies ($n=119$), early CPAP did not result in a significantly lower rate of endotracheal ventilation than rescue CPAP, RR 0.77 (95 % CI 0.43, 1.38) [25]. BPD (supplemental oxygen at 28 days) was only reported in one CPAP study which did not show a significant difference, RR 1.12 (95 % CI 0.08, 16.52).

Very Preterm Infants <32 Weeks' GA

Two studies were included in a 2005 Cochrane review [26], examining the differences between early prophylactic CPAP and supplemental oxygen in very preterm infants (<32 weeks' gestation). In a single-center Canadian study, Han et al. [27] randomized 82 infants <33 weeks' GA, within two hours of birth, to either CPAP or headbox oxygen. This study was done prior to 1986 and neither antenatal steroids nor surfactant were used. One third of the control infants received rescue CPAP. Han et al. reported no difference in the primary outcome of RDS. The Cochrane review additionally reported on the rate of BPD (supplemental oxygen at 28 days), describing a nonsignificant trend to higher rates in the CPAP group, RR 2.27 (95 % CI 0.77, 6.65).

Sandri et al. randomized 230 infants ($28\text{–}31^{+6}$ weeks' GA) at multiple Italian sites, within 30 min of birth, to prophylactic CPAP or supplemental oxygen (oxyhood) with rescue CPAP if oxygen requirement reached 40 %. Surfactant was administered if oxygen requirement reached 40 % while on CPAP in both groups. Over 80 % of mothers received antenatal steroids. Surfactant was given to around 20 % of infants in both groups. More than half of infants in the control group (57 %) eventually also received CPAP (at median age of 109 min). No difference in the primary outcome of need for surfactant was reported. There was a nonsignificant increase in the rate of BPD (supplemental oxygen at 36 weeks' corrected GA or CGA) in the prophylactic CPAP group, RR 2.00 (95 % CI 0.18, 21.75). The Cochrane authors suggested that there was insufficient evidence to evaluate the effectiveness of prophylactic nasal CPAP in very preterm infants and suggested that further randomized trials were required.

A recent study, carried out in Iran [28], evaluated the effects of early versus rescue CPAP on the need for endotracheal ventilation. Seventy-two infants of 25–30 weeks' GA, who were spontaneously breathing but needing respiratory support at 5 min of age, were randomized. CPAP was either commenced at 5 min, or after 30 min of age. The early CPAP group had reduced need for surfactant, intubation, and ventilation, but there was no difference between groups with regard to rates of BPD [2.8 % (early) vs. 5.6 % (rescue), $p=0.5$].

Overall, these data suggest that early CPAP, compared with rescue CPAP, may reduce the need for subsequent additional respiratory support but has little effect on rates of BPD in preterm and very preterm infants.

Early Ventilation Versus Early "Intubation-Surfactant-Extubation to CPAP" (INSURE Technique)

Until relatively recently, extremely premature infants were routinely intubated and ventilated at birth. National guidelines recommended that all infants below a set GA, typically 29 weeks, were intubated in the delivery room and given surfactant via the endotracheal tube [29]. However, by the late 1980s and early 1990s clinicians were already seeking to minimize endotracheal intubation for mechanical ventilation. This resulted in the development of the procedure of brief intubation for surfactant treatment, followed by rapid extubation to CPAP which became known as the INSURE technique. Several randomized studies have compared INSURE versus early intubation, surfactant treatment, and ongoing endotracheal ventilation. Six studies (published between 1994 and 2005) were included in a 2007 meta-analysis [30]. This analysis reported a reduced need for ventilation in the INSURE group, RR 0.67 (95 % CI 0.57, 0.79), as well as less BPD (at 28 days), RR 0.51 (95 % CI 0.26, 0.99).

Observational Studies of CPAP Use from Birth in Extremely Preterm Infants (<28 Weeks' GA)

At around the same time as INSURE was emerging, other data began to accumulate to suggest that not all extremely preterm infants needed to be intubated at birth. In 1987, Avery observed that rates of BPD varied widely across North American nurseries [31], with some centers having much lower BPD rates than others. By the early 1990s, it was noted that when extremely preterm infants were managed with

CPAP from birth, they were less likely to develop BPD. In 1993, Kamper et al. [32] reported results from a cohort of 81 Danish infants <1500 g managed using a strategy of using CPAP to avoid endotracheal intubation and tolerating hypercapnia. Sixty-five infants survived to discharge, of which 61 never required endotracheal intubation. No cases of BPD were reported in the survivors. Another study from Denmark appeared the same year, comparing cohorts born before and after a change to routinely providing CPAP from birth. Although they showed a reduced need for ventilation and lower rates of intracranial hemorrhage, there was no difference in the rate of supplemental oxygen requirement at 28 days [33]. In 1996, Lundstrøm also reported on outcomes of using early prophylactic CPAP, this time showing very low rates of BPD [34]. He called for randomized trials comparing initial intubation and ventilation with CPAP, which he felt were "not only warranted but indeed an absolute necessity to answer the question of which treatment is the best." It was not until 2000 that other sites around the world started to report similar findings. Van Marter et al. [35] reported on a large North American cohort ($n=452$) of infants 500–1500 g, born across three sites in Boston and New York. Columbia, New York predominantly used CPAP from birth, whereas the Boston centers used early intubation and ventilation. Van Marter et al. suggested that variations in ventilatory strategies were the major factors in the difference in rates of BPD (at 36 weeks' CGA) between sites. BPD rates in Columbia, New York were more than 80 % lower than BPD rates in Boston. This and many other reports were encouraging but were all limited by their observational, non-randomized design. It was not until 2004 that the first pilot study randomizing extremely preterm infants to receive CPAP from birth was published [36]. Finer reported on 104 <28-week infants who were randomized to receive CPAP in the delivery room. He showed that 43 % of those randomized to CPAP did not require endotracheal ventilation in the first 7 days of life. No long-term outcomes were reported [36].

In extremely preterm infants (<28 weeks' gestational age), studies have now compared: (1) early CPAP versus initial endotracheal ventilation, (2) early CPAP versus early intubation, surfactant administration, and rapid extubation to CPAP (INSURE technique), and (3) early CPAP versus early nasal intermittent positive pressure ventilation (NIPPV) (addressed later in this chapter).

Early CPAP Versus Early Ventilation for Extremely Preterm Infants

Three studies and a systematic review have now been published addressing this question. The first randomized trial of CPAP versus intubation at birth in extremely preterm infants was the COIN trial [37]. This international trial randomized 610 infants born at 25–28^{+6} weeks' gestation to receive either CPAP or intubation within 5 min of birth. Infants were eligible if they were breathing but required respiratory support. Forty-six percent of infants randomized to CPAP met predefined failure criteria and were intubated in the first 5 days of life. There was no significant difference between the treatment groups in the primary outcome, death, or supplemental oxygen at 36 weeks [OR 0.80 (95 % CI 0.58, 1.12)]. Infants in the CPAP group had a significantly lower rate of BPD at 28 days [OR 0.62 (0.44, 0.86)] but not at 36 weeks [OR 0.76 (95 % CI 0.54–1.09)]. Trends favoring CPAP were noted for other outcomes including median days of respiratory support (21 vs. 26 days, $p=0.24$); median days of supplemental oxygen (42 vs. 49, $p=0.07$) and median days in hospital 74 versus 79 ($p=0.09$). Infants intubated in the delivery room had a significantly lower rate of pneumothorax than those randomized to CPAP (3.0 vs. 9.1 %, $p=0.001$). The authors concluded that CPAP was an acceptable alternative to endotracheal intubation in the delivery room.

In 2010, the results of the SUPPORT trial [38] were published. SUPPORT was a randomized, multicenter trial ($n=1316$), with a 2-by-2 factorial design. Eligible infants were $24–27^{+6}$ weeks' gestation. Infants were randomly assigned to early intubation plus surfactant treatment or to CPAP commencing in the delivery room. Additionally, infants were also randomly assigned to one of two target ranges of oxygen saturation. There was no difference in the primary outcome of death or BPD (at 36 weeks) between the CPAP and intubation groups [47.8 vs. 51.0 %, RR 0.95 (95 % CI 0.85, 1.05)], nor was there a significant difference between groups for the sole outcome of BPD (oxygen requirement at 36 weeks CGA), RR 0.94 (95 % CI 0.82, 1.06). Other outcomes related to BPD which favored the CPAP group included: less need for postnatal corticosteroids for treatment of BPD ($p<0.001$), fewer days of mechanical ventilation ($p=0.03$), and increased survival to day seven without ongoing support via an endotracheal tube ($p=0.01$). The authors of the SUPPORT trial concluded that CPAP should be considered as an alternative to intubation and surfactant from birth in extremely preterm infants.

In 2011, Dunn published the results of a multicenter randomized trial of 648 infants of $26–29^{+6}$ weeks' gestation [39]. This trial compared three approaches to initial respiratory management; group one received intubation, prophylactic surfactant, and ongoing ventilation; group two received intubation, prophylactic surfactant, and rapid extubation to CPAP (INSURE); group three received initial CPAP and selective surfactant treatment only if required. The study was stopped early due to poor recruitment. There were no differences in the primary outcome of the combined rate of death or BPD (at 36 weeks' CGA) for either the CPAP group [RR 0.83 (95 % CI 0.64, 1.09)] or the INSURE group [RR 0.78 (95 % CI 0.59, 1.03)], compared with the ventilation group. In the CPAP group, 48 % never required intubation. The authors concluded that the use of early CPAP leads to a reduction in the number of infants needing intubation and surfactant treatment without adversely affecting respiratory outcomes [39].

A recent meta-analysis [40] included these three trials and a fourth which compared initial CPAP with the INSURE technique [41] (discussed in detail below). None of the three individual trials demonstrate a reduction in BPD rates at 36 weeks' CGA, and the combined outcome (including the fourth trial) shows an RR of BPD at 36 weeks' CGA of 0.91 (95 % CI 0.82, 1.01), with a trend favoring CPAP. The authors of this review rightly point out that caution should be used when generalizing the results of these studies as all required antenatal consent. Reliance on antenatal consent results in the selection of a lower risk population with increased rates of antenatal steroid use and lower incidences of antenatal and neonatal complications. The review also mentions that none of the trials enrolled infants of 23 weeks' gestation and only one trial included infants of 24 weeks' gestation [38], pointing out that these infants are at the highest risk of developing BPD. All three trials used different thresholds for determining CPAP "failure" and subsequent need for surfactant treatment (range 40–60 % oxygen to maintain saturation targets), and all trials were completed at a time when it was standard practice to resuscitate extremely preterm infants using 100 % oxygen. These factors may have influenced the final results [40].

Early CPAP Compared with Early INSURE Technique

As the trials comparing early CPAP with early ventilation were published, concern mounted about managing extremely preterm infants with CPAP alone, i.e., withholding surfactant treatment and therefore potentially leading to an increased risk of pneumothorax [37]. Further studies were then designed to assess whether INSURE was superior to CPAP alone. A small, randomized study ($n=35$), published in 1994, reported a reduced need for mechanical ventilation following INSURE, compared with CPAP alone [42], but no difference in need for supplemental oxygen at 28 days. There have since been two larger randomized trials comparing early CPAP with early INSURE [41, 43] and a third which compared these two treatments to a third arm of intubation, prophylactic surfactant, and ongoing ventilation [39].

The largest trial was carried out in eight Colombian centers, in 279 infants of 27–31^{+6} weeks' gestation. Infants with RDS were randomized within an hour of birth to either INSURE or CPAP. The primary outcome of need for endotracheal ventilation was lower in the INSURE group [26 vs. 39 %, RR 0.69 (95 % CI 0.49–0.97)]; however, BPD (oxygen treatment at 36 weeks' CGA) was not statistically different [49 vs. 59 %, RR 0.84 (95 % CI 0.66–1.05)]. The authors point out that although there were no long-term differences, a lower rate of mechanical ventilation may be an important outcome in resource-limited settings.

The second trial randomized 208 infants born at 25–28^{+6} weeks' gestation, across 24 European sites (the CURPAP Trial). Infants who were not intubated at birth received either INSURE or initial CPAP with selective surfactant replacement only if required [41]. There was no difference in the primary outcome of need for endotracheal ventilation in the first 5 days of life, RR 0.95 (95 % CI 0.64, 1.41). Survival without BPD at 36 weeks' CGA was not different between the groups, RR 0.99 (95 % CI 0.86–1.14). The authors concluded that prophylactic surfactant was not superior to initial CPAP plus early selective surfactant treatment if required in spontaneously breathing extremely preterm infants [41]. The most recent trial, in 648 infants of 26–29^{+6} weeks' gestation, reported similar rates for the combined outcome of death or BPD (at 36 weeks' CGA) between the CPAP (28.5 %) and INSURE (30.5 %) arms but only reported statistical comparisons against the early ventilation group (36.5 %) [39].

A systematic review had previously shown that in infants at high risk of early RDS, early prophylactic surfactant was better than later rescue surfactant, with respect to neonatal mortality and air leak [44]. However, a recent update of this meta-analysis [45] concluded that results vary, depending on whether routine CPAP was used in the selective surfactant treatment group. Two of the 11 studies reviewed used routine application of CPAP in the selective treatment group [38, 39]. Pooled analysis of these two trials, which are reflective of current clinical practice, favored early CPAP with selective use of surfactant in the combined outcome of death and BPD [RR 1.13 (95 % CI 1.02, 1.25)] but not BPD alone [RR1.12 (95 % CI 0.99, 1.26)]. When all 11 studies were evaluated together, the benefits of prophylactic surfactant could no longer be demonstrated. The implication for clinicians from these trials is that CPAP with rescue surfactant is likely to have very similar risks and benefits as prophylactic surfactant using INSURE.

CPAP Weaning and BPD

There are few studies evaluating different strategies for weaning preterm infants from CPAP and even fewer investigating the effects of weaning on rates of BPD. The one randomized clinical trial (RCT) which included BPD as a secondary outcome measure was published in 2012 [46]. This study randomized 177 preterm infants (<30 weeks' GA) to one of three CPAP weaning methods: (A) stopping CPAP with the intention of remaining off CPAP, (B) cycling on and off CPAP with increasing time off CPAP, and (C) cycling on and off CPAP with increasing time off CPAP plus provision of 0.5 L/min of nasal cannula oxygen, delivered during the periods off CPAP. The primary outcome, time to successfully wean from CPAP, was shortest in group A (11 days vs. 17 and 19 days in groups B and C, respectively, $p<0.0001$). Rates of BPD (requiring oxygen at 36 weeks' CGA to maintain oxygen saturations >86 %) were also lowest in group A (12.5 % vs. 42 and 19 % in groups B and C, respectively, $p=0.011$) [46].

Discussion and Recommendations

These results suggest that extubation of preterm infants to CPAP ensures that they have the best chance of avoiding re-intubation, but that there is little long-term effect on BPD.

For preterm infants >28 weeks' GA, prophylactic CPAP may offer no long-term advantages over rescue CPAP. In the extremely preterm group <28 weeks' GA, routine intubation for surfactant administration, with ongoing ventilation, may increase the risk of BPD, and in this population, early CPAP is no worse than early ventilation and has some advantages. So far, there appears little difference in important outcomes between early CPAP with rescue surfactant and prophylactic surfactant using INSURE.

Nasal Intermittent Positive Pressure Ventilation

History of NIPPV

NIPPV was first investigated as a treatment for apnea of prematurity. Initial studies were of short duration (4–6 h) and reported mixed results [47–49]. The technique became less popular after a case-control study highlighted an increased risk of gastrointestinal perforation in infants managed with NIPPV compared with those ventilated via an endotracheal tube [50]. Following an initial RCT that utilized nasopharyngeal prongs to deliver synchronized NIPPV (SNIPPV) [51], two further RCTs using short bi-nasal prongs were able to confirm [52, 53] that extubation failure was significantly reduced when using SNIPPV versus NCPAP. All three RCTs used SNIPPV, and one specifically mentioned the use of an orogastric tube to decompress the stomach [53]. These factors may have contributed to the effectiveness of NIPPV and the absence of previously reported gastrointestinal side effects.

Physiological Effects of SNIPPV

The benefits of using SNIPPV over NCPAP include improved stability of the chest wall, pulmonary mechanics, thoracoabdominal motion synchrony, and decreased airway resistance [54]. In addition, infants on SNIPPV have increased tidal and minute volumes [55] and less apneas [56, 57]. Investigators have also noted improved clinical parameters such as decreased work of breathing and reduced chest wall distortion in infants receiving SNIPPV [58–60]. Probably the most important beneficial effect of SNIPPV is the ability to intermittently increase the distending pressure above positive end expiratory pressure (PEEP), akin to “sigh breaths.” This improves airflow into the upper airways, resulting in “opening-up” of the alveoli with enhancement of the FRC and gas exchange [51, 61–63]. The mechanics of non-synchronized NIPPV are less well studied, with one study reporting increased blood pressure and discomfort but decreased respiratory rate [64].

SNIPPV Pressure Generation and Delivery

NIPPV can be generated using any ventilator that can deliver NCPAP and IPPV, though software adjustments may be required to decrease nuisance alarms [63]. Strategies to compensate for leak around the nasal prongs are important. These are provided by some ventilators and more importantly by the bedside nurses and are crucial in initiating and maintaining effective pressures [63], as per published guidelines [62]. Ventilators capable of delivering SNIPPV include: Infant Star ventilator with the StarSync® module (no longer available in the USA), the Sechrist IV-200 SAVI ventilator (Sechrist Industries, Anaheim, CA) [59], the Giulia ventilator

(Ginevri, Rome, Italy) [65], and the Servo-i ventilator (Maquet Medical Systems, Wayne, NJ) using the neurally adjusted ventilatory assist (NAVA) mode [66].

SiPAP (CareFusion, San Diego, CA), whether synchronized or not, may be considered a variant of NCPAP rather than a SNIPPV mode of respiratory support. The Infant Flow SiPAP Comprehensive ventilator (CareFusion, San Diego, CA) is a bi-level device, providing higher and lower pressures, with much longer inspiratory times, compared to SNIPPV mode. The positive inflation pressures (PIPs) generated by the SiPAP device are typically 9–11 cmH_2O, much lower than those used in published studies of NIPPV. The nasal interfaces available for delivery of SNIPPV are essentially the same as for NCPAP, and short bi-nasal prongs are preferred over the longer, tapered nasopharyngeal prongs. Nasopharyngeal prongs, because of their tapering design, cause an increased airflow resistance and are more likely to be blocked by secretions [62, 67]. While the RAM® (Neotech, Valencia, CA) cannula prongs have been used to deliver NIPPV, they have not been found to be as effective as more commonly used short bi-nasal prongs (Inca®, Argyle®, etc. among others) in infants with moderate respiratory disease [68].

Use of SNIPPV in the Post-extubation Period

A meta-analysis of the first three studies comparing SNIPPV to NCPAP in the post-extubation period [51–53] concluded that SNIPPV provided by the Infant Star ventilator was more effective in preventing failure of extubation within 72 h [RR 0.21 (95 % CI 0.10, 0.45), NNT 3] [69]. Two subsequent RCTs, using different ventilators, confirmed the superiority of SNIPPV over NCPAP for this indication [65, 70]. Two of the studies reported trends to decreased rates of BPD which did not reach statistical significance [52, 53]. Two subsequent retrospective studies reported that infants receiving SNIPPV had significantly lower rates of BPD [71, 72].

One RCT comparing non-synchronized NIPPV with NCPAP in the post-extubation period reported no difference in outcomes [73]. However, there were major limitations in terms of study design (significant differences in the demographics of the infants in the two groups, and ventilator settings were not increased post-extubation) [63, 74]. A recent RCT reported infants randomized to NIPPV had reduced rates of post-extubation atelectasis, re-intubation, and death, compared to the NCPAP group, with no differences in BPD [75]. Another recent RCT reported significantly decreased duration of supplementary oxygen (84.9 ± 92.1 vs. 90.1 ± 140.5 h, $p=0.002$) and BPD (2/29, 6.9 % vs. 9/28, 32.1 %; $p=0.02$) in NIPPV versus NCPAP groups [76].

Studies Using Primary SNIPPV from Birth

The outcomes of death or BPD (20 vs. 52 %; $p=0.03$) and BPD (10 vs. 33 %; $p=0.04$) were significantly decreased in infants who were randomized to immediate extubation to SNIPPV following surfactant administration compared to those continued on conventional ventilation [67]. Infants randomized to receive NIPPV from birth had a significantly lower incidence of BPD, compared with the NCPAP group overall (2 vs. 17 %, $p<0.05$) and in a subgroup with birth weights <1500 g (5 vs. 33 %, $p<0.05$) [77]. In another RCT conducted in preterm neonates with respiratory distress within 6 h of birth, while the failure rate (defined as the need for intubation and mechanical ventilation) at 48 h and 7 days was significantly less among infants randomized to NIPPV, there was no difference in BPD rates [78]. In an RCT comparing NIPPV ($n=100$) to bubble-NCPAP ($n=100$), significantly more infants in the NCPAP group required intubation in the first 24–72 h of life, with no differences in BPD [79]. In a meta-analysis which included the three RCTs noted above, there was no difference between NIPPV and NCPAP groups in the incidence of BPD (RR, 0.56; 95 % CI, 0.09–3.49) [80]. Other RCTs have also reported that infants managed with NIPPV had improved blood gases and/or decreased need for invasive mechanical ventilation [81–83].

Ramanathan et al. reported that early surfactant administration followed by extubation to NIPPV, as compared to extubation to NCPAP, reduced the need for invasive mechanical ventilation at 7 days of age and decreased BPD [84]. In the largest RCT comparing NIPPV to NCPAP, there was no difference in the primary outcome of BPD or death in infants randomized to NIPPV (191 of 497; 38.4 %) versus NCPAP (180 of 490; 36.7 %) [85]. This trial included infants receiving noninvasive ventilation for initial respiratory distress and for post-extubation care. Some infants randomized to NIPPV received bi-level NCPAP or SiPAP. Multiple different ventilators and interfaces were used, and the NIPPV pressures used were markedly lower than earlier studies [62, 63, 74].

A recent meta-analysis which included all SNIPPV studies, whether used as post-extubation or primary modes, reported that SNIPPV significantly reduced extubation failure (OR 0.15, 95 % CI 0.08–0.31) and decreased death and/or BPD (OR 0.57, 95 % CI 0.37–0.88), with a marginal decrease in BPD alone (RR 0.63, 95 % CI 0.39–1.00) [86].

Studies Using Bi-level CPAP

Two studies using bi-level CPAP (whether synchronized or not) suggested that it is better than NCPAP [87, 88], while a third showed no difference [89]. Others reported similar outcomes when compared with SNIPPV [90–92]. A non-randomized sub-analysis of a large RCT reported no significant differences in the composite outcome of BPD/death but significantly increased death alone in the bi-level NCPAP versus NIPPV group; however, there were significant differences in the baseline demographics in the two groups [93].

Discussion and Recommendations

The available data indicate that SNIPPV is superior to NCPAP for management of neonates following extubation. However, there is currently no high-quality evidence to suggest that NIPPV has a significant effect on BPD and/or death rates. Although there is now a substantial body of literature evaluating NIPPV, further studies to determine the optimum settings and mode of synchronization are required [94].

High-Flow Nasal Cannulae

Introduction

High-flow nasal cannulae (HFNC) are an increasingly popular mode of noninvasive respiratory support for preterm and term newborn infants [95–97]. HFNC are small, thin, tapered bi-nasal cannulae that are used to deliver oxygen or blended oxygen and air at gas flows >1 L/min. It is now standard for commercially available systems to heat and humidify the gas. This section will evaluate the evidence from published RCTs of the effect of using HFNC to treat preterm infants on rates of BPD, compared to other forms of noninvasive support.

Only trials that report the outcome of BPD or "chronic lung disease" are discussed. Only one trial [98] included BPD as part of the primary outcome, and no trials were sufficiently powered individually to demonstrate a difference in BPD rates. In some included studies, the definition of BPD used was not clear. Several of the study authors have kindly provided us with unpublished GA subgroup data for the outcome of BPD: where necessary, we have performed statistical analysis of these outcomes.

HFNC Versus Nasal CPAP for Primary Respiratory Support After Birth in Preterm Infants

There are three published randomized trials comparing HFNC to CPAP as primary respiratory support for preterm infants, enrolling over 350 preterm infants in total. None of the three trials included infants born <28 weeks' GA.

Iranpour and colleagues [99] performed a single-center study, published in Persian, which enrolled 70 preterm infants 30–35 weeks' gestation at 24 h of age with ongoing respiratory distress and oxygen requirement. Infants were randomized to HFNC (gas flow 1.5–3 L/min) or to continuing nasal CPAP (6 cmH_2O). Infants who met pre-specified criteria (before or after randomization) received surfactant via the INSURE technique. There were no cases of BPD reported in either group, but it is unclear how this outcome was measured.

Yoder and colleagues [100] performed the largest published clinical trial of HFNC in newborn infants to date: a multicenter study in the USA and China that enrolled 432 term and preterm infants >28 weeks' GA. Noninvasive ventilation was used either as primary support after birth or as post-extubation support. Infants were randomized to receive HFNC (3–5 L/min) or nasal CPAP (5–6 cmH_2O). Several different HFNC and CPAP devices were used. The primary outcome was need for intubation within 72 h of commencing the allocated treatment, based on pre-specified clinical criteria.

Overall, there was no difference in rates of the primary outcome, or in rates of BPD, defined as a supplemental oxygen requirement at 36 weeks' postmenstrual age (PMA): HFNC 20 % versus nasal CPAP 16 %, $p=0.575$. However, infants managed with nasal CPAP had fewer days of any respiratory support (mechanical ventilation, CPAP, or HFNC) (median 4 vs. 6 days, $p<0.001$) as well as a shorter duration of support from their allocated treatment (median 2 vs. 4 days, $p<0.001$). By seven days after study entry, significantly more infants remained on HFNC compared with nasal CPAP (23 vs. 9 %, $p<0.01$). Despite this, there were no differences in the durations of supplemental oxygen or hospitalization or in rates of home oxygen use.

There were 125 preterm infants receiving noninvasive ventilation as primary support. In this subgroup, there was no difference in rates of the primary outcome (HFNC 6/58 vs. CPAP 9/67, $p=0.60$). Rates of BPD favored the CPAP group but did not reach statistical significance: HFNC 5/58 versus CPAP 1/67, $p=0.06$. In very preterm infants born <32 weeks' GA, there was no significant difference: HFNC 3/20 versus CPAP 1/17, $p=0.37$. The HFNC group spent a longer time on respiratory support [mean (SD) 8.3 (8.7) vs. 4.6 (5.3) days, $p=0.004$], but this did not result in a longer duration of supplemental oxygen or hospitalization.

Ciuffini and colleagues [101] reported the interim results of a single-center Italian study that had enrolled 177 of a planned 316 preterm infants 29–36 weeks' GA. These infants had mild to moderate respiratory distress after birth and were randomized to receive HFNC (4–6 L/min) or nasal CPAP (4–6 cmH_2O). The primary outcome was the need for intubation within 72 h of life, based on pre-specified criteria. A trend favoring the CPAP group did not reach statistical significance, 5 % versus 13 % ($p=0.11$). There was no difference in rates of BPD, which were low in both groups (2 infants vs. 1 infant), although the definition of BPD was not provided.

HFNC Versus NIPPV for Primary Respiratory Support After Birth

Only one published study has compared HFNC to NIPPV for the primary respiratory support of preterm infants. Kugelman and colleagues [102] performed a single-center study in Israel that enrolled 76 preterm infants <35 weeks' GA and with birth weight >1000 g, who required primary noninvasive respiratory support. Infants were treated with either HFNC (starting gas flow 1 L/min, increased up to 5 L/min as required) or SNIPPV (positive inflation pressure 14–22 cmH_2O, PEEP 6 cmH_2O, rate 12–30 inflations per minute). The primary outcome was treatment failure according to pre-specified criteria. There was no difference in the primary outcome, or in rates of BPD, defined as supplemental oxygen requirement at 36 weeks' PMA to keep $SpO_2 > 90$ % (HFNC 3 % vs. NIPPV 5 %, $p = 1.0$).

HFNC Versus Nasal CPAP to Prevent Extubation Failure in Preterm Infants

Six randomized trials addressing this topic have enrolled over 900 preterm infants, with the five largest trials all being published in the last 2 years.

Campbell and colleagues [103] performed a single-center study that enrolled 40 intubated preterm infants. Infants in this study had a mean GA of 27 weeks and birth weight 1.0 kg. The authors compared post-extubation humidified, unheated HFNC (mean gas flow rate 1.9 L/min) with variable flow CPAP at 5–6 cmH_2O. Given the comparatively low flows and unheated nature of HFNC support used, the results of this study are difficult to compare with more recent studies. The primary outcome was need for re-intubation, based on pre-specified criteria, and the study found that infants in the HFNC group were more likely to be re-intubated: HFNC 12/20 versus CPAP 3/20, $p = 0.003$. The incidence of BPD was not reported, although the authors state that there was no difference between the groups. The durations of respiratory support and oxygen supplementation were not reported.

Collins and colleagues [104] performed a single-center study in Australia enrolling 132 very preterm infants (<32 weeks' gestation at birth) considered ready for extubation. Infants were randomized to receive either HFNC (initial gas flow 8 L/min) or nasal CPAP via bi-nasal prongs (initial set pressure 8 cmH_2O) after extubation. The primary outcome was extubation failure in the first 7 days after extubation, based on pre-specified criteria, and there was no significant difference between the groups (HFNC 22 % vs. CPAP 34 %, $p = 0.14$). There was also no difference in rates of BPD overall (HFNC 36 % vs. CPAP 43 %, $p = 0.30$), or in the subgroup of extremely preterm infants born <28 weeks' GA (HFNC 47 % vs. CPAP 55 %, $p = 0.69$). There were also no differences in the PMA at which respiratory support or supplemental oxygen ceased.

In the study by Yoder et al. [100], the post-extubation arm included 226 preterm infants. There was no difference in the rate of the primary outcome of intubation within 72 h (HFNC 10 % vs. CPAP 8 %, $p = 0.51$). Rates of BPD were similar between the HFNC and CPAP groups (17 vs. 16 %, $p = 0.93$) and in the subgroup of very preterm infants (22 vs. 20 %, $p = 0.78$).

The "HIPERSPACE" trial [105] was a multicenter, non-inferiority trial conducted in Australia that enrolled 303 very preterm infants (<32 weeks' GA at birth) who were randomized to receive either HFNC (5–6 L/min) or CPAP (7 cmH_2O) after extubation. The primary outcome was treatment failure within 7 days of randomization, based on pre-specified failure criteria. HFNC was found to be "non-inferior" to

CPAP; the risk difference (95 % CI) for treatment failure was 8.4 % (−1.9 %, 18.7 %). There was no difference in rates of BPD (oxygen supplementation at 36 weeks' PMA) overall (HFNC 31 % vs. CPAP 34 %, $p=0.64$), or in surviving extremely preterm infants born <28 weeks' GA (HFNC 52 % vs. CPAP 47 %, $p=0.54$, unpublished data). There were also no differences in the duration of oxygen supplementation, respiratory support, or hospitalization, or in rates of home oxygen use.

Liu and colleagues [98] performed a multicenter study in China that enrolled a total of 255 infants, of which 150 were preterm. Infants were <7 days old at extubation and were randomized to either HFNC (gas flow 3–8 L/min depending on infant weight) or nasal CPAP. The primary outcomes were extubation failure (re-intubation within 7 days), BPD (a requirement for supplemental oxygen after 28 days of life if GA >32 weeks' or at 36 weeks' PMA if GA <32 weeks'), or death in hospital. There was no difference between the groups in rates of BPD: HFNC 7 % vs. CPAP 8 %, $p=0.79$.

Mostafa-Gharehbaghi and Mojabi [106] performed a single-center study in Iran, which enrolled 85 preterm infants with GA 30–34 weeks and birth weight 1250–2000 g. Infants were initially stabilized with nasal CPAP and treated with intubation and surfactant in the NICU (INSURE technique). Infants were extubated after INSURE to either HFNC (6 L/min) or nasal CPAP (5–6 cmH_2O). The primary outcome was re-intubation within 3 days of surfactant administration, according to pre-specified criteria, and there was no difference in this outcome between groups (HFNC 12 % vs. CPAP 19 %, $p=0.58$). BPD, defined as dependence on supplemental oxygen or mechanical respiratory support at day 28, and oxygen dependency at 36 weeks' PMA, occurred in 1/42 infants in the HFNC group and 3/43 in the CPAP group ($p=0.63$).

HFNC for Weaning from CPAP

There are two RCTs that studied whether HFNC was useful to wean preterm infants from CPAP. Abdel-Hady and colleagues [107] performed a single-center study in Egypt that enrolled 60 preterm infants ≥28 weeks' GA who were stable on low levels of noninvasive respiratory support (nasal CPAP 5 cmH_2O and supplemental oxygen ≤30 %). The non-HFNC group was kept on nasal CPAP 5 cmH_2O until they no longer required supplemental oxygen for 24 h, and then CPAP was ceased. If they met failure criteria, nasal CPAP was re-instituted. The HFNC group was changed to HFNC 2 L/min with 30 % oxygen when supplemental oxygen requirement on CPAP was ≤30 %, followed by gradual weaning from oxygen. Infants who failed HFNC were supported on nasal CPAP for 24 h before making a second attempt to wean using HFNC. The primary outcome was the "better approach to weaning from CPAP" (based on duration of supplemental oxygen and respiratory support). The group who remained on CPAP had fewer days receiving supplemental oxygen than the group who received HFNC, median (IQR) 5 [1–8] versus 14 (7.5–19.25) days, $p<0.001$, and a shorter duration of respiratory support, median (IQR) 10.5 [4–21] versus 18 (11.5–29) days, $p=0.03$. There was no difference between groups regarding success of weaning from CPAP. Only one infant in the study (from the HFNC group) was diagnosed with BPD.

Badiee et al. [108] performed a single-center study in Iran that included 88 preterm infants born 28–36 weeks' GA. Eligible infants were stable on nasal bubble CPAP 5 cmH_2O with supplemental oxygen requirement <30 % for at least 6 h. The HFNC group was changed to HFNC 2 L/min with 30 % oxygen and then had a stepwise reduction in oxygen followed by gas flow. The non-HFNC group remained on nasal CPAP 5 cmH_2O and had gradual reduction in oxygen until receiving air, and then CPAP was ceased. The primary outcome was the duration of oxygen requirement after randomization, and this was significantly less in the HFNC group: mean 21 h versus 50 h, $p<0.001$. The HFNC group also had a shorter stay in hospital (mean 11 vs. 15 days, $p=0.04$). However, there was no difference in BPD rates (the definition used was not provided): HFNC 7 % versus non-HFNC 2 %, $p=0.16$.

Discussion and Recommendations

There is accumulating evidence from clinical trials that HFNC may be used to provide respiratory support for preterm infants in a variety of clinical scenarios. HFNC use in preterm infants is increasing around the world, and there is evidence that HFNC is preferred to CPAP by parents [109] and nurses [110] due to its potential advantages over CPAP, including infant comfort [111] and reduced nasal trauma [100, 105, 106, 112]. Most evidence is available for HFNC use as mode of post-extubation support for preterm infants.

With regards to the important outcome of BPD, the limited evidence presented in this chapter suggests that there are no differences in BPD rates when HFNC is compared to CPAP as either primary support after birth or post-extubation support. There was also no difference in one trial comparing HFNC to NIPPV as primary support. However, the number of infants randomized to HFNC as primary therapy remains small, and there is substantial uncertainty about its usefulness in this setting, particularly for the most immature infants.

There are some concerns about HFNC use in preterm infants. Two studies found that the use of HFNC in place of CPAP may result in longer durations of respiratory support, supplemental oxygen, or hospitalization [100, 107]. In addition, the best and quickest way to wean from HFNC remains uncertain. There is little evidence to guide clinicians, but our practice is to wean gas flow in at least 1 L/min decrements and cease HFNC support from 4 L/min. A related question is whether it is "better" for convalescing preterm infants who have minimal oxygen requirement to be treated with HFNC rather than "low flow" or cot oxygen. It has been suggested that the small amount of distending pressure generated with HFNC may be beneficial to some infants and reduce exposure to oxygen.

Further trials of HFNC in extremely preterm infants born <28 weeks' gestation, the population at highest risk of BPD, are required. These studies should be powered to show a difference in rates of BPD in survivors.

Acknowledgments We sincerely thank Professor Bradley Yoder (University of Utah, USA) and Dr. Clare Collins (Mercy Hospital for Women, Melbourne, Australia) for providing unpublished subgroup data for this chapter. We also thank Dr. Ma Li (Hebei Provincial Children's Hospital, Hebei, China), Dr. Manizheh Mostafa-Gharehbaghi (Tabriz University of Medical Sciences, Tabriz, Iran), and Dr. Ramin Iranpour (Isfahan University of Medical Sciences, Isfahan, Iran) for their assistance with translation and clarification of their trial methodology and results. A/Prof. Dominic Wilkinson (University of Oxford, Oxford, UK) assisted with the collection and clarification of data.

References

1. Gregory GA, Kitterman JA, Phibbs RH, Tooley WH, Hamilton WK. Treatment of the idiopathic respiratory-distress syndrome with continuous positive airway pressure. N Engl J Med. 1971;284(24):1333–40.
2. Duke T. CPAP: a guide for clinicians in developing countries. Paediatr Int Child Health. 2014;34(1):3–11.
3. Koyamaibole L, Kado J, Qovu JD, Colquhoun S, Duke T. An evaluation of bubble-CPAP in a neonatal unit in a developing country: effective respiratory support that can be applied by nurses. J Trop Pediatr. 2006;52(4):249–53.
4. Locke R, Greenspan JS, Shaffer TH, Rubenstein SD, Wolfson MR. Effect of nasal CPAP on thoracoabdominal motion in neonates with respiratory insufficiency. Pediatr Pulmonol. 1991;11(3):259–64.
5. Alex CG, Aronson RM, Onal E, Lopata M. Effects of continuous positive airway pressure on upper airway and respiratory muscle activity. J Appl Physiol. 1987;62(5):2026–30.
6. Miller MJ, DiFiore JM, Strohl KP, Martin RJ. Effects of nasal CPAP on supraglottic and total pulmonary resistance in preterm infants. J Appl Physiol. 1990;68(1):141–6.
7. Ohki M, Naito K, Cole P. Dimensions and resistances of the human nose: racial differences. Laryngoscope. 1991;101(3):276–8.
8. Miller MJ, Carlo WA, Martin RJ. Continuous positive airway pressure selectively reduces obstructive apnea in preterm infants. J Pediatr. 1985;106(1):91–4.
9. Kattwinkel J, Nearman HS, Fanaroff AA, Katona PG, Klaus MH. Apnea of prematurity. Comparative therapeutic effects of cutaneous stimulation and nasal continuous positive airway pressure. J Pediatr. 1975;86(4):588–92.
10. Gaon P, Lee S, Hannan S, Ingram D, Milner AD. Assessment of effect of nasal continuous positive pressure on laryngeal opening using fibre optic laryngoscopy. Arch Dis Child Fetal Neonatal Ed. 1999;80(3):F230–2.
11. Saunders RA, Milner AD, Hopkin IE. The effects of continuous positive airway pressure on lung mechanics and lung volumes in the neonate. Biol Neonate. 1976;29(3–4):178–86.
12. Harris H, Wilson S, Brans Y, Wirtschafter D, Cassady G. Nasal continuous positive airway pressure. Improvement in arterial oxygenation in hyaline membrane disease. Biol Neonate. 1976;29(3–4):231–7.
13. Yu VY, Rolfe P. Effect of continuous positive airway pressure breathing on cardiorespiratory function in infants with respiratory distress syndrome. Acta Paediatr Scand. 1977;66(1):59–64.
14. Durand M, McCann E, Brady JP. Effect of continuous positive airway pressure on the ventilatory response to CO2 in preterm infants. Pediatrics. 1983;71(4):634–8.
15. Richardson CP, Jung AL. Effects of continuous positive airway pressure on pulmonary function and blood gases of infants with respiratory distress syndrome. Pediatr Res. 1978;12(7):771–4.
16. Richardson P, Wyman ML, Jung AL. Functional residual capacity and severity of respiratory distress syndrome in infants. Crit Care Med. 1980;8(11):637–40.

17. Cotton RB, Lindstrom DP, Kanarek KS, Sundell H, Stahlman MT. Effect of positive-end-expiratory-pressure on right ventricular output in lambs with hyaline membrane disease. Acta Paediatr Scand. 1980;69(5):603–6.
18. Magnenant E, Rakza T, Riou Y, Elgellab A, Matran R, Lequien P, et al. Dynamic behavior of respiratory system during nasal continuous positive airway pressure in spontaneously breathing premature newborn infants. Pediatr Pulmonol. 2004;37(6):485–91.
19. De Paoli AG, Davis PG, Faber B, Morley CJ. Devices and pressure sources for administration of nasal continuous positive airway pressure (NCPAP) in preterm neonates. Cochrane Database Syst Rev. 2008;1:CD002977.
20. Colaizy TT, Younis UM, Bell EF, Klein JM. Nasal high-frequency ventilation for premature infants. Acta Paediatr. 2008;97(11):1518–22.
21. Lee KS, Dunn MS, Fenwick M, Shennan AT. A comparison of underwater bubble continuous positive airway pressure with ventilator-derived continuous positive airway pressure in premature neonates ready for extubation. Biol Neonate. 1998;73(2):69–75.
22. Davis PG, Henderson-Smart DJ. Nasal continuous positive airways pressure immediately after extubation for preventing morbidity in preterm infants. Cochrane Database Syst Rev. 2003;2:CD000143.
23. Sweet DG, Carnielli V, Greisen G, Hallman M, Ozek E, Plavka R, et al. European consensus guidelines on the management of neonatal respiratory distress syndrome in preterm infants—2013 update. Neonatology. 2013;103(4):353–68.
24. Ho JJ, Subramaniam P, Henderson-Smart DJ, Davis PG. Continuous distending pressure for respiratory distress syndrome in preterm infants. Cochrane Database Syst Rev. 2002; 2:CD002271.
25. Ho JJ, Henderson-Smart DJ, Davis PG. Early versus delayed initiation of continuous distending pressure for respiratory distress syndrome in preterm infants. Cochrane Database Syst Rev. 2002;2:CD002975.
26. Subramaniam P, Henderson-Smart DJ, Davis PG. Prophylactic nasal continuous positive airways pressure for preventing morbidity and mortality in very preterm infants. Cochrane Database Syst Rev. 2005;3:CD001243.
27. Han VK, Beverley DW, Clarson C, Sumabat WO, Shaheed WA, Brabyn DG, et al. Randomized controlled trial of very early continuous distending pressure in the management of preterm infants. Early Hum Dev. 1987;15(1):21–32.
28. Badiee Z, Naseri F, Sadeghnia A. Early versus delayed initiation of nasal continuous positive airway pressure for treatment of respiratory distress syndrome in premature newborns: a randomized clinical trial. Adv Biomed Res. 2013;2:4.
29. British Association of Perinatal Medicine Guidelines. Position statement on Early Care of the Newborn. Statement on current level of evidence (2005): Guidelines for surfactant administration..
30. Stevens TP, Harrington EW, Blennow M, Soll RF. Early surfactant administration with brief ventilation vs selective surfactant and continued mechanical ventilation for preterm infants with or at risk for respiratory distress syndrome. Cochrane Database Syst Rev. 2007;4:CD003063.
31. Avery ME, Tooley WH, Keller JB, Hurd SS, Bryan MH, Cotton RB, et al. Is chronic lung disease in low birth weight infants preventable? A survey of eight centers. Pediatrics. 1987;79(1):26–30.
32. Kamper J, Wulff K, Larsen C, Lindequist S. Early treatment with nasal continuous positive airway pressure in very low-birth-weight infants. Acta Paediatr. 1993;82(2):193–7.
33. Jacobsen T, Gronvall J, Petersen S, Andersen GE. "Minitouch" treatment of very low-birth-weight infants. Acta Paediatr. 1993;82(11):934–8.
34. Lundstrom KE. Initial treatment of preterm infants—continuous positive airway pressure or ventilation? Eur J Pediatr. 1996;155 Suppl 2:S25–9.
35. Van Marter LJ, Allred EN, Pagano M, Sanocka U, Parad R, Moore M, et al. Do clinical markers of barotrauma and oxygen toxicity explain interhospital variation in rates of chronic lung disease? The neonatology committee for the developmental network. Pediatrics. 2000;105(6):1194–201.

36. Finer NN, Carlo WA, Duara S, Fanaroff AA, Donovan EF, Wright LL, et al. Delivery room continuous positive airway pressure/positive end-expiratory pressure in extremely low birth weight infants: a feasibility trial. Pediatrics. 2004;114(3):651–7.
37. Morley CJ, Davis PG, Doyle LW, Brion LP, Hascoet JM, Carlin JB. Nasal CPAP or intubation at birth for very preterm infants. N Engl J Med. 2008;358(7):700–8.
38. Finer NN, Carlo WA, Walsh MC, Rich W, Gantz MG, Laptook AR, et al. Early CPAP versus surfactant in extremely preterm infants. N Engl J Med. 2010;362(21):1970–9.
39. Dunn MS, Kaempf J, de Klerk A, de Klerk R, Reilly M, Howard D, et al. Randomized trial comparing 3 approaches to the initial respiratory management of preterm neonates. Pediatrics. 2011;128(5):e1069–76.
40. Schmolzer GM, Kumar M, Pichler G, Aziz K, O'Reilly M, Cheung PY. Non-invasive versus invasive respiratory support in preterm infants at birth: systematic review and meta-analysis. BMJ. 2013;347:f5980.
41. Sandri F, Plavka R, Ancora G, Simeoni U, Stranak Z, Martinelli S, et al. Prophylactic or early selective surfactant combined with nCPAP in very preterm infants. Pediatrics. 2010;125(6):e1402–9.
42. Verder H, Robertson B, Greisen G, Ebbesen F, Albertsen P, Lundstrom K, et al. Surfactant therapy and nasal continuous positive airway pressure for newborns with respiratory distress syndrome. Danish-Swedish multicenter study group. N Engl J Med. 1994;331(16):1051–5.
43. Rojas MA, Lozano JM, Rojas MX, Laughon M, Bose CL, Rondon MA, et al. Very early surfactant without mandatory ventilation in premature infants treated with early continuous positive airway pressure: a randomized, controlled trial. Pediatrics. 2009;123(1):137–42.
44. Soll RF, Morley CJ. Prophylactic versus selective use of surfactant in preventing morbidity and mortality in preterm infants. Cochrane Database Syst Rev. 2001;2:CD000510.
45. Rojas-Reyes MX, Morley CJ, Soll R. Prophylactic versus selective use of surfactant in preventing morbidity and mortality in preterm infants. Cochrane Database Syst Rev. 2012;3:CD000510.
46. Todd DA, Wright A, Broom M, Chauhan M, Meskell S, Cameron C, et al. Methods of weaning preterm babies <30 weeks gestation off CPAP: a multicentre randomised controlled trial. Arch Dis Child Fetal Neonatal Ed. 2012;97(4):F236–40.
47. Moretti C, Marzetti G, Agostino R, Panero A, Picece-Bucci S, Mendicini M, et al. Prolonged intermittent positive pressure ventilation by nasal prongs in intractable apnea of prematurity. Acta Paediatr Scand. 1981;70(2):211–6.
48. Lin CH, Wang ST, Lin YJ, Yeh TF. Efficacy of nasal intermittent positive pressure ventilation in treating apnea of prematurity. Pediatr Pulmonol. 1998;26(5):349–53.
49. Ryan CA, Finer NN, Peters KL. Nasal intermittent positive-pressure ventilation offers no advantages over nasal continuous positive airway pressure in apnea of prematurity. Am J Dis Child. 1989;143(10):1196–8.
50. Garland JS, Nelson DB, Rice T, Neu J. Increased risk of gastrointestinal perforations in neonates mechanically ventilated with either face mask or nasal prongs. Pediatrics. 1985;76(3):406–10.
51. Friedlich P, Lecart C, Posen R, Ramicone E, Chan L, Ramanathan R. A randomized trial of nasopharyngeal-synchronized intermittent mandatory ventilation versus nasopharyngeal continuous positive airway pressure in very low birth weight infants after extubation. J Perinatol. 1999;19(6 Pt 1):413–8.
52. Barrington KJ, Bull D, Finer NN. Randomized trial of nasal synchronized intermittent mandatory ventilation compared with continuous positive airway pressure after extubation of very low birth weight infants. Pediatrics. 2001;107(4):638–41.
53. Khalaf MN, Brodsky N, Hurley J, Bhandari V. A prospective randomized, controlled trial comparing synchronized nasal intermittent positive pressure ventilation versus nasal continuous positive airway pressure as modes of extubation. Pediatrics. 2001;108(1):13–7.
54. Kiciman NM, Andreasson B, Bernstein G, Mannino FL, Rich W, Henderson C, et al. Thoracoabdominal motion in newborns during ventilation delivered by endotracheal tube or nasal prongs. Pediatr Pulmonol. 1998;25(3):175–81.

55. Moretti C, Gizzi C, Papoff P, Lampariello S, Capoferri M, Calcagnini G, et al. Comparing the effects of nasal synchronized intermittent positive pressure ventilation (nSIPPV) and nasal continuous positive airway pressure (nCPAP) after extubation in very low birth weight infants. Early Hum Dev. 1999;56(2–3):167–77.
56. Lin XZ, Zheng Z, Lin YY, Lai JD, Li YD. Nasal synchronized intermittent positive pressure ventilation for the treatment of apnea in preterm infants. Zhongguo Dang Dai Er Ke Za Zhi. 2011;13(10):783–6.
57. Gizzi C, Montecchia F, Panetta V, Castellano C, Mariani C, Campelli M, et al. Is synchronised NIPPV more effective than NIPPV and NCPAP in treating apnoea of prematurity (AOP)? A randomised cross-over trial. Arch Dis Child Fetal Neonatal Ed. 2015;100(1):F17–23.
58. Aghai ZH, Saslow JG, Nakhla T, Milcarek B, Hart J, Lawrysh-Plunkett R, et al. Synchronized nasal intermittent positive pressure ventilation (SNIPPV) decreases work of breathing (WOB) in premature infants with respiratory distress syndrome (RDS) compared to nasal continuous positive airway pressure (NCPAP). Pediatr Pulmonol. 2006;41(9):875–81.
59. Ali N, Claure N, Alegria X, D'Ugard C, Organero R, Bancalari E. Effects of non-invasive pressure support ventilation (NI-PSV) on ventilation and respiratory effort in very low birth weight infants. Pediatr Pulmonol. 2007;42(8):704–10.
60. Chang HY, Claure N, D'Ugard C, Torres J, Nwajei P, Bancalari E. Effects of synchronization during nasal ventilation in clinically stable preterm infants. Pediatr Res. 2011;69(1):84–9.
61. Jackson JK, Vellucci J, Johnson P, Kilbride HW. Evidence-based approach to change in clinical practice: introduction of expanded nasal continuous positive airway pressure use in an intensive care nursery. Pediatrics. 2003;111(4 Pt 2):e542–7.
62. Bhandari V. Nasal intermittent positive pressure ventilation in the newborn: review of literature and evidence-based guidelines. J Perinatol. 2010;30(8):505–12.
63. Bhandari V. Noninvasive respiratory support in the preterm infant. Clin Perinatol. 2012;39(3):497–511.
64. Kugelman A, Bar A, Riskin A, Chistyakov I, Mor F, Bader D. Nasal respiratory support in premature infants: short-term physiological effects and comfort assessment. Acta Paediatr. 2008;97(5):557–61.
65. Moretti C, Giannini L, Fassi C, Gizzi C, Papoff P, Colarizi P. Nasal flow-synchronized intermittent positive pressure ventilation to facilitate weaning in very low-birthweight infants: unmasked randomized controlled trial. Pediatr Int. 2008;50(1):85–91.
66. Beck J, Reilly M, Grasselli G, Mirabella L, Slutsky AS, Dunn MS, et al. Patient-ventilator interaction during neurally adjusted ventilatory assist in low birth weight infants. Pediatr Res. 2009;65(6):663–8.
67. Bhandari V, Gavino RG, Nedrelow JH, Pallela P, Salvador A, Ehrenkranz RA, et al. A randomized controlled trial of synchronized nasal intermittent positive pressure ventilation in RDS. J Perinatol. 2007;27(11):697–703.
68. Nzegwu NI, Mack T, DellaVentura R, Dunphy L, Koval N, Levit O, et al. Systematic use of the RAM nasal cannula in the Yale-New Haven children's hospital neonatal intensive care unit: a quality improvement project. J Matern Fetal Neonatal Med. 2015;28(6):718–21.
69. De Paoli AG, Davis PG, Lemyre B. Nasal continuous positive airway pressure versus nasal intermittent positive pressure ventilation for preterm neonates: a systematic review and meta-analysis. Acta Paediatr. 2003;92(1):70–5.
70. Gao WW, Tan SZ, Chen YB, Zhang Y, Wang Y. Randomized trial of nasal synchronized intermittent mandatory ventilation compared with nasal continuous positive airway pressure in preterm infants with respiratory distress syndrome. Zhongguo Dang Dai Er Ke Za Zhi. 2010;12(7):524–6.
71. Kulkarni A, Ehrenkranz RA, Bhandari V. Effect of introduction of synchronized nasal intermittent positive-pressure ventilation in a neonatal intensive care unit on bronchopulmonary dysplasia and growth in preterm infants. Am J Perinatol. 2006;23(4):233–40.
72. Bhandari V, Finer NN, Ehrenkranz RA, Saha S, Das A, Walsh MC, et al. Synchronized nasal intermittent positive-pressure ventilation and neonatal outcomes. Pediatrics. 2009;124(2):517–26.

73. Khorana M, Paradeevisut H, Sangtawesin V, Kanjanapatanakul W, Chotigeat U, Ayutthaya JK. A randomized trial of non-synchronized nasopharyngeal intermittent mandatory ventilation (nsNIMV) vs. nasal continuous positive airway pressure (NCPAP) in the prevention of extubation failure in pre-term < 1,500 grams. J Med Assoc Thai. 2008;91 Suppl 3:S136–42.
74. Bhandari V. The potential of non-invasive ventilation to decrease BPD. Semin Perinatol. 2013;37(2):108–14.
75. Kahramaner Z, Erdemir A, Turkoglu E, Cosar H, Sutcuoglu S, Ozer EA. Unsynchronized nasal intermittent positive pressure versus nasal continuous positive airway pressure in preterm infants after extubation. J Matern Fetal Neonatal Med. 2014;27(9):926–9.
76. Jasani B, Nanavati R, Kabra N, Rajdeo S, Bhandari V. Comparison of non synchronized nasal intermittent positive pressure ventilation versus nasal continuous positive airway pressure as post-extubation respiratory support in preterm infants with respiratory distress syndrome: a randomized controlled trial. J Matern Fetal Neonatal Med. 2015:1–22.
77. Kugelman A, Feferkorn I, Riskin A, Chistyakov I, Kaufman B, Bader D. Nasal intermittent mandatory ventilation versus nasal continuous positive airway pressure for respiratory distress syndrome: a randomized, controlled, prospective study. J Pediatr. 2007;150(5):521–6.
78. Sai Sunil Kishore M, Dutta S, Kumar P. Early nasal intermittent positive pressure ventilation versus continuous positive airway pressure for respiratory distress syndrome. Acta Paediatr. 2009;98(9):1412–5.
79. Meneses J, Bhandari V, Alves JG, Herrmann D. Noninvasive ventilation for respiratory distress syndrome: a randomized controlled trial. Pediatrics. 2011;127(2):300–7.
80. Meneses J, Bhandari V, Alves JG. Nasal intermittent positive-pressure ventilation vs. nasal continuous positive airway pressure for preterm infants with respiratory distress syndrome: a systematic review and meta-analysis. Arch Pediatr Adolesc Med. 2012;166(4):372–6.
81. Bisceglia M, Belcastro A, Poerio V, Raimondi F, Mesuraca L, Crugliano C, et al. A comparison of nasal intermittent versus continuous positive pressure delivery for the treatment of moderate respiratory syndrome in preterm infants. Minerva Pediatr. 2007;59(2):91–5.
82. Fu CH, Xia SW. Clinical application of nasal intermittent positive pressure ventilation in initial treatment of neonatal respiratory distress syndrome. Zhongguo Dang Dai Er Ke Za Zhi. 2014;16(5):460–4.
83. Shi Y, Tang S, Zhao J, Shen J. A prospective, randomized, controlled study of NIPPV versus nCPAP in preterm and term infants with respiratory distress syndrome. Pediatr Pulmonol. 2014;49(7):673–8.
84. Ramanathan R, Sekar KC, Rasmussen M, Bhatia J, Soll RF. Nasal intermittent positive pressure ventilation after surfactant treatment for respiratory distress syndrome in preterm infants <30 weeks' gestation: a randomized, controlled trial. J Perinatol. 2012;32(5):336–43.
85. Kirpalani H, Millar D, Lemyre B, Yoder BA, Chiu A, Roberts RS. A trial comparing noninvasive ventilation strategies in preterm infants. N Engl J Med. 2013;369(7):611–20.
86. Tang S, Zhao J, Shen J, Hu Z, Shi Y. Nasal intermittent positive pressure ventilation versus nasal continuous positive airway pressure in neonates: a systematic review and meta-analysis. Indian Pediatr. 2013;50(4):371–6.
87. Lista G, Castoldi F, Fontana P, Daniele I, Cavigioli F, Rossi S, et al. Nasal continuous positive airway pressure (CPAP) versus bi-level nasal CPAP in preterm babies with respiratory distress syndrome: a randomised control trial. Arch Dis Child Fetal Neonatal Ed. 2010;95(2):F85–9.
88. Gao X, Yang B, Hei M, Cui X, Wang J, Zhou G, et al. Application of three kinds of noninvasive positive pressure ventilation as a primary mode of ventilation in premature infants with respiratory distress syndrome: a randomized controlled trial. Zhonghua Er Ke Za Zhi. 2014;52(1):34–40.
89. Lampland AL, Plumm B, Worwa C, Meyers P, Mammel MC. Bi-level CPAP does not improve gas exchange when compared with conventional CPAP for the treatment of neonates recovering from respiratory distress syndrome. Arch Dis Child Fetal Neonatal Ed. 2015; 100(1):F31–4.
90. Ricotti A, Salvo V, Zimmermann LJ, Gavilanes AW, Barberi I, Lista G, et al. N-SIPPV versus bi-level N-CPAP for early treatment of respiratory distress syndrome in preterm infants. J Matern Fetal Neonatal Med. 2013;26(13):1346–51.

91. Thomas PE, LeFlore J. Extubation success in premature infants with respiratory distress syndrome treated with bi-level nasal continuous positive airway pressure versus nasal intermittent positive pressure ventilation. J Perinat Neonatal Nurs. 2013;27(4):328–34. Quiz E3–4.
92. Salvo V, Lista G, Lupo E, Ricotti A, Zimmermann LJ, Gavilanes AW, et al. Noninvasive ventilation strategies for early treatment of RDS in preterm infants: an RCT. Pediatrics. 2015;135(3):444–51.
93. Millar D, Lemyre B, Kirpalani H, Chiu A, Yoder BA, Roberts RS. A comparison of bilevel and ventilator-delivered non-invasive respiratory support. Arch Dis Child Fetal Neonatal Ed. 2016;101:21–5.
94. Roberts CT, Davis PG, Owen LS. Neonatal non-invasive respiratory support: synchronised NIPPV, non-synchronised NIPPV or bi-level CPAP: what is the evidence in 2013? Neonatology. 2013;104(3):203–9.
95. Hough JL, Shearman AD, Jardine LA, Davies MW. Humidified high flow nasal cannulae: current practice in Australasian nurseries, a survey. J Paediatr Child Health. 2012;48:106–13.
96. Nath P, Ponnusamy V, Willis K, Bissett L, Clarke P. Current practices of high and low flow oxygen therapy and humidification in UK neonatal units. Pediatr Int. 2010;52(6):893–4.
97. Hochwald O, Osiovich H. The use of high flow nasal cannulae in neonatal intensive care units: is clinical practice consistent with the evidence? J Neonatal-Perinatal Med. 2010;3(3):187–91.
98. The Collaborative Group for the Multicenter Study on Heated Humidified High flow Nasal Cannula Ventilation. Efficacy and safety of heated humidified high·flow nasal cannula for prevention of extubation failure in neonates. Chin J Pediatr. 2014;52(4):271–6.
99. Iranpour R, Sadeghnia A, Hesaraki M. High-flow nasal cannula versus nasal continuous positive airway pressure in the management of respiratory distress syndrome. J Isfahan Med Sch. 2011;29(143):761–71.
100. Yoder BA, Stoddard RA, Li M, King J, Dirnberger DR, Abbasi S. Heated, humidified high-flow nasal cannula versus nasal CPAP for respiratory support in neonates. Pediatrics. 2013;131(5):e1482–90.
101. Ciuffini F, Pietrasanta C, Lavizzari A, Musumeci S, Gualdi C, Sortino S, et al. Comparison between two different modes of non-invasive ventilatory support in preterm newborn infants with respiratory distress syndrome mild to moderate: preliminary data. Pediatr Med Chir. 2014;36(4):88.
102. Kugelman A, Riskin A, Said W, Shoris I, Mor F, Bader D. A randomized pilot study comparing heated humidified high-flow nasal cannulae with NIPPV for RDS. Pediatr Pulmonol. 2015;50:576–83.
103. Campbell DM, Shah PS, Shah V, Kelly EN. Nasal continuous positive airway pressure from high flow cannula versus infant flow for preterm infants. J Perinatol. 2006;26(9):546–9.
104. Collins CL, Holberton JR, Barfield C, Davis PG. A randomized controlled trial to compare heated humidified high-flow nasal cannulae with nasal continuous positive airway pressure postextubation in premature infants. J Pediatr. 2013;162(5):949–54. e1.
105. Manley BJ, Owen LS, Doyle LW, Andersen CC, Cartwright DW, Pritchard MA, et al. High-flow nasal cannulae in very preterm infants after extubation. N Engl J Med. 2013;369(15): 1425–33.
106. Mostafa-Gharehbaghi M, Mojabi H. Comparing the effectiveness of nasal continuous positive airway pressure (NCPAP) and high flow nasal cannula (HFNC) in prevention of post extubation assisted ventilation. Zahedan J Res Med Sci. 2015;17(6):e984.
107. Abdel-Hady H, Shouman B, Aly H. Early weaning from CPAP to high flow nasal cannula in preterm infants is associated with prolonged oxygen requirement: a randomized controlled trial. Early Hum Dev. 2011;87(3):205–8.
108. Badiee Z, Eshghi A, Mohammadizadeh M. High flow nasal cannula as a method for rapid weaning from nasal continuous positive airway pressure. Int J Prev Med. 2015;6:33.
109. Klingenberg C, Pettersen M, Hansen EA, Gustavsen LJ, Dahl IA, Leknessund A, et al. Patient comfort during treatment with heated humidified high flow nasal cannulae versus nasal continuous positive airway pressure: a randomised cross-over trial. Arch Dis Child Fetal Neonatal Ed. 2014;99(2):F134–7.

110. Roberts CT, Manley BJ, Dawson JA, Davis PG. Nursing perceptions of high-flow nasal cannulae treatment for very preterm infants. J Paediatr Child Health. 2014;50(10):806–10.
111. Osman M, Elsharkawy A, Abdel-Hady H. Assessment of pain during application of nasal-continuous positive airway pressure and heated, humidified high-flow nasal cannulae in preterm infants. J Perinatol. 2015;35(4):263–7.
112. Collins CL, Barfield C, Horne RS, Davis PG. A comparison of nasal trauma in preterm infants extubated to either heated humidified high-flow nasal cannulae or nasal continuous positive airway pressure. Eur J Pediatr. 2014;173(2):181–6.

Chapter 12
Nutrition in Bronchopulmonary Dysplasia: In the NICU and Beyond

Richard A. Ehrenkranz and Fernando R. Moya

Among the challenges facing clinicians caring for preterm infants, especially extremely preterm infants (infants less than 28 weeks' gestation), is the provision of nutritional support that permits an adequate rate of postnatal growth and development. Observational studies have demonstrated that it is common for extrauterine growth restriction to occur during the neonatal intensive care unit (NICU) hospitalization [1–3] and for preterm infants to have a body weight <10th % at their discharge postmenstrual age (PMA). Furthermore, those infants who were small-for-gestational age (SGA) at birth or who had experienced one or more of the common neonatal morbidities, including bronchopulmonary dysplasia (BPD), necrotizing enterocolitis (NEC), or late-onset sepsis, have been shown to grow more slowly than infants who were appropriate-for-gestational age (AGA) at birth and who had not experienced such morbidities [1].

The objective of this chapter is to review the role that nutrition plays in the development and management of BPD. This topic has been recently reviewed [4–7]. BPD is considered to have a multifactorial etiology, and nutrition, both in a general sense or associated with one or more specific nutrients, has long been included as one of those etiologic factors [8–10]. To meet this objective, we will consider the interaction between the receipt of early nutritional support and the development of BPD, the role of specific nutrients in preventing or facilitating the development of BPD, and the importance of post-discharge nutrition on recovery from BPD.

R.A. Ehrenkranz, MD (✉)
Department of Pediatrics/Section of Neonatal-Perinatal Medicine, Yale University School of Medicine, 333 Cedar Street, P.O. Box 208064, New Haven, CT 06520-8064, USA
e-mail: richard.ehrenkranz@yale.edu

F.R. Moya, MD
Betty Cameron Children's Hospital, 2131 South 17th Street, Wilmington, NC 28401, USA

V. Bhandari (ed.), *Bronchopulmonary Dysplasia*, Respiratory Medicine,
DOI 10.1007/978-3-319-28486-6_12

Influence of Nutrition and the Development of BPD

The supportive role that nutrition plays in the process of normal lung growth and its influence on injury and repair have been discussed for years. For example, a workshop [8] held by the National Institutes of Health/National Heart, Lung, and Blood Institute (NIH/NHLBI) in 1986 on "Nutrition and the Respiratory System" concluded that "sufficient evidence is available to recommend that greater clinical priority be given to nutrition as a vigorous part of total support in premature infants." That recommendation was based upon animal and human research which described the adverse effect that undernutrition had on lung growth and maturation as well as on injury and recovery. Additional consequences of undernutrition are listed in Table 12.1; although adapted from publications [9, 10] from the pre-surfactant era, these potential effects of undernutrition are still being discussed and researched today since they contribute to the pathogenesis of BPD.

It remains an all-too-common clinical practice to focus on the acute medical problem at the expense of providing sufficient, early nutritional support to extremely preterm infants, those at greatest risk of developing BPD. Despite studies promoting the benefits of trophic feeding, the initiation of any enteral substrate is often delayed, and only parenteral nutrition is provided until extremely preterm infants are considered "stable" and, especially, after they had recovered from any "acute respiratory illness" [11]. It should be no surprise, therefore, that compared to infants who were treated with prolonged mechanical ventilation (MV) [12] or who developed BPD

Table 12.1 Potential effects of undernutrition in extremely preterm infants with respiratory distress

Variable	Effect
Poor energy reserves at birth	• Early catabolic state
Inadequate postnatal nutritional support	• Cumulative energy, protein, and other nutrient deficits • Slow growth
Respiratory distress syndrome	• Insufficient surfactant synthesis • Decreased respiratory muscle function
Lung growth	• Decreased lung biosynthesis • Decreased cell replication • Decreased structural maturation (alveolarization) • Decreased extracellular matrix formation
Protection from hyperoxia/barotrauma	• Decreased epithelial integrity • Decreased defense against O_2 free radicals and lipid peroxidation • Decreased synthesis of antioxidant enzymes • Decreased lung biosynthesis and cell replication for repair
Lung repair and development of bronchopulmonary dysplasia	• Decreased lung biosynthesis • Decreased replacement of damaged cells • Decreased replacement of damaged extracellular components
Susceptibility to infection	• Decreased cellular and humoral defenses against pathogens • Decreased cell integrity • Decreased mucociliary clearance mechanisms

Adapted from Frank L and Sosenko IR. Am Rev Respir Dis 1988; 138:725–229 and Frank L, in Banaclari & Stocker *Bronchopulmonary Dysplasia*, Aspen Seminars on Pediatric Disease, 1988

[1, 13, 14], infants ventilated for shorter time periods or who did not develop BPD had better growth during the NICU hospitalization. These reports have classified infants by duration of mechanical ventilation or whether they have or have not developed BPD. However, extremely preterm infants are not born with BPD. Following birth, they may experience respiratory insufficiency due to immaturity or respiratory distress syndrome (RDS) and require treatment with supplemental oxygen and mechanical respiratory assistance; the impaired lung development associated with BPD evolves over the next several weeks. Thus, can the growth failure associated with BPD and the incidence and severity of BPD be decreased by making the provision of early nutritional support the "priority" recommended by the 1986 NIH/NHLBI workshop [8]?

Early Nutritional Management of Extremely Preterm Infants and the Development of BPD

A secondary analysis [15] of a dataset derived from a multicenter, randomized controlled trial [16] suggested that the perception of severity of illness, "more critically ill" versus "less critically ill," made within the first several days of life appeared to set in motion practices that might increase the incidence and severity of BPD. For the analysis, infants were stratified by whether or not they received MV for the first 7 days of life; more critically ill infants were defined as having received MV for the first 7 days of life, while less critically ill infants were those who received MV for less than the first 7 days of life. AGA and SGA infants were evaluated separately.

Table 12.2 displays the total daily energy and total daily fluid intakes for the first 3 weeks of life by severity of critical illness for AGA infants enrolled in the trial and alive on day 7. Except for parenteral protein energy during days 1–7, all energy measures were significantly different between the cohorts. Similar results were noted for SGA infants. Specifically, compared with more critically ill infants, less critically ill infants also received significantly more nutritional support during the first 3 weeks of life. In addition, the total daily fluid intake was significantly different between the more and less critically ill cohorts during the first 7 days of life, with less critically ill infants receiving significantly more total daily energy and less total daily fluid than the more critically ill infants. Interestingly, another secondary analysis of this trial's dataset demonstrated that BPD-free survivors received less total daily fluid during the first 10 days of life than infants who died or survived with BPD [17]. Analyses that included a formal mediation framework demonstrated that critical illness status remained an independent and statistically significant predictor of total energy intake.

Table 12.3 displays selected outcome data by severity of critical illness for AGA infants. It is evident that more critically ill infants grew slower, were smaller at 36 weeks' PMA, experienced more morbidities including BPD and late-onset sepsis (but not NEC), achieved nutritional milestones later, and were more likely to have adverse neurodevelopmental outcomes. Similar results were noted for SGA infants. Analyses performed with the mediation framework demonstrated that critical illness was independently and significantly associated with slower growth velocity and with

Table 12.2 Energy and fluid intake by degree of critical illness in AGA infants (unadjusted and adjusted analyses)

	Critically ill		
Energy intake[a] (kcal/kg/day); fluid intake[a] (cc/kg/day)	Less (MV<7days) (n=499)	More (MV day 1–7) (n=646)	p-value[b]
Days 1–7			
Parenteral energy	46.1 (12.5)	41.1 (12.5)	<0.0001
Nonprotein	38.7 (10.8)	33.3 (10.7)	<0.0001
Protein	7.4 (2.5)	7.8 (3.2)	0.34
Enteral energy[c]	3, 5.8 (8.1)	0, 1.6 (3.5)	<0.0001
Total energy	52.0 (13.8)	42.7 (13.1)	<0.0001; <0.0001[d]
Total fluid intake	123 (25)	130 (33)	0.001; 0.09[d]
Days 8–14			
Parenteral energy	62.5 (26.4)	69.5 (18.0)	0.0010
Nonprotein	52.2 (22.3)	56.5 (15.5)	0.047
Protein	10.3 (5.0)	13.0 (4.6)	<0.0001
Enteral energy[c]	24, 32.7 (29.5)	5, 12.1 (17.9)	<0.0001
Total energy	95.2 (17.0)	81.6 (19.5)	<0.0001; <0.0001[d]
Total fluid intake	151 (19)	151 (27)	0.89; 0.48[d]
Days 15–21			
Parenteral energy	41.3 (34.9)	58.5 (28.8)	<0.0001
Nonprotein	34.9 (29.7)	48.3 (24.4)	<0.0001
Protein	6.4 (5.7)	10.2 (5.6)	<0.0001
Enteral energy[c]	52, 58.2 (42.4)	16, 30.7 (35.7)	<.0001
Total energy	99.5 (20.8)	89.2 (21.8)	<0.0001; <0.0001[d]
Total fluid intake	139 (27)	142 (25)	0.068; 0.30[d]

AGA appropriate-for-gestational age, *MV* mechanical ventilation
[a]Presented as mean (standard deviation), except where noted
[b]p-values from Wilcoxon test
[c]Presented as median, mean (standard deviation)
[d]p-value after adjusting for birth weight stratum in GLM procedure
Adapted from Ehrenkranz RA, et al. Pediatr Res 69:522–529, 2011

significantly increased odds ratios (ORs) for BPD, BPD or death, NEC or death, late-onset-sepsis or death, neurodevelopmental impairment (NDI), and NDI or death.

Furthermore, the mediation framework was used to test models containing both critical illness and energy intake variables. For AGA infants, this analysis demonstrated that the effects of critical illness on the magnitude of the ORs for BPD, BPD or death, NEC, NEC or death, late-onset sepsis, and late-onset sepsis or death were all significantly decreased once the total daily energy intake variable was included in the model. Thus, these analyses indicated that critical illness during the first weeks of life and early nutritional practices were both independently associated with morbidity. A significant interaction between critical illness and total daily energy intake during days 1–7 of life for NDI and NDI or death was also noted. The number of SGA infants included in the study population did not permit these analyses to be performed in that patient cohort.

Table 12.3 Outcome variables by degree of critical illness in AGA infants (unadjusted analyses)

Variables	Less critically ill (MV<7days) (n=499)	More critically ill (MV days 1–7) (N=646)	p-value[a]
In-hospital morbidity and mortality			
BPD[b]			<0.0001
None [n (%)]	153 (32.5)	15 (2.8)	
Mild [n (%)]	158 (33.6)	149 (27.4)	
Moderate [n (%)]	109 (23.1)	210 (38.6)	
Severe [n (%)]	51 (10.8)	170 (31.3)	
Duration of positive pressure ventilation (day)	13.5 (16.6)	40.9 (26.6)	<0.0001
Duration of oxygen (day)	46.7 (33.1)	74.6 (34.5)	<0.0001
Postnatal steroids for pulmonary disease [n (%)]	88 (17.6)	331 (51.2)	<0.0001
Severe IVH [n (%)]	42 (8.5)	128 (19.8)	<0.0001
NEC [n (%)]	56 (11.2)	59 (9.1)	0.24
Late-onset sepsis [n (%)]	187 (37.5)	306 (47.4)	0.0008
Death [n (%)]	35 (7.0)	123 (19.0)	<0.0001
Length of hospital stay (day)	82.6 (34.9)	102.6 (57.9)	<0.0001
Feeding outcome measures			
Age when enteral nutrition started (day)	5.4 (3.9)	10.2 (8.3)	<0.0001
Age when enteral nutrition ≥ 110 kcal/kg/day (day)	24.9 (15.4)	35.1 (18.4)	<0.0001
Days parenteral nutrition ≥ 10 % total daily fluid volume (day)	27.5 (20.7)	36.3 (22.0)	<0.0001
Anthropometric outcome measures			
Weight at 36 weeks PMA[c] (g)	1926 (312)	1781 (340)	<0.0001
Weight < 10th % tile at 36 weeks PMA[c] [n (%)]	327 (87.2)	447 (90.7)	0.10
Length at 36 weeks PMA[c] (cm)	41.7 (2.2)	40.7 (2.4)	<0.0001
Head circumference at 36 weeks PMA[c] (cm)	30.8 (1.4)	30.0 (1.7)	<0.0001
Weight gain velocity (g/kg/day), all infants	15.9 (7.5)	13.8 (13.6)	<0.0001
Weight gain velocity[d] (g/kg/day)	15.6 (3.0)	14.0 (3.0)	<0.0001
Follow-up outcomes, 18–22 months CA[e]	416 (83.4)	458 (78.6)	
Bayley MDI < 70 [n (%)]	83 (21.3)	180 (42.7)	<0.0001
Bayley PDI < 70 [n (%)]	34 (8.9)	117 (27.9)	<0.0001
Cerebral palsy [moderate or severe; n (%)]	12 (2.5)	41 (9.1)	0.0002
Bilateral blindness [n (%)]	1 (0.2)	3 (0.7)	0.63
Bilateral deafness [n (%)]	3 (1)	9 (2.4)	0.12
Neurodevelopmental impairment [n (%)]	97 (25.3)	206 (48.6)	<0.0001

AGA appropriate-for-gestational age, *MV* mechanical ventilation, *BPD* bronchopulmonary dysplasia, *IVH* intraventricular hemorrhage, *NEC* necrotizing enterocolitis, *PMA* postmenstrual age, *CA* corrected age, Bayley Bayley Scales of Infant Development (2nd edition), *MDI* mental developmental index, *PDI* psychomotor developmental index

[a] *p*-value from Wilcoxon test for continuous variables; Chi-Square, or Fisher's exact test, where appropriate, for categorical variables

[b] Consensus definition, infants < 32 GA, survived to 36 weeks PMA; not ventilated day of life (DOL) 1–7: $n=472$; ventilated: $n=544$

[c] Infants hospitalized at 36 weeks PMA; not ventilated DOL 1–7: $n=377$; ventilated: $n=496$

[d] Infants surviving to 36 weeks PMA; not ventilated DOL 1–7: $n=472$; ventilated: $n=544$

[e] Infants followed up at 18–22 months CA; not ventilated DOL 1–7: $n=416$; ventilated: $n=458$

Adapted from Ehrenkranz RA, et al. Pediatr Res. 69: 522–529, 2011

Standardized, Evidence-Based Early Nutritional Management Guidelines

Since there is marked practice variation within and between centers related to nutritional practices for extremely preterm infants, the implementation of evidence-based feeding guidelines has been advocated during the past several years in an effort to standardize practice within a center [18–25]. For example, after reviewing the published literature, the neonatal staff at Yale-New Haven Children's Hospital's NICU developed a consensus, evidence-based strategy that provided both early parenteral and enteral nutrition, addressed "feeding intolerance," and aimed to maintain a steady rate of postnatal growth by adjusting nutritional support if growth parameters were not met.

Briefly, for extremely preterm infants, parenteral protein (i.e., as amino acids) is initiated within hours of birth as a component of parenteral fluid support. Specifically, of the 80–100 mL/kg/day of intravenous fluids initially ordered, 50 mL/kg/day would be a "starter" ("vanilla," "off-hours") total parenteral nutrition (TPN) that would be delivered at a rate of 3 g protein/kg/day. Yale's Off-Hours TPN is 10 % glucose that contains 6 g protein/dL, 100 mg calcium/dL, minimal electrolytes, and no vitamins or other minerals. Intravenous lipid (fat) emulsion [(IFE) 20 %] should be initiated within 24 h of birth, at a minimum rate of 1.5 g/kg/day, but may be initiated with starter TPN. TPN support would be optimized to 4 g protein/kg/day and 3 g lipid/kg/day over the next several days, as the transition from trophic or nonnutritive feeds to full enteral nutrition begins and is advanced.

Trophic feeds (~12 mL/kg/day) are initiated with colostrum or donor milk, if possible, within 24 h of birth and usually advanced daily by about 12 mL/kg/day, but may be held at trophic volumes for the first 2–3 days. Given the small enteral volumes provided, gastric residuals are not checked while an infant is on trophic feeds, and enteral volumes are not included in the calculation of total daily fluid volume until ≥24 mL/kg/day. As enteral volumes are increased, TPN is decreased so that the total daily fluid volume (parenteral plus enteral) is maintained at 130–150 mL/kg/day. As the amount of TPN is decreased, the protein concentration is not increased, but maintained at a nil per os ("NPO") concentration, so that about 4–4.5 g protein/kg/day would be provided if enteral feedings were discontinued and only TPN were provided. The IFE is also decreased as enteral volumes are increased to 2 g/kg/day when about 25–30 % of the total daily fluid volume is provided enterally, to 1 g/kg/day when about 50–60 % of the total daily fluid volume is provided enterally, and discontinued when about 100 mL/kg/day is provided enterally. TPN would be discontinued when enteral intake has reached about 100–120 mL/kg/day. By administrating TPN via an umbilical venous catheter until about 14 days of age, the need for a percutaneously inserted central line can often be alleviated.

Evidence-based discussions during the development of the standardized feeding guideline led to a consensus by the healthcare team about nutritional practice strategies and about how to manage "feeding intolerance." Issues considered included exceptions and non-exceptions to initiation of trophic feeds within 24 h of birth, potential contraindications to advancement or continuation of enteral feeds, and reasons for brief (6–12 h) interruptions of feedings. Furthermore, it was decided to no longer routinely check gastric residual volumes, but to consider that assessment as part of the clinical evaluation of feeding intolerance [e.g., significant change in abdominal distension (>2 cm), abdominal discoloration, significant clinical deterioration, grossly bloody stools] performed by a member of the medical team.

Enteral nutrition for extremely preterm infants in the NICU is primarily provided by human milk (mother's own milk or donor human milk) and preterm formula. Since human milk does not meet the recommended nutrient requirements of growing extremely preterm infants, human milk is routinely supplemented with human milk fortifier once an enteral intake of about 100 cc/kg/day has been reached. Similar to the experience in late-onset sepsis and NEC [26–29], human milk intake through 36 weeks' PMA has been shown to be associated with the incidence of BPD [30]. In this study, as the cumulative percentage of enteral feedings as human milk increased over the NICU hospitalization, the incidence of BPD fell; specifically, multivariate logistic regression demonstrated that each 10 mL/kg/day increase in human milk intake was associated with a 12 % reduction in the odds of BPD.

Once full enteral nutrition is achieved, it is essential to monitor growth by plotting measurements on an intrauterine growth curve until 40 weeks' PMA [31, 32] and then on the Centers for Disease Control-World Health Organization (CDC-WHO) 2010 growth curves [33], identify causes of decreased rates of growth, and maintain adequate energy and protein intakes. Infants with evolving BPD have been shown to have increased energy needs due to increased work of breathing [34–37]. Since the caloric requirements for these infants, and others with chronic conditions, range from 120 to 150 kcal/kg/day compared to the 90–120 kcal/kg/day for most growing preterm infants [38], slower growth will occur unless continued attention is paid to energy and protein intake, which may be inadvertently reduced during the fluid restriction commonly imposed on infants with BPD.

Benefits observed following the implementation of feeding guidelines have included regaining birth weight earlier, achieving full enteral nutrition sooner, reducing the need for PN, reducing cumulative energy and protein deficits, decreasing rates of common neonatal morbidities, improving the anthropometrics at 36 weeks' and 40 weeks' PMA, mediating the severity of an infant's illness, and reducing length of stay. However, the degree to which standardized, evidence-based feeding guidelines that emphasize early parenteral and enteral nutritional support and address protein and energy needs promptly and throughout the NICU hospitalization will have on the incidence and severity of BPD remains to be seen. Nonetheless, the incidence of growth failure should be reduced, and impact of undernutrition on lung injury and repair should be lessened.

Role of Specific Nutrients

Use of Fluids

Neonatal lung function is best preserved by avoiding free water overload and exercising close monitoring of weight, urine output, and electrolytes [39]. Pulmonary edema due to fluid overload can decrease pulmonary compliance and increase airway resistance. A relationship between high fluid intake and an increased risk of cardiorespiratory morbidity and NEC has been reported [40]. Nonetheless, a recent systematic review of five randomized controlled trials of restricted versus liberal fluid intake during the neonatal period only showed a trend toward less BPD in spite of marked reductions in patent ductus arteriosus (PDA) and NEC [41]. These studies evaluated different populations as well as volumes for restricted or liberal fluid intake. Therefore, for infants at high risk for BPD, initial fluid intakes not to exceed 80–100 mL/kg/day and progressive increases to a maximum of 120–150 mL/kg/day by day 7 may confer clinical advantages over starting with higher intakes and reaching total volumes above those values during the first week after birth. These recommendations probably cannot be extended to infants weighing less than 750 g at birth since very few of them have been evaluated in these trials.

Carbohydrates

Carbohydrates are the primary source of energy for neonates. Moreover, solutions of glucose in water are used preferentially to administer PN during the first days after birth in extremely low birth weight (ELBW) and very LBW (VLBW) infants. Since oxidation of glucose results in higher production of carbon dioxide (CO_2) than fat oxidation, when energy production is derived mainly from oxidation of carbohydrates, the respiratory quotient (RQ), the ratio between generated CO_2 and consumed oxygen (O_2), is higher than if fats predominate as the energy source.

Normal O_2 consumption of preterm infants without respiratory distress is around 6–7 mL/kg/min, and resting energy expenditure (REE) ranges between 50 and 60 kcal/kg/day. Severe respiratory distress can result in much higher REE during the first several days after birth [42]. The effect of changes in intravenous glucose administration on O_2 consumption, CO_2 production, and REE has been studied among infants evolving to or with established BPD [43, 44]. In these infants, loading with up to 12 mg/kg/min of intravenous glucose results in about a 20 % increase in O_2 consumption and REE. Avoiding high glucose infusion rates over 10–12 mg/kg/min may be of importance among infants who have impaired elimination of CO_2 due to lung disease. Infants with BPD can have an elevated REE, which can contribute to their commonly observed growth failure [34, 36]. Among these infants, respiratory rate is the single most important determinant of energy expenditure [45]. The importance of monitoring the growth of infants with evolving or established BPD so as to ensure adequate energy and protein intake has been discussed above.

Inositol

In humans, inositol is mostly found as part of phosphatidylinositol, which is a phospholipid involved in surfactant synthesis [46]. Infants exhibiting a more significant drop in serum inositol levels after delivery have a more severe course of RDS [47].

A recent systematic review of several small trials of inositol administration after birth [48] showed a decrease in neonatal death [Risk Ratio (RR) 0.53, 95 % confidence interval (CI) 0.31–0.91)], severe retinopathy of prematurity (RR 0.09, 95 % CI 0.01–0.67), and severe intraventricular hemorrhage (RR 0.53, 95 % CI 0.31–0.80), but no effect on BPD at 28 days or 36 weeks corrected gestational age (RR 0.78, 95 % CI 0.54–1.13, and 1.30, 0.64–2.64, respectively). A large multicenter randomized controlled trial is currently being performed by the National Institute of Child Health and Human Development (NICHD) Neonatal Research Network (NCT01954082) to evaluate whether inositol supplementation will reduce the risk of severe retinopathy of prematurity in infants <28 weeks GA; the impact on the incidence of BPD is a secondary outcome.

Protein

Parenteral administration of solutions enriched with branched amino acids like leucine can affect respiration leading to a short-term increase in compliance and decrease of total pulmonary resistance [49, 50]. There may also be a reduction of apneic episodes. In a retrospective study, Porcelli et al. [51] reported less BPD in a small cohort of ELBW infants given up to 4 g/kg/day of parenteral protein compared with historical controls that received a lesser intake [15]. However, in a previous randomized trial of an aggressive nutritional regimen, which included a protein intake up to 3.5 g/kg/day initiated soon after birth, Wilson et al. failed to demonstrate improvements in pulmonary outcomes among preterm infants [52]. A large randomized trial of supplementation of glutamine in parenteral nutrition solutions given to ELBW infants failed to demonstrate beneficial effects on pulmonary outcomes or infectious morbidity [16]. However, as displayed in Table 12.3, less moderate and severe BPD was seen among those infants who received more total nutritional support during the first 3 weeks after birth [15].

Randomized trials comparing protein supplementation of breast milk with protein alone or with multiple components including driving protein supplementation to a high protein intake of up to 4.5 g/kg/day have not shown improvements in pulmonary outcomes. However, these interventions were usually started past a window of time where they could have modified pulmonary outcomes and enrolled infants at lower risk for chronic pulmonary morbidity [53–55].

Triglycerides and Fatty Acids

Long-chain polyunsaturated fatty acids (LCPUFAs) play important pro-inflammatory (n-6) or anti-inflammatory (n-3) roles and can act as immune modulators [56]. However, their role in lung growth or function is not as well known. In mice, addition of docosahexaenoic acid (DHA) to the maternal diet increases surfactant in amniotic fluid and the fetal lung [57], whereas in rats alterations of the lung due to intrauterine growth restriction (IUGR) are improved with maternal supplementation of DHA [58]. Increasing DHA intake in preterm baboons improves surfactant lipid concentrations probably by activation of one of the key enzymes involved in surfactant synthesis [59].

ELBW infants have low levels of DHA at the time of birth, which decrease further during the following weeks, especially with prolonged administration of lipid solutions that do not contain DHA [60]. DHA levels decrease further among infants that develop BPD versus those that do not [61]. Maternal supplementation of tuna oil seeking to increase DHA in breast milk to about 1 % of total fatty acids (six 500 mg of DHA-rich tuna oil capsules per day) lowered the risk of BPD among infants with birth weight <1250 g and in male infants [62]. A recent systematic review of trials of DHA that collectively included over a 1000 infants at <32 weeks' gestation showed a strong trend toward decreasing BPD (RR 0.88, 95 % CI 0.74–1.05) [63]. Infants in these trials started the added LCPUFAs often only several days after delivery and potentially received insufficient amounts of DHA; therefore, it is likely that their DHA levels had already dropped substantially from birth, thereby skipping a critical time period when pulmonary outcomes may have been impacted.

There is no DHA in the most used intravenous source of lipids in the USA, Intralipid®, and its administration can lead to high levels of pro-inflammatory n-6 LCPUFAs. A randomized study of early Intralipid® administration to preterm infants <1000 g suggested an increased risk of death for infants between 600 and 800 g birth weight and no improvements on the incidence of BPD [64]. Also, another study of early parenteral lipid administration to preterm infants reported an increased severity of chronic lung disease [65]. A systematic review of parenteral lipid administration did not show evidence of benefit on neonatal respiratory outcomes with early (within the first several days after birth) versus delayed initiation of intravenous lipid solutions [66]. However, most of these studies utilized parenteral lipid preparations devoid of DHA. Other newer parenteral lipid solutions derived from fish, algae, and other sources, i.e., SMOFlipid® (Fresenius-Kabi, Bad Homburg, Germany), do provide DHA; however, it is unclear whether using them can benefit neonatal lung function.

Whereas definitive data is still lacking, there are strong suggestions that supplementing levels of n-3 LCPUFAs, especially DHA, starting during the early neonatal period may lower the risk of chronic pulmonary problems. Moreover, the postnatal fall of DHA may be avoided or ameliorated by using parenteral lipid formulations that provide n-3 LCPUFAs followed by enteral administration of feedings that contain n-3 LCPUFAs like breast milk, especially if its DHA content is optimized.

Calcium (Ca), Phosphorus (P), and Magnesium (Mg)

Besides bone health, these elements participate in key physiologic and metabolic functions of the cardiovascular, respiratory, and other systems. Hypocalcemia and hypercalcemia can affect myocardial contractility and rhythm. In addition, hypocalcemia has been associated with apnea in preterm infants [67], and laryngospasm can occur with severe hypocalcemia. A relatively recent retrospective study of ELBW infants demonstrated a higher risk for BPD among those with hypocalcemia (serum Ca<5.9–6.3 mg/dL) during the first 48 h after birth [68]. Thoracic instability seen with severe chronic alterations of bone mineralization secondary to inadequate calcium, phosphorus, or vitamin D intake may contribute to ventilatory problems. Recent relatively small clinical trials examining administration of extra calcium to preterm infants did not demonstrate reductions in the incidence of BPD [69, 70]. However, VLBW infants with early BPD can accrete Ca similarly to those without BPD when receiving high caloric density feedings [71].

Phosphorus (P) is needed for intracellular energy storage, and VLBW infants have limited energy reserves in the form of ATP and phosphocreatine measured with nuclear magnetic resonance [72]. Recent data have shown that VLBW infants, particularly those with IUGR, often develop significant hypophosphatemia soon after delivery or during the first week after birth [73, 74], which is associated with higher risks for sepsis, prolonged ventilation, and BPD [74, 75]. Phosphorus is also a component of the phospholipids of pulmonary surfactant. However, it is not known whether the higher risks for prolonged ventilation and BPD shown in infants with early hypophosphatemia are the result of decreased muscle performance, a direct impact to the surfactant system, or other reasons.

Magnesium (Mg) deficiency can enhance the susceptibility to oxidative damage and decreases energy metabolism [76]. A potential role for Mg deficiency in BPD has been suggested [77]. However, lower Mg levels have not been associated with BPD in clinical or epidemiologic studies. Conversely, higher levels of Mg at birth have been associated with a delay in closure of the PDA or decreased responsiveness to indomethacin [78, 79]. However, data from a recent systematic review of antenatal Mg sulfate for preventing preterm birth did not show any differences in BPD or other neonatal morbidities [80].

Monitoring the concentrations of Ca, P, and Mg as well as supplying these elements adequately may be the best approach for sustaining neonatal lung function, especially among those infants at high risk for abnormalities of these elements, e.g., preterm infants with IUGR.

Vitamin A

A deficiency of vitamin A is associated with decreased lung growth and repair. Very preterm infants exhibit lower concentrations of retinol in serum and various tissues, which are associated with increased risk for long-term respiratory morbidity [81]. They also have lower levels of retinol binding protein. Recent evidence has also associated low retinol and retinol binding protein cord blood levels with congenital diaphragmatic hernia [82]. Data from a large, rigorously conducted randomized trial of vitamin A supplementation in ELBW infants sponsored by NICHD as well as a systematic review including several additional trials suggested that postnatal supplementation with intramuscular, not enteral, administration of 5000 IU started within a few days after birth and given three times a week for 4 weeks reduces the risk of BPD by about 7 %. This modest reduction translates into a number needed to treat with vitamin A to prevent one case of BPD of about 14 infants [83, 84]. Administration of such vitamin A regimen results in elevation of serum retinol among AGA but not SGA infants [85]. No specific measures of lung function have been performed in infants supplemented or not with vitamin A from these or other studies. Therefore, the functional mechanisms whereby administration of vitamin A reduces BPD are unclear.

A recent post hoc analysis of infants who received inhaled nitric oxide for prevention of BPD ascribed a potent effect on reduction of BPD as well as improved long-term neurocognitive outcome to the combined use of iNO and vitamin A [86]. The benefits of vitamin A on BPD seem to be confined to the neonatal period given that, in follow-up at 18–22 months corrected age in survivors of the NICHD trial, no reduction in pulmonary problems or rehospitalizations after discharge was observed [87]. Whereas there may be other dosing schemes that may provide additional benefit, those studies have yet to be conducted. In animal models, the potential to administer bioavailable vitamin A intratracheally with surfactant has been shown [88], but, to date, no clinical trials of this method of administration have been reported. In spite of the aforementioned data from clinical trials and systematic reviews, administration of supplemental vitamin A has not been adopted widely [89]. Moreover, because of a national shortage of a commercially available preparation of vitamin A in the USA, this supplement was not provided to ELBW infants at risk for BPD for a prolonged period of time. A large retrospective study described no changes in the outcomes of death or chronic lung disease before and during the vitamin A shortage [90]. Unfortunately, information on doses used and the method of administration was lacking. Smaller retrospective studies, though, have reinforced the notion that supplemental vitamin A administration is worthy of being considered in the management of ELBW infants given its low cost and relative safety in the doses studied [91, 92].

Vitamin E

Vitamin E has antioxidant properties that protect cell membranes. Extensive animal data suggest that a deficiency of vitamin E exacerbates oxygen toxicity. There is a strong correlation between plasma levels of vitamin E in cord blood and day 3 after birth and the occurrence of BPD [93]. More recent studies have continued to show a high prevalence of vitamin E deficiency among preterm infants and in some of them also an association between lower levels of vitamin E with BPD [94, 95]. Earlier trials of vitamin E supplementation given to infants with deficient levels of this vitamin suggested a beneficial effect in decreasing chronic respiratory morbidity [96]. However, subsequent studies when a deficiency of vitamin E was less prevalent did not show benefit [97]. Moreover, excessive administration of vitamin E has been associated with a higher risk of sepsis in preterm neonates, especially if serum levels of vitamin E exceed 3.5 mg/dL [98].

Current recommendations for vitamin E during the neonatal period do not call for additional supplementation over and above intake obtained from a regular diet, unless there is a demonstrated deficiency state. However, this area deserves further study.

Selenium (Se)

This trace mineral plays a role in the activity of selenoproteins, which protect against free radical damage. Two decades ago, lower plasma Se levels were reported among preterm infants who developed BPD [99]. Other studies have correlated low plasma or serum Se at birth or at 1 month of age with the occurrence of BPD [93, 100]. However, a large, randomized trial of Se supplementation among VLBW infants failed to show a reduction of BPD, even though lower pre-randomization Se levels were associated with increased respiratory morbidity [101].

Post-discharge Nutrition and Recovery from BPD

Discharge planning for all extremely preterm infants, especially those infants requiring medications, low-flow nasal oxygen, specialized feedings or feeding methods, and more complex care at home, is essential, and preparations addressing these needs should be started weeks, if not months, prior to discharge. Post-discharge care of the NICU graduate requires a coordinated approach between the primary care pediatrician (PCP) and NICU follow-up programs that supplement the PCP by focusing on growth, development, and nutritional needs and by helping to coordinate care with other pediatric subspecialties, including pulmonology, gastroenterology, neurology, physical therapy, and nutrition. Discharge planning for preterm infants has been the subject of American Academy of Pediatrics Policy Statements [102], and several books have addressed pediatric care of the NICU graduate [103, 104].

Post-discharge nutritional management of VLBW infants has recently been reviewed [105]. The authors stressed the importance of preparing an individualized nutritional management strategy to monitor the growth and development of these infants following discharge so as to reduce the risk of growth failure beyond term equivalent age. Anthropometrics (body weight, length, and head circumference) should be monitored and plotted on the CDC-WHO 2010 gender-specific growth charts for infants from birth to 24 months of age [33].

For infants with BPD, preparation of this nutritional management plan might be more challenging if the infant is fluid restricted, tires easily with oral feeding, is being treated with diuretics and/or low-flow nasal oxygen, or is primarily receiving human milk. Formulas with caloric densities between 24 and 30 calories/ounce may be necessary to ensure adequate energy and protein intake; electrolyte and mineral supplements may also be indicated [4, 106]. But, since the severity-based diagnostic criteria for BPD [107] reflect the continuum of lung injury and repair described in infants with BPD and correlate with growth, pulmonary disease, and pulmonary function during the first 1–2 years of life [108], individualizing nutritional management should allow continued lung growth and repair. This is essential to long-term recovery from BPD and weaning from diuretics and low-flow nasal oxygen. Furthermore, infants with BPD, especially those who have been intubated for prolonged periods of time, may also experience oral aversion, swallowing dysfunction, and gastroesophageal reflux. If appropriate, these conditions should be evaluated prior to discharge, so that management can be implemented and follow-up planned.

Summary

In conclusion, this chapter has reviewed the role that nutrition plays in the development and management of BPD. While specific nutrients, other than n-3 LCPUFAs and vitamin A, have shown limited benefit in reducing the incidence or severity of BPD, increased intake of mother's own milk during the NICU hospitalization has been reported to reduce the incidence of BPD. In addition, standardized, evidence-based early nutritional management guidelines for extremely preterm infants that begin with early, intense parenteral and enteral nutritional support have been shown to reduce the growth failure associated with BPD. Hopefully, this strategy will address some of the adverse effects that undernutrition has had on lung growth, injury, and repair, resulting in a decrease in both the incidence and severity of BPD.

References

1. Ehrenkranz RA, Younes N, Lemons JA, Fanaroff AA, Donovan EF, Wright LL, et al. Longitudinal growth of hospitalized very low birth weight infants. Pediatrics. 1999;104:280–9.
2. Clark RH, Thomas P, Peabody J. Extrauterine growth restriction remains a serious problem in prematurely born neonates. Pediatrics. 2003;111:986–90.
3. Cole TJ, Statnikov Y, Santhakumaran S, Pan H, Modi N. Postnatal weight gain after very preterm birth. A UK population study. Arch Dis Child. 2011;96 Suppl 1:A1–100.
4. Biniwale MA, Ehrenkranz RA. The role of nutrition in the prevention and management of bronchopulmonary dysplasia. Semin Perinatol. 2006;30:200–8.
5. Bhatia J, Parish A. Nutrition and the lung. Neonatology. 2009;95:362–7.
6. Dani C, Poggi C. Nutrition and bronchopulmonary dysplasia. J Matern Fetal Neonatal Med. 2012;25(S3):37–40.
7. Moya F. Preterm nutrition and the lung. In: Koletzko B, Poindexter B, Uauy R, editors. Nutritional care of preterm infants: scientific basis and practical guidelines, World review of nutrition and dietetics, vol. 110. Basel: Karger; 2014. p. 239–52.
8. Edelman NH, Rucker RB, Peavy HH. NIH workshop summary: nutrition and the respiratory system. Chronic obstructive pulmonary disease (COPD). Am Rev Respir Dis. 1986;134:347–52.
9. Frank L. Nutrition: Influence on lung growth, injury and repair, and development of bronchopulmonary dysplasia. In: Bancalari E, Stocker JT, editors. Bronchopulmonary dysplasia. Washington: Hemisphere Publishing Corporation; 1988. p. 78–108.

10. Frank L, Sosenko IRS. Undernutrition as a major contributing factor in the pathogenesis of bronchopulmonary dysplasia. Am Rev Respir Dis. 1988;138:725–9.
11. Ehrenkranz RA. Early, aggressive nutritional management for very low birth weight infants: what is the evidence? Semin Perintaol. 2007;31:48–55.
12. Wright K, Dawson JP, Fallis D, Vogt E, Lorch V. New postnatal growth grids for very low birth weight infants. Pediatrics. 1993;91:922–6.
13. Radmacher PG, Rafail ST, Adamkin DH. Nutrition and growth in VVLBW infants with and without bronchopulmonary dysplasia. Neonatal Intensive Care. 2004;16:22–6.
14. Theile AR, Radmacher PG, Anschutz TW, Davis DW, Adamkin DH. Nutritional strategies and growth in extremely low birth weight infants with bronchopulmonary dysplasia over the past 10 years. J Perinatol. 2012;32:117–22.
15. Ehrenkranz RA, Das A, Wrage LA, Poindexter BB, Higgins R, Stoll BJ, et al. Early nutrition mediates the influence of severity of illness on extremely low birth weight infants. Pediatr Res. 2011;69:522–9.
16. Poindexter BB, Ehrenkranz RA, Stoll BJ, Wright LL, Poole WK, Oh W, et al. Parenteral glutamine supplementation does not reduce the risk of mortality or late-onset sepsis in extremely low birth weight infants. Pediatrics. 2004;113:1209–15.
17. Oh W, Poindexter BB, Perrits R, Lemons JA, Bauer CR, Ehrenkranz RA, et al. Association between fluid intake and weight loss during the first ten days of life and risk of bronchopulmonary dysplasia in extremely low birth weight infants. J Pediatr. 2005;147:786–90.
18. McCallie KR, Lee HC, Mayer O, Cohen RS, Hintz SR, Rhine WD. Improved outcomes with a standardized feeding protocol for very low birth weight infants. J Perinatol. 2011;31: S61–7.
19. Butler TJ, Szekely LJ, Grow JL. A standardized nutrition approach for very low birth weight neonates improves outcomes, reduces cost and is not associated with increased rates of necrotizing enterocolitis, sepsis or mortality. J Perinatol. 2013;33:851–7.
20. Ehrenkranz RA. Ongoing issues in the intensive care for the periviable infant-nutritional management and prevention of bronchopulmonary dysplasia and nosocomial infections. Semin Perinatol. 2014;38:25–30.
21. Ehrenkranz RA. Nutrition, growth and clinical outcomes. In: Koletzko B, Poindexter B, Uauy R, editors. Nutritional care of preterm infants: scientific basis and practical guidelines, World review of nutrition and dietetics, vol. 110. Basel: Karger; 2014. p. 11–26.
22. Torrazza RM, Neu J. Evidence-based guidelines for optimization of nutrition for the very low birthweight infant. NeoReviews. 2013;14:e340–7.
23. Parker LA, Neu J, Torrazza RM, Li Y. Scientifically based strategies for enteral feeding in premature infants. NeoReviews. 2013;14:e350–8.
24. Jadcherla SR, Dail J, Malkar MB, McClead R, Kelleher K, Nelin L. Impact of process optimization and quality improvement measures on neonatal feeding outcomes at an all-referral neonatal intensive care unit. JPEN. 2015;Mar 2. pii:014860711571667 (Epub ahead of print).
25. Dutta S, Singh B, Chessell L, Wilson J, Janes M, McDonald K, et al. Guidelines for feeding very low birth weight infants. Nutrients. 2015;7:423–42.
26. Rønnestad A, Abrahamsen TG, Medbø S, Reigstad H, Lossius K, Kaaresen PI, et al. Late-onset septicemia in a Norwegian national cohort of extremely premature infants receiving very early full human milk feeding. Pediatrics. 2005;115:e269–76.
27. Bigger HR, Fogg LJ, Patel AL, Johnson T, Engstrom JL, Meier PP. Quality indicators for human milk use in very low birthweight infants: are we measuring what we should be measuring? J Perinatol. 2013;34:287–91.
28. Schanler RJ, Lau C, Hurst NM, Smith EO. Randomized trial of donor milk versus preterm formula as substitutes for mothers' own milk in the feeding of extremely premature infants. Pediatrics. 2005;116:400–6.
29. Sisk PM, Lovelady CA, Dillard RG, Gruber KJ, O'Shea TM. Early human milk feeding is associated with a lower risk of necrotizing enterocolitis in very low birth weight infants. J Perinatol. 2007;27:428–33.

30. Patel AL, Robin B, Buchanan A, Christian E, Nandhan V, Shroff A, et al. Beneficial effect of human milk (HM) on chronic lung disease (CLD) in very low birth weight (VLBW) infants. E-PAS. 2015;1601.754.
31. Fenton TR, Kim JH. A systematic review and meta-analysis to revise the Fenton growth chart for preterm infants. BMC Pediatr. 2013;13:59.
32. Olsen IE, Groveman SA, Lawson ML, Clark RH, Zemel BS. New intrauterine growth curves based on United States data. Pediatrics. 2010;125:e214–24.
33. Grummer-Strawn LM, Reinold C, Krebs NF. Use of world health organization and CDC growth charts for children aged 0–59 months in the United States. MMWR. 2010; 59(RR-9):1–15.
34. Weinstein MR, Oh W. Oxygen consumption in infants with bronchopulmonary dysplasia. J Pediatr. 1981;99:958–61.
35. Kurzner SI, Garg M, Bautista DB, Sargent CW, Bowman CM, Keens TG. Growth failure in bronchopulmonary dysplasia: elevated metabolic rates and pulmonary mechanics. J Pediatr. 1988;112:73–80.
36. Kurzner SI, Garg M, Bautista DB, Bader D, Merritt RJ, Warburton D, et al. Growth failure in infants with bronchopulmonary dysplasia: nutrition and elevated resting metabolic expenditure. Pediatrics. 1988;81:379–84.
37. Niermeyer S. Nutrition: nutritional and metabolic problems in infants with bronchopulmonary dysplasia. In: Bancalari E, Stocker JT, editors. Bronchopulmonary dysplasia. Washington: Hemisphere Publishing Corporation; 1988. p. 313–36.
38. Poindexter BB, Ehrenkranz RA. Nutrient requirements and provision of nutritional support in the premature neonate. In: Martin R, Faranoff AA, Walsh M, editors. Neonatal-perinatal medicine. 10th ed. Maryland Heights, MO: Elsevier; 2014. p. 592–612.
39. Oh W. Fluid and electrolyte management of very low birth weight infants. Pediatr Neonatol. 2012;53:329–33.
40. VanMarter LJ, Leviton A, Allred EN, Pagano M, Kuban KC. Hydration during the first days of life and the risk of bronchopulmonary dysplasia in low birth weight infants. J Pediatr. 1990;116(6):942–9.
41. Bell EF, Acarregui MJ. Restricted versus liberal water intake for preventing morbidity and mortality in preterm infants (Review). Cochrane Database Syst Rev. 2010;6:959–80.
42. Hazan J, Chessex P, Piedboeuf B, Bourgeois M, Bard H, Long W. Energy expenditure during synthetic surfactant replacement therapy for neonatal respiratory distress syndrome. J Pediatr. 1992;120(2 Pt 2):S29–33.
43. Yunis KA, Oh W. Effects of intravenous glucose loading on oxygen consumption, carbon dioxide production, and resting energy expenditure in infants with bronchopulmonary dysplasia. J Pediatr. 1989;115:127–32.
44. Chessex P, Belanger S, Piedboeuf B, Pineault M. Influence of energy substrates on respiratory gas exchange during conventional mechanical ventilation of preterm infants. J Pediatr. 1995;126:619–24.
45. De Meer K, Westerterp KR, Houwen RHJ, Brouwers R, Berger R, Okken A. Total energy expenditure in infants with bronchopulmonary dysplasia is associated with respiratory status. Eur J Pediatr. 1997;156:299–304.
46. Hallman M, Gluck L. Formation of acidic phospholipids in rabbit lung during perinatal development. Pediatr Res. 1980;14(11):1250–9.
47. Hallman M, Saugstad OD, Porreco RP, Epstein BL, Gluck L. Role of myoinositol in regulation of surfactant phospholipids in the newborn. Early Hum Dev. 1985;10(3–4):245–54.
48. Howlett A, Ohlsson A, Plakkal N. Inositol for respiratory distress syndrome in preterm infants. Cochrane Database Syst Rev. 2012;3:CD000366.
49. Manner T, Wiese S, Katz DP, Skeie B, Askanazi J. Branched-chain amino acids and respiration. Nutrition. 1992;8(5):311–5.
50. Blazer S, Reinersman GT, Askanazi J, Furst P, Katz DP, Fleischman AR. Branched-chain amino acids and respiratory pattern and function in the neonate. J Perinatol. 1994;14:290–5.

51. Porcelli PJ, Sisk PM. Increased parenteral amino acid administration to extremely low-birth weight infants during early postnatal life. J Pediatr Gastroenterol Nutr. 2002;34:174–9.
52. Wilson DC, Cairns P, Halliday HL, Reid M, McClure G, Dodge JA. Randomised controlled trial of an aggressive nutritional regimen in sick very low birthweight infants. Arch Dis Child. 1997;77:F4–11.
53. O'Connor DL, Jacobs J, Hall R, Adamkin D, Auestad N, Castillo M, et al. Growth and development of premature infants fed predominantly human milk, predominantly premature infant formula, or a combination of human milk and premature formula. J Pediatr Gastroenterol Nutr. 2003;37(4):437–46.
54. Sullivan S, Schanler RJ, Kim JH, Patel AL, Trawöger R, Kiechl-Kohlendorfer U, et al. An exclusively human milk-based diet is associated with a lower rate of necrotizing enterocolitis than a diet of human milk and bovine milk-based products. J Pediatr. 2010;156(4):562–7.
55. Moya F, Sisk PH, Walsh KR, Berseth CL. A new liquid human milk fortifier and linear growth in preterm infants. Pediatrics. 2012;130(4):e928–35.
56. Lapillonne A, Groh-Wargo S, Gonzalez C, Uauy R. Lipid needs of preterm infants: updated recommendations. J Pediatr. 2013;162:S37–47.
57. Blanco PG, Freedman SD, Lopez MC, Ollero M, Comen E, Laposata M, et al. Oral docosahexaenoic acid given to pregnant mice increases the amount of surfactant in lung and amniotic fluid in preterm fetuses. Am J Obstet Gynecol. 2004;190:1369–74.
58. Joss-Moore L, Wang Y, Baack M, Yao L, Norris AW, Yu X, et al. IUGR decreases PPARy and SETD8 Expression in neonatal rat lung and these effects are ameliorated by maternal DHA supplementation. Early Hum Dev. 2010;86:785–91.
59. Chao AC, Ziadeh BI, Diau GY, Wijendran V, Sarkadi-Nagy E, Hsieh AT, et al. Influence of dietary long-chain PUFA on premature baboon lung FA and dipalmitoyl PC composition. Lipids. 2003;38:425–9.
60. Robinson DT, Carlson SE, Murthy K, Frost B, Li S, Caplan M. Docosahexaenoic and arachidonic acid levels in extremely low birth weight infants with prolonged exposure to intravenous lipids. J Pediatr. 2013;162:56–61.
61. Martin CR, Dasilva DA, Cluette-Brown JE, Dimonda C, Hamill A, Bhutta AQ, et al. Decreased postnatal docosahexaenoic and arachidonic acid blood levels in premature infants are associated with neonatal morbidities. J Pediatr. 2011;159(5):743–9.
62. Manley BJ, Makrides M, Collins CT, McPhee AJ, Gibson RA, Ran P, et al. High-dose docosahexaenoic acid supplementation of preterm infants: respiratory and allergy outcomes. Pediatrics. 2011;128:e71–7.
63. Zhang P, Lavoie P, Lacaze-Masmonteil T, Rhainds M, Marc I. Omega-3 long-chain polyunsaturated fatty acids for extremely preterm infants: a systematic review. Pediatrics. 2014;134:120–34.
64. Sosenko IRS, Rodriguez-Pierce M, Bancalari E. Effect of early initiation of intravenous lipid administration on the incidence and severity of chronic lung disease in premature infants. J Pediatr. 1993;123:975–82.
65. Hammerman C, Aramburo MJ. Decreased lipid intake reduces morbidity in sick premature neonates. J Pediatr. 1988;113(6):1083–8.
66. Simmer K, Rao SC. Early introduction of lipids to parenterally-fed preterm infants. Cochrane Database Syst Rev. 2005;18(2):CD005256.
67. Gershanik JJ, Levkoff AH, Duncan R. The association of hypocalcemia and recurrent apnea in premature infants. Am J Obstet Gynecol. 1972;113(5):646–52.
68. Altirkawi K, Rozycki H. Hypocalcemia is common in the first 48 h of life in ELBW infants. J Perinat Med. 2008;36:348–53.
69. Pereira-da-Silva L, Costa AB, Pereira L, Filipe AF, Virella D, Leal E, et al. Early high calcium and phosphorus intake by parenteral nutrition prevents short-term bone strength decline in preterm infants. J Pediatr Gastroenterol Nutr. 2011;52(2):203–9.
70. Carroll WF, Fabres J, Nagy TR, Frazier M, Roane C, Pohlandt F, et al. Results of extremely-low-birth-weight infants randomized to receive extra enteral calcium supply. J Pediatr Gastroenterol Nutr. 2011;53(3):339–45.

71. Hicks P, Rogers S, Hawthorne K, Chen Z, Abrams S. Calcium absorption in very low birth weight infants with and without bronchopulmonary dysplasia. J Pediatr. 2011;158:885–90.
72. Bertocci LA, Mize CE, Uauy R. Muscle phosphorus energy state in very-low-birth-weight infants: effect of exercise. Am J Physiol. 1992;262:E289–94.
73. Ichikawa G, Watabe Y, Suzumura H, Sairenchi T, Muto T, Arisaka O. Hypophosphatemia in small for gestational age extremely low birth weight infants receiving parenteral nutrition in the first week after birth. J Pediatr Endocr Met. 2012;25(3–4):317–21.
74. Ross JR, Finch C, Ebeling M, Taylor SN. Refeeding syndrome in very-low-birth-weight intrauterine growth-restricted neonates. J Perinatol. 2013;33:717–20.
75. Moltu SJ, Strommen K, Blakstad EW, Almaas AN, Westerberg AC, Brække E, et al. Enhanced feeding in very-low-birth-weight infants may cause electrolyte disturbances and septicemia – a randomized, controlled trial. Clin Nutr. 2013;32:207–12.
76. Caddell J. Evidence for magnesium deficiency in the pathogenesis of bronchopulmonary dysplasia. Magnes Res. 1996;9:205–16.
77. Fridman E, Linder N. Magnesium and bronchopulmonary dysplasia. Harefuah. 2013;152: 158–61.
78. Stigson L, Kjellmer I. Serum levels of magnesium at birth related to complications of immaturity. Acta Paediatr. 1997;86:991–4.
79. Katayama Y, Minami H, Enomoto M, Takano T, Hayashi S, Lee Y. Antenatal magnesium sulfate and the postnatal response of the ductus arteriosus to indomethacin in extremely preterm neonates. J Perinatol. 2011;31:21–4.
80. Crowther C, Brown J, McKinlay C, Middleton P. Magnesium sulphate for preventing preterm birth in threatened preterm labour. Cochrane Database Syst Rev. 2014;8:CD001060.
81. Spears K, Cheney C, Zerzan J. Low plasma retinol concentrations increase the risk of developing bronchopulmonary dysplasia and long-term respiratory disability in very-low-birth-weight infants. Am J Clin Nutr. 2004;80:1589–94.
82. Beurskens L, Tibboel D, Lindemnas J, Duvekot JJ, Cohen-Overbeek TE, Veenma DC, et al. Retinol status of newborn infants is associated with congenital diaphragmatic hernia. Pediatrics. 2010;126:712–20.
83. Tyson JE, Wright LL, Oh W, Kennedy KA, Mele L, Ehrenkranz RA, et al. Vitamin A supplementation for extremely-low-birth-weight infants. A national institute of child health and human development neonatal research network. N Engl J Med. 1999;340:1962–8.
84. Darlow BA, Graham PJ. Vitamin A supplementation for preventing morbidity and mortality in very low birthweight infants. Cochrane Database Syst Rev. 2002;4:CD000501.
85. Londhe V, Nolen T, Das A, Higgins RD, Tyson JE, Oh W, et al. Vitamin A supplementation in extremely low-birth-weight infants: subgroup analysis in small-for-gestational-age infants. Am J Perinatol. 2013;30:771–80.
86. Gadhia M, Cutter G, Abman S, Kinsella J. Effects of early inhaled nitric oxide therapy and vitamin A supplementation on the risk of bronchopulmonary dysplasia in premature newborns with respiratory failure. J Pediatr. 2014;164:744–8.
87. Ambalavanan N, Tyson JE, Kennedy KA, Hansen NI, Vohr BR, Wtright LL, et al. Vitamin A supplementation for extremely low birth weight infants: outcome at 18 to 22 months. Pediatrics. 2005;115:e249–54.
88. Singh A, Bronshtein V, Khashu M, Lee K, Potts JE, Friel J, et al. Vitamin A is systemically bioavailable after intratracheal administration with surfactant in an animal model of newborn respiratory distress. Pedaitr Res. 2010;67:619–23.
89. Kaplan H, Tabangin M, McClendon D, Meinzen-Derr J, Margolis P, Donovan E. Understanding variation in vitamin A supplementation among NICUs. Pediatrics. 2010;126:e367–73.
90. Tolia V, Murthy K, McKinley P, Bennett M, Clark R. The effect of national shortage of vitamin A on death or chronic lung disease in extremely low-birth-weight infants. JAMA Pediatr. 2014;168:1039–44.
91. Moreira A, Caskey M, Fonseca R, Malloy M, Geary C. Impact of providing vitamin A to the routine pulmonary care of extremely low birth weight infants. J Matern Fetal Neonatal Med. 2012;25:84–8.

92. Peluso A, Hair A, Hawthorne K, Abrams S. Vitamin A and chronic lung disease in infants: what happened when there wasn't any? Am J Respir Crit Care Med. 2003;168:356–96.
93. Falciglia HS, Johnson JR, Sullivan J, Hall CF, Miller JD, Reichmann GC. Role of antioxidant nutrients and lipid peroxidation in premature infants with respiratory distress syndrome and bronchopulmonary dysplasia. Am J Perinatol. 2003;20:97–107.
94. Kositamongkol S, Suthutvoravut U, Chongviriyaphan N, Feungpean B, Nuntnarumit P. Vitamin A and E status in very low birth weight infants. J Perinatol. 2011;31:471–6.
95. Abdel Ghany E, Alsharany W, Ali A, Younass E, Hussein J. Anti-oxidant profiles and markers of oxidative stress in preterm neonates. Paediatr Int Child Health. 2015, May 4 (Epub ahead of print).
96. Ehrenkranz RA, Bonta BW, Ablow RC, Warshaw JB. Amelioration of bronchopulmonary dysplasia after vitamin E administration. A preliminary report. N Engl J Med. 1978;299: 564–9.
97. Ehrenkranz RA, Ablow RC, Warshaw JB. Effect of vitamin E on the development of oxygen-induced lung injury in neonates. Ann N Y Acad Sci. 1982;393:452–66.
98. Brion LP, Bell EF, Raghuveer TS. Vitamin E supplementation for prevention of morbidity and mortality in preterm infants. Cochrane Database Syst Rev. 2003;4:CD003665.
99. Darlow B, Inder T, Graham P, Sluis KB, Malpas TJ, Taylor BJ, et al. The relationship of selenium status to respiratory outcome in the very low birth weight infant. Pediatrics. 1995;96:314–9.
100. Mostafa-Gharehbaghi M, Mostafa-Gharahbaghi P, Ghanbari F, Abdolmohammad-Zadeh H, Sadeghi GH, Jouyban A. Determination of selenium in serum samples of preterm newborn infants with bronchopulmonary dysplasia using a validated hydride generation system. Biol Trace Elem Res. 2012;147:1–7.
101. Darlow B, Winterbourn C, Inder T, Graham PJ, Harding JE, Weston PJ, et al. The effect of selenium supplementation on outcome in very low birth weight infants: a randomized controlled trial. The New Zealand neonatal study group. J Pediatr. 2000;136:473–80.
102. American Academy of Pediatrics Committee on Fetus and Newborn. Hospital discharge of the high-risk neonate. Pediatrics. 2008;122:1119–26.
103. Ballard RA. Pediatric care of the ICN Graduate. Philadelphia: WB Saunders; 1988.
104. Brodsky D, Oullette MA. Primary care of the premature infant. Philadelphia: Saunders/ Elsevier; 2008.
105. Nzegwu NI, Ehrenkranz RA. Post-discharge nutrition and the VLBW infant: to supplement or not supplement? A review of the current evidence. Clin Perinatol. 2014;41:463–74.
106. Allen J, Zwerdling, Ehrenkranz R, Gaultier C, Geggel R, Greenough A, et al. Statement on the care of the child with chronic lung disease of infancy and childhood. Am J Respir Crit Care Med. 2003;168:356–96.
107. Jobe AH, Bancalari E. Bronchopulmonary dysplasia. Am J Respir Crit Care Med. 2001;163:1723–9.
108. Ehrenkranz RA, Walsh MC, Vohr BR, Jobe AC, Wright LL, Fanaroff AA, et al. Validation of the National Institutes of Health consensus definition of bronchopulmonary dysplasia. Pediatrics. 2005;116:1353–60.

Chapter 13
Radiology of Bronchopulmonary Dysplasia: From Preterm Birth to Adulthood

Outi Tammela and Päivi Korhonen

The Original Description of BPD

The new syndrome termed bronchopulmonary dysplasia (BPD), first introduced in 1967, represented a prolonged healing phase of respiratory distress syndrome (RDS) associated with pulmonary oxygen (O_2) toxicity. The clinical, pathologic, and radiographic course of BPD was described in premature infants with a mean gestational age of 34 weeks and mean birth weight of 2235 g, who had had severe RDS and exposure to intermittent positive pressure ventilation and 80–100 % O_2 for longer than 6 days [1]. Of the original 32 patients with severe RDS who required continuous mechanical ventilation with high concentrations of O_2 for 24 h or more, three were excluded as a result of congenital anomalies or hypophosphatasia. Thirteen of the remaining patients were treated with high concentrations of O_2 for longer than 150 h. Nine of these patients lived beyond 2 weeks of age and suffered pulmonary disease beyond 4 weeks' age. Five of them died and four survived with chronic lung disease. Development of the chronic pulmonary disease was categorized into four sequential stages according to the clinical, pathologic, and radiographic course [1].

Stage I—the period of acute respiratory distress at the age of 2–3 days was identical to severe RDS. Chest X-rays showed a generalized granular pattern in the lung parenchyma and a positive air bronchogram (Fig. 13.1). Pathological findings at autopsy included hyaline membranes, atelectasis, and lymphatic dilatation.

O. Tammela, MD, PhD (✉)
Adjunct Professor in Neonatology, Department of Pediatrics,
Tampere University Hospital, Teiskontie 35, P.O. Box 2000, Tampere 33521, Finland
e-mail: Outi.Tammela@uta.fi

P. Korhonen, MD, PhD
Department of Pediatrics, Tampere University Hospital, Teiskontie 35,
P.O. Box 2000, Tampere 33521, Finland
e-mail: paivi.h.korhonen@uta.fi

V. Bhandari (ed.), *Bronchopulmonary Dysplasia*, Respiratory Medicine,
DOI 10.1007/978-3-319-28486-6_13

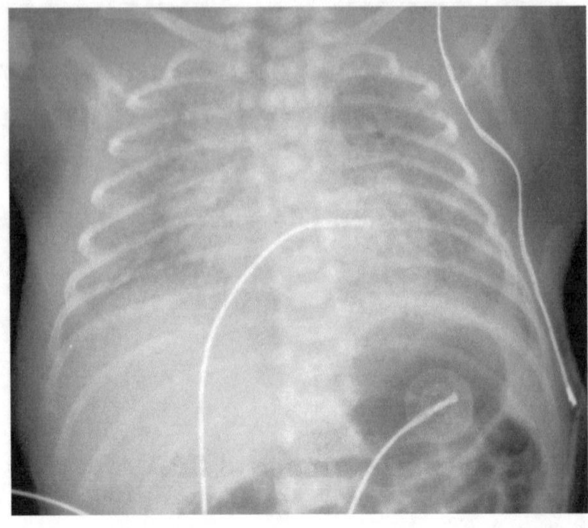

Fig. 13.1 Chest radiograph of a 1-day-old boy born at 29 weeks of gestation showing a generalized granular pattern in the lung parenchyma and a positive air bronchogram typical of Northway stage I [1]

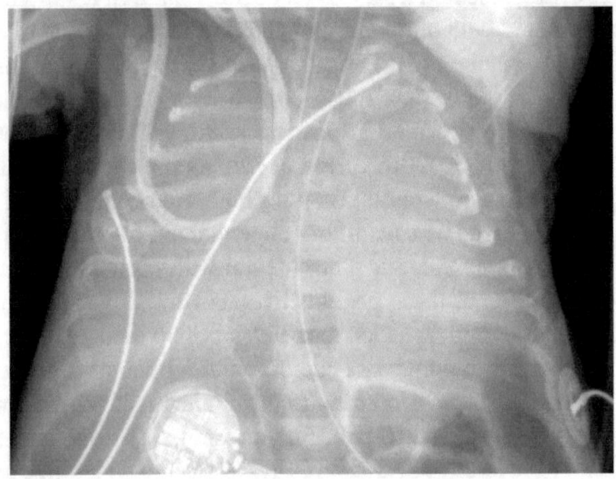

Fig. 13.2 Chest radiograph of a 3-week-old boy born at 24 weeks of gestation showing complete opacification of the lung fields and indistinguishable cardiac borders typical of leaky lung syndrome [2] and Northway stage II [1]

Stage II—a period of regeneration occurred at the age of 4–10 days. At that time most of the patients had been weaned from ventilators and O_2 supplementation, but again became cyanotic. High concentrations of O_2 treatment were needed, and chest X-ray examination revealed complete opacification of the lung fields, where cardiac borders were often indistinguishable (Fig. 13.2). Necrosis and healing of alveolar epithelium, persisting hyaline membranes, coalescence of the alveoli, bronchiolar necrosis, and a thick eosinophilic exudate in the bronchiolar lumen were found in lung tissue specimens.

Stage III—the period of transition to chronic disease, at the age of 10–20 days; lung opacification had disappeared and changed to a honeycomb or spongelike appearance throughout the lungs. Small rounded radiolucent areas resembled bullae, which alternated with areas of irregular density (Fig. 13.3). The air bronchogram had disappeared. All but two of the patients had been weaned from the

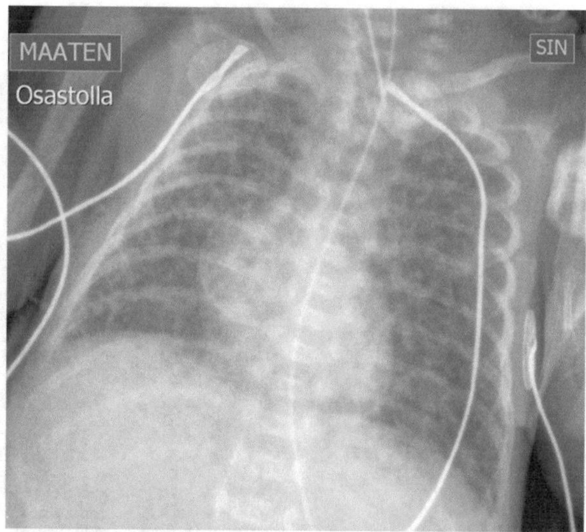

Fig. 13.3 Chest radiograph of an 11-day-old boy born at 25 weeks of gestation showing a honeycomb or spongelike appearance throughout the lungs typical of bubbly lung [2] and Northway stage III [1]. The labels in Finnish contain technical information

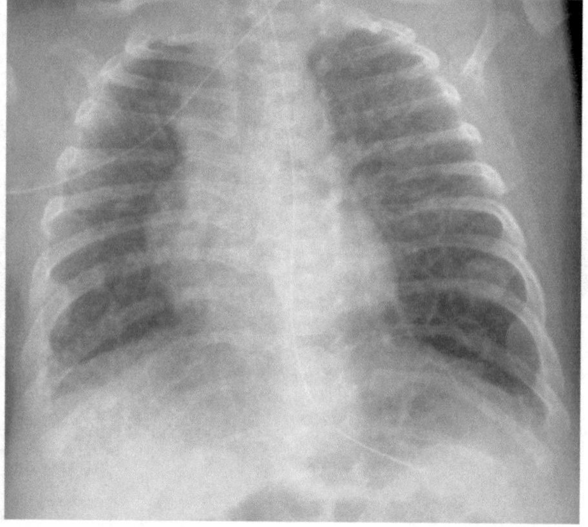

Fig. 13.4 Chest radiograph of a 3-month-old boy born at 25 weeks of gestation showing enlarged lucent areas alternating with strands of density typical of bubbly lung [2] and Northway stage IV [1]

ventilator. Histopathologic examination revealed persisting alveolar epithelial injury, fewer hyaline membranes, and abundant mucous secretion. Alveolar coalescence had progressed to emphysematous alveoli with atelectatic surrounding alveoli. Thin strands of interseptal collagen and coarse focal thickening in the basement membranes were present.

Stage IV—the period of chronic disease, present beyond 1 month of age. In chest X-ray images the previously lucent areas were enlarged, alternating with strands of density (Fig. 13.4). Cardiomegaly was detected, and in some cases it was associated with right-sided congestive heart failure and death. Eleven infants were hospitalized, having breathing difficulty and cyanosis when not being administered high concentrations of O_2. Groups of emphysematous alveoli with peribronchiolar

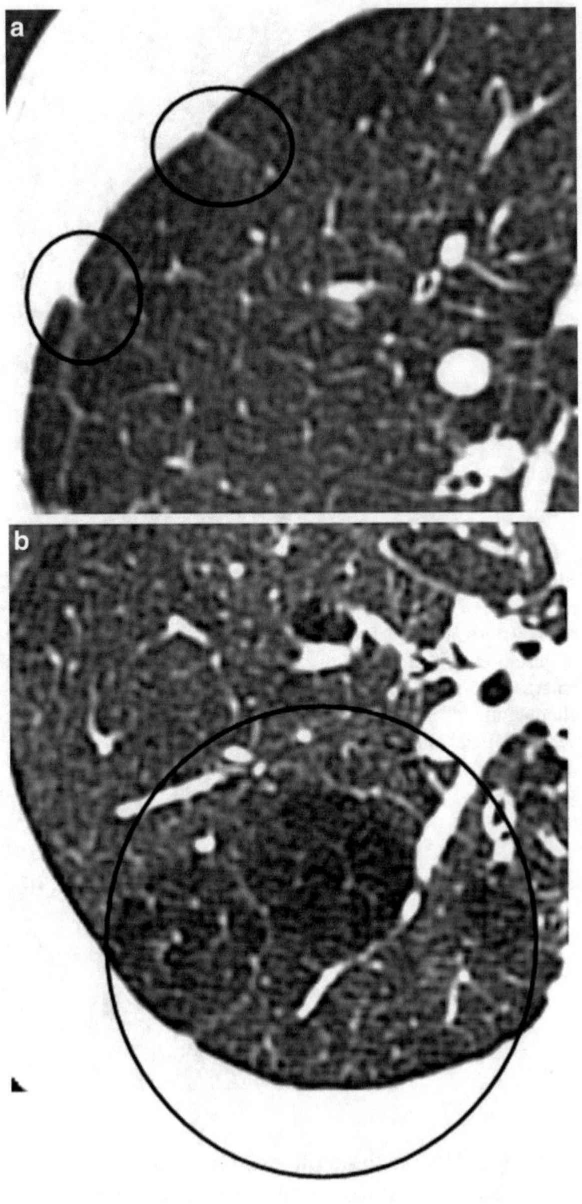

Fig. 13.5 High-resolution CT findings in an 11-year-old boy showing (**a**) linear and subpleural triangular opacities and (**b**) a hypoattenuated area. Aukland et al. [39], with permission

smooth muscle hypertrophy and atelectatic areas with more ordinary-appearing bronchioles were detected on pathologic examination. Perimucosal fibrosis, generalized focal thickening of the basement membranes, fine collagen and elastin fibers in the septal walls, as well as tortuous lymphatics were also seen in the lung fields. Pulmonary vascular medial hypertrophy suggestive of pulmonary hypertension was present.

Chest Radiographs

Chest radiographs had an important role in the initial description of BPD. Although not included in the current consensus definition of BPD [3], radiographic findings continue to have a role in the clinical evaluation of BPD infants, especially in terms of pulmonary complications and differential diagnosis [4]. Chest radiographs are more feasible but not as sensitive to structural changes in the lung as high-resolution computed tomography [5].

The Evolution of Chest X-ray Findings Typical of BPD

Radiographic development of BPD seems to be more insidious than originally described [6], and the chronologic sequence proposed by Northway is not always present [7–9]. Furthermore, the evaluation of radiographs is hampered by interobserver variation [10, 11]. Several scoring systems have been suggested in order to create uniformity in the assessment of radiographs, to study their role in the diagnosis of BPD, and to enable comparison between different centers [2, 6, 12–19].

Four of the most prominent features of radiographic BPD, i.e., interstitial disease/fibrosis, focal emphysema, overall lung expansion, and cardiovascular effects, combined with a subjective impression of severity were scored by Edwards and associates [13, 20]. Hyde and associates suggested BPD classification of type 1 and type 2 diseases, with type 1 presenting bilateral, ill-defined predominantly perihilar homogeneous or patchy pulmonary opacities and type 2 presenting coarse reticulation with streaky densities interspersed with small cystic translucencies, sometimes due to air cysts [12]. Yuksel and associates presented a radiographic score system that included the volume of the thorax, the degree of inflation of lung fields, opacification, air bronchogram, pulmonary interstitial emphysema, interstitial changes (coarse shadowing), and cystic elements, including the size of the largest cyst [14]. The Weinstein score included evaluation of the presence, type, and size of opacities [17]. Greenough and associates proposed a simple chest radiograph score in which the degree of hyperexpansion of the lungs (according to the number of ribs visible), the number of zones with fibrosis/interstitial change, and the presence of cystic elements were scored [16]. Despite some associations with clinical parameters, none of the scoring systems have been universally accepted so far [21]. Analysis of digital chest X-ray images by calculating chest X-ray thoracic areas after free hand tracing of the perimeters of the thoracic area has also been suggested [22].

With advances in peri- and neonatal care, including surfactant and antenatal corticosteroid therapy and gentler ventilation techniques, the survival of very preterm infants has improved and the clinical, pathologic, and radiologic findings in cases of BPD have changed [6, 21, 23]. The immature lung is exposed to the extrauterine environment at an earlier stage of lung development, thus causing the various pathological features of "new BPD" such as impaired alveolar and pulmonary vascular development, less airway epithelial damage, and less interstitial fibrosis [21, 23, 24].

In the surfactant era, the initially clear or slightly abnormal chest radiographs of very premature infants seem to show a gradual progression from a hazy ground-glass appearance to a relatively uniform pattern of coarse interstitial opacities without cysts [21]. If cystic lucencies develop, they are usually smaller and more uniform than in Northway stage IV BPD and found in both lungs [21]. Two radiographic patterns of BPD have been suggested by Swischuk and associates [2]. Leaky lung syndrome (LLS), i.e., hazy-to-opaque findings resembling Northway stages I–II (Figs. 13.1 and 13.2), is thought to be caused by capillary leakage due to damage by hyperoxia. The cystic findings resembling Northway stages III–IV, referred to as "bubbly lung" (Figs. 13.3 and 13.4), seem to represent more severe lung injury [2] with a heterogeneous pattern of opaque strands, cystic lucencies of varying size, and regional air trapping [21].

Chest Radiographic Findings from Infancy to Adulthood

In a study population of 75 premature infants managed with rescue surfactant therapy, positive pressure ventilation, and O_2 supplementation, the initial granular opacities cleared by the second day in 45 % of cases [2]. In 31 % of the infants, the initial clearing was followed by "hazy-to-opaque" lungs by day 7 to day 14. Of these, 35 % cleared and 65 % progressed to bubbly lungs [2]. The remaining 24 % of the whole population had hazy-to-opaque lungs for 2–5 weeks, and 89 % of them developed bubbly lungs at 10 days to 3 weeks. The two radiographic patterns may emerge irrespective of each other [21, 25]. In a population of 82 very-low-birth-weight infants, 54 % showed radiographic evidence of BPD from the sixth day of life until term; 31 % of these had LLS and 23 % bubbly lung [25]. In 11 of the 19 cases with bubbly lung, cystic findings appeared before 15 days of life [25]. In eight infants LLS progressed to bubbly lungs.

In a population of 100 infants with birth weight ≤1750 g born before the surfactant era, chest radiographic findings tended to normalize by 3–6 months of age [26]. Hakulinen and associates found minor fibrotic changes in the chest radiographs at 6–9 years of age in four of 10 BPD survivors [27]. In another study including 14 children with a history of BPD (Northway stage III or IV), 11 presented with chest radiographic abnormalities at 4–6 years of age, nine of these with hyperinflation, and six with interstitial changes [28]. Ten BPD survivors from the same population were reexamined at 8–10 years of age, and 80 % showed abnormal radiographs [29]. Generalized hyperinflation was present in all, and four also had local areas of hyperinflation. Mild perihilar fibrosis was found in five children [29]. In 26 adolescents and young adults (mean age 18.3 years) who were born between 1964 and 1973 and had BPD in infancy, chest X-rays showed mild hyperexpansion, blebs, interstitial thickening, peribronchial cuffing, and pleural thickening [30].

The findings were mild, but more severe in BPD survivors compared with age-matched prematurely born controls without neonatal mechanical ventilation and normal subjects [30].

Radiographic Differential Diagnosis of BPD

Radiographic findings of pulmonary edema, pulmonary interstitial emphysema, meconium aspiration syndrome, and pneumonia (especially cytomegalovirus) may resemble those found in BPD [6]. Therefore, combining clinical data with radiographic information is important. Other radiographic differential diagnoses include pulmonary lymphangiectasia, total anomalous pulmonary venous return, recurrent pneumonitis or aspiration (immune deficiency, gastroesophageal reflux, tracheo-esophageal fistula, cystic fibrosis), and Wilson–Mikity syndrome [6]. Wilson–Mikity syndrome was first described in 1960 in premature infants without severe initial respiratory problems who developed areas of cystic emphysema in the first month of life, with progression to chronic lung disease [31]. Although the validity of this diagnosis has not been clear, the earliest pathology has been suggested to be alveolar air leak [32].

High-Resolution Computed Tomography Imaging

High-resolution computed tomography (HRCT) is the most preferred method for the morphological imaging of the pulmonary parenchyma with excellent spatial resolution [33]. The typical effective radiation dose is about 1 mSv in all age groups and ranges in adults between 1.8 and 4.3 mSv depending on HRCT techniques, while the typical radiation dose in bidirectional chest X-ray examination is around 0.03 mSv [34, 35]. Thus, while HRCT is not suitable for routine evaluation of patients with BPD, it provides important information regarding both the underlying pathology and the long-term course of BPD [4]. It detects lung abnormalities typical of BPD with a greater sensitivity than chest radiographs, especially in older survivors of BPD [21]. Chest HRCT examination may be of use in patients with severe BPD, especially when home O_2 therapy is needed [36]. In most clinical studies on BPD patients, HRCT findings have been correlated with the severity of BPD according to NIH criteria [37], the duration of O_2 supplementation and assisted ventilation, and with concomitant abnormalities in lung function.

HRCT findings in BPD patients were first systematically described in 1994 [38]. Twenty-three children of median age 3.3 years (range 2 months to 13 years) with a history of BPD and current signs of respiratory dysfunction underwent chest X- ray and chest HRCT examinations. The chest radiographs revealed hyperexpansion in 17, hyperlucent areas in 11, and linear opacities in 10 of the images, whereas in four cases the chest X-rays were normal. On the other hand, HRCT scans showed abnormalities in all 23 cases. Multifocal areas of hyperaeration and unevenly distributed hypoattenuated areas with pulmonary vascular thinning and pruning were detected in 22 of the 23 patients. These areas were suggested to correspond to emphysema, caused by obstructed small airways. The CT scans also revealed linear opacities, radiating from the external lung toward the hilum, and atelectatic lung segments or lobes. The opacities were suggested to reflect strands of atelectasis, extending to the pleura and forming pleural grooves. All 23 CT scans contained triangular subpleural opacities, usually observed on several consecutive sections. It was concluded that CT scans can detect lesions in the lungs of BPD survivors better than chest radiographs.

Typical HRCT Findings in Patients with BPD

Typical chest HCRT findings in BPD patients include linear and subpleural triangular opacities, reduced lung attenuation both on inspiration and expiration, bullae or blebs, emphysema, collapse, consolidation, bronchial wall thickening, bronchiectasis, and inverse bronchopulmonary artery diameter ratios [36, 39–43].

Scoring systems have been created in order to assess the severity, distribution, and quantity of chest HRCT abnormalities in BPD patients. The first was introduced in 2008 at the end of the primary hospitalization period (Table 13.1, [36]). The main variables in the scoring system included hyperexpansion, emphysema, fibrous and

Table 13.1 Scoring of chest CT scan for BPD

		Score		
Category	Variable	0	1	2
Hyperexpansion	Hyperexpansion	None	Focal	Global
	Mosaic pattern of lung attenuation	None	Unclear	Obvious
	Intercostal bulging	None	Unclear	Obvious
Emphysema	Number of bullae or blebs	None	Single	Multiple
	Size of bullae or blebs	None	≤5 mm	>5 mm
Fibrous/interstitial	Triangular subpleural opacities	None	1–3 lobes	4–6 lobes
	Distortion and thickening of bronchovascular bundle	Mild	Moderate	Severe
	Consolidation	None	Unclear	Obvious
Subjective impression		Mild	Moderate	Severe

A mosaic pattern of lung attenuation is indicated by visible attenuation differences in the lung fields; intercostal bulging suggests pulmonary overexpansion into the intercostal space. Focal hyperexpansion is expressed as the mosaic pattern of lung attenuation and global hyperexpansion as a diffuse low-attenuation image of the lung field with intercostal bulging. Bullae and blebs are defined as sharply demarcated areas of emphysema. Triangular subpleural opacities are classified according to the number of involved lobes, with the lingual segment accounted for separately to correlate with the right middle lobe. Consolidation is expressed as an increase in lung opacity resulting in the obstruction of underlying vessels

Ochiai et al. [36], with permission

Table 13.2 Revised high-resolution CT scoring system with nine different parameters and a total score of 50

	Scoring per lobe
1. Linear or triangular subpleural opacities	0 = absent, 1 = present
	Maximum score = 6
2. Decreased pulmonary attenuation	0 = absent, 1 = one lobe
Hypoattenuation ("mosaic perfusion") in inspiration	Maximum = 6
3. Decreased pulmonary attenuation	0 = absent, 1 = one lobe
Hypoattenuation ("air trapping") in expiration	Maximum = 6
4. Bronchus/bronchiole: artery diameter ratio	0 = absent, 1 = one lobe
	Maximum = 6
5. Bronchiectasies	0 = absent, 1 = one lobe
	Maximum = 6
6. Peribronchial thickening	0 = absent, 1 = one lobe
	Maximum = 6
7. Bullae	0 = absent, 1 = one lobe
	Maximum = 6
8. Emphysema	0 = absent, 1 = one lobe
	Maximum = 6
9. Collapse/consolidation	0 = absent, 1 = subsegmental, 2 = segmental

Aukland et al. [39], with permission

interstitial findings, and subjective impression. A year later, another scoring system was used in a study on two cohorts of survivors of extremely preterm birth (Table 13.2, [39]). Subpleural opacities, decreased pulmonary attenuation in inspiration and expiration, bronchial/artery diameter ratio, bronchiectasis, peribronchial thickening, bullae, emphysema, and collapse/consolidation were scored per lobe in order to evaluate the distribution of the abnormalities. The scoring system seems to be of use in decreasing interobserver variability [36].

Chest HRCT from Preterm Birth to Adulthood

Infancy and Early Childhood

Forty-two infants [36] with BPD underwent chest HRCT examinations at hospital discharge. The infants were born at a median of 26 (range 22–33) weeks of gestational age and had a median birth weight of 829 (range 484–1430) g. The CT scans were scored and correlations of the scores to the clinical severity of BPD [37] were assessed. The patients with more severe BPD had higher HRCT scores (Fig. 13.6). The HRCT score correlated with the clinical scores at 36 week's postmenstrual age and the duration of O_2 therapy. Patients with a need of home O_2 treatment had higher HRCT scores than those without.

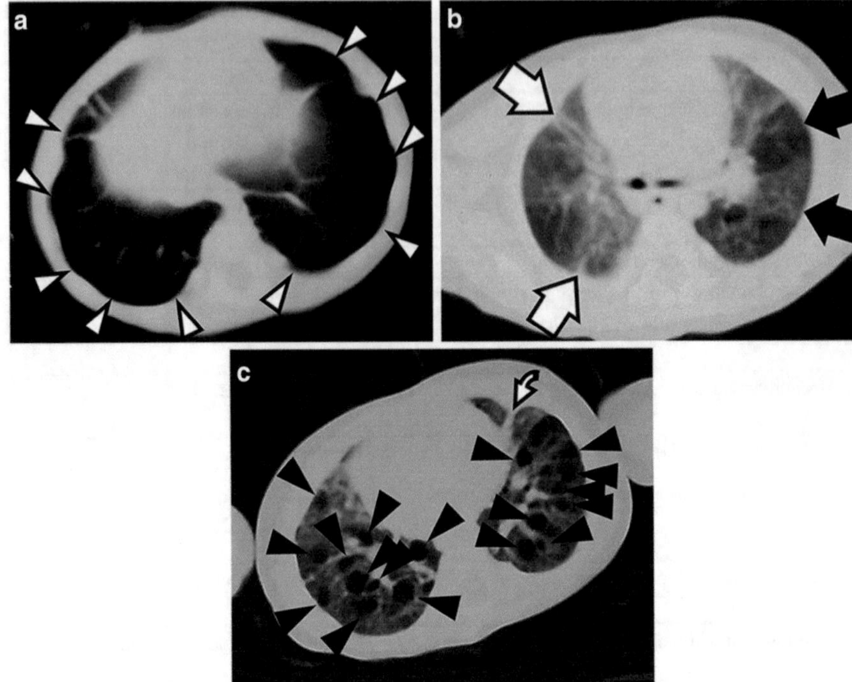

Fig. 13.6 Representative CT findings in BPD. (**a**) Intercostal bulging suggesting pulmonary overexpansion into the intercostal space (*open arrowhead*). Global hyperexpansion is seen as a diffuse low-attenuation image of lung fields with bulging intercostals. (**b**) Mosaic pattern of lung attenuation indicated by visible attenuation differences in the lung fields (*solid straight arrow*). Triangular subpleural opacities are seen as external base and internal apex involvement (*open straight arrow*). (**c**) Bullae and blebs, defined as sharply demarcated areas of emphysema (*solid arrowhead*). Consolidation is seen as an increase in lung opacity resulting from obstruction of underlying vessels (*open curved arrow*). Ochiai et al. [36], with permission

Nineteen premature infants, of whom six had moderate and 13 severe BPD according to NIH criteria [37], underwent chest CT scans at a median age of 14.6 (range 1.5–53.7) months. Abnormalities were detected in all images. Bronchial wall thickening was found in all and linear and subpleural opacities in 17 (90 %) patients. Areas of decreased attenuation were seen in 69 %, emphysema in 26 %, and bronchiectasis in four (21 %) of the cases. Four patients had more than one scan (10.6–43.2 months apart). The abnormalities neither resolved nor worsened in these cases. Decreased attenuation was seen more frequently in the cases with severe BPD than in those with moderate BPD, whereas occurrences of other radiological abnormalities were similar regardless of the severity of BPD. The positive predictive values of the radiological items used to predict BPD severity were as follows: subpleural and linear opacities 70.6 %, bronchiectasis 100 %, emphysema 80.0 %, and attenuation 84.6 %. The presence or absence of each abnormality was recorded in every lung lobe. Thus, the worst score would be 36, where all abnormalities were seen in all six lobes. In the moderate BPD group, the median composite score was 12 (range 9–27) and in the severe BPD group 18 (range 8–24). It was concluded that chest CT can be useful in assessment of the severity of BPD, but not in prediction of the course of BPD.

Chest HRCT scans were obtained from 39 infants and toddlers with BPD at a mean of 11.9 (range 5–18) months of age and in 41 full-term controls at a mean of 16.7 (range 4–33) months [42]. The severity of BPD was mild in 11 (28 %), moderate in five (13 %), and severe in 23 (59 %) of the preterm participants. The CT scans were used for quantitative assessment of lung structure. Airway size of the trachea, airway generation of the right lower lobe, lung volume, and lung tissue density were measured. The relationship between airway generation and airway size in taller BPD cases and control subjects was similar. However, in the shorter BPD cases, the sizes of the first and second airway generations were larger than in the shorter control subjects. The longer duration of mechanical ventilation during the first period of hospitalization was correlated with increased airway size and the longer duration of O_2 supplementation with smaller lung volumes. The subjects with BPD had greater lung density than the full-term controls.

From Early Teenage to Adolescence

Two Norwegian cohorts of survivors born in 1982–1985 and 1991–1992 at gestational ages of 28 weeks or less or with birth weights less than 1000 g were invited for chest HRCT scanning examinations and pulmonary function tests [39]. The examinations were performed less than 2 weeks apart in 74 of 86 eligible subjects at mean age of 18 and 10 years, respectively, in the two cohorts. A structured scoring system was used in interpretation of the HRCT scans (Table 13.2). Abnormal results were detected in 64 (86 %) of the cases. Linear and subpleural triangular opacities were seen in 83 %, hypoattenuated areas in inspiration in 14 %, and hypoattenuated areas in expiration in 26 % of the scans (Fig. 13.5) [39]. The earlier-born birth cohort had higher scores than the cohort born in the 1990s. The median total HRCT score for the whole group was 3.0 (interquartile range 1.75–5.0 points). Of the neonatal variables, the duration of mechanical ventilation and O_2 supplementation was significantly associated with the HRCT scores. The number of days with O_2 supplementation turned out to be the strongest variable explaining the high HRCT scores, and an increase of 100 days of O_2 treatment increased the HRCT score by 3.8 points. Worse pulmonary function test results were associated with linear/triangular opacities and higher total HRCT scores. Participants with hypoattenuated areas had significantly lower forced expiratory volumes in 1 s (FEV_1) than those without.

In another study, chest HRCT findings were correlated with pulmonary function test results at a median of 10 (range 5–18) years of age in 26 patients, of whom 25 had a history of BPD [44]. The extent of air trapping, i.e., areas of persistent lung parenchymal radiolucency during expiration in both lobes, was graded in percentages of each CT slice. HRCT at inspiration revealed abnormalities in 22 cases, including areas of decreased density in lung parenchyma, compressing the adjacent lung in nine subjects. Two patients had bronchiectasis, 22 showed reticular opacities, and 18 had areas of architectural distortion. In the expiratory scans, 24 patients had air trapping. Pulmonary findings of obstruction correlated significantly with the number of cells with decreased density and with the expiratory CT air trapping scores. The duration of O_2 supplementation correlated both with the severity of HRCT findings and worse pulmonary function test results. Air trapping and architectural distortion in HRCT scans best predicted abnormal pulmonary function.

Adulthood

The first report on the appearance of chest HRCT scans in adult BPD survivors was published in 2000 [40]. Five preterm-born patients with BPD diagnosed during their first period of hospitalization underwent chest HRCT scans at a mean of 25 (range 20–26) years of age. Ten healthy age- and sex-matched nonsmoking subjects at a mean age of 26 (range 18–30) years, without a history of lung disease, gave their consent to be control cases in the study. Hypoattenuated areas, where the numbers and sizes of the vessels were decreased in both lungs, were detected in all BPD cases, the areas being larger than one lung segment. Small focal areas of low lung attenuation were also found in six of the control cases. Bullae were seen in the lungs of two BPD patients. Bilateral bronchial wall thickening was observed in the scans of all BPD subjects; the involvement was either diffuse or concentrated in the lower lung lobes. The bronchus-to-pulmonary artery diameter ratio was much higher in the BPD patients than in the controls [mean 0.81 (SD 0.08) vs. 0.45 (0.04)]. Pulmonary function tests were performed within 1 day of the HRCT examination in the BPD subjects. Air trapping, i.e., increased residual volume to total lung capacity, was seen in all and hyperinflation in two participants. Maximal expiratory flow at 50 % of vital capacity represented a significant airflow obstruction in four cases with BPD.

Wong et al. [43] described structural pulmonary abnormalities in 51 adult (median age 20, range 18–33 years) survivors of BPD by means of inspiratory and expiratory chest HRCT. Abnormalities were detected in 50 (98 %) cases, the most common being subpleural triangular (94 %) and linear (90 %) opacities, air trapping (65 %), and emphysema (47 %). Mosaic perfusion, defined as foci of radiolucency or radiodensity in lung lobes or segments, was seen in 31 %, bullae in 18 %, peribronchial thickening in 12 %, bronchiectasis in 8 %, mucous plugging in 6 %, and interlobar septal thickening in 5 % of the scans. These findings were regarded as being compatible with histological features, including septal fibrosis and small vessel and airway disease.

Magnetic Resonance Imaging

The strength of magnetic resonance imaging (MRI) is the lack of radiation exposure. However, the technique is expensive and time-consuming. It is useful for evaluation of vascular and mediastinal structures, but its role in the assessment of lung

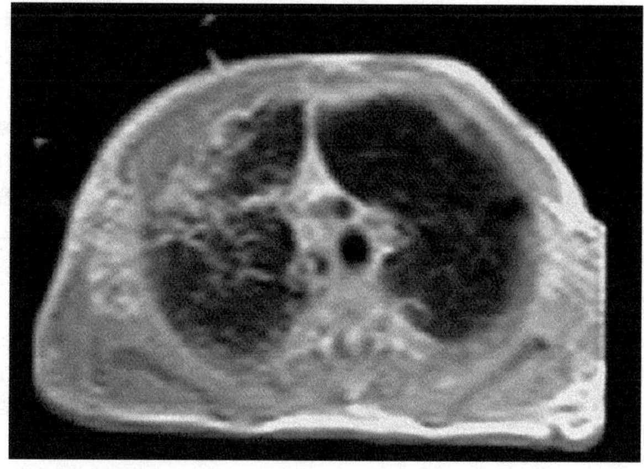

Fig. 13.7 Transverse T1-weighted image of a 26-week-gestation infant with severe BPD 76 days after delivery. Focal high-density regions, which have a reticular appearance and extended toward the periphery, are seen on the *left*. Adams et al. [46], with permission

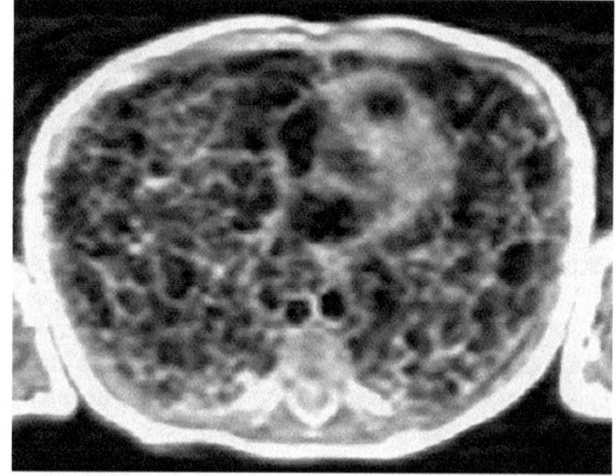

Fig. 13.8 Transverse T1-weighted image of an infant born at 27 weeks of gestation with severe BPD 54 days after delivery. Multiple low-density focal abnormalities of a cyst-like appearance are seen throughout both lungs. Adams et al. [46], with permission

parenchyma is limited [33]. In the imaging of BPD, MRI has the potential to give functional information [4], and it is sensitive in detection of early changes in cases of emphysema [45].

In one study, lung MRI was used in 35 preterm infants born at 23–33 weeks of gestation [46]. Fifteen of the cases had developed severe BPD, 13 mild BPD, and 7 were without BPD. Relative proton density, reflecting water content, was calculated by combining T1-weighted and proton density-weighted images. High-density focal reticulated areas, extending toward the periphery (Fig. 13.7), and low-density cyst-like focal abnormalities of 0.3–0.5 cm in diameter were noted (Fig. 13.8). Focal high-signal intensities were graded as follows: 0 (none detected), 1 (<50 % of the area affected), and 2 (>50 % of the area affected), and cyst-like abnormalities were graded as 0 (no cysts), 1 (≤5 cysts < 0.5 cm in diameter), 2 (<50 % of the area affected), and 3 (>50 % of the area affected). Average proton density was higher in the dependent lung and greater in the infants with severe BPD compared with those without. The dependence of changes in water content on gravity was presented in images where the patients were scanned both in supine and prone positions. The infants with severe BPD had significantly higher scores for cyst-like lesions and focal densities than the infants with mild BPD or without it. The cases with severe BPD had significantly higher scores in the dorsal than in the ventral regions, but no difference was seen either in the cephalocaudal or left-right distribution of the abnormalities. The number of days of assisted ventilation significantly predicted both cyst-like and signal-intensity abnormalities. In conclusion, these lung MRI examinations showed that infants with BPD have increased water content leading to a tendency toward alveolar collapse in the dependent lung, according to gravity, and that focal abnormalities in the lung are not distributed homogeneously.

Conclusion

The appearance of chest radiographs of the "new" BPD in infancy/childhood range from LLS to a heterogeneous pattern of opaque strands, cystic lucencies of varying size (bubbly lung), and regional air trapping. During adolescence/adulthood, they show mild hyperexpansion, blebs, interstitial thickening, peribronchial cuffing, and pleural thickening. HRCT scans are more informative and show bronchial wall thickening, linear and subpleural opacities with areas of decreased attenuation, and emphysema in early childhood. In older patients, features of subpleural triangular and linear opacities, air trapping, and emphysema predominate. There is good correlation of abnormal pulmonary function with air trapping and architectural distortion noted in HRCT scans. More recently, MRI is increasingly being used given the lack of radiation exposure. The images are characterized by high-density focal reticulated areas, extending toward the periphery, and low-density cyst-like focal abnormalities.

Acknowledgments We thank very much Päivi Savikurki, MD, pediatric radiologist, Tampere University Hospital, for valuable comments on the manuscript and help in choosing and editing the radiographs and Päivi Laarne, PhD, Medical Physicist, Tampere University Hospital, for help in the interpretation of radiation doses.

References

1. Northway Jr WH, Rosan RC, Porter DY. Pulmonary disease following respirator therapy of hyaline membrane disease. Bronchopulmonary dysplasia. N Engl J Med. 1967;276(7): 357–68.
2. Swischuk LE, Shetty BP, John SD. The lungs in immature infants: how important is surfactant therapy in preventing chronic lung problems? Pediatr Radiol. 1996;26(8):508–11.
3. Jobe AJ. The new BPD: an arrest of lung development. Pediatr Res. 1999;46:641–3.

4. Wilson AC. What does imaging of the chest tell us about bronchopulmonary dysplasia. Pediatr Respir Rev. 2010;11:158–61.
5. Bhandari A, Panitch HB. Pulmonary outcomes in bronchopulmonary dysplasia. Semin Perinatol. 2006;30:219–26.
6. Edwards DK. Radiology of hyaline membrane disease, transient tachypnea of the newborn, and bronchopulmonary dysplasia. In: Farrell PM, editor. Lung development: biological and clinical perspectives, vol. 2. New York: Academic; 1982. p. 47–89.
7. Oppermann HC, Wille L, Bleyl U, Obladen M. Bronchopulmonary dysplasia in premature infants. A radiological and pathological correlation. Pediatr Radiol. 1977;5(3):137–41.
8. Heneghan MA, Sosulski R, Baquero JM. Persistent pulmonary abnormalities in newborns: the changing picture of bronchopulmonary dysplasia. Pediatr Radiol. 1986;16(3):180–4.
9. Fitzgerald P, Donoghue V, Gorman W. Bronchopulmonary dysplasia: a radiographic and clinical review of 20 patients. Br J Radiol. 1990;63(750):444–7.
10. Fitzgerald DA, Van Asperen PP, Lam AH, De Silva M, Henderson-Smart DJ. Chest radiograph abnormalities in very low birth weight survivors of chronic neonatal lung disease. J Paediatr Child Health. 1996;32:491–4.
11. Moya MP, Bisset GS, Auten Jr RL, Miller C, Hollingworth C, Frush DP. Reliability of CXR for the diagnosis of bronchopulmonary dysplasia. Pediatr Radiol. 2001;31:339–42.
12. Hyde I, English RE, Williams JD. The changing pattern of chronic lung disease of prematurity. Arch Dis Child. 1989;64:448–51.
13. Toce SS, Farrell PM, Leavitt LA, Samuels DP, Edwards DK. Clinical and roentgenographic scoring systems for assessing bronchopulmonary dysplasia. Am J Dis Child. 1984;138: 581–5.
14. Yuksel B, Greenough A, Karani J, Page A. Chest radiograph scoring system for use in pre-term infants. Br J Radiol. 1991;64:1015–8.
15. Greenough A, Dimitriou G, Johnson AH, Calvert S, Peacock J, Karani J. The chest radiograph appearances of very premature infants at 36 weeks post-conceptional age. Br J Radiol. 2000;73:366–9.
16. Greenough A, Kavvadia V, Johnson AH, Calvert S, Peacock J, Karani J. A simple radiograph score to predict chronic lung disease in prematurely born infants. Br J Radiol. 1999;72: 530–3.
17. Weinstein MR, Peters ME, Sadek M, Palta M. A new radiographic scoring system for bronchopulmonary dysplasia. Pediatr Pulmonol. 1994;18:284–9.
18. Maconochie I, Greenough A, Yuksel B, Page A, Karani J. A chest radiograph scoring system to predict chronic oxygen dependency in low birth weight infants. Early Hum Dev. 1991;26(1):37-43.
19. Noack G, Mortensson W, Robertson B, Nilsson R. Correlations between radiological and cytological findings in early development of bronchopulmonary dysplasia. Eur J Pediatr. 1993; 152(12):1024-9.
20. Edwards DK. Radiographic aspects of bronchopulmonary dysplasia. J Pediatr. 1979;95(5): 823-9.
21. Agrons GA, Courtney SE, Stocker JT, Markowitz RI. From the archives of AFIP. Lung disease in premature neonates: radiologic-pathologic correlation. Radiographics. 2005;25:1047–73.
22. May C, Prendergast M, Salman S, Rafferty GF, Greenough A. Chest radiograph thoracic areas and lung volumes in infants developing bronchopulmonary dysplasia. Pediatr Pulmonol. 2009;44:80–5.
23. Eber E, Zach MS. Long term pulmonary sequelae of bronchopulmonary dysplasia (chronic lung disease of infancy). Thorax. 2001;56:317–23.
24. Husain AN, Siddiqui NH, Stocker JT. Pathology of arrested acinar development in postsurfactant bronchopulmonary dysplasia. Hum Pathol. 1998;29(7):710–7.
25. Hyödynmaa E, Korhonen P, Ahonen S, Luukkaala T, Tammela O. Frequency and clinical correlates of radiographic patterns of bronchopulmonary dysplasia in very low birth weight infants by term age. Eur J Pediatr. 2012;171:95–102.
26. Lanning P, Tammela O, Koivisto M. Radiological incidence and course of bronchopulmonary dysplasia in 100 consecutive low birth weight neonates. Acta Radiol. 1995;36(4):353–7.

27. Hakulinen AL, Heinonen K, Lansimies E, Kiekara O. Pulmonary function and respiratory morbidity in school-age children born prematurely and ventilated for neonatal respiratory insufficiency. Pediatr Pulmonol. 1990;8:226–32.
28. Lindroth M, Mortensson W. Long term follow-up of ventilator treated low birthweight infants. I. Chest X-ray, pulmonary mechanics, clinical lung disease and growth. Acta Paediatr Scand. 1986;75:819–26.
29. Andreasson B, Lindroth M, Mortensson W, Svenningsen NW, Jonson B. Lung function eight years after neonatal ventilation. Arch Dis Child. 1989;64:108–13.
30. Northway Jr WH, Moss RB, Carlisle KB, Parker BR, Popp RL, Pitlick PT, Eichler I, Lamm RL, Brown BW. Late pulmonary sequelae of bronchopulmonary dysplasia. N Engl J Med. 1990;323:1793–9.
31. Wilson M, Mikity V. A new form of respiratory disease in premature infants. Am J Dis Child. 1960;99:489–99.
32. Hoepker A, Seear M, Petrocheilou A, Hayes Jr D, Nair A, Deodhar J, Kadam S, O'Toole J. Wilson-Mikity syndrome: updated diagnostic criteria based on nine cases and a review of the literature. Pediatr Pulmonol. 2008;43:1004–12.
33. Rossi UG, Owens CM. The radiology of chronic lung disease in children. Review Arch Dis Child. 2005;90:601–7.
34. Bankier AA, Tack D. Dose reduction strategies for thoracic multidetector computed tomography. Background, current issues, and recommendations. J Thorac Imaging. 2010;25:278–88.
35. Christner JA, Kofler JM, McCollough CH. Estimating effective dose for CT using dose-length product compared with using organ doses: consequences of adopting international commission on radiological protection publication 103 or dual-energy scanning. AJR Am J Roentgenol. 2010;194:881–9.
36. Ochiai M, Hikino S, Yabuuchi H, Nakayama H, Sato K, Ohga S, et al. A new scoring system for computed tomography of the chest for assessing the clinical status of bronchopulmonary dysplasia. J Pediatr. 2008;152:90–5.
37. Jobe AH, Bancalari E. NICHD/NHLRI workshop summary: bronchopulmonary dysplasia. Am J Respir Crit Care Med. 2001;163:1723–9.
38. Oppenheim C, Mamou-Mani T, Sayegh N, de Blic J, Scheinmann P, Lallemand D. Bronchopulmonary dysplasia: value of identifying pulmonary sequelae. AJR Am J Roentgenol. 1994;193:169–72.
39. Aukland SM, Rosendahl K, Owens CM, Fosse KR, Eide GE, Halvorsen T. Neonatal bronchopulmonary dysplasia predicts abnormal pulmonary HRCT scans in long-term survivors of extreme preterm birth. Thorax. 2009;64:405–10.
40. Howling SJ, Northway Jr WH, Hansell DM, Moss RB, Ward S, Műller NL. Pulmonary sequelae of bronchopulmonary dysplasia survivors: high resolution CT findings. Am Respir J. 2000;174:1323–6.
41. La Tour AT, Spadola L, Sayegh Y, Comescure C, Pfister R, Argiroffo CB, et al. Chest CT in bronchopulmonary dysplasia: clinical and radiological correlations. Pediatr Pulmonol. 2013;48:693–8.
42. Sarria EE, Mattiello R, Rao L, Tiller CJ, Pointdexter B, Applegate KE, et al. Quantitative assessment of chronic lung disease of infancy using computed tomography. Eur Respir J. 2012;39:992–9.
43. Wong P, Murray C, Louw J, French N, Chambers D. Adult bronchopulmonary dysplasia: computed tomography pulmonary findings. J Med Imaging Radiat Oncol. 2011;55:373–8.
44. Aquino SL, Schechter MS, Chilers C, Ablin DS, Chills B, Webb WR. High-resolution inspiratory and expiratory CT in older children and adults with BPD. AJR Am J Roentgenol. 1999;173:963–7.
45. Yablonsky DA, Suskianskii A, Woods JC, Gierada DS, Quick JD, Hogg JC, et al. Quantification of lung microstructure with hyperpolarized 3He diffusion MRI. J Appl Physiol. 2009; 107:1258–65.
46. Adams EW, Harrison MC, Counsell SJ, Allsop JM, Kenea NL, Hainal JV, et al. Increased lung water and tissue damage in bronchopulmonary dysplasia. J Pediatr. 2004;145:503–7.

Chapter 14
Pulmonary Hypertension in Bronchopulmonary Dysplasia

Charitharth Vivek Lal and Namasivayam Ambalavanan

Introduction

Bronchopulmonary dysplasia (BPD) is a chronic lung disease of premature infants characterized by impaired lung development [1, 2]. Approximately 1.5 % of all births in the USA (64,000/year) are of very low birth weight (VLBW) infants, of whom 15,000 develop BPD. BPD ranks among the top three chronic respiratory diseases of childhood along with asthma and cystic fibrosis with a cost burden in the USA of over $2.4 billion per year. BPD was first described by Northway et al. in 1967 [3], and in 1976, Bonikos et al. described symptoms or signs of cardiac atrial or ventricular stress, including cor pulmonale in 6 of 21 patients who died of BPD [4]. Since then, pulmonary hypertension (PH) and resulting cor pulmonale have been described in many case reports, case series, and retrospective and prospective studies. In addition, the phenotype of BPD has changed over the past four decades with increasing survival of smaller and more immature infants. PH contributes significantly to morbidity and mortality of chronic lung disease of infancy. Despite many recent clinical advances, pulmonary vascular disease (PVD) remains an important contributor to poor outcomes in preterm infants with BPD [5, 6]. Substantial challenges persist, especially with regard to understanding mechanisms and the clinical approach to PVDs.

C.V. Lal, MBBS, FAAP (✉) • N. Ambalavanan, MBBS, MD, FAAP
Division of Neonatology, Department of Pediatrics, University of Alabama, 176F, Suite 9380, Birmingham, AL, USA

Women and Infant Center, University of Alabama, Birmingham, AL, USA

Childrens Hospital of Alabama, Birmingham, AL, USA
e-mail: clal@peds.uab.edu; nambalavanan@peds.uab.edu

V. Bhandari (ed.), *Bronchopulmonary Dysplasia*, Respiratory Medicine,
DOI 10.1007/978-3-319-28486-6_14

PH is usually defined as mean pulmonary artery pressure measurement via catheterization, equal to or greater than 25 mmHg at rest or 30 mmHg on exercise [7], although this definition may not apply to young infants. On echocardiography, PH is generally defined as estimated systolic pulmonary artery pressure of greater than or equal to 40 mmHg [7].

The Epidemiology and Importance of Pulmonary Hypertension in Bronchopulmonary Dysplasia

We believe that prevalence of PH in BPD is underestimated. In observational studies, PH occurs in up to 17–43 % of preterm infants with BPD [8–11], and BPD with severe PH is associated with significantly increased mortality rate [10]. Preterm infants with PH spent at least three additional weeks in the hospital [8], indicating substantial additional healthcare costs involved in management of these infants. PH is relatively common, affecting at least one in six extremely LBW (ELBW) infants, and persists to discharge in most survivors [12]. A recent study from Denmark showed the prevalence of PH among the entire sample of preterm infants with BPD to be 23 % [13]. As per the Tracking Outcomes and Practices in Pediatric Pulmonary Hypertension (TOPP) registry, 12 % of PH was associated with respiratory disease. Of the respiratory diseases, BPD was the most common cause. Other reasons for this underestimation could be the absence of an existing ICD-9 code for this diagnosis. In addition, the accurate diagnosis of PH in preterm infants is difficult, and hence many cases might be missed. There are not many large prospective studies on this subject, and the first published large prospective study found that around 18 % of infants (1 in 6) were diagnosed with PH before discharge from the hospital [12]. This study evaluated 145 ELBW infants by screening echocardiography at 4 weeks of age and subsequently if signs of cardiac failure or severe lung disease were present [12]. Overall, 18 % were diagnosed with PH, with 6 % diagnosed at the initial screening (median age of 31 days; interquartile range or IQR 29–41), and 12 % subsequently (median age of 112 days; IQR 93–122), indicating that PH can be a late finding even with previously negative echocardiograms. Of the infants with severe BPD (oxygen requirement at 36 weeks postmenstrual age), 50 % had PH [12]. Infants with PH were more likely to have lower BW for a given gestational age (GA) than infants without PH and were more likely to receive higher oxygen supplementation or ventilator support on day 28. Mortality and length of stay were increased in infants with PH, after adjusting for other variables. PH persisted to discharge in many infants (5 of 9 with early PH and 10 of 17 with late PH) [12]. Consistent with these findings, another recent prospective study found that early PVD is associated with the development of BPD and with late PH in preterm infants [14]. In this study, the authors concluded that echocardiograms at 7 days of age may be a useful tool to identify infants at high risk for BPD and PH [14]. As these studies have been single-center studies, it is not clear how well these results can be generalized, for marked center variation in rates of BPD are known, even after adjustment for patient characteristics [15], and it is possible that rates of PH secondary to BPD will also vary by center.

Risk Factors for the Development of Pulmonary Hypertension in Bronchopulmonary Dysplasia

Small for GA (SGA) or growth-restricted infants have been reported to have higher risk of developing PH as compared to appropriate for GA infants [8, 9, 12, 16], the exact mechanisms for which are not well known but may be secondary to impaired lung development associated with intrauterine growth restriction. Maternal factors such as preeclampsia [17], oligohydramnios, and premature rupture of membranes leading to pulmonary hypoplasia have all been associated with development of PH. Concomitant lung disease such as surfactant disorders or interstitial lung diseases may contribute to development of PH in addition to other factors which hinder lung growth and recovery such as positive pressure ventilation, respiratory infections, and suboptimal nutrition [18]. Other possible factors include intra- or extra-cardiac shunts including patent ductus arteriosus (PDA) or collateral vessels, which would increase pulmonary circulation. Future studies are required to identify risk factors such as specific upper respiratory tract infections, aspiration, reflux disease, etc., which may potentially exacerbate PH in preterm infants.

Pathophysiology of Pulmonary Vascular Disease in Bronchopulmonary Dysplasia

Although the exact pathophysiological mechanisms of PH in BPD are unknown, several mechanisms have been proposed [19]. The pathogenesis of PH in BPD is complex, often resulting from interactions between genetic and epigenetic susceptibility and environmental or acquired factors, including hyperoxia, hypoxia, hemodynamic stress, infection, inflammation, and others [5]. The key principle leading to PH is a loss in the balance between factors contributing to vasodilation and vasoconstriction of pulmonary blood vessels, thus leading to an elevation in pulmonary artery pressures. Multiple growth factors and signaling have been implicated in normal lung vascular growth. Various noxious stimuli such as hyperoxia, inflammation, infection, and ventilator-induced lung injury affect the immature pulmonary circulation in various ways thus influencing the structure, function, and growth of the lungs. Smooth muscle hyperplasia, fibroblast incorporation, and adventitial thickening are some of the structural changes seen in PVD that may contribute to impaired vasodilation, increased hypoxic constriction, enhanced myogenic response, and abnormal metabolic function in these lungs. These lungs may have fewer pulmonary arteries leading to decreased pulmonary vascular surface area and hence reduced alveolarization [19, 20]. Coalson et al. [21] showed in animal models that impaired alveolarization and capillary development can occur in immature lungs, even in the absence of marked hyperoxia and high ventilation settings [21]. Hence, the mechanisms underlying PVD are still speculative.

The damage and thickening of pulmonary circulation in BPD may induce hypoxia and thus cause further vessel constriction and worsening PH. Hence, a vicious cycle of hypoxia, vasoconstriction, and increased vascular remodeling may be initiated. Studies have shown that PH itself can inhibit vascular growth and impair alveolarization in the developing lung, suggesting that hemodynamic stress may be an additional mechanism for abnormal lung structure in BPD [22]. Pulmonary blood vessels actively promote and contribute to alveolar growth throughout postnatal life [23, 24]. However, a recent study also shows that the pulmonary vasculature may develop even in the absence of lung development [25]. Furthermore, it is possible that disruption of either the emerging distal air sacs or the pulmonary vasculature could result in an alteration in the normal morphogenesis of each other, due to the significant cross talk between the two (Fig. 14.1).

Multiple vascular growth factors have a marked impact on pulmonary cell populations during pulmonary vascular morphogenesis. Over the years, vascular endothelial growth factor (VEGF) has been mainly implicated in the pathogenesis of PVD [26]. VEGF and its receptors VEGFR1 and VEGFR2 are essential for vascular development and embryonic survival [27, 28], as modulators of endothelial differentiation, blood vessel formation, and morphogenesis [29]. VEGFR2 is also directly involved in the expansion and propagation of the lymphatic network in the body [30]. Several known mediators of VEGF signaling are also present during lung morphogenesis. For example, endothelial monocyte-activating polypeptide II (EMAP II) an anti-angiogenic protein known to downregulate VEGFR2 phosphorylation, is prevalent in early lung development at the epithelial-mesenchymal interface with its expression being inversely correlated to periods of vascularization. EMAP II which is a potent anti-angiogenic and proinflammatory cytokine functions as a likely director of pulmonary vascular development and has been implicated in the pathogenesis of BPD [31–35]. EMAP II's intricate role in pulmonary vessel

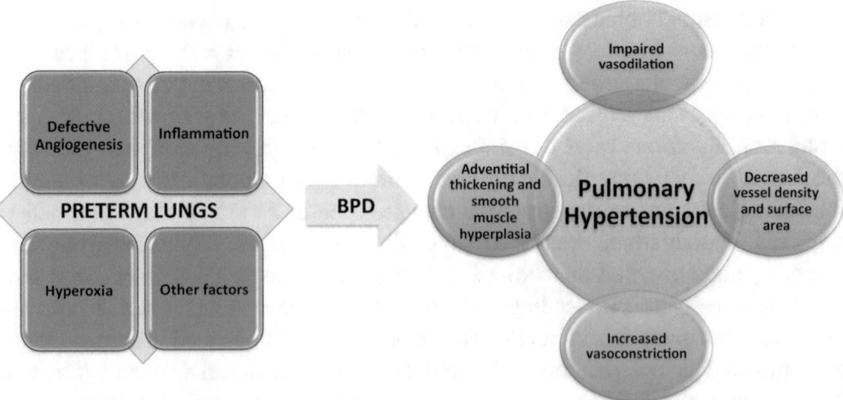

Fig. 14.1 Schematic depicting the possible pathophysiology of development of pulmonary hypertension in patients with bronchopulmonary dysplasia (BPD)

formation makes it a very likely contributor to the development of vascular complications of BPD, studies regarding which are currently underway. Similarly, endothelin-1 (ET-1), known as a potent vasoconstrictor and smooth muscle cell mitogen, is increased in human infants with BPD and has been shown to have striking anti-angiogenic effects in the developing lung, which may further contribute to PVD in BPD [36].

Other factors like nuclear factor kappa B (NF-κB) have also been described in the regulation of neonatal pulmonary vasculature and in transcriptional regulation of VEGF [37]. In addition, the oxygen-sensing mechanism that stimulates endothelial nitric oxide (NO) production, hypoxia-inducible factor-1alpha (HIF-1alpha), can contribute to the development of PH [38]. HIFs are oxygen-responsive transcription factors known to influence VEGF and VEGFR expression. Tsao et al. [39] recently showed that prenatal hypoxia insults, at least in late gestation, influence pulmonary VEGF and VEGF receptor expression through the downregulation of HIF pathways. Identification of those factors such as HIF that promote normal alveolar development may be useful targets for alveolar regeneration [40] and hence help in lung dysplasia-induced PH. Studies have also revealed alterations in endothelial progenitor cells and mesenchymal progenitor cells in experimental models of BPD, and cell-based therapy holds promise in the treatment of BPD [41, 42]. In addition to VEGF-mediated vessel growth, endothelial cells (ECs) themselves generate factors that contribute to their behavior during vessel formation. The angiopoietin (ANG)/Tie-2 ligand/receptor system is known to interact with the VEGF pathway to determine the fate of blood vessels during angiogenesis [43–47]. ANG-1 protein, a mediator of reciprocal interactions between the matrix, mesenchyme, and endothelium, is likely to be required for pulmonary vessel integrity and quiescence. Combination of VEGF + ANG-1 gene transfer corrects VEGF-induced vessel leakiness [48]. ANG-1 also serves as the ligand to the tyrosine kinase Tie2 receptor, responsible for communication between the endothelial and smooth muscle cells in venous morphogenesis by phosphorylating Tie2 on tyrosine residues [49]. Importantly, the Tie2 antagonist, angiopoietin 2 (ANG-2), shares the same Tie2 receptor. ANG-2 decreases Tie2 signaling, thereby preparing vascular ECs for enhanced responsiveness to factors that cause destabilization of the endothelial barrier [50]. Implicated in many aspects of angiogenesis, the canonical Wnt/β-catenin pathway mediates vascular remodeling and differentiation in various species and organ systems. Recent studies show that the Wnt/β-catenin pathway influences vascular sprouting, remodeling, and arteriovenous specification and growing evidence also points to a role of the Wnt pathway in vascular development by regulating VEGF availability [51–54]. Other studies have examined the role of microRNA (miR) in lung development. Mujahid et al. [55] examined how anti-angiogenic miR-221 and pro-angiogenic miR-130a affect airway and vascular development. Fetal lungs treated with anti-miR 221 had more distal branch generations with increased Hoxb5 and VEGFR2 gene expression around airways, whereas anti-miR 130a treatment led to a reduction in airway branching associated with increased Hoxa5 and decreased VEGFR2 in the mesenchyme.

In addition to the various vascular growth factors, other proteins have been shown to extend their influence on pulmonary vasculature. One example is endothelial nitric oxide synthase (eNOS). Han et al. [56] showed that eNOS deficiency resulted in capillary hypoperfusion, misaligned pulmonary veins, and a paucity of distal alveolar branches [56]. It has been demonstrated that there is marked diminution in both basal and acetylcholine (Ach)-stimulated NO production in the lungs of chronically hypoxic piglets [57] and targeted deletion of eNOS in mice is associated with capillary hypoperfusion, misaligned pulmonary veins, and a paucity of distal alveolar branches [56], closely resembling alveolar capillary dysplasia in humans, a universally fatal form of persistent PH of the newborn [58]. Studies by the Shaul laboratory [59–64] also demonstrated decreased content of eNOS in this model. Indeed, replacement with inhaled NO improved physiologic and structural parameters in the baboon model [59–64]. Although routine use of NO in preterm infant with PH is not recommended, selected use may still be beneficial [65], and an imbalance between arginase II and eNOS may partially account for the development of PH in the preterm infant [66]. In addition to factors that have endothelial-specific receptors, growth factors secreted from other cell types like the fibroblast growth factors (FGFs) influence vascular integrity and hence distal alveolar formation [67]. Scientists have also tried to predict neonatal lung dysplasias and its complications by using levels of circulating angiogenic cells. They found that there was no correlation between the levels of these circulating angiogenic cells with the future development of BPD [68].

Appropriate physical properties of lung tissue are necessary for physiological postnatal lung development, and deregulation of this mechanism contributes to postnatal lung developmental disorders. Mammotto et al. [69] first reported that low-density lipoprotein receptor-related protein 5 (LRP5)-Tie2 signaling controls postnatal lung development by modulating angiogenesis and more recently showed that tissue stiffness modulated by the ECM cross-linking enzyme, lysyl oxidase (LOX), regulates postnatal lung development through LRP5-Tie2 signaling. Interactions between lung epithelium and mesenchyme mediated by peroxisome proliferator-activated receptor-γ are critical for normal lung development and homeostasis. Very recently, rosiglitazone, a peroxisome proliferator-activated receptor-γ agonist, has been shown to restore alveolar development and vascular growth in a rat model of BPD [70].

In this section, we have tried to outline how multiple growth factors have been described to work in a very complex and coordinated manner through various pathways to form the pulmonary vasculature, which is critical in alveologenesis and gas exchange. Aberration in one or more of these pathways may be responsible for the development of pulmonary hypertension in BPD. Deviation from the normal pulmonary development due to any inciting factor could lead to aberrant lungs and disease states. A better understanding of the genetic and pathophysiological basis for the development of vascular disease in lung dysplasia is needed which would allow for identification of diagnostic and therapeutic possibilities.

Diagnosis of Pulmonary Hypertension in Bronchopulmonary Dysplasia

Clinical features of PH in BPD are often difficult to recognize, and the clinician needs to maintain a high degree to suspicion in high-risk patients. Some patients such as infants with BPD who have disproportionately high oxygen requirements and/or poor growth and infants who require supplemental oxygen and/or need positive pressure ventilation beyond 2 months of age need special attention. Obvious physical findings of parasternal lift and evidence of right heart failure may not always be present until very late in the clinical course. Chest X-ray may reveal cardiomegaly and enlarged central arteries. The electrocardiogram (EKG) might reveal right axis deviation and right ventricular hypertrophy.

Some clinical conditions can mimic PH, one of which is pulmonary vein stenosis—a rare but important diagnosis to make in the setting of BPD [71]. It is mostly an acquired condition and often has poor survival outcomes. Pulmonary vein stenosis has strong associations with prematurity and BPD. In a study by Drossner et al. [72], 11 (42 %) of the 26 subjects were treated for BPD before being diagnosed with pulmonary vein stenosis, and preterm birth was strongly associated with this diagnosis [72]. Factors involved in pathophysiology of BPD could also contribute to the intimal proliferation seen in this disease. Conversely, it is possible that pulmonary vein stenosis may produce venous congestion, interstitial edema, and elevated pulmonary artery pressures that may be indistinguishable from PH in BPD.

Another diagnosis to consider in infants with worsening BPD is left ventricular diastolic dysfunction (LVDD). Infants with BPD can have a clinical course complicated by LVDD, mechanisms for which remain unclear [73]. This diagnosis is important because it brings to light a potentially treatable cardiac complication of late BPD not responding to regular therapy. Echocardiography might miss subtle findings of LVDD, but cardiac catheterization may show increased pulmonary capillary wedge pressures in the absence of left ventricular systolic dysfunction and volume overload. LVDD is characterized by increased stiffness and abnormal relaxation of the ventricle, which leads to elevated LV filling pressures and abnormal early diastolic filling. Hence, afterload reduction might help in this setting.

Echocardiogram Echocardiography is one of the most commonly used modalities to access PH in neonates, but no guidelines exist about its use to detect PH in the setting of BPD [5, 9, 10]. Methods to assess pulmonary artery pressure usually include determination of tricuspid regurgitation jet velocity (TRJV) and velocity of flow through the PDA. Various qualitative measures such as evaluation for ventricular septal flattening, right atrial enlargement, right ventricular hypertrophy/dilation, pulmonary artery dilation, and directions of flow through shunts are also employed by the cardiologist. Studies have also used right ventricular outflow patterns or time intervals obtained with echocardiography to estimate pulmonary artery pressures and to diagnose PH in BPD, but with limited success [74–76] (Table 14.1).

Table 14.1 Echocardiographic diagnosis of PH in BPD

Echocardiographic diagnosis of PH in BPD
When pulmonary artery (PA) pressure ≥ half systemic pressure → PH
When PA pressure above 2/3 systemic pressure → moderate to severe pulmonary hypertension
Methods to assess PA pressure
1. Tricuspid regurgitation jet velocity (TRJV)[a]
2. Velocity of flow through PDA
Qualitative measures
Ventricular septal flattening
Right atrial enlargement
Right ventricular hypertrophy/dilation
PA dilation
Direction of flow through shunts

[a] *TRJV calculated by Modified Bernoulli equation*
Modified Bernoulli equation $P = 4\,V^2$
$RVP - RAP = 4 \times (TRJV)^2$

Although echocardiography is widely used in the determination of PH in chronic lung disease, estimates of pulmonary artery pressure are not obtained consistently and are not reliable for determining the severity of PH [75]. A major limitation of echocardiographic evaluation of TRJV is that it relies on adequately analyzable TR regurgitant jet, which might not be present in all patients. In a study by Mourani et al. [75], 58 % of children without a measureable TRJV were found to have PH by cardiac catheterization, and overall echocardiogram was accurate in determining severity of PH in just 47 % of cases. The authors found that qualitative measures of PH had worse predictive value for subsequent diagnosis of PH during catheterization [75]. Hill et al. [77] recently found a poor correlation between transthoracic echocardiographic estimates of right ventricular systolic pressure based on TRJV and cardiac catheterization in patients undergoing cardiac catheterization for a suspected diagnosis of PH. In that study [77], the echo and catheterization data were not simultaneously obtained, and general anesthesia administered to all patients could have played a role in affecting pulmonary vasoreactivity. In essence, the lack of a measurable TRJV on echocardiogram should not be interpreted as absence of PH.

Cardiac Catheterization Despite its limited use in infants, cardiac catheterization remains the gold standard for diagnosis of pulmonary hypertension through which one can retrieve definitive and comprehensive information about cardiopulmonary hemodynamics. There are no fixed guidelines for the use of cardiac catheterization in infants with BPD, and the exact proportion of infants undergoing this study varies from center to center. In one study, 31 % of formerly premature infants with BPD and PH underwent cardiac catheterization [10].

Lesions such as alveolar capillary dysplasias, pulmonary vein stenosis, and collaterals that may occur in BPD and may mimic PH can also be detected by cardiac catheterization. Cardiac catheterization is usually performed in infants with BPD and PH who fail to respond to oxygen or inhaled NO (iNO) and in those in whom there is suspicion of associated anatomic cardiac lesions or systemic-pulmonary collaterals, pulmonary venous obstruction, or myocardial dysfunction [78]. Acute hemodynamic responses to pulmonary vasodilators can be assessed and can inform decision-making about long-term use of vasodilators. There are no widely accepted guidelines that indicate which patients with BPD and PH should be catheterized, but it is probably appropriate to do cardiac catheterization before initiation of a third or fourth agent if there is insufficient improvement or worsening with first- and second-line therapy. Cardiac catheterizations could also be of help in infants with severe BPD who deteriorate over time despite adequate therapy and in whom echocardiography is not helpful [78]. However, the risks of cardiac catheterization are significant, especially in a sick preterm infant on high cardiorespiratory support. It is a procedure requiring general anesthesia and hence is not always feasible in preterm infant population. One registry study showed that cardiac catheterization could be performed for pediatric PH patients with few (mostly technical) adverse events and zero mortality, but another retrospective study from a single center showed that resuscitation or death occurred in almost 6 % of cases [77, 79]. Hence, a decision to perform a cardiac catheterization in a patient with BPD and PH should be discussed in a multidisciplinary setting and the risks and benefits carefully weighed.

Risk of Anesthesia Infants with BPD with PH are at increased risk for PH crises while under anesthesia or sedation [18]. Various physiological changes could occur during anesthesia such as hypercarbia, hypoxia, increased catecholamine surge, and acidosis—which can all change the vascular reactivity of the pulmonary capillaries and cause a crisis [80]. A retrospective review showed a nearly sixfold increase in risk of perioperative/periprocedural cardiac arrest in children with PH [81]. This study showed a 1.3 % mortality rate and a 4.5 % risk of major complications in patients with PH, and most complications occurred in patients that had suprasystemic pulmonary artery pressures documented preoperatively [81]. Judicious preoperative sedative premedication can decrease the risk of sympathetic stimulation during anesthetic induction, and continuation of vasodilator therapies such as sildenafil and NO may prevent a PH crisis in the operating room [81]. Management considerations during the critical induction period include the placement of all standard monitors, maintenance of adequate alveolar and arterial oxygenation, ample minute ventilation, protection of systemic blood pressure by careful administration of IV fluids and slow infusion of vasoactive induction agents, and availability of adequate vascular access and inotropic support [82]. For optimal anesthetic maintenance in PH, a balanced technique incorporating inhalational agents, narcotics, and neuromuscular blockade is recommended. Controlled ventilation is indicated in order to reduce hypoventilation and the resultant hypoxia that may occur during spontaneous ventilation; however, adequate anesthetic depth must be ensured prior to placement of an endotracheal tube. Finally, postoperative care should incorporate PH therapy that is compatible with the need for continued nil per os (NPO) status [83].

Additional Imaging Tracheobronchomalacia is also commonly seen in children with BPD [84]. In addition, Del Cerro et al. [85] evaluated 29 patients with PH and

BPD without major congenital heart disease, and cardiovascular anomalies were noted in approximately two-thirds of patients: aortopulmonary collaterals ($n=9$), pulmonary vein stenosis ($n=7$), atrial septal defect (ASD; $n=4$), and PDA ($n=9$). High-resolution computerized tomography (CT) scanning/CT angiogram may be helpful as an adjunct investigation in some infants (e.g., intractable PH) to evaluate the airway, lung parenchyma, and the vasculature.

Biomarkers of PH in BPD The use of B-type natriuretic peptide (BNP) or NT-pro-BNP for evaluation of PH in BPD is becoming increasingly common [86], particularly as we have shown an association with increased risk for PH and death [12]. However, some infants have elevations of BNP in whom echocardiography does not suggest significant elevations of right ventricular pressure, and conversely, other infants have low BNP values despite echocardiography suggesting PH. BNP is a marker of cardiac ventricular strain that is not specific to the right ventricle, and infants with systemic hypertension (frequently seen in BPD, especially during corticosteroid therapy), PDA [87, 88], or left ventricular dysfunction for other reasons may also have elevations of BNP. Clinical improvement (or lack thereof) may be followed using serial echocardiography combined with BNP measurements. Currently, there are not many published reports of the utility of serial BNP measurements in neonatal PH, but Cuna et al. have found [89] that BNP elevation and magnitude of PH are positively correlated and that it is associated with increased risk for mortality. The frequency of these repeat measurements generally depends upon the severity of the PH and underlying clinical illness. In general, we obtain echocardiograms and/or BNP twice a week for unstable infants with an acute pulmonary hypertensive crisis or those undergoing weaning of PH therapies such as iNO and once or twice a month for infants who are more stable.

Treatment of Pulmonary Hypertension in Bronchopulmonary Dysplasia

In addition to marked vasoconstriction due to acute hypoxia, the pulmonary circulation in BPD is further characterized by altered lung structure and growth. Hence, it is very difficult to have standardized clinical guidelines for the treatment of PH in infants and children with BPD. In this disease, impaired gas exchange results in hypoxemic vasoconstriction and eventually structural remodeling of the vasculature, but there are very few studies looking at clinical outcomes of patients with BPD and PH. Various pulmonary vasodilators have been tried over the years, and there has been an increasing off-label use of these drugs with little evidence to support their use [18]. Many preterm infants with BPD could have some degree of PH [12], and the most common triggers for this have been thought to include aspiration, respiratory infections, or anesthesia for surgery [81, 90]. The PH in BPD consists of a fixed component, secondary to a reduction of cross-sectional area of the pulmonary vasculature due to impaired lung development and nonresponsive remodeling of pulmonary arteries and a responsive component presumably due to pulmonary vascular smooth muscle that is capable of relaxation in response to vasodilator stimuli [78]. Historically, the mainstay of treatment has been optimization of BPD management to promote normal lung development and use of pulmonary vasorelaxation. The therapeutic agents used are generally vasodilators (e.g., oxygen, iNO, sildenafil, prostacyclin analogs) or inhibitors of vasoconstrictors (e.g., endothelin-receptor antagonists). The major unanswered question in this regard remains whether aggressive pulmonary management and vasodilator therapy attenuate morbidity and mortality. There are a limited number of clinical outcome studies and little published literature regarding vasodilator therapy in preterm infants. In addition, preterm infants with BPD have diverse phenotypes and may have highly variable responses to treatment.

Pulmonary Vasodilators

Oxygen In the 1980s, it was considered that oxygen therapy may not be effective for pulmonary vasoreactivity [91], but over the years supplemental oxygen therapy has become the standard therapy for patients with BPD with intermittent or chronic hypoxia [92]. Nevertheless major controversies still exist in the literature regarding the use of oxygen in preterm infants [93]. Abman et al. [94] demonstrated in 1985 that the pulmonary vascular resistance in infants with BPD was responsive to oxygen, with a greater than 10 mmHg reduction in mean pulmonary artery pressure on exposure to high concentrations of oxygen ($FiO_2 > 0.8$). However, Farrow et al. [95, 96] have shown in animal studies that hyperoxia-induced oxidant stress increases phosphodiesterase 5 (PDE5), an enzyme that degrades cyclic guanosine monophosphate (cGMP), hence decreasing NO bioavailability. Lakshminrusimha et al. [97] showed that 100 % oxygen increases pulmonary vascular contractility and attenuates response to iNO in the PH sheep model [97]. Therefore, although oxygen works as a vasodilator, there may be potential harm in using excess oxygen long term in preterm infants, and no clear evidence exists on whether supplemental oxygen to maintain baseline oxygen saturations at 95 % should be considered in preterm infants with PH and BPD.

Nitric Oxide Pathway *Inhaled Nitric Oxide* (*iNO*): NO produced by endothelial cells stimulates soluble guanylate cyclase to increase intracellular cGMP which relaxes smooth muscle cells, and alteration in NO signaling has been described in the baboon BPD model [63]. In patients with primary PH, it has been suggested that iNO may be useful for long-term therapy [98], but few studies have evaluated its role in BPD. As increased pulmonary vascular tone and heightened vasoreactivity persist in older patients with BPD, Mourani et al. [99] demonstrated the pulmonary vascular effects of iNO and oxygen in this population. The authors found that although acute hyperoxia caused modest pulmonary vasodilatation above normoxic baseline values, iNO augmented the vasodilator response of oxygen and that the combination of supplemental oxygen and iNO often reduced mean pulmonary arterial pressure to near normal values for age [99]. Chronic management with iNO is not yet practical in the outpatient setting due to the logistics and cost, but efficacy of iNO may indicate that other vasodilators could likely be effective. No clinical trial has evaluated the use of iNO in systematic fashion in this population looking at long-term outcomes, and the benefit of prolonged treatment with iNO in PH associated with BPD is unknown.

Sildenafil: cGMP is a secondary intracellular messenger that mediates NO activity and vascular contractility. High concentrations of cyclic nucleotide PDE5 isoenzyme can rapidly degrade cGMP through hydrolysis. Sildenafil is a PDE5 inhibitor that increases cGMP concentrations, thus allowing for improved pulmonary vasodilation [100]. Oral sildenafil was approved by the US Food and Drug Administration (FDA) in 2005 for the treatment of PH in adults and has become widely used in neonates and infants with PH [101]. Its use for this indication is off-label. Various case reports and small studies have looked at the use of sildenafil in persistent PH in neonates (PPHN), but the evidence for the use of sildenafil in preterm infants is minimal and multiple clinical trials are currently active. Sildenafil did not improve short-term respiratory outcomes in a pilot trial of mechanically ventilated extremely preterm infants less than 7 days of age, suggesting that its earlier use may not be beneficial [102]. In a retrospective study, 25 infants <2 years of age with BPD-associated PH received sildenafil at different doses, and it was reported to be safe and effective [103]. In a more recent retrospective study by Nyp et al. [104], sildenafil use in patients with BPD and PH reduced estimated pulmonary artery pressures, but this reduction was not reflected in improved gas exchange within the first 48 h. The STARTS-2 study noted higher mortality in older children taking a higher dose (>3 mg/kg/day) of sildenafil as compared to those taking a lower dose [105], and thus the US FDA has issued a warning against the use of sildenafil in children between 1 and 17 years of age. While acknowledging and respecting the FDA's decision, the Scientific Leadership Council of the Pulmonary Hypertension Association provided some perspectives, arguing that results do not account for the differences in disease severity at the time of enrollment or subgroup differences. With respect to survival, there was no control group. The overall survival for the sildenafil-treated patients was favorable compared to historical controls [101]. The FDA has recently also warned about hearing loss and vision abnormalities in patients treated with sildenafil. The information from FDA for healthcare professionals can be found at http://www.fda.gov/drugs/drugsafety/postmarketdrugsafetyinformationforpatientsandproviders/ucm124841.htm. Based on the most recent evidence on adverse effects available for adults, caution should be exercised while treating infants with sildenafil, and special attention should be paid to dosing and response measures. On the other hand, it is also important to understand that these FDA warnings might not represent the potential efficacy or safety of sildenafil for infants with BPD.

Endothelin Pathway Endothelin 1 (ET-1) which is a potent vasoconstrictor produced by endothelial cells acts via two G protein-coupled receptors, ET_A and ET_B [106]. ET_A promotes smooth muscle cells proliferation and vasoconstriction, and ET_B in addition to proliferation and vasoconstriction mediates vasodilation by release of NO and prostacyclin (also known as prostaglandin I2 or PGI2) from endothelial cells [106]. Bosentan, a nonselective antagonist of both ET_A and ET_B receptors, has potent vasodilator effects and has been shown to reverse endothelin-induced smooth muscle constriction, hypertrophy, and hyperplasia [107, 108]. In retrospective cohort studies, bosentan has been shown to have clinical and hemodynamic efficacy in children with pulmonary arterial hypertension (idiopathic, associated with congenital heart, or connective tissue disease) [107, 109, 110]. In a small randomized controlled trial, bosentan administration improved oxygenation and reduced pulmonary arterial pressures in neonates with PPHN [111]. The evidence regarding the use of bosentan in neonates is scarce and its efficacy not well established in this population, although in pediatric patients with PH the use of bosentan has improved outcomes [112, 113]. A specific pediatric formulation of bosentan was recently approved for use in children by the European authorities [106]. The use of bosentan in BPD, usually in combination with either prostacyclin analogs or sildenafil, has been reported in only some case reports and case series [114, 115]. Also, bosentan being hepatotoxic can potentially induce liver injury in preterm patients and being teratogenic mandates careful handling by caregivers. Further studies are needed to evaluate the benefit of this medication for treating PH in infants with BPD.

Prostacyclin Derivatives Prostacyclin (PGI2) is produced by the vascular endothelium and promotes vasodilation by stimulating the cyclic adenosine monophosphate or cAMP-dependent relaxation of pulmonary smooth muscle cells [100]. PGI2 treatment should be initiated with caution, as it may also cause systemic hypotension, and given its very short half-life, it must be given continuously, without interruptions in delivery [116]. Analogues of PGI2 may be aerosolized or given by either intravenous or subcutaneous infusion [117, 118]. Epoprostenol (prostacyclin) was approved by the FDA in 1995 for the treatment of severe chronic pulmonary arterial hypertension. Due to its very short half-life, the medication must be given continuously, and unplanned interruptions in delivery may be dangerous [106]. Iloprost is a prostacyclin analog with a half-life of 20–30 min, and inhaled iloprost has been effective at reducing pulmonary pressures in pediatric patients, including some with BPD-associated PH [119, 120]. It may however cause acute bronchoconstriction, which potentially limits its utility. Treprostinil is another long-acting analog of PGI and can be administered via inhaled or subcutaneous routes. Subcutaneous treprostinil has been used to transition some children who were chronically stable on intravenous epoprostenol and may improve the clinical course in children as an add-on therapy [120, 121]. Additional studies in infants with BPD-associated PH are needed, as the evidence for these medications in this disease is limited.

Approach to Management of Pulmonary Hypertension in Bronchopulmonary Dysplasia

We recommend the use of a multidisciplinary team approach in managing such patients, with frequent discussions between neonatology, cardiology, and pulmonology teams. Optimization of ventilation and minimization of hypoxia, hypercarbia, and acidosis are of utmost importance in these patients. Some infants may need higher end expiratory pressures and longer inspiratory times for proper lung expansion, whereas others may need modest mean airway pressures to allow adequate preload, with the goal to provide adequate functional residual capacity (FRC). It is important to avoid sudden dips in saturation to 85 % or below to avoid hypoxic pulmonary vasoconstriction, as well as hyperoxia with saturations of 97 % or greater. Therapies such as diuretics, inhaled corticosteroids, and bronchodilators have not been well studied in children with BPD and PH; however, they could be used in the short term for temporary relief and for possible reduction in ventilation perfusion mismatch. Adequate nutrition is necessary as it may help optimize pulmonary vascular bed growth secondary to adequate lung growth.

Tracheobronchomalacia is also commonly seen in children with BPD [84]. Bronchoscopy is the gold standard for the diagnosis of this condition but may be difficult in children who are still at less than term GA or who are still ventilated; hence, advanced CT techniques could prove useful. The patients with tracheobronchomalacia might benefit from higher end expiratory pressures to keep the airway distended. Gastroesophageal reflux can sometime cause micro aspirations, which can lead to worsening of PH associated with lung disease. Such patients may require treatment and possibly fundoplication in severe cases.

Echocardiograms and/or BNP may be obtained weekly or twice weekly for very unstable infants and twice a month for infants who are more stable. Currently, there are limited published reports of the utility of serial BNP measurements in neonates, but recently it has been found that BNP estimation may be a useful prognostic marker of all-cause mortality in ELBW infants with BPD-associated PH [89]. In the setting of established PH by echocardiographic evidence, iNO may possibly be considered a first line of therapy and is the only pulmonary vasodilator with good available safety data in infants. iNO is typically administered at an initial dose of 20 ppm, as this dose provides optimal reduction of pulmonary arterial pressure with less risk of methemoglobinemia than higher doses [122]. iNO is gradually weaned off over days to weeks, with careful clinical monitoring and evaluation of oxygen requirement. If there is partial or no response to iNO, a second-line agent such as sildenafil (0.5–1 mg/kg/dose every 8 h) may be added for chronic therapy. Minimal sildenafil dosage should be started, and subsequently doses should be increased as needed. Chronic therapy in these patients may also include the use of endothelin-1 (ET-1) receptor antagonist bosentan. We use bosentan as a third-line agent in infants with persistent PH despite treatment with first- and second-line drugs. Prostacyclin analogs like intravenous epoprostenol (Flolan), inhaled iloprost (Ventavis), or subcutaneous or intravenous treprostinil (Remodulin) may be considered as second- or third-line agents although there is very limited data on their use in neonates. We recommend considering cardiac catheterization if the first- and second-line treatments are ineffective and if the patient is stable. Clinical improvement (or lack thereof) may be followed using serial echocardiography that may be combined with BNP measurements (Fig. 14.2).

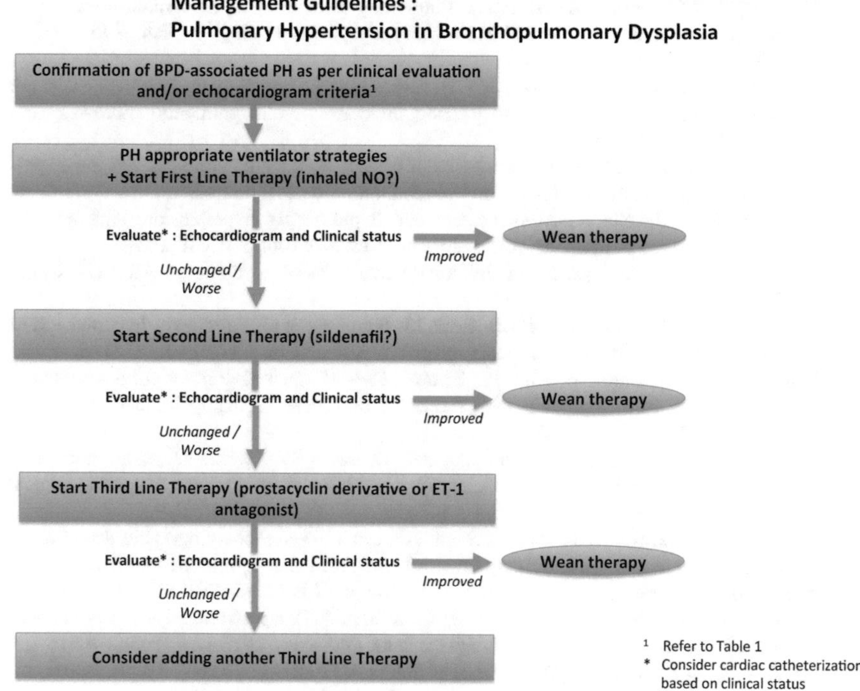

Fig. 14.2 Management guidelines for patients with pulmonary hypertension secondary to bronchopulmonary dysplasia (BPD) (*NO* nitric oxide, *ET-1* endothelin-1)

Conclusion

Our understanding of the pathophysiology and management of PH in preterm infants with BPD is rapidly evolving, but further efforts are needed to better characterize the prevalence, clinical course, and response to therapy. The heterogeneity and variability in each clinical phenotype of this disease are vast, and hence generalized guidelines for management are not always applicable. Due to the complexity of this disease, we recommend that a multidisciplinary approach be employed to formulate a tailor-made, patient-specific management strategy.

References

1. Ambalavanan N, Carlo WA. Bronchopulmonary dysplasia: new insights. Clin Perinatol. 2004;31(3):613–28.
2. Coalson JJ. Pathology of bronchopulmonary dysplasia. Semin Perinatol. 2006;30(4): 179–84.

3. Northway Jr WH, Rosan RC, Porter DY. Pulmonary disease following respirator therapy of hyaline-membrane disease. Bronchopulmonary dysplasia. N Engl J Med. 1967;276(7): 357–68.
4. Bonikos DS, Bensch KG, Northway Jr WH, Edwards DK. Bronchopulmonary dysplasia: the pulmonary pathologic sequel of necrotizing bronchiolitis and pulmonary fibrosis. Hum Pathol. 1976;7(6):643–66.
5. Mourani PM, Abman SH. Pulmonary vascular disease in bronchopulmonary dysplasia: pulmonary hypertension and beyond. Curr Opin Pediatr. 2013;25(3):329–37.
6. Steinhorn RH, Kinsella JP, Abman SH. Beyond pulmonary hypertension: sildenafil for chronic lung disease of prematurity. Am J Respir Cell Mol Biol. 2013;48(2):3–5.
7. Haworth SG. The management of pulmonary hypertension in children. Arch Dis Child. 2008;93(7):620–5.
8. An HS, Bae EJ, Kim GB, Kwon BS, Beak JS, Kim EK, et al. Pulmonary hypertension in preterm infants with bronchopulmonary dysplasia. Korean Circ J. 2010;40(3):131–6.
9. Kim DH, Kim HS, Choi CW, Kim EK, Kim BI, Choi JH. Risk factors for pulmonary artery hypertension in preterm infants with moderate or severe bronchopulmonary dysplasia. Neonatology. 2012;101(1):40–6.
10. Khemani E, McElhinney DB, Rhein L, Andrade O, Lacro RV, Thomas KC, et al. Pulmonary artery hypertension in formerly premature infants with bronchopulmonary dysplasia: clinical features and outcomes in the surfactant era. Pediatrics. 2007;120(6):1260–9.
11. Slaughter JL, Pakrashi T, Jones DE, South AP, Shah TA. Echocardiographic detection of pulmonary hypertension in extremely low birth weight infants with bronchopulmonary dysplasia requiring prolonged positive pressure ventilation. J Perinatol. 2011;31(10):635–40.
12. Bhat R, Salas AA, Foster C, Carlo WA, Ambalavanan N. Prospective analysis of pulmonary hypertension in extremely low birth weight infants. Pediatrics. 2012;129(3):e682–9.
13. Ali Z, Schmidt P, Dodd J, Jeppesen DL. Predictors of bronchopulmonary dysplasia and pulmonary hypertension in newborn children. Dan Med J. 2013;60(8):A4688.
14. Mourani PM, Sontag MK, Younoszai A, Miller JI, Kinsella JP, Baker CD, et al. Early pulmonary vascular disease in preterm infants at risk for bronchopulmonary dysplasia. Am J Respir Crit Care Med. 2015;191(1):87–95.
15. Ambalavanan N, Walsh M, Bobashev G, Das A, Levine B, Carlo WA, et al. Intercenter differences in bronchopulmonary dysplasia or death among very low birth weight infants. Pediatrics. 2011;127(1):e106–16.
16. Check J, Gotteiner N, Liu X, Su E, Porta N, Steinhorn R, et al. Fetal growth restriction and pulmonary hypertension in premature infants with bronchopulmonary dysplasia. J Perinatol. 2013;33(7):553–7.
17. Hansen AR, Barnes CM, Folkman J, McElrath TF. Maternal preeclampsia predicts the development of bronchopulmonary dysplasia. J Pediatr. 2010;156(4):532–6.
18. Collaco JM, Romer LH, Stuart BD, Coulson JD, Everett AD, Lawson EE, et al. Frontiers in pulmonary hypertension in infants and children with bronchopulmonary dysplasia. Pediatr Pulmonol. 2012;47(11):1042–53.
19. Abman SH. Monitoring cardiovascular function in infants with chronic lung disease of prematurity. Arch Dis Child Fetal Neonatal Ed. 2002;87(1):F15–8.
20. Pulmonary hypertension in infants with bronchopulmonary dysplasia. Korean J Pediatr. 2010;53(6):688–93.
21. Coalson JJ, Winter VT, Siler-Khodr T, Yoder BA. Neonatal chronic lung disease in extremely immature baboons. Am J Respir Crit Care Med. 1999;160(4):1333–46.
22. Grover TR, Parker TA, Balasubramaniam V, Markham NE, Abman SH. Pulmonary hypertension impairs alveolarization and reduces lung growth in the ovine fetus. Am J Physiol Lung Cell Mol Physiol. 2005;288(4):L648–54.
23. Ding BS, Nolan DJ, Guo P, Babazadeh AO, Cao Z, Rosenwaks Z, et al. Endothelial-derived angiocrine signals induce and sustain regenerative lung alveolarization. Cell. 2011;147(3): 539–53.

24. Thebaud B, Abman SH. Bronchopulmonary dysplasia: where have all the vessels gone? Roles of angiogenic growth factors in chronic lung disease. Am J Respir Crit Care Med. 2007;175(10):978–85.
25. Peng T, Tian Y, Boogerd CJ, Lu MM, Kadzik RS, Stewart KM, et al. Coordination of heart and lung co-development by a multipotent cardiopulmonary progenitor. Nature. 2013;500(7464):589–92.
26. Abman SH. Impaired vascular endothelial growth factor signaling in the pathogenesis of neonatal pulmonary vascular disease. Adv Exp Med Biol. 2010;661:323–35.
27. Carmeliet P, Mackman N, Moons L, Luther T, Gressens P, Van Vlaenderen I, et al. Role of tissue factor in embryonic blood vessel development. Nature. 1996;383(6595):73–5.
28. Carmeliet P, Ferreira V, Breier G, Pollefeyt S, Kieckens L, Gertsenstein M, et al. Abnormal blood vessel development and lethality in embryos lacking a single VEGF allele. Nature. 1996;380(6573):435–9.
29. Ferrara N, Gerber HP, LeCouter J. The biology of VEGF and its receptors. Nat Med. 2003;9(6):669–76.
30. Dellinger MT, Meadows SM, Wynne K, Cleaver O, Brekken RA. Vascular endothelial growth factor receptor-2 promotes the development of the lymphatic vasculature. PLoS One. 2013;8(9):e74686.
31. Kao J, Ryan J, Brett G, Chen J, Shen H, Fan YG, et al. Endothelial monocyte-activating polypeptide II. A novel tumor-derived polypeptide that activates host-response mechanisms. J Biol Chem. 1992;267(28):20239–47.
32. Schwarz M, Lee M, Zhang F, Zhao J, Jin Y, Smith S, et al. EMAP II: a modulator of neovascularization in the developing lung. Am J Physiol. 1999;276(2 Pt 1):L365–75.
33. Schwarz MA, Zhang F, Gebb S, Starnes V, Warburton D. Endothelial monocyte activating polypeptide II inhibits lung neovascularization and airway epithelial morphogenesis. Mech Dev. 2000;95(1–2):123–32.
34. Schwarz MA, Zhang F, Lane JE, Schachtner S, Jin Y, Deutsch G, et al. Angiogenesis and morphogenesis of murine fetal distal lung in an allograft model. Am J Physiol Lung Cell Mol Physiol. 2000;278(5):L1000–7.
35. Schwarz MA, Wan Z, Liu J, Lee MK. Epithelial-mesenchymal interactions are linked to neovascularization. Am J Respir Cell Mol Biol. 2004;30(6):784–92.
36. Gien J, Tseng N, Seedorf G, Roe G, Abman SH. Endothelin-1 impairs angiogenesis in vitro through Rho-kinase activation after chronic intrauterine pulmonary hypertension in fetal sheep. Pediatr Res. 2013;73(3):252–62.
37. Iosef C, Alastalo TP, Hou Y, Chen C, Adams ES, Lyu SC, et al. Inhibiting NF-kappaB in the developing lung disrupts angiogenesis and alveolarization. Am J Physiol Lung Cell Mol Physiol. 2012;302(10):L1023–36.
38. Cornfield DN. Developmental regulation of oxygen sensing and ion channels in the pulmonary vasculature. Adv Exp Med Biol. 2010;661:201–20.
39. Tsao PN, Wei SC. Prenatal hypoxia downregulates the expression of pulmonary vascular endothelial growth factor and its receptors in fetal mice. Neonatology. 2013;103(4):300–7.
40. Vadivel A, Alphonse RS, Etches N, van Haaften T, Collins JJ, O'Reilly M, et al. Hypoxia inducible factors promotes alveolar development and regeneration. Am J of Respir Cell Mol Biol. 2014;50(1):96–105.
41. van Haaften T, Byrne R, Bonnet S, Rochefort GY, Akabutu J, Bouchentouf M, et al. Airway delivery of mesenchymal stem cells prevents arrested alveolar growth in neonatal lung injury in rats. Am J Respir Crit Care Med. 2009;180(11):1131–42.
42. O'Reilly M, Thebaud B. Cell-based strategies to reconstitute lung function in infants with severe bronchopulmonary dysplasia. Clin Perinatol. 2012;39(3):703–25.
43. Eklund L, Olsen BR. Tie receptors and their angiopoietin ligands are context-dependent regulators of vascular remodeling. Exp Cell Res. 2006;312(5):630–41.
44. Witzenbichler B, Maisonpierre PC, Jones P, Yancopoulos GD, Isner JM. Chemotactic properties of angiopoietin-1 and -2, ligands for the endothelial-specific receptor tyrosine kinase Tie2. J Biol Chem. 1998;273(29):18514–21.

45. Hayes AJ, Huang WQ, Mallah J, Yang D, Lippman ME, Li LY. Angiopoietin-1 and its receptor Tie-2 participate in the regulation of capillary-like tubule formation and survival of endothelial cells. Microvasc Res. 1999;58(3):224–37.
46. Maisonpierre PC, Suri C, Jones PF, Bartunkova S, Wiegand SJ, Radziejewski C, et al. Angiopoietin-2, a natural antagonist for Tie2 that disrupts in vivo angiogenesis. Science. 1997;277(5322):55–60.
47. Suri C, Jones PF, Patan S, Bartunkova S, Maisonpierre PC, Davis S, et al. Requisite role of angiopoietin-1, a ligand for the TIE2 receptor, during embryonic angiogenesis. Cell. 1996;87(7):1171–80.
48. Thebaud B, Ladha F, Michelakis ED, Sawicka M, Thurston G, Eaton F, et al. Vascular endothelial growth factor gene therapy increases survival, promotes lung angiogenesis, and prevents alveolar damage in hyperoxia-induced lung injury: evidence that angiogenesis participates in alveolarization. Circulation. 2005;112(16):2477–86.
49. Fiedler U, Augustin HG. Angiopoietins: a link between angiogenesis and inflammation. Trends Immunol. 2006;27(12):552–8.
50. Fiedler U, Reiss Y, Scharpfenecker M, Grunow V, Koidl S, Thurston G, et al. Angiopoietin-2 sensitizes endothelial cells to TNF-alpha and has a crucial role in the induction of inflammation. Nat Med. 2006;12(2):235–9.
51. Reis M, Liebner S. Wnt signaling in the vasculature. Exp Cell Res. 2013;319(9):1317–23.
52. Goodwin AM, D'Amore PA. Wnt signaling in the vasculature. Angiogenesis. 2002;5(1–2):1–9.
53. Kazanskaya O, Ohkawara B, Heroult M, Wu W, Maltry N, Augustin HG, et al. The Wnt signaling regulator R-spondin 3 promotes angioblast and vascular development. Development. 2008;135(22):3655–64.
54. Cornett B, Snowball J, Varisco BM, Lang R, Whitsett J, Sinner D. Wntless is required for peripheral lung differentiation and pulmonary vascular development. Dev Biol. 2013;379(1):38–52.
55. Mujahid S, Nielsen HC, Volpe MV. MiR-221 and miR-130a regulate lung airway and vascular development. PLoS One. 2013;8(2):e55911.
56. Han RN, Babaei S, Robb M, Lee T, Ridsdale R, Ackerley C, et al. Defective lung vascular development and fatal respiratory distress in endothelial NO synthase-deficient mice: a model of alveolar capillary dysplasia? Circ Res. 2004;94(8):1115–23.
57. Tulloh RM, Hislop AA, Boels PJ, Deutsch J, Haworth SG. Chronic hypoxia inhibits postnatal maturation of porcine intrapulmonary artery relaxation. Am J Physiol. 1997;272(5 Pt 2):H2436–45.
58. Han RN, Stewart DJ. Defective lung vascular development in endothelial nitric oxide synthase-deficient mice. Trends Cardiovasc Med. 2006;16(1):29–34.
59. Shaul PW. Nitric oxide in the developing lung. Adv Pediatr. 1995;42:367–414.
60. Shaul PW, Yuhanna IS, German Z, Chen Z, Steinhorn RH, Morin 3rd FC. Pulmonary endothelial NO synthase gene expression is decreased in fetal lambs with pulmonary hypertension. Am J Physiol. 1997;272(5 Pt 1):L1005–12.
61. Sherman TS, Chen Z, Yuhanna IS, Lau KS, Margraf LR, Shaul PW. Nitric oxide synthase isoform expression in the developing lung epithelium. Am J Physiol. 1999;276(2 Pt 1):L383–90.
62. Shaul PW, Afshar S, Gibson LL, Sherman TS, Kerecman JD, Grubb PH, et al. Developmental changes in nitric oxide synthase isoform expression and nitric oxide production in fetal baboon lung. Am J Physiol Lung Cell Mol Physiol. 2002;283(6):L1192–9.
63. Afshar S, Gibson LL, Yuhanna IS, Sherman TS, Kerecman JD, Grubb PH, et al. Pulmonary NO synthase expression is attenuated in a fetal baboon model of chronic lung disease. Am J Physiol Lung Cell Mol Physiol. 2003;284(5):L749–58.
64. Steinhorn RH, Shaul PW, de Regnier RA, Kennedy KA. Inhaled nitric oxide and bronchopulmonary dysplasia. Pediatrics. 2011;128(1):e255–6. Author reply e6–7.
65. Kumar VH, Hutchison AA, Lakshminrusimha S, Morin 3rd FC, Wynn RJ, Ryan RM. Characteristics of pulmonary hypertension in preterm neonates. J Perinatol. 2007;27(4):214–9.

66. Ryoo S, Lemmon CA, Soucy KG, Gupta G, White AR, Nyhan D, et al. Oxidized low-density lipoprotein-dependent endothelial arginase II activation contributes to impaired nitric oxide signaling. Circ Res. 2006;99(9):951–60.
67. Murakami M, Nguyen LT, Zhuang ZW, Moodie KL, Carmeliet P, Stan RV, et al. The FGF system has a key role in regulating vascular integrity. J Clin Invest. 2008;118(10):3355–66.
68. Borghesi A, Massa M, Campanelli R, Garofoli F, Longo S, Cabano R, et al. Different subsets of circulating angiogenic cells do not predict bronchopulmonary dysplasia or other diseases of prematurity in preterm infants. Int J Immunopathol Pharmacol. 2013;26(3):809–16.
69. Mammoto T, Jiang E, Jiang A, Mammoto A. ECM structure and tissue stiffness control postnatal lung development through the LRP5-Tie2 signaling system. Am J Respir Cell Mol Biol. 2013;49(6):1009–18.
70. Lee HJ, Lee YJ, Choi CW, Lee JA, Kim EK, Kim HS, et al. Rosiglitazone, a peroxisome proliferator-activated receptor-gamma agonist, restores alveolar and pulmonary vascular development in a rat model of bronchopulmonary dysplasia. Yonsei Med J. 2014;55(1): 99–106.
71. Breinholt JP, Hawkins JA, Minich LA, Tani LY, Orsmond GS, Ritter S, et al. Pulmonary vein stenosis with normal connection: associated cardiac abnormalities and variable outcome. Ann Thorac Surg. 1999;68(1):164–8.
72. Drossner DM, Kim DW, Maher KO, Mahle WT. Pulmonary vein stenosis: prematurity and associated conditions. Pediatrics. 2008;122(3):e656–61.
73. Mourani PM, Ivy DD, Rosenberg AA, Fagan TE, Abman SH. Left ventricular diastolic dysfunction in bronchopulmonary dysplasia. J Pediatr. 2008;152(2):291–3.
74. Newth CJ, Gow RM, Rowe RD. The assessment of pulmonary arterial pressures in bronchopulmonary dysplasia by cardiac catheterization and M-mode echocardiography. Pediatr Pulmonol. 1985;1(1):58–62.
75. Mourani PM, Sontag MK, Younoszai A, Ivy DD, Abman SH. Clinical utility of echocardiography for the diagnosis and management of pulmonary vascular disease in young children with chronic lung disease. Pediatrics. 2008;121(2):317–25.
76. Skinner JR, Stuart AG, O'Sullivan J, Heads A, Boys RJ, Hunter S. Right heart pressure determination by Doppler in infants with tricuspid regurgitation. Arch Dis Child. 1993;69(2):216–20.
77. Hill KD, Lim DS, Everett AD, Ivy DD, Moore JD. Assessment of pulmonary hypertension in the pediatric catheterization laboratory: current insights from the Magic registry. Catheter Cardiovasc Interv. 2010;76(6):865–73.
78. Ambalavanan N, Mourani P. Pulmonary hypertension in bronchopulmonary dysplasia. Birth Defects Res A Clin Mol Teratol. 2014;100(3):240–6.
79. Taylor CJ, Derrick G, McEwan A, Haworth SG, Sury MR. Risk of cardiac catheterization under anaesthesia in children with pulmonary hypertension. Br J Anaesth. 2007;98(5): 657–61.
80. Shukla AC, Almodovar MC. Anesthesia considerations for children with pulmonary hypertension. Pediatr Crit Care Med. 2010;11(2 Suppl):S70–3.
81. Carmosino MJ, Friesen RH, Doran A, Ivy DD. Perioperative complications in children with pulmonary hypertension undergoing noncardiac surgery or cardiac catheterization. Anesth Analg. 2007;104(3):521–7.
82. van der Griend BF, Lister NA, McKenzie IM, Martin N, Ragg PG, Sheppard SJ, et al. Postoperative mortality in children after 101,885 anesthetics at a tertiary pediatric hospital. Anesth Analg. 2011;112(6):1440–7.
83. Gorenflo M, Gu H, Xu Z. Peri-operative pulmonary hypertension in paediatric patients: current strategies in children with congenital heart disease. Cardiology. 2010;116(1):10–7.
84. Doull IJ, Mok Q, Tasker RC. Tracheobronchomalacia in preterm infants with chronic lung disease. Arch Dis Child Fetal Neonatal Ed. 1997;76(3):F203–5.
85. Del Cerro MJ, Sabate Rotes A, Carton A, Deiros L, Bret M, Cordeiro M, et al. Pulmonary hypertension in bronchopulmonary dysplasia: clinical findings, cardiovascular anomalies and outcomes. Pediatr Pulmonol. 2014;49(1):49–59.

86. Kim GB. Pulmonary hypertension in infants with bronchopulmonary dysplasia. Korean J Pediatr. 2010;53(6):688–93.
87. Kim JS, Shim EJ. B-type natriuretic peptide assay for the diagnosis and prognosis of patent ductus arteriosus in preterm infants. Korean Circ J. 2012;42(3):192–6.
88. Sanjeev S, Pettersen M, Lua J, Thomas R, Shankaran S, L'Ecuyer T. Role of plasma B-type natriuretic peptide in screening for hemodynamically significant patent ductus arteriosus in preterm neonates. J Perinatol. 2005;25(11):709–13.
89. Cuna A, Kandasamy J, Sims B. B-type natriuretic peptide and mortality in extremely low birth weight infants with pulmonary hypertension: a retrospective cohort analysis. BMC Pediatr. 2014;14:68.
90. Farquhar M, Fitzgerald DA. Pulmonary hypertension in chronic neonatal lung disease. Paediatr Respir Rev. 2010;11(3):149–53.
91. Berman Jr W, Yabek SM, Dillon T, Burstein R, Corlew S. Evaluation of infants with bronchopulmonary dysplasia using cardiac catheterization. Pediatrics. 1982;70(5):708–12.
92. Hudak BB, Allen MC, Hudak ML, Loughlin GM. Home oxygen therapy for chronic lung disease in extremely low-birth-weight infants. Am J Dis Child. 1989;143(3):357–60.
93. Fleck BW, Stenson BJ. Retinopathy of prematurity and the oxygen conundrum: lessons learned from recent randomized trials. Clin Perinatol. 2013;40(2):229–40.
94. Abman SH, Wolfe RR, Accurso FJ, Koops BL, Bowman CM, Wiggins Jr JW. Pulmonary vascular response to oxygen in infants with severe bronchopulmonary dysplasia. Pediatrics. 1985;75(1):80–4.
95. Farrow KN, Wedgwood S, Lee KJ, Czech L, Gugino SF, Lakshminrusimha S, et al. Mitochondrial oxidant stress increases PDE5 activity in persistent pulmonary hypertension of the newborn. Respir Physiol Neurobiol. 2010;174(3):272–81.
96. Farrow KN, Groh BS, Schumacker PT, Lakshminrusimha S, Czech L, Gugino SF, et al. Hyperoxia increases phosphodiesterase 5 expression and activity in ovine fetal pulmonary artery smooth muscle cells. Circ Res. 2008;102(2):226–33.
97. Lakshminrusimha S, Russell JA, Steinhorn RH, Ryan RM, Gugino SF, Morin 3rd FC, et al. Pulmonary arterial contractility in neonatal lambs increases with 100% oxygen resuscitation. Pediatr Res. 2006;59(1):137–41.
98. Ivy DD, Parker D, Doran A, Parker D, Kinsella JP, Abman SH. Acute hemodynamic effects and home therapy using a novel pulsed nasal nitric oxide delivery system in children and young adults with pulmonary hypertension. Am J Cardiol. 2003;92(7):886–90.
99. Mourani PM, Ivy DD, Gao D, Abman SH. Pulmonary vascular effects of inhaled nitric oxide and oxygen tension in bronchopulmonary dysplasia. Am J Respir Crit Care Med. 2004;170(9):1006–13.
100. Porta NF, Steinhorn RH. Pulmonary vasodilator therapy in the NICU: inhaled nitric oxide, sildenafil, and other pulmonary vasodilating agents. Clin Perinatol. 2012;39(1):149–64.
101. Bhatt-Mehta V, Donn SM. Sildenafil for pulmonary hypertension complicating bronchopulmonary dysplasia. Expert Rev Clin Pharmacol. 2014;7(4):393–5.
102. Konig K, Barfield CP, Guy KJ, Drew SM, Andersen CC. The effect of sildenafil on evolving bronchopulmonary dysplasia in extremely preterm infants: a randomised controlled pilot study. J Matern Fetal Neonatal Med. 2014;27(5):439–44.
103. Mourani PM, Sontag MK, Ivy DD, Abman SH. Effects of long-term sildenafil treatment for pulmonary hypertension in infants with chronic lung disease. J Pediatr. 2009;154(3):379–84, 84 e1–2.
104. Nyp M, Sandritter T, Poppinga N, Simon C, Truog WE. Sildenafil citrate, bronchopulmonary dysplasia and disordered pulmonary gas exchange: any benefits? J Perinatol. 2012;32(1):64–9.
105. Barst RJ, Ivy DD, Gaitan G, Szatmari A, Rudzinski A, Garcia AE, et al. A randomized, double-blind, placebo-controlled, dose-ranging study of oral sildenafil citrate in treatment-naive children with pulmonary arterial hypertension. Circulation. 2012;125(2):324–34.
106. Berkelhamer SK, Mestan KK, Steinhorn RH. Pulmonary hypertension in bronchopulmonary dysplasia. Semin Perinatol. 2013;37(2):124–31.

107. Rosenzweig EB, Ivy DD, Widlitz A, Doran A, Claussen LR, Yung D, et al. Effects of long-term bosentan in children with pulmonary arterial hypertension. J Am Coll Cardiol. 2005;46(4):697–704.
108. Wilkins MR, Paul GA, Strange JW, Tunariu N, Gin-Sing W, Banya WA, et al. Sildenafil versus endothelin receptor antagonist for pulmonary hypertension (SERAPH) study. Am J Respir Crit Care Med. 2005;171(11):1292–7.
109. Ivy DD, Rosenzweig EB, Lemarie JC, Brand M, Rosenberg D, Barst RJ. Long-term outcomes in children with pulmonary arterial hypertension treated with bosentan in real-world clinical settings. Am J Cardiol. 2010;106(9):1332–8.
110. Hislop AA, Moledina S, Foster H, Schulze-Neick I, Haworth SG. Long-term efficacy of bosentan in treatment of pulmonary arterial hypertension in children. Eur Respir J. 2011; 38(1):70–7.
111. Mohamed WA, Ismail M. A randomized, double-blind, placebo-controlled, prospective study of bosentan for the treatment of persistent pulmonary hypertension of the newborn. J Perinatol. 2012;32(8):608–13.
112. Beghetti M. Current treatment options in children with pulmonary arterial hypertension and experiences with oral bosentan. Eur J Clin Invest. 2006;36 Suppl 3:16–24.
113. Maiya S, Hislop AA, Flynn Y, Haworth SG. Response to bosentan in children with pulmonary hypertension. Heart. 2006;92(5):664–70.
114. Krishnan U, Krishnan S, Gewitz M. Treatment of pulmonary hypertension in children with chronic lung disease with newer oral therapies. Pediatr Cardiol. 2008;29(6):1082–6.
115. Rugolotto S, Errico G, Beghini R, Ilic S, Richelli C, Padovani EM. Weaning of epoprostenol in a small infant receiving concomitant bosentan for severe pulmonary arterial hypertension secondary to bronchopulmonary dysplasia. Minerva Pediatr. 2006;58(5):491–4.
116. Baker CD, Abman SH, Mourani PM. Pulmonary hypertension in preterm infants with bronchopulmonary dysplasia. Pediatr Allergy Immunol Pulmonol. 2014;27(1):8–16.
117. Brown AT, Gillespie JV, Miquel-Verges F, Holmes K, Ravekes W, Spevak P, et al. Inhaled epoprostenol therapy for pulmonary hypertension: Improves oxygenation index more consistently in neonates than in older children. Pulm Circ. 2012;2(1):61–6.
118. Melnick L, Barst RJ, Rowan CA, Kerstein D, Rosenzweig EB. Effectiveness of transition from intravenous epoprostenol to oral/inhaled targeted pulmonary arterial hypertension therapy in pediatric idiopathic and familial pulmonary arterial hypertension. Am J Cardiol. 2010;105(10):1485–9.
119. Ewert R, Schaper C, Halank M, Glaser S, Opitz CF. Inhalative iloprost – pharmacology and clinical application. Expert Opin Pharmacother. 2009;10(13):2195–207.
120. Doran AK, Ivy DD, Barst RJ, Hill N, Murali S, Benza RL, et al. Guidelines for the prevention of central venous catheter-related blood stream infections with prostanoid therapy for pulmonary arterial hypertension. Int J Clin Pract Suppl. 2008;160:5–9.
121. Levy M, Celermajer DS, Bourges-Petit E, Del Cerro MJ, Bajolle F, Bonnet D. Add-on therapy with subcutaneous treprostinil for refractory pediatric pulmonary hypertension. J Pediatr. 2011;158(4):584–8.
122. Davidson D, Barefield ES, Kattwinkel J, Dudell G, Damask M, Straube R, et al. Inhaled nitric oxide for the early treatment of persistent pulmonary hypertension of the term newborn: a randomized, double-masked, placebo-controlled, dose-response, multicenter study. The I-NO/PPHN study group. Pediatrics. 1998;101(3 Pt 1):325–34.

Chapter 15
Pulmonary Function in Survivors of Bronchopulmonary Dysplasia

Jennifer S. Landry and Simon P. Banbury

Introduction

Bronchopulmonary dysplasia (BPD) and the long-term respiratory consequences of prematurity are unfamiliar and under-recognized entities to adult clinicians. Well described by the pediatric scientific community, these young adults who were born prematurely and suffered respiratory complications are joining the ranks of a growing population of adults with chronic lung disease.

BPD is a chronic respiratory disease that develops as a consequence of neonatal lung injury and is one of the most important sequelae of preterm birth [1]. It occurs most commonly in preterm infants who have needed mechanical ventilation and oxygen therapy for respiratory distress syndrome of the newborn (RDS) [2]. BPD was first described four decades ago in children born slightly preterm with severe RDS who were exposed to aggressive mechanical ventilation and high concentrations of inspired oxygen [3]. Over time, this has been largely replaced by a new form of the condition occurring in more extreme preterm infants, often with less severe RDS following pulmonary surfactant administration [4].

J.S. Landry, MD, MSc, FRCP(C) (✉)
Montreal Chest Institute, McGill University Health Center,
1001, boul Décarie, Bureau D 05.2044, Montréal, QC, Canada H4A 3J1
e-mail: Jennifer.landry@mcgill.ca

S.P. Banbury, BSc, PhD
Psychology Department, C3 Human Factors Consulting,
2828 Laurier Ave Suite 700, Quebec City, QC, Canada G1B 0V1
e-mail: Simon.banbury@c3hf.com

V. Bhandari (ed.), *Bronchopulmonary Dysplasia*, Respiratory Medicine,
DOI 10.1007/978-3-319-28486-6_15

Despite notable advances in prenatal and neonatal care, BPD remains an important complication of preterm births, frequently resulting in mortality as well as short-term and long-term morbidities, including airflow limitations and bronchial hyperresponsiveness [5]. With high rates of preterm birth worldwide, and more notably in North America [6], and with the improved survival associated with preterm birth, numerous young adults who were born prematurely and suffered respiratory complications are now manifesting chronic obstructive lung disease at a much younger age than their contemporaries with smoking-related chronic obstructive pulmonary disease (COPD). Their relative contribution to the growing adult populations with chronic pulmonary diseases has clinical and healthcare resources implications.

After the initial description of BPD in 1967 by Northway [7], many advances have been made in our understanding of the pathophysiology of this disease. With advances in neonatal care over the last three decades, a greater proportion of preterm infants are surviving the initial complications of prematurity and are now reaching adulthood in ever increasing numbers. Furthermore, the improved survival of very preterm infants has led to increasing incidence of pulmonary complications among these infants [2] and increased numbers of adolescents and young adults with sequelae of BPD [8]. This has clinical implications because their course, prognosis, and treatment are largely unknown and health system implications because of increased resource utilization.

Old BPD Versus New BPD

The form originally described in 1967 by Northway is now commonly referred to as "old BPD." Lung histology of "old BPD" showed prominent signs of barotraumas with fibroproliferative reaction. These findings were reminiscent of the histopathology observed in adults suffering from the acute respiratory distress syndrome (ARDS) when high ventilatory pressures were used during mechanical ventilation [9, 10] for the management of acute lung injury.

However, the form of BPD seen nowadays ("new BPD") often develops in more extreme preterm or very low birth weight (VLBW) newborns who received surfactant and needed less initial ventilator support or supplemental oxygen in their early days for the treatment of respiratory distress or apnea of prematurity [6]. It is increasingly recognized that the new BPD has a different underlying pathology and clinical course than was first described three decades ago. The lung histology of "new BPD" shows signs of truncated lung growth with abnormal alveolarization and dysmorphic vascular growth with a dysregulated pulmonary microvasculature. There is more uniform inflation, less fibrosis, little or no metaplasia of small and large airways, and only minimal smooth muscle hypertrophy [11]. These changes in histology may reflect the routine use of exogenous surfactants and the advances in mechanical ventilation techniques that were introduced in order to prevent barotrauma. It is to be expected that both forms of BPD will result in different phenotypes in the long-term and that they cannot be expected to behave the same way and, thus, should be considered as different entities.

Definition of BPD

In 2000, the National Institute of Child Health and Human Development (NICHD) sponsored a workshop to arrive at a consensus definition of BPD [12]. The final definition was that an infant requiring at least 28 days of supplemental oxygen should be considered to have BPD and that infants should be reassessed at 36 weeks postmenstrual date (or 56 days of life if born after 32 weeks) to establish the disease severity.

Long-Term Respiratory Outcomes of BPD Survivors

In the last 10 years, several studies have described the long-term sequelae of survivors of preterm births as these subjects reach adolescence and young adulthood [1, 13–20]. Most of these studies focused on pulmonary and neurological outcomes, the two systems most affected by prematurity and low birth weight [21, 22].

Early Childhood

Respiratory morbidity is common in infants and young children who were born prematurely, especially if they had developed BPD. Up to 50 % of children with BPD are readmitted in their first year of life for respiratory illnesses [18]. Lower respiratory tract infections contribute to this high rate of readmission. Rates of readmission and episodes of respiratory distress fall after the first year of life, as lung growth and remodeling of the airway take place, resulting in progressive improvement of pulmonary function [23]. Few children remain dependent on oxygen after 2 years of age [24].

BPD is associated with persistent pulmonary function abnormality in preschool children. In a cohort of 28 children diagnosed with BPD during their infancy, lung function testing before the age of 3 in a subset of seven asymptomatic children showed mild to moderate obstruction and air trapping [25]. In this same study, the 21 symptomatic children (with wheezing) had moderate to severe expiratory flow limitation, hyperinflation, and airway hyperresponsiveness.

Late Childhood and Adolescence

In most children who survive BPD, pulmonary function will improve, permitting normal activities, although increased airway resistance and hyperreactivity can remain present until adolescence [26]. Compared to controls matched for age and size, children with BPD have reduced absolute and size-corrected flow rates, a finding consistent with poor airway growth and persistent airflow limitation [27]. Among school age children, those who were born prematurely, particularly if they had BPD, were more likely to be symptomatic than their classroom colleagues who had been born at term. In a cohort of 125 children aged 7–8 years old, wheezing was present in 30 % of those who had had preterm birth and BPD, 24 % of those with preterm birth but did not develop BPD, and only 7 % of children born at term. This study ascertained symptoms, but did not measure lung function [23]. In a second study composed of 300 children, those who had had VLBW and who were aged 8–9 years old were significantly more likely to use inhalers, have school absences, or have a history of hospital admission for respiratory illness than 590 classroom controls with a normal birth weight. This study did not comment on the presence or absence of BPD among those born with VLBW [28].

One other study has reported 10 % lower forced expiratory volume in 1 s (FEV_1 % predicted) in 12 survivors of moderate to severe BPD (mean age: 17.7 years) when compared to preterm infants with either mild or no BPD [29].

Adulthood

There are few published data from comprehensive longitudinal studies of patients followed into adulthood and few data on pulmonary function of adults with a history of preterm birth and BPD. One case–control study included 26 subjects with a history of preterm birth and BPD born between 1964 and 1973 and two control groups [15]. The first group was composed of 26 controls matched for gestational age and weight at birth that did not undergo mechanical ventilation, and the second group was composed of 53 age-matched subjects who were born at term. In this study, 76 % of 26 young adults with prior BPD had measurable pulmonary dysfunction (increased bronchial resistance, bronchial hyperreactivity, and hyperinflation) compared to none of the 53 controls that had been born at term. The cases also had significantly more frequent wheezing and need for long-term medication than subjects born prematurely (p-value: 0.047) and normal controls (p-value: 0.0001) [15].

A second study compared 690 19-year-old subjects, all of whom were born prematurely (prior to 32 weeks of gestation) and with VLBW (less than 1 500 g), to a control group of Dutch participants in the European Community Respiratory Health Survey. In this study, females with a history of BPD were more likely to report shortness of breath on exertion (43 vs. 16 %) and wheezing without a cold (35 vs. 13 %) and have doctor-diagnosed asthma (24 vs. 5 %) The prevalence of symptoms in the males with prior BPD was comparable to the controls [30].

Pulmonary Lung Function and Bronchial Hyperresponsiveness

In a more recent prospective cohort study, young adults (mean age of 22 years) born between 1987 and 1993 and who were living in the province of Quebec at the time of the study were included in one of four groups based on their hospital discharge diagnosis at birth: (1) preterm subjects (born at less than 37 weeks of gestation) with no respiratory complications (preterm), (2) preterm subjects with RDS but without BPD (RDS), (3) preterm subjects with BPD (with or without preceding RDS) (BPD), and (4) subjects born at term without respiratory complications following birth (term).

In the majority of subjects, the hospital discharge diagnosis data at birth were obtained from the Régie de l'assurance maladie du Québec (RAMQ) using the ICD-9 diagnostic codes for preterm birth (765.**) & RDS (769.*), and BPD (770.7). These data were obtained as part of a previously published cross-sectional study that surveyed the population of BPD and RDS and a portion of the preterm subjects born in the province of Quebec during the same period of time [31, 32]. The cohort study took place between 2011 and 2014 and consisted in two distinct visits at a research center (Montreal, Canada).

A study questionnaire was used to assess medical and smoking history, Medical Research Council (MRC) dyspnea score, and education level. The SF-36v2 and Saint George's Respiratory (SGRQ) questionnaires were completed by participants to respectively evaluate their quality of life and their respiratory health.

Full pulmonary function tests were performed following the American Thoracic Society (ATS) guidelines [33–35]. Reversibility to bronchodilator was tested independently of the lung function test results, and a methacholine challenge test was also performed using the 2-min tidal breathing dosing protocol [36].

The BPD group was composed of 31 subjects, whereas the RDS group had 31, the preterm group had 26, and the term group had 35 subjects. Table 15.1 summarized the demographic and clinical information as well as the medical history across the four groups.

The mean age of the cohort participants was between 21 and 22 years and male subjects composed 35 % of the BPD and the term groups. The degree of dyspnea and the highest level of education achieved did not differ across the four groups. There were significantly more diagnoses of asthma, attention deficit hyperactivity disorder (ADHD), and learning disabilities in the preterm subjects who suffered respiratory complications at birth (RDS and BPD) compared to preterm and term controls.

Lung Functions, Bronchodilator Response, and Bronchial Hyperresponsiveness to Methacholine

BPD participants had mild but significant airflow obstruction compared to the others, defined using a FEV_1/forced vital capacity (FVC) ratio of 70 or less. The group with BPD also had significantly more gas trapping with a mean residual volume of 158 % of predicted. The diffusion capacity was also diminished compared to the other groups but was still within the lower limit of normal (Table 15.2). These findings are similar to those reported in another study looking at young adults, aged between 18 and 25 years, following a preterm birth complicated by BPD,

Table 15.1 Demographic and clinical information of participants in a cohort study comparing four groups of young adults (preterm with BPD, preterm with RDS, preterm with no respiratory complications, and term subjects)

	BPD ($n=31$)	RDS ($n=31$)	Preterm ($n=26$)	Term ($n=35$)	p-value
Demographic and clinical information					
Age, mean (SD)	22 (2)	21 (2)	22 (2)	22 (2)	0.041
Male, *n* (%)	11 (35)	18 (58)	6 (23)	11 (31)	0.037
BMI, mean (%)	24 (6)	23 (3)	24 (5)	23 (3)	0.223
Current smoker, *n* (%)	5 (16)	2 (6)	1 (4)	3 (9)	0.450
MRC dyspnea score, mean (SD)	1.45 (0.68)	1.32 (0.54)	1.46 (0.71)	1.11 (0.32)	0.054
Education (completed high school level)	15 (48)	17 (55)	18 (69)	25 (71)	0.179
Birth weight, kg (SD)	1.06 (0.37)	1.96 (0.78)	2.17 (0.80)	3.45 (0.42)	<0.001
ELBW (≤1 kg), *n* (%)	15 (48)	3 (10)	4 (15)	–	<0.001
VLBW (≤1.5 kg), *n* (%)	27 (87)	12 (39)	5 (19)	–	<0.001
GA, days (SD)	192 (18)	224 (25)	230 (23)	277 (10)	<0.001
APGAR score 1′ (SD)	5 (2)	5 (3)	7 (2)	8 (1)	<0.001
APGAR score 5′ (SD)	6 (2)	7 (2)	8 (1)	9 (1)	<0.001
Multiple gestations, *n* (%)	1 (3)	1 (3)	–	1 (3)	–
Cesarean section, *n* (%)	18 (58)	14 (45)	9 (35)	6 (17)	0.006
Maternal smoking during pregnancy, *n* (%)	6 (19)	3 (10)	–	1 (3)	0.027
Medical history					
Childhood asthma, *n* (%)	12 (39)	10 (32)	6 (23)	10 (29)	0.641
Asthma, *n* (%)	9 (29)	5 (16)	3 (12)	1 (3)	0.024
Anxiety disorder, *n* (%)	3 (10)	4 (13)	3 (12)	1 (3)	0.433
Obesity[a], *n* (%)	3 (10)	1 (3)	4 (15)	3 (9)	0.468
ADHD, *n* (%)	9 (29)	4 (13)	–	1 (3)	0.001
Learning disability[b], *n* (%)	6 (19)	6 (19)	–	–	0.001
Atopy[c], *n* (%)	9 (29)	7 (23)	12 (46)	8 (23)	0.175
Familial asthma[d], *n* (%)	8 (26)	8 (26)	7 (27)	15 (43)	0.349
Maternal asthma, *n* (%)	2 (6)	2 (6)	3 (12)	2 (6)	0.850

[a]Obesity refers to a BMI > 30
[b]As reported by participant
[c]Atopy refers to respiratory allergies: dust, animals, pollen, seasonal allergies, etc.
[d]Familial asthma if brother/sister, father, mother, or grandparents suffer from asthma
BPD bronchopulmonary dysplasia, *RDS* respiratory distress syndrome, *BMI* body mass index, *MRC* medical research council, *ELBW* extremely low birth weight, *VLBW* very low birth weight, *GA* gestational age, *ADHD* attention deficit hyperactivity disorder, *SD* standard deviation

which revealed a significant reduction in FEV_1 when compared to control subjects born at term [37].

Forty-six percent of the BPD subjects had a significant bronchodilator response compared to RDS (18 %), preterm (12 %), and term (6 %) participants (p-value < 0.0001).

Table 15.2 Results of pulmonary function tests of participants in a cohort study comparing four groups of young adults (preterm with BPD, preterm with RDS, preterm with no respiratory complications, and term subjects)

	BPD ($n=31$)	RDS ($n=31$)	Preterm ($n=26$)	Term ($n=35$)	p-value
FEV_1, % predicted (SD)	80 (18)	94 (12)	94 (14)	98 (9)	<0.001
FVC, % predicted (SD)	100 (15)	99 (9)	104 (14)	109 (10)	0.006
FEV1/FVC	70 (12)	81 (9)	79 (7)	79 (7)	<0.001
FEF_{25-75}, % predicted (SD)	68 (26)	92 (19)	89 (26)	96 (18)	<0.001
IC, % predicted (SD)	108 (20)	97 (14)	109 (16)	108 (20)	0.04
FRC, % predicted (SD)	121 (22)	119 (18)	114 (15)	120 (16)	0.447
TLC, % predicted (SD)	114 (13)	107 (9)	111 (9)	113 (12)	0.069
VC, % predicted (SD)	97 (13)	96 (10)	101 (15)	107 (13)	0.002
RV, % predicted (SD)	158 (43)	138 (31)	134 (34)	125 (26)	0.001
RV/TLC	157 (43)	137 (31)	133 (34)	123 (26)	0.001
D_LCO, % predicted (SD)	86 (11)	93 (19)	98 (18)	99 (10)	0.002
VA, % predicted (SD)	95 (11)	93 (11)	96 (11)	98 (8)	0.24
DLCO/VA, mean (SD)	5.54 (0.31)	5.45 (0.33)	5.59 (0.27)	5.49 (0.29)	0.328
RAW, % predicted (SD)	186 (93)	124 (45)	130 (45)	124 (34)	<0.001

FEV_1 forced expiratory volume in 1 s, *FVC* forced vital capacity, *FEF_{25-75}* forced expiratory flow 25–75 %, *IC* inspiratory capacity, *FRC* functional residual capacity, *TLC* total lung capacity, *VC* vital capacity, *RV* residual volume, *DLCO* diffusing capacity of the lung for carbon monoxide, *VA* alveolar volume, *RAW* airway resistance

Table 15.3 Results of methacholine challenge[a] in participants in a cohort study comparing four groups of young adults (preterm with BPD, preterm with RDS, preterm with no respiratory complications, and term subjects)

	BPD ($n=21$)	RDS ($n=29$)	Preterm ($n=26$)	Term ($n=33$)	p-value
PC_{20}, mean (in mg/ml) (SD)	2.68 (2.72)	2.54 (2.85)	3.65 (3.15)	4.11 (3.76)	0.369
$PC_{20} \leq 8$ mg/ml, n (%)	15 (71)	18 (62)	18 (69)	15 (45)	0.169
Not done $FEV_1 < 60$ %, n (%)[b]	7 (25)	–	–	–	<0.001

PC_{20} = concentration of methacholine required to decrease FEV_1 by 20 %
[a]Methacholine challenge was only performed in subjects with a FEV_1 > than 60 % predicted
[b]Percentage calculated over number of participants that performed the methacholine challenge + number of participants that could not do it because FEV_1 was <60 % predicted

Results of methacholine challenge can be seen in Table 15.3. Seventy-one percent of the BPD subjects had evidence of bronchial hyperresponsiveness, but it was not found to be significantly different than the RDS group and the preterm group with 62 % and 69 %, respectively, although 25 % of the BPD subjects could not undergo the challenge because of a FEV_1 that was less than 60 % of predicted.

With regard to their respiratory health and quality of life, the symptoms, activity, and impact scores of the SGRQ were not found to be significantly different across the four groups or different when compared to the general population. The total score on the SGRQ was 11 [standard deviation (SD): 12], 8 (SD: 8), 10 (SD: 12), and 5 (SD: 5) for the BPD, RDS, preterm, and term subjects, respectively (p-value: 0.06).

Similar findings were found with the SF-36v2 health survey questionnaire where the physical component summary and mental component summary scores were not different across the four groups.

In this study, the presence of mild airflow obstruction and a mean FEV_1 value at the lower limit of normal in the BPD subjects at the age of 21–22 is somewhat of a worrisome finding, especially since 25 % of subjects in the BPD group were found to have an FEV_1 less than 60 % of predicted, placing them in the category of moderate airflow obstruction. It is well known that the FEV_1 value peaks at age 25 and then assumes a steady decline over time, ranging between 30 ml per year in non-smokers to 60 ml per year in susceptible smokers [38, 39].

The annual rate of decline of the FEV_1 in BPD subjects over time has still not yet been clearly defined, and there is a theoretical risk that the BPD subjects will have an accelerated loss of lung function with time, similar to what is seen in the COPD population.

The high prevalence of bronchial hyperresponsiveness in all preterm subjects that was found in this study is well supported by population studies that describe a fourfold increase in the incidence of asthma in preterm populations [40–42]. This raises an interesting issue of delineating the phenotypic features of a preterm lung from true asthma and a possible overlap between the two conditions.

Despite the abnormalities found in the pulmonary function, it is encouraging to see that the respiratory health and health-related quality of life do not differ significantly among the four groups, despite higher incidence of ADHD and learning difficulties in the BPD and RDS groups.

The Initial Severity of BPD and Its Impact on Long-Term Lung Function

BPD has undergone a radical change in its pathogenesis and its presentation over the past three decades since it was initially described. This prompted a consensus conference in order to better define the disease in 2000, as mentioned earlier. It combined two existing BPD definitions—oxygen dependency at 28 days of life and at 36 weeks of postmenstrual age. The new definition divided BPD into three forms: mild, moderate, and severe and clearly delineated criteria for judging severity. However, these criteria to differentiate mild from moderate disease or moderate from severe disease were chosen arbitrarily and were not based on analysis of factors associated with differences in outcome [12]. Knowing that the severity of BPD is associated with long-term outcomes would greatly add to the validity of the definition.

In a study looking at postnatal risk factors according to the new BPD definition, a chart review of 244 cases of VLBW preterm infants born between 1999 and 2004 showed that the frequency of BPD in VLBW neonates was high (76 %) but in the majority of cases the disease was mild (67 %). The authors concluded that severe BPD was more common in neonates with late onset sepsis and intraventricular hemorrhage grade III or IV and that the BPD risk factors were low gestational age, low birth weight, as well as late onset sepsis, late pneumonia, and patent ductus arteriosus [43].

In a retrospective study conducted to provide a detailed description of the long-term clinical characteristics of a cohort of preterm subjects who developed BPD of varying degrees of severity, as defined using the National Institutes of Health (NIH) consensus criteria, the initial severity of BPD was found to have an impact on the long-term lung function [41].

This cohort consisted of preterm infants admitted to the Montreal Children's Hospital between the year 1980 and 1992 that were identified as suffering from BPD using the NIH consensus definition. The objective of this study was to provide a detailed description of the long-term consequences of BPD and to examine the association of initial BPD disease severity with these outcomes.

The inclusion criteria for the study population was a diagnosis of BPD, as defined by the NIH consensus [2] in subjects born before 37 weeks gestational age and admitted between January 1, 1980 and December 31, 1992 to a tertiary pediatric hospital with specialized neonatal care that serves as a referral center for the province of Quebec (Canada).

The presence of BPD was defined as the need for supplemental oxygen for at least 28 days [44]. Disease severity was graded based on an assessment done at 36 weeks postmenstrual age (or 56 days of life if born after 32 weeks). Mild disease was defined as breathing room air at that time (FiO_2 of 0.21), moderate disease as requiring a FiO_2 less than 0.30, and severe disease was defined as needing FiO_2 of 0.30 or more or requiring positive pressure ventilation. Infants with BPD, who died of respiratory causes before the assessment date, were considered to have severe disease. These definitions are based on the NIH consensus definition of BPD established in 2000 [45].

Infants were grouped into three categories of disease severity (mild, moderate, and severe as defined above). Baseline and follow-up characteristics were compared between severity categories and/or age groups and differences between these groups tested for statistical significance. The statistical significance for trend across levels of disease severity was assessed using regression analysis.

Three hundred and twenty-two preterm infants with BPD identified during their hospital course were admitted over the 12-year study period. Of the 322 infants, 60 had mild, 123 had moderate, and 107 had severe disease. For 32 subjects (9.9 %), their disease severity was not assessed, mostly because they were transferred to other medical institutions before the severity assessment date but after having met the criterion for diagnosis of BPD of 28 days of oxygen treatment. Fifty-three infants died in the hospital. Among all infants discharged alive, 62 (26 %) were discharged on oxygen. The mean (± standard deviation) gestational age at discharge was 334.4 ± 117.7 days. The severity of BPD was associated with 1-min APGAR score, gestational age, presence of VLBW, and the occurrence of neonatal pneumonia/sepsis [41]. The duration of invasive and noninvasive mechanical ventilation as well as the total duration of oxygen therapy was significantly greater in more severe BPD cases, as seen in Table 15.4.

Table 15.4 Clinical characteristics of BPD subjects associated with their initial hospitalization—by BPD severity

	All BPD	Mild	Moderate	Severe	*p*-value[a]
Neonatal factors					
N (% of total)	322	60 (20.7)	123 (42.4)	107 (36.9)	–
Birth weight (kg) (mean, SD)	1.11 (0.46)	1.17 (0.41)	1.14 (0.53)	1.08 (0.43)	0.1
Gestational age (days) (mean, SD)	195.7 (21.1)	196.9 (22.3)	195.6 (19.9)	196.9 (21.6)	0.46
Male gender (*n*, %)	190 (59.0)	32 (53.3)	66 (53.6)	70 (65.4)	0.04
1-min APGAR score (mean, SD)	4.06 (2.36)	5.17 (2.24)	3.95 (2.24)	3.83 (2.39)	0.001
Mortality (*n*, %)	53 (16.7)	1 (1.7)	4 (3.3)	48 (44.9)	<0.0001
Length of hospital stay (median)	108	78	117	145	<0.0001
Traditional mechanical ventilation during initial admission					
Mechanical ventilation (*n*, %)	301 (96.5)	56 (93.3)	112 (94.2)	107 (100)	0.008
Maximal FiO_2 (mean, SD)	0.84 (2.3)	0.80 (0.23)	0.83 (0.25)	0.88 (0.22)	0.06
Duration (days) (median)	42	27	29	72	<0.0001
Noninvasive positive pressure ventilation during initial admission					
NIPPV (*n*, %)	122 (37.9)	34 (56.7)	49 (39.8)	38 (35.5)	0.27
Duration (days) (median)	4	4	4	7	0.28
Supplemental oxygen therapy					
Duration (days)[b] (median)	56	18	75	96	<0.0001
Discharge home on O_2 (*n*, %)	62 (26.1)	1 (1.7)	33 (27.7)	25 (42.4)	<0.0001

Values expressed in: *n* (%) or mean (± standard deviation)

[a]*p*-value for trend

[b]The duration of supplemental oxygen consists of the entire duration of therapy, both in and out of the hospital

BPD bronchopulmonary dysplasia, *n* numbers, *NIPPV* noninvasive positive pressure ventilation, *SD* standard deviation

FEV_1, FVC, and their ratio were significantly associated with the initial BPD severity as shown in Table 15.5. Of all lung function indices, only the FEV_1 was associated with another parameter—the total duration of oxygen therapy (*p*-value: 0.02). No other parameters of lung function were associated with mechanical ventilation parameters (maximum pressure, positive end-expiratory pressure (PEEP), use of traditional mechanical ventilation versus nasal continuous positive airway pressure (CPAP), or level of FiO_2 used.

This study described the post-hospitalization course of a retrospective cohort of infants with preterm birth who suffered the complication of BPD. Its major findings were the association of the initial BPD severity with numerous morbidities such as hospital readmissions in the first 2 years of life, the presence of developmental delay, and lung function abnormalities later in childhood. These findings have implications for the care of preterm infants and for planning of healthcare services.

In this cohort, 83 % of infants who were discharged alive had at least one admission in the first 2 years of their life. This is substantially higher than the 50 % readmission rate reported previously [24]. Oxygen therapy was discontinued after a

Table 15.5 Lung function measurements of BPD subjects—by BPD severity

	Mild BPD	Moderate BPD	Severe BPD	p-value[a]
n	6	10	9	–
Mean age (SD)	14.0 (2.8)	13.8 (1.9)	13.7 (1.8)	0.62
FEV_1 (%) (SD)	93.5 (9.7)	53.0 (19.0)	52.2 (12.5)	0.006
FVC (%) (SD)	103.0 (2.5)	72.0 (15.8)	64.5 (12.1)	0.19
FEV_1/FVC (SD)	83.8 (12.8)	68.8 (23.7)	76.3 (19.0)	0.06
$FEF_{25–75}$ (%) (SD)	83.3 (17.0)	43.2 (33.6)	34.2 (18.5)	0.001
TLC (%) (SD)	105.7 (23.8)	113.3 (35.3)	110.5 (9.2)	0.37
FRC (%) (SD)	104.0 (71.2)	148.0 (76.9)	163.0 (24.0)	0.07
RV (%) (SD)	121.3 (96.8)	248.5 (73.6)	294.0 (59.4)	0.29
D_LCO (%) (SD)	–	78.0 (5.0)	55.5 (6.4)	–

Values expressed in mean or % predicted (± standard deviation)
[a]Comparison between values across severity categories
FEV_1 force expiratory capacity at 1 s, *FVC* forced vital capacity, *$FEF_{25–75}$* forced expiratory flow 25–75 %, *SD* standard deviation, *TLC* total lung capacity, *FRC* functional residual capacity, *RV* residual volume, *D_LCO* diffusing capacity of the lung for carbon monoxide, *n* numbers

mean duration of 20 weeks, but severe cases were maintained on oxygen for an average of 40 weeks, which, when considering their corrected gestational age at discharge, meant that subjects with severe BPD were weaned off oxygen after an average of 1 year and 2 months. More than half of the children (54 %) received inhaled short-acting beta-agonist in their first few years of life, presumed to represent the occurrence of wheezing episodes. Inhaled corticosteroids were used in 20.4 % of subjects, but their use was not associated with disease severity. Although not associated with disease severity, 68 % of BPD survivors had persistent radiological abnormalities compatible with chronic changes of BPD. Others have reported that radiological abnormalities improve with time [18], which was not observed in our dataset, a phenomenon possibly attributable to a selection bias, since chest X-rays were available for only a small proportion of subjects.

In previous studies, lung function abnormalities were not related to severity of neonatal respiratory illness [18, 46, 47], in contrast to our finding of a clear association between greater severity of BPD and greater abnormalities of FEV_1, the FEV_1/FVC ratio, forced expiratory flow from 25 to 75 % of vital capacity ($FEF_{25–75}$), and FRC. This finding is supported by another study showing a trend toward lower FEV (% predicted) in moderate to severe BPD subjects among former preterm infants born between 1982 and 1985 [29]. These findings are in agreement with the principle of "disynaptic" or unequal lung growth previously described, which means normal growth of lung volume but not of airway size [18]. When comparing to Northway's earlier report of "old" BPD subjects born between 1964 and 1973, the overall airway obstruction and hyperinflation found in our study were more severe, likely to represent an evolving phase of the pathophysiology of BPD between "old" and "new," accounting for the effects of greater prematurity and lower birth weight [15].

In one earlier study, infants with BPD had higher risk of cerebral palsy and delays in cognitive and motor function compared with controls matched for gestational age at birth [24]. A NICHD review on neurological developmental outcome of extreme low birth weight infants reported abnormal outcomes in 50–60 % of infants with BPD. Findings in these reports are comparable to our BPD cohort, of whom 52 % were found to have development delay and 20 % had neurological impairment during childhood [24]. Poor developmental outcomes were previously associated with prolonged hospital admissions and prolonged mechanical ventilation [24]. In our study, we found an association between the presence of a developmental delay and the following variables: length of the initial hospital admission, duration of mechanical ventilation, and birth weight when correcting for BPD severity. Other associations were found between neurological impairment and the presence of neonatal seizures or a history of anoxic encephalopathy. In another study, the risks of impaired neurological development, cerebral palsy, and/or low intellectual quotient were more than doubled in infants with severe BPD compared with infants with mild BPD [48]; however, this trend of neurological impairment with BPD of increased severity was not found in our study. The prevalence of ADHD in our BPD population was also significantly different than the general population (6.5 vs. 5.3 %) [49, 50], an observation previously reported in preterm infants [51] but never linked to chronic lung disease or its treatment. In our study, ADHD was associated with smaller gestational age and the use of steroids postnatally, but not with the degree of BPD severity.

This study described an association between the initial BPD severity and hospital readmission rate, long-term lung function, and developmental delay. Severity of BPD was not associated with greater long-term use of inhalers or with persistent radiological abnormalities. In addition, the duration of mechanical ventilation and oxygen therapy was associated with developmental delay during childhood, and the use of postnatal corticosteroids was associated with the development of ADHDs. Initial BPD severity was an important predictor of pulmonary function abnormality and healthcare utilization during childhood. These findings contribute to a better description of the impact of BPD and its severity on long-term outcomes and will help sensitize the adult caregivers to the long-term consequences of preterm birth.

Conclusion

The impact of preterm birth and its respiratory complications have lasting consequences on respiratory health. Clinicians have to be better informed of its manifestation and the long-term consequences in order to better assist their young patients in maintaining their health and lung function. Prevention and education focusing on smoking avoidance or smoking cessation, health lifestyle, and physical activity will be key factors in ensuring that our young patients born prematurely will maintain an optimal respiratory health and quality of life.

The long-term effect of BPD on the evolution of FEV_1 is unclear, particularly whether adults who had BPD as children will have normal, early, or accelerated decline in respiratory function [21]. Some investigators have expressed concern that survivors of preterm birth and BPD may be susceptible to COPD in later life, underlying the need for longer follow-up data [15, 18, 20, 21, 29, 52].

References

1. Wohl ME. Bronchopulmonary dysplasia in adulthood. N Engl J Med. 1990;323(26):1834–6.
2. Bancalari E, Claure N, Sosenko IR. Bronchopulmonary dysplasia: changes in pathogenesis, epidemiology and definition. Semin Neonatol. 2003;8(1):63–71.
3. Bancalari E, Abdenour GE, Feller R, Gannon J. Bronchopulmonary dysplasia: clinical presentation. J Pediatr. 1979;95(5 Pt 2):819–23.
4. Russell RB, Green NS, Steiner CA, Meikle S, Howse JL, Poschman K, et al. Cost of hospitalization for preterm and low birth weight infants in the United States. Pediatrics. 2007;120(1):e1–9.
5. Jobe AH. The new bronchopulmonary dysplasia. Curr Opin Pediatr. 2011;23(2):167–72.
6. Bhandari A, McGrath-Morrow S. Long-term pulmonary outcomes of patients with bronchopulmonary dysplasia. Semin Perinatol. 2013;37(2):132–7.
7. Northway Jr WH, Rosan RC, Porter DY. Pulmonary disease following respirator therapy of hyaline-membrane disease. Bronchopulmonary dysplasia. N Engl J Med. 1967;276(7):357–68.
8. Hulsmann AR, van den Anker JN. Evolution and natural history of chronic lung disease of prematurity. Monaldi Arch Chest Dis. 1997;52(3):272–7.
9. Lessard MR. New concepts in mechanical ventilation for ARDS. Can J Anaesth. 1996;43(5 Pt 2):R42–54.
10. Malhotra A. Low-tidal-volume ventilation in the acute respiratory distress syndrome. N Engl J Med. 2007;357(11):1113–20.
11. Bhandari A, Bhandari V. Pitfalls, problems, and progress in bronchopulmonary dysplasia. Pediatrics. 2009;123(6):1562–73.
12. Jobe AH, Bancalari E. Bronchopulmonary dysplasia. Am J Respir Crit Care Med. 2001;163(7):1723–9.
13. Churg A, Golden J, Fligiel S, Hogg JC. Bronchopulmonary dysplasia in the adult. Am Rev Respir Dis. 1983;127(1):117–20.
14. Samuels MP, Warner JO. Bronchopulmonary dysplasia: the outcome. Arch Dis Child. 1987;62(11):1099–101.
15. Northway Jr WH, Moss RB, Carlisle KB, Parker BR, Popp RL, Pitlick PT, et al. Late pulmonary sequelae of bronchopulmonary dysplasia. N Engl J Med. 1990;323(26):1793–9.
16. Northway Jr WH. Bronchopulmonary dysplasia: twenty-five years later. Pediatrics. 1992; 89(5 Pt 1):969–73.
17. Parat S, Moriette G, Delaperche MF, Escourrou P, Denjean A, Gaultier C. Long-term pulmonary functional outcome of bronchopulmonary dysplasia and premature birth. Pediatr Pulmonol. 1995;20(5):289–96.
18. Eber E, Zach MS. Long term sequelae of bronchopulmonary dysplasia (chronic lung disease of infancy). Thorax. 2001;56(4):317–23.
19. Greenough A. Bronchopulmonary dysplasia—long term follow up. Paediatr Respir Rev. 2006;7 Suppl 1:S189–91.
20. Vrijlandt EJ, Gerritsen J, Boezen HM, Grevink RG, Duiverman EJ. Lung function and exercise capacity in young adults born prematurely. Am J Respir Crit Care Med. 2006; 173(8):890–6.
21. Baraldi E, Filippone M. Chronic lung disease after premature birth. N Engl J Med. 2007;357(19):1946–55.
22. Fanaroff AA, Stoll BJ, Wright LL, Carlo WA, Ehrenkranz RA, Stark AR, et al. Trends in neonatal morbidity and mortality for very low birthweight infants. Am J Obstet Gynecol. 2007;196(2):147.e1–8.
23. Greenough A. Long-term pulmonary outcome in the preterm infant. Neonatology. 2008;93(4):324–7.
24. Kinsella JP, Greenough A, Abman SH. Bronchopulmonary dysplasia. Lancet. 2006; 367(9520):1421–31.
25. Robin B, Kim YJ, Huth J, Klocksieben J, Torres M, Tepper RS, et al. Pulmonary function in bronchopulmonary dysplasia. Pediatr Pulmonol. 2004;37(3):236–42.

26. Koumbourlis AC, Motoyama EK, Mutich RL, Mallory GB, Walczak SA, Fertal K. Longitudinal follow-up of lung function from childhood to adolescence in prematurely born patients with neonatal chronic lung disease. Pediatr Pulmonol. 1996;21(1):28–34.
27. Filippone M, Sartor M, Zacchello F, Baraldi E. Flow limitation in infants with bronchopulmonary dysplasia and respiratory function at school age. Lancet. 2003;361(9359):753–4.
28. McLeod A, Ross P, Mitchell S, Tay D, Hunter L, Hall A, et al. Respiratory health in a total very low birthweight cohort and their classroom controls. Arch Dis Child. 1996;74(3):188–94.
29. Halvorsen T, Skadberg BT, Eide GE, Roksund OD, Carlsen KH, Bakke P. Pulmonary outcome in adolescents of extreme preterm birth: a regional cohort study. Acta Paediatr. 2004;93(10):1294–300.
30. Vrijlandt EJ, Gerritsen J, Boezen HM, Duiverman EJ. Gender differences in respiratory symptoms in 19-year-old adults born preterm. Respir Res. 2005;6:117.
31. Landry JS, Croitoru D, Menzies D. Validation of ICD-9 diagnostic codes for bronchopulmonary dysplasia in Quebec's provincial healthcare databases. Chronic Dis Inj Can. 2012;33(1):47–52.
32. Beaudoin S, Tremblay GM, Croitoru D, Benedetti A, Landry JS. Healthcare utilization and health-related quality of life of adult survivors of preterm birth complicated by bronchopulmonary dysplasia. Acta Paediatr. 2013;102(6):607–12.
33. Macintyre N, Crapo RO, Viegi G, Johnson DC, van der Grinten CP, Brusasco V, et al. Standardisation of the single-breath determination of carbon monoxide uptake in the lung. Eur Respir J. 2005;26(4):720–35.
34. Miller MR, Hankinson J, Brusasco V, Burgos F, Casaburi R, Coates A, et al. Standardisation of spirometry. Eur Respir J. 2005;26(2):319–38.
35. Wanger J, Clausen JL, Coates A, Pedersen OF, Brusasco V, Burgos F, et al. Standardisation of the measurement of lung volumes. Eur Respir J. 2005;26(3):511–22.
36. Crapo RO, Casaburi R, Coates AL, Enright PL, Hankinson JL, Irvin CG, et al. Guidelines for methacholine and exercise challenge testing-1999. This official statement of the American Thoracic Society was adopted by the ATS Board of Directors, July 1999. Am J Respir Crit Care Med. 2000;161(1):309–29.
37. Vollsaeter M, Roksund OD, Eide GE, Markestad T, Halvorsen T. Lung function after preterm birth: development from mid-childhood to adulthood. Thorax. 2013;68(8):767–76.
38. Mangham LJ, Petrou S, Doyle LW, Draper ES, Marlow N. The cost of preterm birth throughout childhood in England and Wales. Pediatrics. 2009;123(2):e312–27.
39. Lam HS, Wong SP, Liu FY, Wong HL, Fok TF, Ng PC. Attitudes toward neonatal intensive care treatment of preterm infants with a high risk of developing long-term disabilities. Pediatrics. 2009;123(6):1501–8.
40. Kirkby S, Greenspan JS, Kornhauser M, Schneiderman R. Clinical outcomes and cost of the moderately preterm infant. Adv Neonatal Care. 2007;7(2):80–7.
41. Landry JS, Menzies D. Occurrence and severity of bronchopulmonary dysplasia and respiratory distress syndrome after a preterm birth. Paediatr Child Health. 2011;16(7):399–403.
42. Landry JS, Chan T, Lands L, Menzies D. Long-term impact of bronchopulmonary dysplasia on pulmonary function. Can Respir J. 2011;18(5):265–70.
43. Woynarowska M, Rutkowska M, Szamotulska K. Risk factors, frequency and severity of bronchopulmonary dysplasia (BPD) diagnosed according to the new disease definition in preterm neonates. Med Wieku Rozwoj. 2008;12(4 Pt 1):933–41.
44. Lavoie PM, Pham C, Jang KL. Heritability of bronchopulmonary dysplasia, defined according to the consensus statement of the national institutes of health. Pediatrics. 2008;122(3):479–85.
45. Ehrenkranz RA, Walsh MC, Vohr BR, Jobe AH, Wright LL, Fanaroff AA, et al. Validation of the National Institutes of Health consensus definition of bronchopulmonary dysplasia. Pediatrics. 2005;116(6):1353–60.
46. Chan KN, Noble-Jamieson CM, Elliman A, Bryan EM, Silverman M. Lung function in children of low birth weight. Arch Dis Child. 1989;64(9):1284–93.

47. Kitchen WH, Olinsky A, Doyle LW, Ford GW, Murton LJ, Slonim L, et al. Respiratory health and lung function in 8-year-old children of very low birth weight: a cohort study. Pediatrics. 1992;89(6 Pt 2):1151–8.
48. Vohr BR, Coll CG, Lobato D, Yunis KA, O'Dea C, Oh W. Neurodevelopmental and medical status of low-birthweight survivors of bronchopulmonary dysplasia at 10 to 12 years of age. Dev Med Child Neurol. 1991;33(8):690–7.
49. Greenbaum RL, Stevens SA, Nash K, Koren G, Rovet J. Social cognitive and emotion processing abilities of children with fetal alcohol spectrum disorders: a comparison with attention deficit hyperactivity disorder. Alcohol Clin Exp Res. 2009;33(10):1656–70.
50. Merrill RM, Lyon JL, Baker RK, Gren LH. Attention deficit hyperactivity disorder and increased risk of injury. Adv Med Sci. 2009;54:20–6.
51. Delobel-Ayoub M, Arnaud C, White-Koning M, Casper C, Pierrat V, Garel M, et al. Behavioral problems and cognitive performance at 5 years of age after very preterm birth: the EPIPAGE Study. Pediatrics. 2009;123(6):1485–92.
52. Doyle LW, Faber B, Callanan C, Freezer N, Ford GW, Davis NM. Bronchopulmonary dysplasia in very low birth weight subjects and lung function in late adolescence. Pediatrics. 2006;118(1):108–13.

Part IV
BPD: Novel Therapeutic Options

Chapter 16
Stem Cells for the Prevention of Bronchopulmonary Dysplasia

Won Soon Park

Introduction

Bronchopulmonary dysplasia (BPD), a chronic lung disease of premature infants receiving prolonged ventilator and oxygen therapy, is a serious complication of preterm birth [1]. BPD remains an important cause of mortality and long-term respiratory morbidities, such as airway hyperreactivity, poor lung function, and low exercise capacity [2, 3], and neurologic morbidities, such as developmental delay and cerebral palsy, in preterm survivors [4]. Moreover, as the risk for developing BPD is correlated with the extent of immaturity [5], recent improvements in the survival of very preterm infants through advances in neonatal medicine have made the task of protecting extremely immature lungs against BPD increasingly challenging. Currently, few effective therapies are available to prevent or ameliorate this common and serious disorder. Therefore, the development of new safe and effective therapeutic modalities to improve the prognosis of BPD in preterm infants is an urgent issue.

Recently, it has been shown that exogenous administration of stem cells significantly attenuates neonatal hyperoxic lung injuries in newborn animal models [6–14], and phase I clinical trial has shown that human stem cell transplantation to prevent and/or treat BPD is safe, feasible, and potentially efficacious [15]. Taken together, these findings suggest that exogenous stem cell transplantation might be a promising new therapeutic modality for the treatment of hyperoxic neonatal lung injury or BPD. This chapter will summarize recent advances in stem cell research for preventing and/or treating BPD with a particular focus on preclinical data relevant to issues essential for clinical translation, such as mechanism of action, optimal cell type, route, dose, and timing of stem cell transplantation, as well as successful phase I clinical trial results of stem cell therapies for BPD.

W.S. Park, MD, PhD (✉)
Department of Pediatrics, Sungkyunkwan University School of Medicine, Samsung Medical Center, 81 Irwon-Ro, Kangnam Gu, Seoul 135-710, South Korea
e-mail: wonspark@skku.edu

V. Bhandari (ed.), *Bronchopulmonary Dysplasia*, Respiratory Medicine,
DOI 10.1007/978-3-319-28486-6_16

Preclinical Data

Therapeutic Potential of Stem Cell Transplantation for BPD

The histopathological characteristics of BPD include impaired alveolarization, vascular growth, and minimal interstitial fibrosis [16]. Although its etiology is not completely understood, oxidative stress and inflammatory responses due to diverse adverse stimuli, including hyperoxia, volutrauma, barotrauma, and intrauterine or postnatal infection, are believed to play key roles in the lung injury process leading to the development of BPD [5]. Prolonged exposure of newborn murine pups results in decreased alveolarization, impaired vascular growth, and increased lung fibrosis, simulating the histopathology of human BPD [17, 18]. Furthermore, the saccular stage of term newborn rat pups is comparable to the lung development of very preterm human premature infants at ~25 weeks of gestation. Hence, the newborn rodent model of BPD is both convenient and effective for studying various therapeutic strategies, and recent studies using this model to simulate clinical BPD have highlighted its importance in investigating cell-based therapies to prevent or repair lung injury in BPD [6, 8, 9, 12, 14, 19–23].

The therapeutic efficacy of cell-based therapies has been tested in the hyperoxia-induced neonatal rodent model of BPD, and these studies have demonstrated that stem cell therapy aids in ameliorating neonatal hyperoxic injuries such as oxidative stress, lung inflammation, impaired alveolar growth, vascular injuries, fibrosis, and associated pulmonary hypertension [6–9, 14, 20, 23–30].

The observed reduction in lung mesenchymal stem cells (MSCs), endothelial progenitor cells (EPCs), and endothelial colony-forming cells (ECFCs) in the hyperoxic newborn rat model [20, 31, 32] or in clinical BPD of premature infants [33, 34] and the increase in bronchoalveolar stem cells observed after MSC treatment in a mouse model of BPD [35] also provide a strong rationale for exogenous stem/progenitor cell supplementation for the prevention or repair of lung injury in BPD. Overall, these findings support the assumption that stem cell transplantation shows promise as a novel therapeutic approach for BPD.

Protective Mechanisms of Stem Cell Transplantation for BPD

Engraftment and Differentiation

Several studies have shown that donor stem cells can reconstitute lung parenchymal cells, such as type I or II pneumocytes or fibroblasts, both in vitro and in vivo [6, 36–39]. Therefore, the beneficial effects have been initially ascribed to the transdifferentiation of donor cells into lung parenchymal cells such as type II pneumocytes [6, 37]. However, this is a very rare event in vivo [6], and the numbers of engrafted cells observed are extremely low [12]. These findings suggest that direct donor cell engraftment, transdifferentiation, and therapeutic replacement of the damaged lung tissue with exogenously transplanted stem cells might not be the primary mechanism of lung protection [40, 41].

Paracrine Effects

Conditioned media has been observed to show equal or better therapeutic efficacy than stem cells for preventing or reversing established BPD [6, 8, 12–14, 21, 42, 43]. More recently, Lee et al. reported that microvesicles released by MSCs (exosomes) are the major paracrine anti-inflammatory and therapeutic mediators of MSCs in hypoxia-induced pulmonary hypertension [44]. Taken together, these findings suggest that the protective effects of stem cell transplantation might be predominantly mediated by paracrine rather than regenerative mechanisms [6, 8, 10, 23, 28, 40, 41, 45, 46]. The use of the MSC secretome rather than stem cells shows excellent promise as a new therapeutic approach for BPD, as it bypasses theoretical concerns, such as tumor formation, associated with live cell treatments.

Paracrine Mediators

It has been reported that paracrine factors, such as keratinocyte growth factor [47, 48], interleukin (IL) 1 receptor antagonist [49], IL-10 [50, 51], angiopoietin-1 [52], and prostaglandin E2 [53], that are secreted by transplanted MSCs could decrease inflammation, reduce permeability of the alveolar capillary membrane, and enhance tissue repair in acute respiratory distress syndrome [54, 55]. However, the specific humoral substances secreted by the transplanted stem cells that mediate the protective paracrine anti-inflammatory, anti-oxidative, and antiapoptotic activities in BPD have not yet been elucidated.

Growth factors secreted by donor cells, such as vascular endothelial growth factor (VEGF) and hepatocyte growth factor (HGF), are known to be the key paracrine mediators that protect against neonatal hyperoxic lung injuries such as increased inflammation, oxidative stress and apoptosis, and impaired alveolarization and angiogenesis [8, 10, 56]. In previous studies, it has been observed that growth factors that are significantly reduced in BPD, such as VEGF and HGF, were significantly increased by MSC transplantation [7, 8]; the extent to which MSCs protected against BPD was positively correlated with the paracrine potency of the transplanted donor cells [11, 57, 58]. Moreover, knockdown of the VEGF secreted by MSCs, via transfection with small interfering RNAs specific for human VEGF, abolished the protective effects of MSCs in hyperoxic lung injury (i.e., attenuation of impaired alveolarization and angiogenesis, reduction in apoptotic cells and alveolar macrophages, and downregulation of proinflammatory cytokine levels) [10]. Overall, these findings suggest that growth factors, including VEGF, that are secreted by transplanted MSCs are critical paracrine factors mediating the protective effects of MSCs against hyperoxic lung injuries.

Growth factors secreted by transplanted stem cells are a crucial paracrine mediator in facilitating recovery not only in BPD [10] but also in various animal models of disease, such as myocardial injury [59], acute kidney injury [60], and stroke [61]. These findings suggest that growth factors secreted by transplanted stem cells, such as VEGF and HGF, might be universal paracrine mediators responsible for the protective effects of stem cell transplantation in various diseases [62] and that these factors could also be used as potential biomarkers of the potency of transplanted stem cells [10, 56, 59, 63].

Although levels of growth factors such as VEGF and HGF were significantly improved in BPD by MSC transplantation, their levels remained much lower than those in the control group. Overexpression of VEGF in MSCs has been reported to significantly enhance stem cell-mediated therapeutic efficacy in neural and cardiac repair [64, 65]. Therefore, further studies will be necessary to investigate whether overexpression of growth factors in transplanted MSCs enhances their beneficial effects in the BPD model.

Determining the Optimal Cell Type for Stem Cell Transplantation

Determining the most appropriate cell types and sources is critical for successful clinical translation of cell-based therapies into protection against BPD. However, it is very difficult to choose among the various types and sources of stem cells and to identify those that ultimately exhibit the best therapeutic efficacy in protecting against BPD [35].

Mesenchymal Stem Cells

MSCs have several unusual characteristics, including their fibroblast-like morphology, plastic-adherent cultured cells, expression of defined surface marker profiles (positive expression of CD73, 90, and 105 and negative expression of CD45, CD34, CD14, or CD11b surface molecules), and capacity for differentiation into different cell types including adipocytes, chondrocytes, and osteoblasts [66]. Because they are more ethically and socially acceptable than embryonic stem cells (ESCs) and because they lack MHC II antigens and are therefore immune privileged, MSCs have been extensively investigated for their potential for transplantation in experimental models of BPD.

MSCs are broadly distributed in the body and can be isolated from adult tissues such as bone marrow (BM) and adipose tissue (AT), as well as from gestational tissues such as placenta, amniotic fluid, Wharton's jelly, and umbilical cord blood (UCB). BM is the best-characterized source of MSCs, and all studies using BM-derived MSCs have demonstrated improvements in survival, impaired alveolar and vascular growth, lung inflammation, fibrosis, lung function, and ensuing pulmonary hypertension in the newborn rat model of hyperoxic lung injury [13, 14, 21–23, 27, 35, 43, 67]. Despite the beneficial effects of BM-derived MSCs in protecting against neonatal hyperoxic lung injuries, their clinical translation is limited due to the very invasive and painful harvesting procedure and the extremely low numbers of MSCs that can be obtained [68]. AT might be a potential alternative source of MSCs, as they can be harvested from AT less invasively and in larger quantities than from BM. However, the in vivo therapeutic efficacy of AT-derived MSCs in protecting against neonatal hyperoxic lung injury has not yet been tested.

As umbilical cord and placental tissue are medical waste that is usually discarded at birth, MSCs obtained from gestational tissues are particularly attractive due to the lack of significant ethical concerns; in addition to their easy obtainability, MSCs derived from gestational tissues show lower immunogenicity [69, 70] and higher proliferative capacity [71, 72] and paracrine potency than adult tissue-derived MSCs [73]. These findings suggest that gestational tissue might be another promising source for human MSCs.

Donor age has been shown to have a negative impact on the expansion and differentiation potential of MSCs, even when they originate from the same adult tissue of origin, AT [74, 75] or BM [76]. MSCs obtained from gestational tissues, such as UCB [77], Wharton's jelly, or umbilical cord [73], exhibit higher cell proliferation and increased secretion of chemokines, proinflammatory proteins, and growth factors than MSCs derived from adult AT or BM. Moreover, in a recent study comparing the in vivo therapeutic efficacy of AT- and UCB-derived MSCs in protecting against hyperoxic lung injury in newborn rats, UCB-derived MSCs exhibited better therapeutic efficacy in attenuating hyperoxia-induced lung injuries (i.e., impaired angiogenesis, increased cell death and pulmonary macrophages, and elevated lung cytokines) and increased paracrine potency in secreting vascular growth factor and HGF than AT-derived MSCs in newborn rats [11]. Taken together, these findings suggest that donor age must be considered in the development of successful stem cell therapies and that MSCs derived from birth-associated tissues, such as UCB or Wharton's jelly, might be the optimal source for future clinical uses in protecting against BPD in premature infants [78].

Other Cell Types

UCB is a rich source of mononuclear cells (MNCs), and it contains high levels of primitive multipotent stem/progenitor cells [79]. Due to the long period (4 weeks) required for isolation, ex vivo expansion, and characterization of MSCs [80], the relatively short therapeutic window for treatment of BPD could easily be missed [8, 15]. Moreover, in the clinical setting for the prevention of BPD, autologous UCB MNCs, collected at birth, could be given instead of allogeneic UCB-derived MSCs. UCB MNCs could thus be a good alternative source for MSCs for therapies designed to protect against BPD [81] because of the short period required for obtaining the cells. However, although they can easily and rapidly be obtained, the quantity of

UCB MNCs obtained from each patient and the amount of therapeutically effective stem cells in each batch of MNCs are variable and heterogeneous. Therefore, it would be virtually impossible to standardize the therapeutically effective optimal doses of UCB MNCs. Moreover, UCB MNCs do not require a manufacturing license, to ensure good manufacturing practices, which is essential for human trials [15, 82]. UCB-derived MSCs were recently found to show better therapeutic efficacy and paracrine potency, both in vitro and in vivo, than UCB-derived MNCs in attenuating hyperoxic lung injuries in newborn rats [11]. Taken together, these findings suggest that human UCB MNCs might not be an ideal source for "off-the-shelf" clinical applications of cell-based therapies for treating/preventing BPD.

EPCs, ECFCs [23, 26, 30, 83], and human amnion cells sourced from human placenta [24, 26, 84, 85] are garnering increasing interest and have shown promise as alternative cell-based therapeutic agents for BPD. However, as few reports detailing their therapeutic benefits have been published, compared to those on MSCs, extensive further study will be necessary to verify their therapeutic efficacy.

ESCs are pluripotent cells capable of generating cells from all three germ layers. However, their high tumorigenicity and the ethical concerns related to destruction of embryos for their acquisition have limited their availability for research and clinical applications.

Determining the Optimal Route for Stem Cell Transplantation

Determining the optimal route for MSC transplantation is a key issue to be resolved for future successful clinical translation of stem cell therapies for protection against BPD. Currently, MSC transplantation is performed via local intratracheal (IT) [6, 14], systemic intraperitoneal (IP) [6], or intravenous (IV) [13] administration. Injured lung tissue produces chemotactic factors that cause MSCs to proliferate and migrate toward the injury [86]. Furthermore, systemically administered MSCs have been shown to localize to an injured lung [39]. The systemic IV or IP approach, which is most convenient and minimally invasive, shows distinct therapeutic advantages compared with the more invasive local IT approach, especially in very unstable preterm infants with BPD. However, some animal studies have suggested that the IV route is not optimal for treating local pulmonary lesions because transplanted cells might be retained not only in the pulmonary capillaries but also in other organs such as the liver, spleen, and kidney [13]. Furthermore, the IT approach is more clinically relevant, as most preterm infants at high risk of developing BPD are intubated to receive ventilator therapy, and MSCs could be administered in the same manner as surfactant [15]. In previous studies [6], although the dosage of MSCs administered by IT was only one-quarter that administered by IP or IV, engraftment of donor cells, attenuation of hyperoxia-induced lung injury, and paracrine potency were found to be higher with local IT transplantation of MSCs than with systemic IP or IV administration [6]. Overall, these findings suggest that local IT rather than systemic IV or IP transplantation of MSCs is the optimal delivery route for treating premature infants with BPD.

Determining the Optimal Dose for MSC Transplantation

Determining the optimal dose for MSC transplantation is another important issue to be addressed for successful clinical translation. A previous study showed that the therapeutically effective dose for MSC transplantation could be reduced more than fourfold by choosing local IT over systemic IV or IP administration [6]. Another previous study [7] tested the therapeutic efficacy of three different doses of human UCB-derived MSCs (5×10^3, 5×10^4, and 5×10^5 cells) given intratracheally to hyperoxic newborn rat pups with an average weight of 8 g at postnatal day (P) 5. The intratracheal transplantation of human UCB-derived MSCs dose-dependently attenuated hyperoxia-induced lung injury, such as decreased alveolarization; a dosage of 5×10^5 cells produced the best protection, and at least 5×10^4 cells were necessary to achieve effective anti-inflammatory, anti-fibrotic, and anti-oxidative effects. These findings demonstrate that IT transplantation of appropriate doses of MSCs might attenuate hyperoxic lung injuries through active involvement of these cells in modulating host inflammatory responses and oxidative stress in neonatal rats. In light of these findings, further studies to determine the optimal dose of human UCB-derived MSCs for their potential clinical benefit in human preterm neonates with BPD are anticipated.

Determining the Optimal Timing for MSC Transplantation

Although the therapeutic efficacy of MSC transplantation for BPD has already been shown [6], the optimal timing for their administration is a key issue that remains to be clarified. Pierro et al. [12] reported that MSC transplantation not only prevented but also rescued hyperoxic arrested alveolar growth. A previous study attempted to determine the optimal timing by comparing the therapeutic efficacy of early (at P3) versus late (at P10) intratracheal transplantation of MSCs [8]. Hyperoxia-induced lung injuries, such as impaired alveolarization, increased apoptosis, oxidative stress, inflammation, fibrosis, and reduced VEGF and HGF levels, were significantly attenuated by early but not by late transplantation of MSCs. No synergies were observed with combined early and late MSCs transplantation. These findings suggest that the therapeutic time window for MSC transplantation for BPD is narrow and occurs only during the early phase of inflammatory responses. In concordance with this study, van Haaften et al. [14] have shown that IT transplantation of MSCs at P4 for prevention, but not at P14 for regeneration, significantly attenuated neonatal hyperoxic lung injuries. Thus, in a clinical setting, the early identification of preterm infants at the highest risk for developing BPD, who are therefore potential candidates for stem cell therapy, is essential [87].

Long-Term Safety and Outcomes of MSC Transplantation

Several clinical studies have demonstrated that BPD produces long-term respiratory complications such as wheezing, asthma, or bronchial hyperresponsiveness [88] and that persistent detrimental pulmonary function is correlated with BPD severity at diagnosis [89]; these effects extend beyond childhood and into adult life. Therefore, long-term studies in experimental models are needed. Long-term research using the rat model is feasible in a short timeframe, due to its short life span. In two long-term studies in rats up to 70 days [9] and 6 months of age [12], comparable to human adolescence and mid-adulthood, respectively, hyperoxic lung injuries persisted even after a prolonged recovery period, and the protective effects of stem cell transplantation as evidenced by improved alveolarization and angiogenesis were sustained. Overall, these findings support the assumption that transplantation of MSCs to prevent and/or treat BPD in premature infants at a critical early time point might improve the long-term respiratory morbidities of BPD.

Some clinical studies have also identified BPD as an independent risk factor for the development of neuro-functional deficits, such as cerebral palsy and developmental retardation, even in the absence of catastrophic brain injuries, such as intraventricular hemorrhage or hypoxic ischemic encephalopathy, in premature infants [90–93]. A study done by our group/laboratory showed that IT transplantation of MSCs significantly improved not only hyperoxic lung injuries, including impaired alveolarization and increased lung inflammatory cytokines, but also brain injuries, including reduced myelin basic protein (MBP) and increased TUNEL-positive cells; the extent of attenuation of both injuries was synchronized (unpublished data). These findings suggest that IT transplantation of MSCs in preterm infants at a critical early time point might improve not only the long-term respiratory but also the neurologic morbidities associated with BPD. The results of the long-term follow-up safety and efficacy study, up to 5 years of age, for the phase I (NCT01632475, NCT02023788) and II (NCT01897987) clinical trials are keenly anticipated.

The long-term safety of MSC transplantation is not yet known. In two long-term studies [9, 12], the transplanted MSCs rapidly disappeared, and no abnormal gross or histological findings, such as tumors, were observed in various organs. Moreover, no adverse outcomes, including tumorigenicity, have been reported in the more than 350 clinical studies of MSC transplantation conducted worldwide. The data indicating the sustained long-term protective effects of IT transplantation of MSCs without any long-term adverse effects warrant the translation of MSC transplantation into clinical studies for the treatment of BPD in premature infants.

Phase I Clinical Trial of MSCs for BPD

In previous preclinical translational studies to determine the therapeutic efficacy [6], optimal route [6], dose and timing [7, 8], and long-term effects [9] of human UCB-derived MSC transplantation in a neonatal hyperoxic lung injury model in rat pups, MSCs were found to provide persistent protection against neonatal hyperoxic lung injury, without long-term toxicity or tumorigenicity. Based on the promising evidence from these preclinical studies in the experimental BPD model, a phase I dose-escalating clinical study on the safety and feasibility of human UCB-derived MSC transplantation in preterm infants with BPD was designed and conducted [15].

This study was an open-label, single-center clinical trial to assess the safety and feasibility of a single IT transplantation of allogeneic human UCB-derived MSCs for BPD. The MSCs were transplanted to nine very preterm infants at high risk for developing BPD, with a mean gestational age of 25.3 ± 0.9 weeks (24–26 weeks) and a birth weight of 793 ± 127 g (630–1030 g) at a mean age of 10.4 ± 2.6 days (7–14 days) after birth. The preterm infants were all on ventilator support that could not be decreased due to significant respiratory distress. The first three patients were given a low dose (1×10^7 cells/kg in 2 ml/kg of saline), and the next six patients were given a high dose (2×10^7 cells/kg in 4 ml/kg of saline). The MSCs were administered intratracheally in two fractions, using the method for administering surfactant. The treatment was well tolerated, without any serious adverse effects or dose-limiting toxicity up to 84 days following transplantation. No significant differences in serious adverse effects were observed between the low- and high-dose groups, and BPD severity was lower in transplant recipients than in a gestational age-, birth weight-, and respiratory severity score-matched control group. Levels of IL-6, IL-8 matrix metalloproteinase (MMP)-9, tumor necrosis factor-alpha (TNF-α), and transforming growth factor beta1 (TGFß1) in tracheal aspirates at day 7 were significantly reduced compared with those at baseline or at day 3 posttransplantation. Overall, these findings suggest that IT transplantation of allogeneic human UCB-derived MSCs in very preterm infants at highest risk for developing BPD is safe and feasible. Long-term follow-up studies, up to 2 years of age (NCT01632475) and 5 years of age (NCT02023788), are currently underway to assess the long-term safety of these phase I MSC-treated preterm infants. Moreover, a phase II double-blind, randomized, multicenter, controlled trial is currently underway to assess the therapeutic efficacy and safety of low-dose MSC transplantation compared with a control group for the treatment of BPD (NCT0182957). A long-term follow-up study of these patients, up to 5 years of age, is also underway to assess the long-term safety and efficacy of the phase II clinical trial (NCT01897987). Favorable results from these current clinical trials are greatly anticipated and are expected to pave the way for future clinical introduction of stem cell transplantation for a currently intractable disease, BPD.

Conclusions

Various translational studies have broadened the knowledge and understanding of stem cell therapy for neonatal lung injury, and clinical trials are harnessing the therapeutic potential of stem cell therapies for BPD. The exciting progress in both animal and clinical research has brought human stem cell therapy for BPD one step closer to clinical translation. However, a better understanding of the potential mechanism of stem cells in BPD and the resolution of clinical issues such as clinical indication, timing, dose, and multiple modes of action are required to permit safe clinical translation of stem cell therapy for BPD.

References

1. Bhandari A, Panitch HB. Pulmonary outcomes in bronchopulmonary dysplasia. Semin Perinatol. 2006;30(4):219–26. doi:10.1053/j.semperi.2006.05.009. S0146-0005(06)00074-7 [pii].
2. Narang I, Rosenthal M, Cremonesini D, Silverman M, Bush A. Longitudinal evaluation of airway function 21 years after preterm birth. Am J Respir Crit Care Med. 2008;178(1):74–80. doi:10.1164/rccm.200705-701OC.
3. Avery ME, Tooley WH, Keller JB, Hurd SS, Bryan MH, Cotton RB, Epstein MF, Fitzhardinge PM, Hansen CB, Hansen TN, et al. Is chronic lung disease in low birth weight infants preventable? A survey of eight centers. Pediatrics. 1987;79(1):26–30.
4. Bregman J, Farrell EE. Neurodevelopmental outcome in infants with bronchopulmonary dysplasia. Clin Perinatol. 1992;19(3):673–94.
5. Walsh MC, Szefler S, Davis J, Allen M, Van Marter L, Abman S, Blackmon L, Jobe A. Summary proceedings from the bronchopulmonary dysplasia group. Pediatrics. 2006;117(3 Pt 2):S52–6. doi:10.1542/peds.2005-0620I.
6. Chang YS, Oh W, Choi SJ, Sung DK, Kim SY, Choi EY, Kang S, Jin HJ, Yang YS, Park WS. Human umbilical cord blood-derived mesenchymal stem cells attenuate hyperoxia-induced lung injury in neonatal rats. Cell Transplant. 2009;18(8):869–86. doi:10.3727/096368909X471189. CT-1859 [pii].
7. Chang YS, Choi SJ, Sung DK, Kim SY, Oh W, Yang YS, Park WS. Intratracheal transplantation of human umbilical cord blood-derived mesenchymal stem cells dose-dependently attenuates hyperoxia-induced lung injury in neonatal rats. Cell Transplant. 2011;20(11–12):1843–54. doi:10.3727/096368911X565038.
8. Chang YS, Choi SJ, Ahn SY, Sung DK, Sung SI, Yoo HS, Oh WI, Park WS. Timing of umbilical cord blood derived mesenchymal stem cells transplantation determines therapeutic efficacy in the neonatal hyperoxic lung injury. PLoS One. 2013;8(1):e52419. doi:10.1371/journal.pone.0052419.
9. Ahn SY, Chang YS, Kim SY, Sung DK, Kim ES, Rime SY, Yu WJ, Choi SJ, Oh WI, Park WS. Long-term (postnatal day 70) outcome and safety of intratracheal transplantation of human umbilical cord blood-derived mesenchymal stem cells in neonatal hyperoxic lung injury. Yonsei Med J. 2013;54(2):416–24. doi:10.3349/ymj.2013.54.2.416.
10. Chang YS, Ahn SY, Jeon HB, Sung DK, Kim ES, Sung SI, Yoo HS, Choi SJ, Oh WI, Park WS. Critical role of vascular endothelial growth factor secreted by mesenchymal stem cells in hyperoxic lung injury. Am J Respir Cell Mol Biol. 2014;51(3):391–9. doi:10.1165/rcmb.2013-0385OC.
11. Ahn SY, Chang YS, Sung DK, Yoo HS, Sung SI, Choi SJ, Park WS. Cell type-dependent variation in paracrine potency determines therapeutic efficacy against neonatal hyperoxic lung injury. Cytotherapy. 2015;17(8):1025–35. doi:10.1016/j.jcyt.2015.03.008.

12. Pierro M, Ionescu L, Montemurro T, Vadivel A, Weissmann G, Oudit G, Emery D, Bodiga S, Eaton F, Peault B, Mosca F, Lazzari L, Thebaud B (2012) Short-term, long-term and paracrine effect of human umbilical cord-derived stem cells in lung injury prevention and repair in experimental bronchopulmonary dysplasia. Thorax. doi:10.1136/thoraxjnl-2012-202323
13. Aslam M, Baveja R, Liang OD, Fernandez-Gonzalez A, Lee C, Mitsialis SA, Kourembanas S. Bone marrow stromal cells attenuate lung injury in a murine model of neonatal chronic lung disease. Am J Respir Crit Care Med. 2009;180(11):1122–30. doi:10.1164/rccm.200902-0242OC. 200902-0242OC [pii].
14. van Haaften T, Byrne R, Bonnet S, Rochefort GY, Akabutu J, Bouchentouf M, Rey-Parra GJ, Galipeau J, Haromy A, Eaton F, Chen M, Hashimoto K, Abley D, Korbutt G, Archer SL, Thebaud B. Airway delivery of mesenchymal stem cells prevents arrested alveolar growth in neonatal lung injury in rats. Am J Respir Crit Care Med. 2009;180(11):1131–42. doi:10.1164/rccm.200902-0179OC.
15. Chang YS, Ahn SY, Yoo HS, Sung SI, Choi SJ, Oh WI, Park WS. Mesenchymal stem cells for bronchopulmonary dysplasia: phase 1 dose-escalation clinical trial. J Pediatr. 2014;164(5):966–72. doi:10.1016/j.jpeds.2013.12.011. e966.
16. Coalson JJ. Pathology of bronchopulmonary dysplasia. Semin Perinatol. 2006;30(4):179–84. doi:10.1053/j.semperi.2006.05.004.
17. Warner BB, Stuart LA, Papes RA, Wispe JR. Functional and pathological effects of prolonged hyperoxia in neonatal mice. Am J Physiol. 1998;275(1 Pt 1):L110–7.
18. deLemos RA, Coalson JJ. The contribution of experimental models to our understanding of the pathogenesis and treatment of bronchopulmonary dysplasia. Clin Perinatol. 1992;19(3):521–39.
19. O'Reilly M, Thebaud B. Animal models of bronchopulmonary dysplasia. The term rat models. Am J Physiol Lung Cell Mol Physiol. 2014;307(12):L948–58. doi:10.1152/ajplung.00160.2014.
20. Alphonse RS, Vadivel A, Fung M, Shelley WC, Critser PJ, Ionescu L, O'Reilly M, Ohls RK, McConaghy S, Eaton F, Zhong S, Yoder M, Thebaud B. Existence, functional impairment, and lung repair potential of endothelial colony-forming cells in oxygen-induced arrested alveolar growth. Circulation. 2014;129(21):2144–57. doi:10.1161/CIRCULATIONAHA.114.009124.
21. Waszak P, Alphonse R, Vadivel A, Ionescu L, Eaton F, Thebaud B. Preconditioning enhances the paracrine effect of mesenchymal stem cells in preventing oxygen-induced neonatal lung injury in rats. Stem Cells Dev. 2012;21(15):2789–97. doi:10.1089/scd.2010.0566.
22. Zhang H, Fang J, Su H, Yang M, Lai W, Mai Y, Wu Y. Bone marrow mesenchymal stem cells attenuate lung inflammation of hyperoxic newborn rats. Pediatr Transplant. 2012;16(6):589–98. doi:10.1111/j.1399-3046.2012.01709.x.
23. Zhang H, Fang J, Wu Y, Mai Y, Lai W, Su H. Mesenchymal stem cells protect against neonatal rat hyperoxic lung injury. Expert Opin Biol Ther. 2013;13(6):817–29. doi:10.1517/14712598.2013.778969.
24. Vosdoganes P, Lim R, Koulaeva E, Chan ST, Acharya R, Moss TJ, Wallace EM. Human amnion epithelial cells modulate hyperoxia-induced neonatal lung injury in mice. Cytotherapy. 2013;15(8):1021–9. doi:10.1016/j.jcyt.2013.03.004.
25. Batsali AK, Kastrinaki MC, Papadaki HA, Pontikoglou C. Mesenchymal stem cells derived from Wharton's Jelly of the umbilical cord: biological properties and emerging clinical applications. Curr Stem Cell Res Ther. 2013;8(2):144–55.
26. Hodges RJ, Lim R, Jenkin G, Wallace EM. Amnion epithelial cells as a candidate therapy for acute and chronic lung injury. Stem Cells Int. 2012;2012:709763. doi:10.1155/2012/709763.
27. Zhang X, Wang H, Shi Y, Peng W, Zhang S, Zhang W, Xu J, Mei Y, Feng Z. Role of bone marrow-derived mesenchymal stem cells in the prevention of hyperoxia-induced lung injury in newborn mice. Cell Biol Int. 2012;36(6):589–94. doi:10.1042/CBI20110447.
28. Fung ME, Thebaud B. Stem cell-based therapy for neonatal lung disease: it is in the juice. Pediatr Res. 2014;75(1–1):2–7. doi:10.1038/pr.2013.176.
29. Park HK, Cho KS, Park HY, Shin DH, Kim YK, Jung JS, Park SK, Roh HJ. Adipose-derived stromal cells inhibit allergic airway inflammation in mice. Stem Cells Dev. 2010;19(11):1811–8. doi:10.1089/scd.2009.0513.

30. Balasubramaniam V, Ryan SL, Seedorf GJ, Roth EV, Heumann TR, Yoder MC, Ingram DA, Hogan CJ, Markham NE, Abman SH. Bone marrow-derived angiogenic cells restore lung alveolar and vascular structure after neonatal hyperoxia in infant mice. Am J Physiol Lung Cell Mol Physiol. 2010;298(3):L315–23. doi:10.1152/ajplung.00089.2009.
31. Yee M, Vitiello PF, Roper JM, Staversky RJ, Wright TW, McGrath-Morrow SA, Maniscalco WM, Finkelstein JN, O'Reilly MA. Type II epithelial cells are critical target for hyperoxia-mediated impairment of postnatal lung development. Am J Physiol Lung Cell Mol Physiol. 2006;291(5):L1101–11. doi:10.1152/ajplung.00126.2006.
32. Bozyk PD, Popova AP, Bentley JK, Goldsmith AM, Linn MJ, Weiss DJ, Hershenson MB. Mesenchymal stromal cells from neonatal tracheal aspirates demonstrate a pattern of lung-specific gene expression. Stem Cells Dev. 2011;20(11):1995–2007. doi:10.1089/scd.2010.0494.
33. Borghesi A, Massa M, Campanelli R, Bollani L, Tzialla C, Figar TA, Ferrari G, Bonetti E, Chiesa G, de Silvestri A, Spinillo A, Rosti V, Stronati M. Circulating endothelial progenitor cells in preterm infants with bronchopulmonary dysplasia. Am J Respir Crit Care Med. 2009;180(6):540–6. doi:10.1164/rccm.200812-1949OC. 200812-1949OC [pii].
34. Baker CD, Balasubramaniam V, Mourani PM, Sontag MK, Black CP, Ryan SL, Abman SH. Cord blood angiogenic progenitor cells are decreased in bronchopulmonary dysplasia. Eur Respir J. 2012;40(6):1516–22. doi:10.1183/09031936.00017312.
35. Tropea KA, Leder E, Aslam M, Lau AN, Raiser DM, Lee JH, Balasubramaniam V, Fredenburgh LE, Alex Mitsialis S, Kourembanas S, Kim CF. Bronchioalveolar stem cells increase after mesenchymal stromal cell treatment in a mouse model of bronchopulmonary dysplasia. Am J Physiol Lung Cell Mol Physiol. 2012;302(9):L829–37. doi:10.1152/ajplung.00347.2011.
36. Abe S, Lauby G, Boyer C, Rennard SI, Sharp JG. Transplanted BM and BM side population cells contribute progeny to the lung and liver in irradiated mice. Cytotherapy. 2003;5(6):523–33. doi:10.1080/14653240310003576.
37. Berger MJ, Adams SD, Tigges BM, Sprague SL, Wang XJ, Collins DP, McKenna DH. Differentiation of umbilical cord blood-derived multilineage progenitor cells into respiratory epithelial cells. Cytotherapy. 2006;8(5):480–7. doi:10.1080/14653240600941549.
38. Grove JE, Lutzko C, Priller J, Henegariu O, Theise ND, Kohn DB, Krause DS. Marrow-derived cells as vehicles for delivery of gene therapy to pulmonary epithelium. Am J Respir Cell Mol Biol. 2002;27(6):645–51. doi:10.1165/rcmb.2002-0056RC.
39. Ortiz LA, Gambelli F, McBride C, Gaupp D, Baddoo M, Kaminski N, Phinney DG. Mesenchymal stem cell engraftment in lung is enhanced in response to bleomycin exposure and ameliorates its fibrotic effects. Proc Natl Acad Sci USA. 2003;100(14):8407–11. doi:10.1073/pnas.1432929100. 1432929100 [pii].
40. Weiss DJ. Concise review: current status of stem cells and regenerative medicine in lung biology and diseases. Stem Cells. 2014;32(1):16–25. doi:10.1002/stem.1506.
41. Ahn SY, Chang YS, Park WS. Stem cell therapy for bronchopulmonary dysplasia: bench to bedside translation. J Korean Med Sci. 2015;30(5):509–13. doi:10.3346/jkms.2015.30.5.509.
42. Abman SH, Matthay MA. Mesenchymal stem cells for the prevention of bronchopulmonary dysplasia: delivering the secretome. Am J Respir Crit Care Med. 2009;180(11):1039–41. doi:10.1164/rccm.200909-1330ED.
43. Hansmann G, Fernandez-Gonzalez A, Aslam M, Vitali SH, Martin T, Mitsialis SA, Kourembanas S. Mesenchymal stem cell-mediated reversal of bronchopulmonary dysplasia and associated pulmonary hypertension. Pulm Circ. 2012;2(2):170–81. doi:10.4103/2045-8932.97603.
44. Lee C, Mitsialis SA, Aslam M, Vitali SH, Vergadi E, Konstantinou G, Sdrimas K, Fernandez-Gonzalez A, Kourembanas S. Exosomes mediate the cytoprotective action of mesenchymal stromal cells on hypoxia-induced pulmonary hypertension. Circulation. 2012;126(22):2601–11. doi:10.1161/CIRCULATIONAHA.112.114173.
45. Ahn SY, Chang YS, Sung DK, Sung SI, Yoo HS, Lee JH, Oh WI, Park WS. Mesenchymal stem cells prevent hydrocephalus after severe intraventricular hemorrhage. Stroke. 2013;44(2):497–504. doi:10.1161/STROKEAHA.112.679092.

46. Niver D. Bronchopulmonary dysplasia: structural challenges and stem cell treatment potential. Adv Neonatal Care. 2014;14(1):E1–11. doi:10.1097/ANC.0000000000000050.
47. Borok Z, Lubman RL, Danto SI, Zhang XL, Zabski SM, King LS, Lee DM, Agre P, Crandall ED. Keratinocyte growth factor modulates alveolar epithelial cell phenotype in vitro: expression of aquaporin 5. Am J Respir Cell Mol Biol. 1998;18(4):554–61. doi:10.1165/ajrcmb.18.4.2838.
48. Atabai K, Ishigaki M, Geiser T, Ueki I, Matthay MA, Ware LB. Keratinocyte growth factor can enhance alveolar epithelial repair by nonmitogenic mechanisms. Am J Physiol Lung Cell Mol Physiol. 2002;283(1):L163–9. doi:10.1152/ajplung.00396.2001.
49. McCarter SD, Mei SH, Lai PF, Zhang QW, Parker CH, Suen RS, Hood RD, Zhao YD, Deng Y, Han RN, Dumont DJ, Stewart DJ. Cell-based angiopoietin-1 gene therapy for acute lung injury. Am J Respir Crit Care Med. 2007;175(10):1014–26. doi:10.1164/rccm.200609-1370OC.
50. Gupta N, Su X, Popov B, Lee JW, Serikov V, Matthay MA. Intrapulmonary delivery of bone marrow-derived mesenchymal stem cells improves survival and attenuates endotoxin-induced acute lung injury in mice. J Immunol. 2007;179(3):1855–63. 179/3/1855 [pii].
51. Folkesson HG, Pittet JF, Nitenberg G, Matthay MA. Transforming growth factor-alpha increases alveolar liquid clearance in anesthetized ventilated rats. Am J Physiol. 1996;271(2 Pt 1):L236–44.
52. Fang X, Neyrinck AP, Matthay MA, Lee JW. Allogeneic human mesenchymal stem cells restore epithelial protein permeability in cultured human alveolar type II cells by secretion of angiopoietin-1. J Biol Chem. 2010;285(34):26211–22. doi:10.1074/jbc.M110.119917.
53. Nemeth K, Leelahavanichkul A, Yuen PS, Mayer B, Parmelee A, Doi K, Robey PG, Leelahavanichkul K, Koller BH, Brown JM, Hu X, Jelinek I, Star RA, Mezey E. Bone marrow stromal cells attenuate sepsis via prostaglandin E(2)-dependent reprogramming of host macrophages to increase their interleukin-10 production. Nat Med. 2009;15(1):42–9. doi:10.1038/nm.1905.
54. Li J, Huang S, Wu Y, Gu C, Gao D, Feng C, Wu X, Fu X. Paracrine factors from mesenchymal stem cells: a proposed therapeutic tool for acute lung injury and acute respiratory distress syndrome. Int Wound J. 2014;11(2):114–21. doi:10.1111/iwj.12202.
55. Lee JW, Fang X, Krasnodembskaya A, Howard JP, Matthay MA. Concise review: mesenchymal stem cells for acute lung injury: role of paracrine soluble factors. Stem Cells. 2011;29(6):913–9. doi:10.1002/stem.643.
56. Deuse T, Peter C, Fedak PW, Doyle T, Reichenspurner H, Zimmermann WH, Eschenhagen T, Stein W, Wu JC, Robbins RC, Schrepfer S. Hepatocyte growth factor or vascular endothelial growth factor gene transfer maximizes mesenchymal stem cell-based myocardial salvage after acute myocardial infarction. Circulation. 2009;120(11 Suppl):S247–54. doi:10.1161/CIRCULATIONAHA.108.843680.
57. Khubutiya MS, Vagabov AV, Temnov AA, Sklifas AN. Paracrine mechanisms of proliferative, anti-apoptotic and anti-inflammatory effects of mesenchymal stromal cells in models of acute organ injury. Cytotherapy. 2014;16(5):579–85. doi:10.1016/j.jcyt.2013.07.017.
58. Henning RJ, Sanberg P, Jimenez E. Human cord blood stem cell paracrine factors activate the survival protein kinase Akt and inhibit death protein kinases JNK and p38 in injured cardiomyocytes. Cytotherapy. 2014;16(8):1158–68. doi:10.1016/j.jcyt.2014.01.415.
59. Markel TA, Wang Y, Herrmann JL, Crisostomo PR, Wang M, Novotny NM, Herring CM, Tan J, Lahm T, Meldrum DR. VEGF is critical for stem cell-mediated cardioprotection and a crucial paracrine factor for defining the age threshold in adult and neonatal stem cell function. Am J Physiol Heart Circ Physiol. 2008;295(6):H2308–14. doi:10.1152/ajpheart.00565.2008.
60. Togel F, Zhang P, Hu Z, Westenfelder C. VEGF is a mediator of the renoprotective effects of multipotent marrow stromal cells in acute kidney injury. J Cell Mol Med. 2009;13(8B):2109–14. doi:10.1111/j.1582-4934.2008.00641.x.
61. Horie N, Pereira MP, Niizuma K, Sun G, Keren-Gill H, Encarnacion A, Shamloo M, Hamilton SA, Jiang K, Huhn S, Palmer TD, Bliss TM, Steinberg GK. Transplanted stem cell-secreted vascular endothelial growth factor effects poststroke recovery, inflammation, and vascular repair. Stem Cells. 2011;29(2):274–85. doi:10.1002/stem.584.

62. Song SY, Chung HM, Sung JH. The pivotal role of VEGF in adipose-derived-stem-cell-mediated regeneration. Expert Opin Biol Ther. 2010;10(11):1529–37. doi:10.1517/14712598.2010.522987.
63. Lehman N, Cutrone R, Raber A, Perry R, Van't Hof W, Deans R, Ting AE, Woda J. Development of a surrogate angiogenic potency assay for clinical-grade stem cell production. Cytotherapy. 2012;14(8):994–1004. doi:10.3109/14653249.2012.688945.
64. Lee HJ, Kim KS, Park IH, Kim SU. Human neural stem cells over-expressing VEGF provide neuroprotection, angiogenesis and functional recovery in mouse stroke model. PLoS One. 2007;2(1), e156. doi:10.1371/journal.pone.0000156.
65. Zisa D, Shabbir A, Suzuki G, Lee T. Vascular endothelial growth factor (VEGF) as a key therapeutic trophic factor in bone marrow mesenchymal stem cell-mediated cardiac repair. Biochem Biophys Res Commun. 2009;390(3):834–8. doi:10.1016/j.bbrc.2009.10.058.
66. Spencer ND, Gimble JM, Lopez MJ. Mesenchymal stromal cells: past, present, and future. Vet Surg. 2011;40(2):129–39. doi:10.1111/j.1532-950X.2010.00776.x.
67. Sutsko RP, Young KC, Ribeiro A, Torres E, Rodriguez M, Hehre D, Devia C, McNiece I, Suguihara C. Long-term reparative effects of mesenchymal stem cell therapy following neonatal hyperoxia-induced lung injury. Pediatr Res. 2013;73(1):46–53. doi:10.1038/pr.2012.152.
68. Mosna F, Sensebe L, Krampera M. Human bone marrow and adipose tissue mesenchymal stem cells: a user's guide. Stem Cells Dev. 2010;19(10):1449–70. doi:10.1089/scd.2010.0140.
69. Rocha V, Wagner Jr JE, Sobocinski KA, Klein JP, Zhang MJ, Horowitz MM, Gluckman E. Graft-versus-host disease in children who have received a cord-blood or bone marrow transplant from an HLA-identical sibling. Eurocord and international bone marrow transplant registry working committee on alternative donor and stem cell sources. N Engl J Med. 2000;342(25):1846–54. doi:10.1056/NEJM200006223422501. MJBA-422501 [pii].
70. Le Blanc K. Immunomodulatory effects of fetal and adult mesenchymal stem cells. Cytotherapy. 2003;5(6):485–9. doi:10.1080/14653240310003611. XLQTCMQP660JW0LU [pii].
71. Kern S, Eichler H, Stoeve J, Kluter H, Bieback K. Comparative analysis of mesenchymal stem cells from bone marrow, umbilical cord blood, or adipose tissue. Stem Cells. 2006;24(5):1294–301. doi:10.1634/stemcells.2005-0342.
72. Yang SE, Ha CW, Jung M, Jin HJ, Lee M, Song H, Choi S, Oh W, Yang YS. Mesenchymal stem/progenitor cells developed in cultures from UC blood. Cytotherapy. 2004;6(5):476–86. doi:10.1080/14653240410005041. W4J80FJ7EV8TWW9R [pii].
73. Amable PR, Teixeira MV, Carias RB, Granjeiro JM, Borojevic R. Protein synthesis and secretion in human mesenchymal cells derived from bone marrow, adipose tissue and Wharton's jelly. Stem Cell Res Ther. 2014;5(2):53. doi:10.1186/scrt442.
74. Choudhery MS, Badowski M, Muise A, Pierce J, Harris DT. Donor age negatively impacts adipose tissue-derived mesenchymal stem cell expansion and differentiation. J Transl Med. 2014;12:8. doi:10.1186/1479-5876-12-8.
75. Dos-Anjos Vilaboa S, Navarro-Palou M, Llull R. Age influence on stromal vascular fraction cell yield obtained from human lipoaspirates. Cytotherapy. 2014;16(8):1092–7. doi:10.1016/j.jcyt.2014.02.007.
76. Kretlow JD, Jin YQ, Liu W, Zhang WJ, Hong TH, Zhou G, Baggett LS, Mikos AG, Cao Y. Donor age and cell passage affects differentiation potential of murine bone marrow-derived stem cells. BMC Cell Biol. 2008;9:60. doi:10.1186/1471-2121-9-60.
77. Jin HJ, Bae YK, Kim M, Kwon SJ, Jeon HB, Choi SJ, Kim SW, Yang YS, Oh W, Chang JW. Comparative analysis of human mesenchymal stem cells from bone marrow, adipose tissue, and umbilical cord blood as sources of cell therapy. Int J Mol Sci. 2013;14(9):17986–8001. doi:10.3390/ijms140917986.
78. Pievani A, Scagliotti V, Russo FM, Azario I, Rambaldi B, Sacchetti B, Marzorati S, Erba E, Giudici G, Riminucci M, Biondi A, Vergani P, Serafini M. Comparative analysis of multilineage properties of mesenchymal stromal cells derived from fetal sources shows an advantage of mesenchymal stromal cells isolated from cord blood in chondrogenic differentiation potential. Cytotherapy. 2014;16(7):893–905. doi:10.1016/j.jcyt.2014.02.008.

79. Mayani H, Alvarado-Moreno JA, Flores-Guzman P. Biology of human hematopoietic stem and progenitor cells present in circulation. Arch Med Res. 2003;34(6):476–88. doi:10.1016/j.arcmed.2003.08.004.
80. Kogler G, Critser P, Trapp T, Yoder M. Future of cord blood for non-oncology uses. Bone Marrow Transplant. 2009;44(10):683–97. doi:10.1038/bmt.2009.287.
81. Monz D, Tutdibi E, Mildau C, Shen J, Kasoha M, Laschke MW, Roolfs T, Schmiedl A, Tschernig T, Bieback K, Gortner L. Human umbilical cord blood mononuclear cells in a double-hit model of bronchopulmonary dysplasia in neonatal mice. PLoS One. 2013;8(9):e74740. doi:10.1371/journal.pone.0074740.
82. Bieback K, Kinzebach S, Karagianni M. Translating research into clinical scale manufacturing of mesenchymal stromal cells. Stem Cells Int. 2011;2010:193519. doi:10.4061/2010/193519.
83. Thebaud B, Abman SH. Bronchopulmonary dysplasia: where have all the vessels gone? Roles of angiogenic growth factors in chronic lung disease. Am J Respir Crit Care Med. 2007;175(10):978–85. doi:10.1164/rccm.200611-1660PP.
84. Vosdoganes P, Hodges RJ, Lim R, Westover AJ, Acharya RY, Wallace EM, Moss TJ. Human amnion epithelial cells as a treatment for inflammation-induced fetal lung injury in sheep. Am J obstet Gynecol. 2011;205(2):156.e126–33. doi:10.1016/j.ajog.2011.03.054.
85. Hodges RJ, Jenkin G, Hooper SB, Allison B, Lim R, Dickinson H, Miller SL, Vosdoganes P, Wallace EM. Human amnion epithelial cells reduce ventilation-induced preterm lung injury in fetal sheep. Am J Obstet Gynecol. 2012;206(5):448.e8–15. doi:10.1016/j.ajog.2012.02.038.
86. Rojas M, Xu J, Woods CR, Mora AL, Spears W, Roman J, Brigham KL. Bone marrow-derived mesenchymal stem cells in repair of the injured lung. Am J Respir Cell Mol Biol. 2005;33(2):145–52. doi:10.1165/rcmb.2004-0330OC. 2004-0330OC [pii].
87. Laughon M, Allred EN, Bose C, O'Shea TM, Van Marter LJ, Ehrenkranz RA, Leviton A, Investigators ES. Patterns of respiratory disease during the first 2 postnatal weeks in extremely premature infants. Pediatrics. 2009;123(4):1124–31. doi:10.1542/peds.2008-0862.
88. Northway Jr WH, Moss RB, Carlisle KB, Parker BR, Popp RL, Pitlick PT, Eichler I, Lamm RL, Brown Jr BW. Late pulmonary sequelae of bronchopulmonary dysplasia. N Engl J Med. 1990;323(26):1793–9. doi:10.1056/NEJM199012273232603.
89. Landry JS, Chan T, Lands L, Menzies D. Long-term impact of bronchopulmonary dysplasia on pulmonary function. Can Respir J. 2011;18(5):265–70.
90. Ratner V, Kishkurno SV, Slinko SK, Sosunov SA, Sosunov AA, Polin RA, Ten VS. The contribution of intermittent hypoxemia to late neurological handicap in mice with hyperoxia-induced lung injury. Neonatology. 2007;92(1):50–8. doi:10.1159/000100086.
91. Stoll BJ, Hansen NI, Bell EF, Shankaran S, Laptook AR, Walsh MC, Hale EC, Newman NS, Schibler K, Carlo WA, Kennedy KA, Poindexter BB, Finer NN, Ehrenkranz RA, Duara S, Sanchez PJ, O'Shea TM, Goldberg RN, Van Meurs KP, Faix RG, Phelps DL, Frantz 3rd ID, Watterberg KL, Saha S, Das A, Higgins RD, Eunice Kennedy Shriver National Institute of Child H, Human Development Neonatal Research Network. Neonatal outcomes of extremely preterm infants from the NICHD neonatal research network. Pediatrics. 2010;126(3):443–56. doi:10.1542/peds.2009-2959.
92. Anderson PJ, Doyle LW. Neurodevelopmental outcome of bronchopulmonary dysplasia. Semin Perinatol. 2006;30(4):227–32. doi:10.1053/j.semperi.2006.05.010.
93. Dammann O, Leviton A, Bartels DB, Dammann CE. Lung and brain damage in preterm newborns. Are they related? How? Why? Biol Neonate. 2004;85(4):305–13. doi:10.1159/000078175.

Chapter 17
Less Invasive Surfactant Administration (LISA) for the Prevention of Bronchopulmonary Dysplasia

Wolfgang Göpel, Angela Kribs, and Egbert Herting

The Problem: CPAP or Surfactant

Epidemiological data of single centers reporting extremely low bronchopulmonary dysplasia (BPD) rates while using continuous positive airway pressure (CPAP) support of preterm infants [1, 2] stimulated researchers to investigate if primary CPAP treatment is effective in preventing BPD [3, 4]. However, these trials were not successful. Infants who were treated with CPAP and rescue intubation had no significant benefit with regard to survival without BPD when compared to infants who were intubated at birth and received surfactant immediately. Only in a meta-analysis of four randomized controlled trials, CPAP had a significant protective effect with regard to death or BPD (number needed to treat with CPAP = 25 infants to prevent one case of BPD/death [5]). What was the reason for this moderate effect of CPAP treatment? One important difference between the CPAP and intubation group in all of these trials was the percentage of surfactant treatment in the study arms. In all trials, infants who were randomized to CPAP only received surfactant if rescue intubation was necessary, whereas infants who were randomized to the intubation group received surfactant earlier and more frequently and sometimes even prophylactically. Since surfactant is the only effective medication for respiratory distress syndrome (RDS), the lack of surfactant treatment in preterm infants stabilized with CPAP might be one reason for the lower than expected benefit of CPAP.

W. Göpel, MD (✉) • E. Herting, MD, PhD
Department of Pediatrics, University Hospital Schleswig Holstein, Campus Lübeck, Ratzeburger Allee 160, Lübeck 23538, Germany
e-mail: wolfgang.goepel@uksh.de; Egbert.herting@uksh.de

A. Kribs, MD
Department of Pediatrics, University Hospital Cologne, Kerpener Str. 62, Cologne 50924, Germany
e-mail: angela.kribs@uk-koeln.de

V. Bhandari (ed.), *Bronchopulmonary Dysplasia*, Respiratory Medicine,
DOI 10.1007/978-3-319-28486-6_17

To circumvent this disadvantage, some Scandinavian centers developed the "INSURE" (intubation–surfactant treatment–extubation) method of surfactant administration [6, 7]. This was also tested in a number of randomized controlled trials [8, 9]. However, the INSURE technique was not able to reduce BPD/death rates when compared to CPAP treatment [9], which might be due to the approach itself. For INSURE, infants are intubated with a standard endotracheal tube. Sedation and analgesia is frequently provided to ensure that infants tolerate this procedure. Furthermore, surfactant is often "distributed" with bag ventilation. In animal experiments, even a few high-pressure and high-volume ventilation breaths are able to induce significant lung injury [10, 11]. Finally, many infants who are treated with INSURE are not extubated immediately after the procedure, due to lack of respiratory drive and other problems [8, 12].

As early as 1990, a report from the Mideast described successful surfactant replacement therapy to spontaneously breathing preterm infants. This was done because no mechanical ventilators were available [13]. Two years later, a Danish group described surfactant application via a small diameter gastric tube into the trachea while the infant was breathing spontaneously. However, this approach was not investigated further since this group was more interested in exploring the INSURE technique [7].

A New Approach: Less Invasive Surfactant Administration

In 2001, the technique of surfactant administration via a thin tube while the preterm infant is breathing spontaneously was rediscovered by a research group from Cologne [14]. They now describe the method as "less invasive surfactant administration or LISA" [15–17]. For the LISA technique, the larynx is visualized with a laryngoscope and a small diameter tube (outer diameter 1.2–1.5 mm) is placed into the trachea by a Magill forceps. The laryngoscope is removed and surfactant is instilled into the trachea via the thin diameter tube while the infant is breathing spontaneously. CPAP is provided during the whole procedure. If the infant is apneic, which sometimes occurs when surfactant is instilled, inspiration is supported by a short increase of inspiratory pressure via the CPAP device. The tip of the small diameter tube is usually placed 1–2 cm beyond the vocal cords, to ensure that surfactant can spread into both lungs. Many physicians who use the LISA technique mark the catheter 1–2 cm proximal to the tip, to ensure proper placement. Catheters with a single hole at the tip are preferable. The Cologne group usually used a soft thin diameter tube which is handled by a Magill forceps and can be introduced via the nasal or oral route. Other groups prefer the oral route and used stiffer tubes (16G vascular catheters) which can be placed intratracheally without the Magill forceps [18]. Sedation or premedication with atropine (which was described in the first clinical publications on LISA) is usually not necessary. A number of videos which are available on the internet illustrate the LISA technique (e.g., https://www.youtube.com/watch?v=OUvgJ57FQR8).

The small diameter of the surfactant replacement tube, which enables the infant to breath spontaneously and disallows the physician to apply high airway pressure and high tidal volumes during the procedure, is the main advantage of the LISA procedure. This is due to the small cross-sectional area which is occluded by a small catheter. A 5-French (1.5 mm diameter) tube occludes a cross-sectional area of approximately 1.8 mm^2. A standard endotracheal tube (inner diameter 2.5 mm, outer diameter 4.1 mm) has a total cross-sectional area of 13.2 mm^2. It must be emphasized that only 4.9 mm^2 of this area is available for respiration. The rest (8.3 mm^2) is occluded by the wall of the endotracheal tube. Therefore, it might be much more difficult for infants breathing spontaneously during the INSURE procedure to achieve sufficient tidal volumes through the endotracheal tube. In contrast to INSURE and surfactant treatment of infants who are on mechanical ventilation, even the laryngeal function is preserved during LISA surfactant replacement. Surfactant overspill into the pharynx/esophagus is minimal in most infants if the LISA tube is properly placed 1–2 cm below the vocal cords.

In Germany, the LISA technique was disseminated rapidly throughout the country. As mentioned above, in 2001, only a single center used LISA. In 2014, according to data from the German Neonatal Network (GNN, a cohort study enrolling about one third of all very low birth weight or VLBW infants born in Germany), 47 % of all VLBW infants who were treated with surfactant received LISA and 47 of 53 (89 %) participating study sites use the method.

LISA and Mechanical Ventilation

The main short-term effect of LISA is to mitigate dyspnea in spontaneously breathing preterm infants with RDS. Significantly more infants can be stabilized with CPAP if the LISA technique is used. This was demonstrated in single and multiple center observational studies [14, 15, 18–26], but also in three recently published randomized controlled trials (Table 17.1) [12, 17, 27, 28]. The effect with regard to prevention of any mechanical ventilation is closely linked to gestational age (Fig. 17.1).

Table 17.1 Randomized controlled LISA trials

Study/references	Gestational age (weeks)	Mechanical ventilation until discharge (%)	BPD or death (%)
Göpel et al. [27]			
Control group: CPAP and rescue intubation, LISA prohibited, $n=112$	27.5 ± 0.8	**73**	14
Intervention group: CPAP and rescue intubation, LISA allowed, $n=108$	27.6 ± 0.8	**33**	15
Kanmaz et al. [12]			
Control group: INSURE, $n=100$	28.3 ± 2	49	32
Intervention group: LISA, $n=100$	28.0 ± 2	40	22
Kribs et al. [17]			
Control group: intubation and surfactant treatment, $n=104$	25.2 ± 0.9	**99**	41
LISA, $n=107$	25.3 ± 1.1	**75**	33

Data are given as mean ± SD (gestational age) and (%); significant values are given in bold ($p<0.05$ chi-square test)

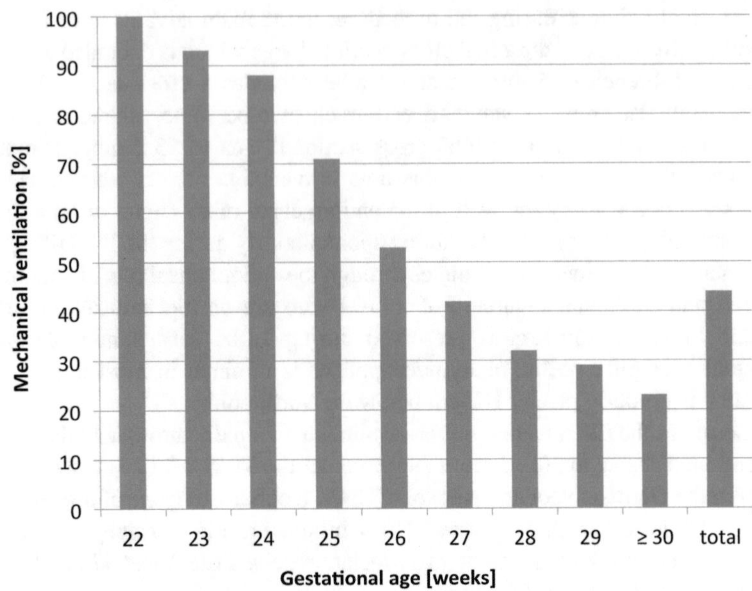

Fig. 17.1 Mechanical ventilation during the stay in the hospital in VLBW infants treated with LISA. Data stratified to gestational age (GNN 2009–2014, $n=2414$)

If surfactant is given with LISA to infants below 25 weeks of gestation, about 90 % of these infants will finally require intubation and mechanical ventilation during their stay in the hospital. In these infants mechanical ventilation is often necessary due to severe apnea. In infants between 25 and 27 weeks of gestation, the percentage of infants who need intubation and mechanical ventilation is closely linked to the severity of RDS and complications of prematurity (e.g., intubations due to surgery). In VLBW infants above 27 weeks of gestation who are treated with LISA mechanical ventilation is necessary in less than 30 % (Fig. 17.1). It should be mentioned that most infants in Fig. 17.1 were treated with LISA due to the severity of RDS (i.e., instead of rescue intubation and surfactant treatment via an endotracheal tube), since few centers in the GNN apply LISA prophylactically. The total rate of mechanical ventilation in VLBW infants treated with LISA was 44 %. This confirms the impression of many centers who introduced LISA that they were able to reduce their rate of mechanical ventilation in VLBW infants by 30–50 % [22, 23, 26].

LISA and BPD

Although LISA has a distinct effect on the rate of mechanical ventilation, the effect of the method on the incidence of BPD is less clear. One of the randomized controlled trials was able to demonstrate a significant reduction of BPD, but the

Table 17.2 Selected observational LISA studies and reported BPD/death rates

Study/references	Gestational age (weeks)	Mechanical ventilation until discharge (%)	BPD or death (%)
Kribs et al. [26]			
Control group[a], $n = 1222$	**27.9 ± 1.9**	**58**	**20**
LISA $n = 319$	**27.3 ± 1.9**	**42**	**13**
Dargaville et al. [22],			
Control group[a], $n = 41$	27 (26–27)	73	37
LISA $n = 38$	27 (26–28)	53	32
Dargaville et al. [22],			
Control group[a], $n = 56$	31 (30–31)	46	5
LISA $n = 23$	30 (29–31)	26	0
Klebermass-Schrehof et al. [23]			
Control group[a], $n = 182$	25.4 ± 1.3	**78**	**51**
LISA $n = 224$	25.3 ± 1.3	**59**	**40**
Aguar et al. [19]			
Control group[a](INSURE), $n = 31$	30.7 ± 3.0	25	10
LISA $n = 44$	30.6 ± 2.7	33	9
Göpel et al. [15]			
Control group[b], $n = 1103$	28 ± 1.3	**62**	**21**
LISA $n = 1103$	28 ± 1.3	**41**	**14**

[a]Historical control groups
[b]Matched pairs
Gestational age is given as mean (IQR) [22] or mean ± SD (all other studies). All other data are given as (%). Significant values are given in bold ($p < 0.05$ chi-square or t-test)

control group in this trial had an unusually high BPD rate with regard to the mean gestational age and the combined endpoint BPD/death was not significantly different [12] (Table 17.1). Another recently published trial failed to demonstrate a significant effect on BPD/death rate in LISA-treated infants with a gestational age between 23 and 26 weeks. In this trial, the control group had an unexpected low BPD/death rate. The trial was powered on the assumption that BPD/death will occur in 50 % of control group infants (which was in accordance to other recently published trials) and that BPD/death will occur in only 30 % of the LISA intervention group. Although the ambitious target in the intervention group was met (33 % BPD/death-rate), the 8 % higher rate of BPD/death in the control group was statistically not significantly different [17] (Table 17.1). However, observational data and matched pairs analyses support the view that LISA might be able to reduce the rate of BPD/death by 5–10 % (Table 17.2).

Large-scale meta-analysis indicates that any intervention which is able to reduce mechanical ventilation in preterm infants reduces the risk for BPD [29]. The recently published NINSAPP trial gives some clues why the LISA method might be protective for extremely immature infants, although the total rate of mechanical ventilation was not reduced in the most immature infants (23 and 24 weeks of gestation). The median duration of mechanical ventilation in the LISA group of the NINSAPP trial was 5 days (interquartile range, IQR: 0–17 days) which was only 2 days shorter

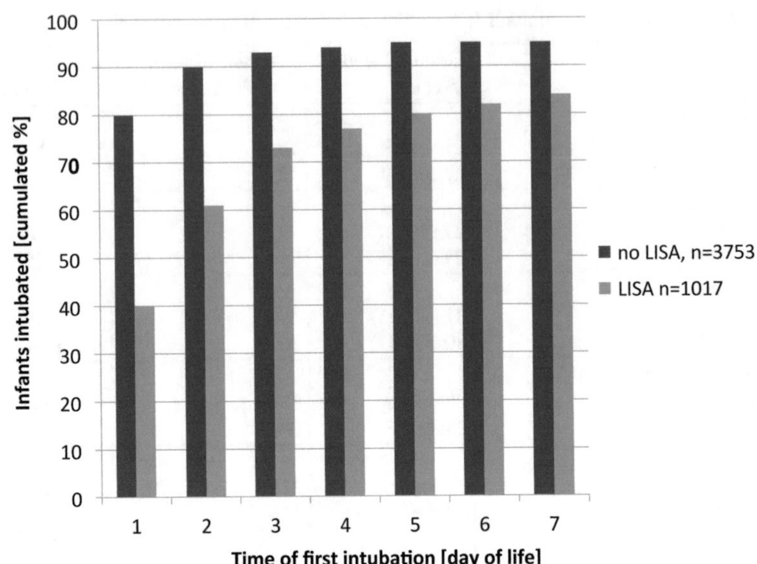

Fig. 17.2 Time of first intubation (cumulative %) of 4770 VLBW infants who were intubated during the first 28 days of life. Gestational age was 26.9±2.2 weeks in the LISA group and 27.3±2.4 weeks in the non-LISA group (GNN 2009–2014)

if compared to the control group of the NINSAPP trial (median 7 days IQR 2.5–19.5 days). However, a large amount of this difference was due to a marked reduction of mechanical ventilation during the first 72 h of life [17]. The same is true if observational data from the GNN are analyzed. Most preterm infants who are intubated during the first 28 days of life receive their first intubation on day one (dark blue bars, Fig. 17.2). In contrast to that, LISA-treated infants are often not intubated during the first 3 days of life, which is the most dangerous period for VLBW infants due to the high risk of intraventricular hemorrhage (IVH) and other severe complications of prematurity.

A delayed first intubation also offers some advantages with regard to BPD. Even if LISA-treated infants receive mechanical ventilation, this external stress is applied to more stable and mature lungs, and a possible chronic inflammatory response will be less severe. The concept of lung protection by CPAP treatment during the first days of life is also supported by clinical and animal data concerning the timing of the first extubation [30, 31].

LISA was also tested in an animal model. Surfactant treatment of spontaneously breathing preterm lambs induced PaO_2 values similar to intubated animals, although surfactant deposition was less in LISA-treated animals [32]. This data indicates that LISA might be associated with a more physiologic (and more effective) distribution of surfactant if compared to surfactant replacement under mechanical ventilation.

Long-term pulmonary outcome data of LISA-treated infants are scarce [16, 33, 34]. This is regrettable since it has been shown in preterm infants treated with high-frequency oscillation that modifications of postnatal treatment which have no significant effects on parameters like BPD can be very important with regard to long-term outcome data like forced expiratory volume in 1 s (FEV_1) [35].

Safety of LISA

Short periods of desaturation and even bradycardia are frequently observed during the LISA procedure. Therefore, only physicians who are proficient in endotracheal intubation should consider to give surfactant to a spontaneously breathing infant. Other complications include misplacement of the small diameter tube into the esophagus or into one main bronchus. Esophageal placement of the tube and surfactant application to the gastrointestinal tract will result in persistent respiratory distress. Some centers therefore use an additional feeding tube which is positioned in the stomach and continuously aspirate the tube during the LISA procedure, to recognize if the thin surfactant catheter is positioned in the esophagus. In this case, the instilled surfactant can be aspirated from the stomach immediately. Surfactant administration will then be interrupted and the position of the thin surfactant catheter can be corrected. If the thin surfactant catheter is inserted too deep (usually in the right main bronchus), surfactant distribution to both lungs will be reduced. Even completely unilateral surfactant distribution has been reported. Although suboptimal, such unequal distribution of surfactant may also occur with an endotracheal tube in place.

Other complications are rarely reported in LISA-treated infants. In contrast, most observational and some randomized trials report lower rates of IVH and other serious short-term complications of prematurity. Furthermore, LISA-treated infants received significantly less dexamethasone in observational studies [15]. This might be due to the reduced total rate of mechanical ventilation and delayed intubation in LISA infants which was already mentioned above. VLBW infants who were treated with LISA can usually be stabilized with CPAP—at least during the first days of life. This enables the neonatal intensive care unit (NICU) team to provide "minimal handling care" during the most vulnerable time period.

LISA was introduced in a single center in 2001. Therefore, few long-term outcome data of LISA-treated infants are available so far. Porath et al. reported data from 31 LISA-treated infants who were assessed at a median age of 6 5/12 years. If compared to a historical control cohort, no significant differences with regard to IQ and other long-term outcome measures were observed [34]. Since ongoing cohort studies with large numbers of LISA-treated preterm infants like the GNN are designed for routine assessment at 5 years, large-scale long-term outcome data of LISA-treated infants will be hopefully available soon.

Future of LISA

In summary, data from observational and randomized studies suggest that LISA is a promising new therapy which might reduce BPD/death in VLBW infants by 5–10 %. However, large-scale randomized controlled trials [36] and long-term outcome data are lacking. One very important aspect for future studies will be the initial cardiorespiratory stabilization (or resuscitation) phase. In the multicenter randomized controlled LISA trials reported in Table 17.1 (AMV and NINSAPP), the percentage of infants who were successfully stabilized with CPAP and could be enrolled was very different between study sites. This is also observed in the GNN dataset. In 2014, 47 % of all VLBW infants who were treated with surfactant received LISA. However, 6 of 53 study sites used LISA in more than 80 % of surfactant-treated infants, indicating that LISA is their routine way of surfactant replacement. Future randomized trials will have to address the question of optimal initial stabilization of preterm infants, including the prophylactic use of LISA.

References

1. Avery ME, Tooley WH, Keller JB, Hurd SS, Bryan MH, Cotton RB, et al. Is chronic lung disease in low birth weight infants preventable? A survey of eight centers. Pediatrics. 1987;79:26–30.
2. Vanpée M, Walfridsson-Schultz U, Katz-Salamon M, Zupancic JA, Pursley D, Jónsson B. Resuscitation and ventilation strategies for extremely preterm infants: a comparison study between two neonatal centers in Boston and Stockholm. Acta Paediatr. 2007;96:10–6.
3. Finer NN, Carlo WA, Walsh MC, Rich W, Gantz MG, Laptook AR, et al. Early CPAP versus surfactant in extremely preterm infants. N Engl J Med. 2010;362:1970–9.
4. Morley CJ, Davis PG, Doyle LW, Brion LP, Hascoet JM, Carlin JB, COIN Trial Investigators. Nasal CPAP or intubation at birth for very preterm infants. N Engl J Med. 2008;358:700–8.
5. Schmölzer GM, Kumar M, Pichler G, Aziz K, O'Reilly M, Cheung PY. Non-invasive versus invasive respiratory support in preterm infants at birth: systematic review and meta-analysis. BMJ. 2013;347:f5980.
6. Blennow M, Bohlin K. Surfactant and noninvasive ventilation. Neonatology. 2015;107:330–6.
7. Verder H, Agertoft L, Albertsen P, Christensen NC, Curstedt T, Ebbesen F, et al. Surfactant treatment of newborn infants with respiratory distress syndrome primarily treated with nasal continuous positive air pressure. A pilot study. Ugeskr Laeger. 1992;154:2136–9.
8. Dunn MS, Kaempf J, de Klerk A, et al. Randomized trial comparing 3 approaches to the initial respiratory management of preterm neonates. Pediatrics. 2011;128:e1069–76.
9. Isayama T, Chai-Adisaksopha C, McDonald SD. Noninvasive ventilation with vs. without early surfactant to prevent chronic lung disease in preterm infants: a systematic review and meta-analysis. JAMA Pediatr. 2015. doi:10.1001/jamapediatrics.2015.0510 (Epub ahead of print).
10. Björklund LJ, Ingimarsson J, Curstedt T, John J, Robertson B, Werner O, et al. Manual ventilation with a few large breaths at birth compromises the therapeutic effect of subsequent surfactant replacement in immature lambs. Pediatr Res. 1997;42:348–55.
11. Dreyfuss D, Saumon G. Ventilator-induced lung injury: lessons from experimental studies. Am J Respir Crit Care Med. 1998;157:294–323.
12. Kanmaz HG, Erdeve O, Canpolat FE, Mutlu B, Dilmen U. Surfactant administration via thin catheter during spontaneous breathing: randomized controlled trial. Pediatrics. 2013;131:e502–9.

13. Victorin LH, Deverajan LV, Curstedt T, Robertson B. Surfactant replacement in spontaneously breathing babies with hyaline membrane disease--a pilot study. Biol Neonate. 1990;58: 121–6.
14. Kribs A, Pillekamp F, Hünseler C, Vierzig A, Roth B. Early administration of surfactant in spontaneous breathing with nCPAP: feasibility and outcome in extremely premature infants (postmenstrual age </=27 weeks). Paediatr Anaesth. 2007;17:364–9.
15. Göpel W, Kribs A, Härtel C, Avenarius S, Teig N, Groneck P, et al. German Neonatal Network (GNN). Less invasive surfactant administration is associated with improved pulmonary outcomes in spontaneously breathing preterm infants. Acta Paediatr. 2015;104:241–6.
16. Herting E. Less invasive surfactant administration (LISA) – ways to deliver surfactant in spontaneously breathing infants. Early Hum Dev. 2013;89:875–80.
17. Kribs A, Roll C, Göpel W, Wieg C, Groneck P, Laux R, et al. NINSAPP trial investigators. Nonintubated surfactant application vs. conventional therapy in extremely preterm infants: a randomized clinical trial. JAMA Pediatr. 2015; 169:723–80.
18. Dargaville PA, Aiyappan A, Cornelius A, Williams C, De Paoli AG. Preliminary evaluation of a new technique of minimally invasive surfactant therapy. Arch Dis Child Fetal Neonatal Ed. 2011;96:F243–8.
19. Aguar M, Cernada M, Brugada M, Gimeno A, Gutierrez A, Vento M. Minimally invasive surfactant therapy with a gastric tube is as effective as the intubation, surfactant, and extubation technique in preterm babies. Acta Paediatr. 2014;103:e229–33.
20. Bao Y, Zhang G, Wu M, Ma L, Zhu J. A pilot study of less invasive surfactant administration in very preterm infants in a Chinese tertiary center. BMC Pediatr. 2015;15:21.
21. Canals Candela FJ, Vizcaíno Díaz C, Ferrández Berenguer MJ, Serrano Robles MI, Vázquez Gomis C, Quiles Durá JL. Surfactant replacement therapy with a minimally invasive technique: experience in a tertiary hospital. An Pediatr (Barc). 2015 May 28 doi:10.1016/j.anpedi.2015.04.013.
22. Dargaville PA, Aiyappan A, De Paoli AG, Kuschel CA, Kamlin CO, Carlin JB, et al. Minimally-invasive surfactant therapy in preterm infants on continuous positive airway pressure. Arch Dis Child Fetal Neonatal Ed. 2013;98:F122–6.
23. Klebermass-Schrehof K, Wald M, Schwindt J, Grill A, Prusa AR, Haiden N, et al. Less invasive surfactant administration in extremely preterm infants: impact on mortality and morbidity. Neonatology. 2013;103:252–8.
24. Krajewski P, Chudzik A, Strzałko-Głoskowska B, Górska M, Kmiecik M, Więckowska K, et al. Surfactant administration without intubation in preterm infants with respiratory distress syndrome – our experiences. J Matern Fetal Neonatal Med. 2014;14:1–4.
25. Kribs A, Vierzig A, Hünseler C, Eifinger F, Welzing L, Stützer H, et al. Early surfactant in spontaneously breathing with nCPAP in ELBW infants—a single centre four year experience. Acta Paediatr. 2008;97:293–8.
26. Kribs A, Härtel C, Kattner E, Vochem M, Küster J, Möller J, et al. Surfactant without intubation in preterm infants with respiratory distress: first multi-center data. Klin Padiatr. 2010;222:13–7.
27. Göpel W, Kribs A, Ziegler A, et al. Avoidance of mechanical ventilation by surfactant treatment of spontaneously breathing preterm infants (AMV): an open-label, randomised, controlled trial. Lancet. 2011;378:1627–34.
28. More K, Sakhuja P, Shah PS. Minimally invasive surfactant administration in preterm infants: a meta-narrative review. JAMA Pediatr. 2014;168:901–8.
29. Fischer HS, Bührer C. Avoiding endotracheal ventilation to prevent bronchopulmonary dysplasia: a meta-analysis. Pediatrics. 2013;132:e1351–60.
30. Berger J, Mehta P, Bucholz E, Dziura J, Bhandari V. Impact of early extubation and reintubation on the incidence of bronchopulmonary dysplasia in neonates. Am J Perinatol. 2014; 31:1063–72.
31. Thomson MA, Yoder BA, Winter VT, Giavedoni L, Chang LY, Coalson JJ. Delayed extubation to nasal continuous positive airway pressure in the immature baboon model of bronchopulmonary dysplasia: lung clinical and pathological findings. Pediatrics. 2006;118:2038–50.

32. Niemarkt HJ, Kuypers E, Jellema R, Ophelders D, Hütten M, Nikiforou M, et al. Effects of less-invasive surfactant administration on oxygenation, pulmonary surfactant distribution, and lung compliance in spontaneously breathing preterm lambs. Pediatr Res. 2014;76:166–70.
33. Herting E, Kribs A, Roth B, Härtel C, Göpel W, German Neonatal Network. Less invasive surfactant administration (LISA) is safe: two-year follow-up of 476 infants [abstract]. Neonatology. 2015;107:372–3.
34. Porath M, Korp L, Wendrich D, Dlugay V, Roth B, Kribs A. Surfactant in spontaneous breathing with nCPAP: neurodevelopmental outcome at early school age of infants ≤ 27 weeks. Acta Paediatr. 2011;100:352–9.
35. Zivanovic S, Peacock J, Alcazar-Paris M, Lo JW, Lunt A, Marlow N, et al. United Kingdom Oscillation Study Group. Late outcomes of a randomized trial of high-frequency oscillation in neonates. N Engl J Med. 2014;370:1121–30.
36. Dargaville PA, Kamlin CO, De Paoli AG, Carlin JB, Orsini F, Soll RF, et al. The OPTIMIST-A trial: evaluation of minimally-invasive surfactant therapy in preterm infants 25–28 weeks gestation. BMC Pediatr. 2014;14:213.
37. Herting E, Kribs A, Roth B, et al. Growth and development of VLBW-infants after less invasive surfactant administration during spontaneous breathing: two-year follow-up of the AMV-trial [abstract]. Neonatology. 2013;103:349–50.

Chapter 18
Anti-inflammatory Agents for the Prevention of Bronchopulmonary Dysplasia

Sneha Taylor and Virender K. Rehan

Background

Bronchopulmonary dysplasia (BPD), the most common form of chronic lung disease (CLD) in infancy, is a consequence of exposure to a variety of risk factors on the backdrop of an immature lung. It is a major consequence of prematurity that leads to significant morbidity and mortality. The long-term health consequences of BPD include, but are not limited to, detrimental effects on somatic growth, altered respiratory function persisting into adulthood, increased susceptibility to pulmonary infections, repeated hospitalizations, pulmonary hypertension, asthma, and neurodevelopmental impairment causing a major financial burden in health care [1, 2].

Since its first description around 50 years back, the epidemiology and pathophysiology of BPD has changed. The "new" BPD primarily affects infants born less than 1500 g and 32 weeks gestation, characterized by "arrested alveolarization" with minimal large or small airway disease, and relatively *little* inflammation and fibrosis compared to the "old BPD" [3–6]. With the widespread use of antenatal steroids and postnatal surfactant, we have achieved improved survival among very low birth weight (VLBW) infants; however, it has led to an overall increase in the prevalence of BPD [3]. Based on the Vermont Oxford Network's 2000–2009 data, the incidence of BPD among VLBW infants remains up to 26–30 %; however, there is a wide range among centers and variable use of the definition of BPD [3].

Despite intense research, the pathogenesis of BPD remains incompletely understood. Currently we have no definite measures to prevent or cure BPD except preventing prematurity, a daunting challenge, which is unlikely to be resolved for decades. However, it is known that the etiology of BPD is multifactorial, i.e., "multiple hit" hypothesis, combined with a genetically predisposed premature lung

---

S. Taylor, MBBS, MD, FAAP (✉) • V.K. Rehan, MD, MRCP (UK), MRCPI (Dublin) (✉)
Department of Neonatology, Pediatrics, Harbor-UCLA Medical Center,
1124 West Carson Street, Torrance, CA 90502, USA
e-mail: staylor@labiomed.org

V. Bhandari (ed.), *Bronchopulmonary Dysplasia*, Respiratory Medicine,
DOI 10.1007/978-3-319-28486-6_18

[7] and the impact of a variety of antenatal and postnatal factors [8–10]. Though single nucleotide polymorphisms of various pro- and anti-inflammatory mediators have been proposed to predict BPD, these data lack generalization due to limitations in study design for most of these studies [11, 12]. In animal models, gender as well as epigenetics has been shown to affect BPD susceptibility [13–15]. Along with this, other prenatal modulators such as the fetal inflammatory response syndrome, characterized as an elevated interleukin-6 (IL-6) concentration in fetal blood, has been shown to initiate significant pro-inflammatory changes, which play a critical role not only in the onset of premature labor but also in the subsequent increased risk of severe neonatal morbidities, especially BPD [16].

As seen in the Fig. 18.1, along with genetic predisposition, various pre- and postnatal inflammatory modulators initiate a cascade mediated by inflammation-specific cells and various cytokines [11, 17]. It leads to cell apoptosis and lung injury, which results in either resolution of injury and restoration of normal lung architecture or repair and remodeling, consistent with the BPD phenotype, i.e., impaired alveolar-

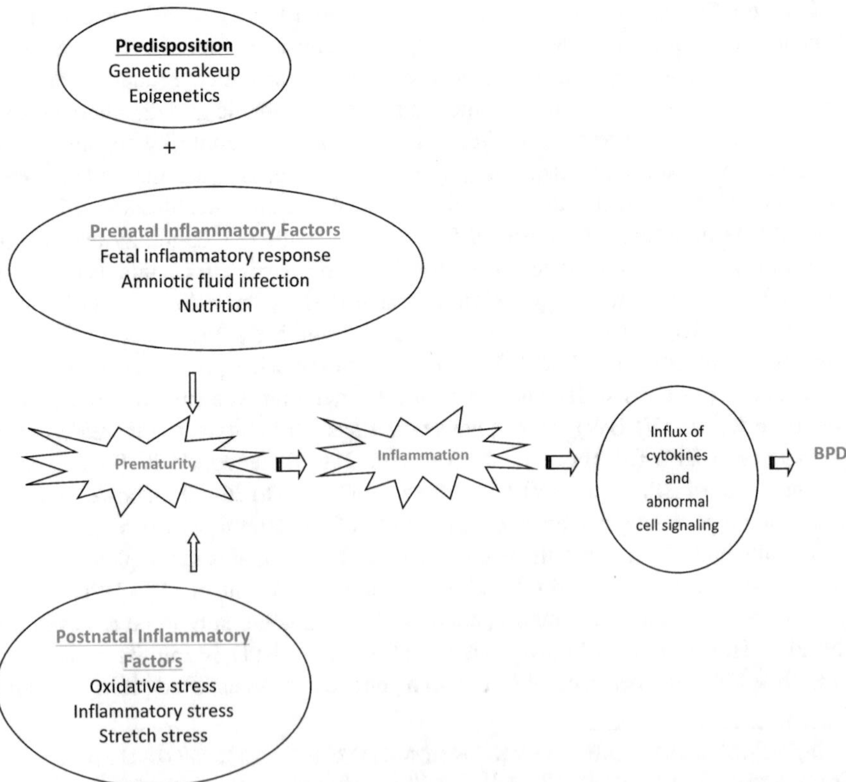

Fig. 18.1 Proposed pathogenesis of BPD involving "multiple hit" phenomena. Genetically predisposed premature lung when exposed to various antenatal and postnatal inflammatory factors elicits inflammation-induced influx of cytokines and abnormal cell signaling leading to the development of BPD

ization and vasculogenesis, features that are the "hallmark" of "new" BPD [10, 17]. Other antenatal (e.g., antenatal steroids) and postnatal (e.g., prompt stabilization of infant, exposure to hyperoxia, intubation, and ventilatory and nutritional support strategies, etc.) factors play a significant role in modulating the influence of inflammation in the pathogenesis of BPD. Detailed review of selective mediators and inflammatory molecules is discussed elsewhere [11, 17].

Approach to Prevent/Treat BPD Based on Specific Inciting Mechanisms

Oxidative Stress and Role of Antioxidants

Within the relatively hypoxic in utero environment, the fetus does not need significant antioxidant defense. Hence, the fetus has low levels of antioxidant enzymes (AOEs) [18]. It is known that there is a strong association between inflammation and oxidative stress, which increases the susceptibility to BPD. The premature lung is more prone to being affected by oxidative stress due to an inadequate antioxidant defense system, increased susceptibility to postnatal inflammation, and the presence of free iron. Oxidative stress triggers apoptosis, which acts as a second messenger and modulates transcription factors, which in turn activate and release nuclear factor kappa B (NF-κB), a critical modulator of inflammation and apoptosis [19]. Hence, it makes sense to use antioxidants in the prevention of BPD. But unfortunately, none of the potential antioxidant interventions such as using allopurinol [20], erythropoietin [21], *n*-acetyl cysteine (NAC) [22], vitamin E [23], or AOEs such as superoxide dismutase (SOD) [24, 25] have shown a benefit in reducing BPD in clinical trials. So far, only vitamin A has shown benefit in decreasing BPD [26–29], but its availability and route of administration make its use inconsistent.

Surfactant as an Antioxidant/Anti-inflammatory Agent

Along with its property to reduce alveolar surface tension and improve lung mechanics, there is evidence that surfactant contains a complex of anti-inflammatory and antioxidant properties [30–34]. Some exogenous surfactants also contain AOEs, such as SOD and catalase, and nonenzymatic antioxidant molecules such as plasmalogens and polyunsaturated phospholipids. Tracheal aspirates of surfactant-treated preterm neonates had lower levels of oxidative stress markers versus controls [35]. Moreover, surfactant protein A (SP-A) and SP-D not only act as collectins, clearing alveolar pathogens [36, 37], but also suppress the pro-inflammatory pathway mediated by NF-κB [38], inhibit cytokine secretion, and modulate lymphocyte proliferation [39]. It is important to note that there is an association between lower levels of SP-D in tracheal aspirates of preterm infants and the development of BPD versus age-matched non-BPD controls [40]. The antioxidant effect of surfactant seems promising; however, its role in vivo needs to be confirmed [41–43].

Infection/Sepsis

Although chorioamnionitis (CA) may have a protective role in BPD, it is clear that postnatal sepsis is associated with a progression of BPD [44, 45]; moreover, postnatal infection/inflammation might also attenuate the protective effect of chorioamnionitis and BPD. One study showed that infants at highest risk for BPD had experienced sepsis but not histologic CA [46]. Similarly, late-onset sepsis also increases the risk of BPD [47, 48]. It is suggested that irrespective of the timing, the inflammatory exposure from sepsis plays an important role in the development of BPD [11] which needs to be treated promptly and completely.

Stretch Stress

Much has been learned about molecular mechanisms involved in stretch-induced inflammation. The mechanical signal of stretch is transduced in part by the mitogen-activated protein kinase (MAPK) signaling cascade, and possibly the NF-κB pathway, causing the activation of transcription factors that bind stretch response elements in the promoter regions of genes, such as the chemokine IL-8 [49]. Animal studies using different ventilator strategies have shown that stretch-induced inflammation is reversible by inhibiting NF-κB [11]. Moreover, parathyroid hormone-related protein (PTHrP), a stretch-sensitive gene, transduces homeostatic peroxisome proliferator-activated receptor γ (PPARγ) signaling in alveolar mesenchyme, promoting alveolar health and optimal gas exchange [50]. However, cell-stretch stress, i.e., alveolar overdistension, results in PPARγ downregulation and alveolar dyshomeostasis seen in BPD, setting the stage for PPARγ agonists as a possible intervention for BPD, as reviewed later.

It is also known that high tidal volume ventilation along with hyperoxia causes increased microvascular permeability, neutrophil infiltration, macrophage inflammatory protein-2 (MIP-2) and plasminogen activator inhibitor-1 (PAI-1) production, Src activation, nicotinamide adenine dinucleotide phosphate (NADPH) oxidase activity, malaldehyde (MDA) levels, and release of high-mobility group box-1 (HMGB1) [51, 52]. Based on these mechanisms, a few potential preventive treatments such as ethyl pyruvate, enoxaparin, unfractionated heparin and induced pluripotent stem cells have been used in various mouse models of adult CLDs; however, their validity in neonatal lung injury remains to be tested [51–54].

We have good data suggesting the use of a noninvasive ventilation approach to reduce stretch-induced inflammatory stress and the incidence of BPD, especially when surfactant is used in a timely manner. In 2007, the Cochrane Review showed that early surfactant replacement with extubation to nasal continuous positive airway pressure (NCPAP) within 1 h, compared to later selective surfactant replacement and continued mechanical ventilation and extubation from low ventilator settings, was associated with a lower incidence of BPD [55]. A more recent Cochrane Review in 2012 showed that selective surfactant use decreased BPD and BPD/death compared to prophylactic use [56]. These findings suggest that initial stabilization on NCPAP, followed by early selective surfactant replacement, might be the ideal approach. Despite promising results using NCPAP, the respiratory failure rate remains high, requiring intubation [57], which has prompted the use of nasal intermittent positive pressure ventilation (NIPPV) to improve the rates of successful extubation within first 72 h of life, this strategy being more beneficial than NCPAP alone [58, 59]. Recently, two major randomized controlled trials (RCTs) showed that early extubation to NIPPV might be beneficial in BPD, even if the total duration of mechanical ventilation is the same [60, 61]. Overall, it would be best to avoid intubation altogether, if possible; however, if intubated, it is recommended to give "early" selective surfactant followed by rapid extubation, ideally within 1 h, to NIPPV, use a low tidal volume strategy, and permissive hypercapnia to decrease the chance of developing BPD [44, 57, 62].

Current Anti-inflammatory Treatments

Inhaled Nitric Oxide

The anti-inflammatory properties of inhaled nitric oxide (iNO) are likely mediated via the inhibition of canonical, inflammatory, and oxidant stress-induced NF-κB activation [11]. However, NO cannot be strictly classified as an anti- or pro-inflammatory molecule [63]. In the use of iNO for preventing BPD, when give ≥7 days after birth, it was associated with worse outcomes compared to controls; it especially increased risk of severe BPD or death [64]. In 2011, an individual-patient data meta-analysis of 12 randomized trials, including 3298 infants of <37 week gestational age (GA), showed no significant effect of iNO on death, CLD ($P=0.11$), or neurologic events ($P=0.09$). However, although one trial suggested that a higher starting dose >5 ppm might be associated with improved outcome, because of differences in the study design of the trials, no definite recommendations could be made regarding the routine use of iNO for the treatment of respiratory failure in preterm infants [65]. An earlier 2010 Cochrane meta-analysis of 14 RCTs of iNO in preterm infants also concluded no significant reduction in death or BPD [66]. The latest multicenter randomized trial involving the prophylactic use of noninvasive iNO in VLBW infants within 72 h of life also showed that it neither decreased the incidence or severity of BPD nor the need for mechanical ventilation [67]. A recent report of late treatment (up to five doses) of surfactant in ventilated preterm infants receiving iNO did not improve survival without BPD at 36 or 40 weeks [68]. Therefore, despite possessing potential anti-inflammatory properties, current data do not support the routine use of iNO in VLBW infants for reduction of BPD.

Azithromycin

Ureaplasma urealyticum (*Uu*) has been implicated in the development of BPD. Azithromycin, a macrolide and anti-inflammatory agent, suppresses activation of NF-κB and the synthesis of pro-inflammatory cytokines IL-6 and IL-8, making it a potential therapy for preventing BPD [69]. However, the data are not very promising regarding the routine prophylactic use of azithromycin for preventing BPD.

In 2007, a double-blind pilot RCT showed that azithromycin prophylaxis in extremely low birth weight (ELBW) infants' effectively decreased postnatal use of steroids and mechanical ventilation days, but did not affect the incidence of BPD or death. In further studies, the same group, using 10 mg/kg/day for 1 week and then 5 mg/kg/day for 6 weeks in the treatment group found no difference in BPD or death in the treatment versus placebo groups; however, early treatment in the *Uu*-positive patients decreased the incidence of BPD ($P=0.03$) [70]. A meta-analysis in 2013 showed conflicting results in terms of prophylactic use of macrolides and the reduction in BPD [71]. Overall, although there are data supporting the tolerance of azithromycin in <28 week GA infants without any significant adverse effects, and a suggestion that a multiple-dose regimen might be efficacious for microbial clearance, the effect on BPD remains yet to be proven [72].

Pentoxifylline

Pentoxifylline, a synthetic methylxanthine and a phosphodiesterase inhibitor, has unique immunomodulatory properties—it downregulates the production of powerful inflammatory cytokines such as IL-6, tumor necrosis factor (TNF)-α, and interferon (IFN) γ, all of which have been implicated in the pathogenesis of BPD. Only one RCT has evaluated the prophylactic use of nebulized pentoxifylline in the reduction of BPD, showing no difference between intervention versus placebo in the prevention of BPD (at 36 weeks GA), or on death. In addition, there were no significant effects on the incidences of intraventricular hemorrhage (IVH), periventricular leukomalacia (PVL), sepsis, or patent ductus arteriosus (PDA) requiring ligation. However, validation of these results remains limited due to risk of bias as this study was non-blinded [73]. The same group in 2015 published a double-blinded RCT evaluating efficacy and safety of nebulized pentoxifylline in <28 week gestation infants, showing that it is safe, but it does not reduce the duration of oxygen supplementation at 40 weeks corrected age in high-risk BPD infants [74]. Therefore, a better study design, with various doses and durations and routes of administration of pentoxifylline is needed prior to making any recommendation. Overall, currently, there is insufficient evidence to determine the safety and efficacy of pentoxifylline for prevention of BPD in preterm neonates.

Steroids

The critical role of inflammation during both antenatal and postnatal stages of preterm infant development has led neonatologists to use steroids for a long time. Much has been learned in the last few decades in terms of the beneficial effects of antenatal steroids for pulmonary maturation and the long-term neurodevelopmental adverse effects associated with the early and prolonged postnatal use of systemic steroids [4].

Treatment with antenatal corticosteroids improves lung maturation in preterm infant, but does not reduce the incidence of BPD [75]. The 2011Cochrane Review, comparing multiple courses of antenatal steroids with a single course, showed reduced respiratory distress syndrome (RDS), but no decrease in BPD with multiple courses [76]. The 2013 Cochrane Review showed that there is no clear evidence that either one particular steroid such as dexamethasone or betamethasone, or one particular regimen, including dosing frequency and route of delivery has advantages over the other [77]. These data suggest that there is a need to better identify the most effective steroid with a regimen that has the potential benefit of reduction in BPD.

In terms of postnatal systemic steroids, once the adverse effects of early regimens were recognized, researchers began studying different timings and durations to prevent BPD. Recent studies are mainly divided into early (≤7 days after birth) or late (>7 days after birth), based on the timing of steroid (mainly dexamethasone) administration [78, 79]. The 2010 Cochrane Review and a revision in 2014 showed that early administration of postnatal steroid facilitated extubation and decreased risk of CLD at both 28 days and 36 weeks post-menstrual age (PMA), death or CLD, PDA, and retinopathy of prematurity (ROP). There were no significant differences in the rates of mortality, infection, severe IVH, PVL, necrotizing enterocolitis (NEC), or pulmonary hemorrhage. Some trials found growth failure and adverse neurological effects such as abnormal neurological examination, neurodevelopmental delays, and cerebral palsy associated with the use of early systemic steroids. In subgroup analyses based on the type of corticosteroid, it was found that most of the beneficial and harmful effects were seen with dexamethasone; hydrocortisone had almost no impact on any outcomes except for an increase in intestinal perforation and a marginal decrease in PDA [78, 80].

The 2014 Cochrane Review showed that postnatal systemic steroid administration at >7 days of life produces short-term benefits in reducing the need for assisted ventilation and the rate of CLD, perhaps also reducing death in the first 28 days of life. However, high doses in particular were associated with short-term side effects such as bleeding from the stomach or bowel, higher blood pressure, and glucose intolerance [79]. There was no significant increase in NEC, but there was a trend toward decreased IVH in a few studies. Thus, late postnatal steroids might decrease mortality without significantly increasing the risk of long-term adverse neurodevelopmental outcomes. However, overall, the benefits of late corticosteroid therapy may not outweigh actual or potential adverse effects. In particular, at least in some cases, the methodological quality of the studies determining the long-term outcome was limited; for example, in some studies, the surviving children have only been assessed before school age, when some important neurological outcomes cannot be determined with certainty, and no study was sufficiently powered to detect increased rates of important adverse long-term neurosensory outcomes. Given the evidence of both benefits and harms of treatment, and the limitations of the evidence at present, it appears prudent to reserve the use of late corticosteroids only for infants who cannot be weaned from mechanical ventilation and to minimize the dose and duration of their use [79].

Systemic hydrocortisone has also been used in preterm infants for primary adrenal insufficiency, and its role in the prevention of BPD is not proven. A meta-analysis in 2010 evaluating the effect of hydrocortisone administration in the first week of life of VLBW infants for hypotension showed no significant reduction in mortality, BPD, or cerebral palsy; in fact, there was a significant increase in the incidence of gastrointestinal perforations when used concurrently with indomethacin [81].

Systemic and neurodevelopmental side effects of systemic steroids have led to study the role of inhaled postnatal steroids in BPD; however, currently there is no evidence that early/late inhaled steroids have any significant beneficial effect on BPD or death at 36 weeks PMA or on longer-term pulmonary function [82–84]. On the contrary, there is also a possibility for its systemic absorption and subsequent side effects such as adrenal suppression, growth inhibition, etc. [85]. In the recently reported results of the Neonatal European Study of Inhaled Steroids (NEUROSIS) study, while the incidence of BPD was lower among those who received early inhaled budesonide versus placebo, there is concern of increased mortality in the treatment group [86].

In summary, the antenatal use of corticosteroids is recommended for fetal lung maturation. Late (>7 days after birth) postnatal steroid treatment is suggested for use with caution mainly to facilitate extubation, and the role of hydrocortisone and inhaled steroids is not yet clear in preventing BPD.

On the Horizon: Potential Bench to Bedside Therapies for BPD

Docosahexaenoic Acid

Long-chain polyunsaturated fatty acids (LCPUFA) are inflammatory and immune response mediators. Docosahexaenoic acid (DHA), an *n*-3 LCPUFA, was initially studied for its efficacy in affecting neurodevelopmental outcomes. However, its anti-inflammatory properties sparked interest in studying its role in BPD. Animal data suggest that DHA inhibits hyperoxia-induced lung injury by blocking inflammatory cytokines IL-6 and C-X-C motif ligand 1 (CXCL1)/keratinocyte-derived chemokine (KC) along with restoration of NF-κB inhibitor levels, a mediator in inflammation-induced BPD [87]. A multicenter RCT, examining the role of DHA supplementation in BPD in <33 week GA infants receiving via breast milk through mothers consuming high DHA versus standard DHA diet, found that DHA supplementation decreased the incidence of BPD in infants with BW <1250 g and also decreased the incidence of hay fever in boys at either 12 or 18 months. The translational value of these findings and safety remains to be determined [88].

Cell-Based Therapy

Recent preclinical data have shown the potential for the use of stem/progenitor cells in the prevention of lung injury and also for promoting lung growth [89]. In animal models of both lipopolysaccharide (LPS)- and hyperoxia-induced neonatal lung injury, bone marrow-derived mesenchymal stem cells (MSCs) have shown protection from lung injury, as evidenced by the prevention of inflammation, vascular damage and alveolar impairment, preservation of lung structure, and inhibition of lung fibrosis without long-term adverse effects [89, 90]. A variety of progenitor cells have been studied in neonatal lung injury and a detailed review can be found elsewhere [90]. Cell-based therapies function by their paracrine effect, mediating the beneficial effects rather than stem cells themselves [90]. Promising results from stem cell-based therapy has prompted its translation from the bench to the bedside. In 2014, A phase I dose-escalation trial studied the safety and feasibility of a single, intratracheal transplantation of allogeneic human umbilical cord blood (hUCB)-derived MSCs in ELBW infants at high risk for BPD [91]. Comparing low- and high-dose MSCs with case-matched controls, there was decreased severity of BPD in the transplanted group versus control group without any adverse outcomes. Although this study suggested hUCB-MSC to be safe and feasible in preterm infants, it requires a larger, multicenter RCT before its translational value can be fully ascertained.

Vitamin D

Vitamin D (VD) is a key molecule known to modulate alveolar epithelial-mesenchymal interactions via its autocrine/paracrine effects. In animal models, $1\alpha,25(OH)_2D_3$ (1,25D), the physiologically active form of VD, has been shown to modulate perinatal lung maturation by stimulating surfactant protein and phospholipid synthesis, and modulating alveolar septation by regulating alveolar lipofibroblast apoptosis [92–94]. 1,25D and its active metabolite 3,epi-1, 25D have also been shown to protect against hyperoxia-induced neonatal lung injury in a rat model [90]. In the last decade, VD deficiency among women of childbearing age and an association of lower VD levels during gestation with pulmonary comes such as childhood asthma has been demonstrated [95, 96]. Recently, in an experimental rat model, VD supplementation effectively blocked the asthma phenotype associated with perinatal VD deficiency, providing a strong rationale for clinical trials to prevent VD deficiency-associated childhood lung morbidity [97]. Overall, promising bench data, combined with its efficacy in treating neonatal lung injury in experimental models, render VD as a potential therapy for translation to bedside.

Peroxisome Proliferator-Activated Receptor gamma Agonists

The nuclear transcription factor PPARγ plays an important role in lipofibroblast (LIF) differentiation, a specialized alveolar fibroblast population that, by enhancing epithelial-mesenchymal signaling, has been unequivocally demonstrated to modulate lung homeostasis and injury repair [4]. However, unlike LIFs, myofibroblasts that proliferate in BPD cannot promote alveolar type II (ATII) cell growth and differentiation, resulting in an impairment in alveolarization, characteristic of "new" BPD [98]. PPARγ agonists such as rosiglitazone (RGZ), pioglitazone, and prostaglandin J_2 can effectively block myofibroblast differentiation and promote LIF function. In a neonatal rat model, systemically administered RGZ significantly enhanced lung maturation without any demonstrable systemic side effects. Not only that, in a hyperoxia-induced neonatal rat lung injury model, both systemic and inhaled RGZ blocked lung injury/inflammation and protected lung structure [99–102]. Therefore, PPARγ agonists appear to be compelling candidates for a potential therapy for preventing BPD. However, detailed pharmacodynamic, pharmacokinetic, and safety studies using potent novel PPARγ agonists in human neonates are needed before the translational value of this line of work can be realized.

Curcumin

Curcumin is a potent anti-inflammatory and antioxidant agent which modulates PPARγ signaling, as outlined above, an important molecular pathway in the pathophysiology of BPD [103, 104]. In a neonatal rat model, curcumin, by stimulating key alveolar epithelial-mesenchymal interactions, enhanced lung maturation and protected against hyperoxia-induced neonatal lung injury under both in vivo and in vitro conditions; this protection was possibly mediated by blocking hyperoxia-induced transforming growth factor (TGF)-β activation [103]. Additionally, in this model, curcumin administration, by activating Erk1/2, an important extracellular signaling pathway, had long-term structural and cytoprotective effects on lung injury [104]. Recent data have also shown that the curcumin analog c26 has more stability and significant protective effects on LPS-induced acute lung injury (ALI) in rats, and its actions were mediated via inhibition of the production of inflammatory cytokines (IL-6, TNF-α), again through the ERK pathway [105]. These data are promising and suggest curcumin to be a strong translational candidate for BPD.

Phosphodiesterase Inhibitors

Available data suggest that preterm birth, lung injury, and neonatal pulmonary hypertension disrupt the NO-cyclic guanosine monophosphate (cGMP) pathway [106]. An animal model of hyperoxia-induced BPD has shown that impaired vascular endothelial growth factor (VEGF) signaling and decreased NO production inhibits alveolar and vascular growth in the developing lung [107]. Sildenafil is a selective cGMP-specific phosphodiesterase inhibitor (PI) that was recently approved for the treatment of adult pulmonary arterial hypertension (PAH) [108]. It has been studied for prevention of persistent pulmonary hypertension (PPHN) in term neonates, but recent studies are looking at its role in preventing BPD-induced pulmonary hypertension. It has been shown that sildenafil preserves lung angiogenesis and alveolar growth and decreases pulmonary vascular resistance, right ventricular hypertrophy (RVH), and medial wall thickness [107]. Sildenafil, when given simultaneously with hyperoxia, improves survival, increases pulmonary cGMP levels, and decreases the pulmonary inflammatory response and RVH; it also enhances alveolarization in experimental BPD [109]. Hypoxia-inducible factors (HIFs) are the key regulators of the transcriptional response to hypoxia. Several downstream targets of HIF play a role in abnormal lung development in animal models of BPD, especially via VEGF, in preterm infants. Sildenafil improves lung growth and alveolarization by restoration of HIF and VEGF levels and provides interesting mechanistic insights into its potential role in improving lung development along with angiogenesis [110]. Small clinical retrospective studies reviewing the efficacy of sildenafil in BPD-induced PAH have shown that it improves PAH based on significant improvement in echocardiographic markers for PAH, and a decreased need for oxygen, but with only modest clinical benefits, yet without any side effects [111, 112].

In summary, we have good experimental evidence that sildenafil has beneficial effects for both lung angiogenesis and alveolar growth in BPD, along with improvement in BPD-induced PAH. However, to assess it as a clinical therapy, we need more prospective, larger trials to confirm its efficacy and safety.

Recombinant Human Clara Cell 10 Protein

Clara Cell 10 Protein (CC10) inhibits phospholipase A2 and possesses potent anti-inflammatory and immunomodulatory properties [113]. CC10 is normally abundant in the respiratory tract but is deficient in premature infants leading to respiratory morbidities [114]. In various animal models of neonatal lung injury, CC10 has been shown to reduce lung inflammation and injury, improve pulmonary function, and upregulate surfactant protein and VEGF expression [113–115], rendering intratracheally administered CC10 protein a promising agent in preventing BPD. So far, one pilot multicenter RCT, performed to evaluate the safety and efficacy of intratracheal Recombinant Human Clara Cell 10 Protein (rhCC10) in 22 preterm infants 700–1300 g birth weight with RDS requiring surfactant administration [116, 117], did not find a significant difference in CLD (at 36 weeks PMA or 28 days), death, sepsis, or any other major prematurity-related morbidity compared to placebo-administered controls. However, a single dose of intratracheally administered rhCC10 was well-tolerated and led to a significant reduction in tracheal aspirate neutrophil and total cell count, and lung protein concentration, but without a significant difference in tracheal aspirate cytokine levels. Currently, a larger RCT with similar doses, assessing its efficacy after single dose administration in infants 24–29 weeks with primary outcome being survival without chronic respiratory morbidity at 12 months corrected GA (NCT01941745, clinical trial.gov), is under way [118].

In addition to above-reviewed anti-inflammatory agents, as shown in Table 18.1, there are many other agents that have been tried or are being tested for treating BPD [123–141]; despite the long list, there are only a few such as vitamin A [26–29], caffeine [119], and dexamethasone [78–80] that have demonstrated a reduction in

Table 18.1 Current treatment in use for BPD and its effect in reduction of BPD

Drug	Decreases BPD
Vitamin A [26–29]	Yes
Caffeine [119]	Yes
Dexamethasone [78–80]	Yes
Inositol [120, 121]	Yes
Clarithromycin [122]	Yes
DHA [88]	Yes
Surfactant [41–43]	No
Inhaled nitric oxide [66, 67]	No
Hydrocortisone [81]	No
Allopurinol [20]	No
Selenium [124–127]	No
N-acetylcysteine [22]	No
Inhaled steroid [82–84]	No
Azithromycin [70]	No
Estrogen/progesterone [128]	No
α-1-Antitrypsin [129]	No
Superoxide dismutase [24, 25]	No
Melatonin [130]	No
Cromolyn sodium [131–133]	No
Thyroxine [134]	No
Zinc [135]	No
Diuretics [136–138]	No
Bronchodilators [139, 140]	No
Recombinant human Clara cell secretory protein (rhCC10) [116]	No
Pentoxifylline [73, 74]	No
Montelukast [141]	No
Erythropoietin [21]	No
Vitamin E [23]	No

BPD; in addition, small studies using inositol [120, 121], clarithromycin [122], and DHA [88] have shown some benefit in decreasing the incidence of BPD. Other recent reviews have also discussed drug therapy in BPD [1, 85, 123, 142]. These reviews also support that even after decades of intense research in understanding BPD, we still have a long way to find better options to prevent or cure BPD.

Conclusion

BPD is a multifactorial disease process, with inflammation playing a major role. Despite numerous data regarding potential mechanisms and inventions of novel molecules/mediators involved in the pathogenesis of BPD, we currently do not have any proven preventive or curative treatment. The nature of this research field (changing definition and epidemiology of BPD, a lack of access to human lung tissue from BPD patients, a lack of an affordable animal model of BPD, etc.) and the lack of adequate funding have hampered bringing novel ideas from the bench to the bedside. It is important to target upstream mechanisms/molecules fundamental to the process of BPD rather than aiming for individual molecules involved in the pathogenesis because we know that it is a complex and multifactorial condition with a wide range of molecular intermediates involved in its pathogenesis. Thus far, we know that prevention of prematurity is the best, yet most challenging, approach to prevent BPD. The current practice of promoting growth; avoiding hyperoxia and mechanical ventilation, possibly altogether; and preventing and/or promptly treating infection is the best approach to prevent BPD. Available extensive data and their limitations also raise a question about the working definition of BPD. Is it time to rethink it? Unfortunately, as yet, there is no specific anti-inflammatory therapy we have that benefits BPD. Cell-based therapies, DHA, vitamin D, PPARγ agonists, curcumin, and sildenafil seem promising, but much work needs to be done to find the answer for this challenging condition, especially in the current climate of reduced funding.

References

1. Ghanta S, Leeman KT, Christou H. An update on pharmacologic approaches to bronchopulmonary dysplasia. Semin Perinatol. 2013;37(2):115–23.
2. Hilgendorff A, O'reilly MA. Bronchopulmonary dysplasia early changes leading to long-term consequences. Front Med (Lausanne). 2015;2:2.
3. Jensen EA, Schmidt B. Epidemiology of bronchopulmonary dysplasia. Birth Defects Res A Clin Mol Teratol. 2014;100(3):145–57. doi:10.1002/bdra.23235.
4. Cerny L, Torday JS, Rehan VK. Prevention and treatment of bronchopulmonary dysplasia: contemporary status and future outlook. Lung. 2008;186(2):75–89.
5. Northway Jr WH, Rosan RC, Porter DY. Pulmonary disease following respirator therapy of hyaline-membrane disease. Bronchopulmonary dysplasia. N Engl J Med. 1967;276:357–68.
6. Jobe AH, Bancalari E. Bronchopulmonary dysplasia. Am J Respir Crit Care Med. 2001;163:1723–9.

7. Parker RA, Lindstrom DP, Cotton RB. Evidence from twin study implies possible genetic susceptibility to bronchopulmonary dysplasia. Semin Perinatol. 1996;20:206–9.
8. Bland R. Neonatal chronic lung disease in the post-surfactant era. Biol Neonate. 2005;88:181–91.
9. Thomas W, Speer CP. Chorioamnionitis is essential in the evolution of bronchopulmonary dysplasia—the case in favour. Paediatr Respir Rev. 2014;15(1):49–52.
10. Mcevoy CT, Jain L, Schmidt B, Abman S, Bancalari E, Aschner JL. Bronchopulmonary dysplasia: NHLBI workshop on the primary prevention of chronic lung diseases. Ann Am Thorac Soc. 2014;11 Suppl 3:S146–53.
11. Wright CJ, Kirpalani H. Targeting inflammation to prevent bronchopulmonary dysplasia: can new insights be translated into therapies? Pediatrics. 2011;128(1):111–26.
12. Shaw GM, O'brodovich HM. Progress in understanding the genetics of bronchopulmonary dysplasia. Semin Perinatol. 2013;37(2):85–93.
13. Hagood JS. Beyond the genome: epigenetic mechanisms in lung remodeling. Physiology (Bethesda). 2014;29(3):177–85.
14. Hamvas A, Deterding R, Balch WE, et al. Diffuse lung disease in children: summary of a scientific conference. Pediatr Pulmonol. 2014;49(4):400–9.
15. Joss-Moore LA, Wang Y, Ogata EM, Sainz AJ, Yu X, Callaway CW, McKnight RA, Albertine KH, Lane RH. IUGR differentially alters MeCP2 expression and H3K9Me3 of the PPARgamma gene in male and female rat lungs during alveolarization. Birth Defects Res A Clin Mol Teratol. 2011;91:672–81.
16. Romero R, Espinoza J, Kusanovic JP, Gotsch F, Hassan S, Erez O, et al. The preterm parturition syndrome. BJOG. 2006;113 Suppl 3:17–42. doi:10.1111/j.1471-0528.2006.01120.x.
17. Bhandari V. Postnatal inflammation in the pathogenesis of bronchopulmonary dysplasia. Birth Defects Res A Clin Mol Teratol. 2014;100(3):189–201.
18. Russell GA. Antioxidants and neonatal lung disease. Eur J Pediatr. 1994;153(9 Suppl 2):S36–41.
19. Saugstad OD. Bronchopulmonary dysplasia-oxidative stress and antioxidants. Semin Neonatol. 2003;8(1):39–49.
20. Russell GA, Cooke RW. Randomised controlled trial of allopurinol prophylaxis in very preterm infants. Arch Dis Child Fetal Neonatal Ed. 1995;73:F27–31.
21. Aher SM, Ohlsson A. Early versus late erythropoietin for preventing red blood cell transfusion in preterm and/or low birth weight infants. Cochrane Database Syst Rev. 2012;10:CD004865.
22. Ahola T, Lapatto R, Raivio KO, Selander B, Stigson L, Jonsson B, et al. N-acetylcysteine does not prevent bronchopulmonary dysplasia in immature infants: a randomized controlled trial. J Pediatr. 2003;143:713–9.
23. Watts JL, Milner R, Zipursky A, et al. Failure of supplementation with vitamin E to prevent bronchopulmonary dysplasia in infants less than 1,500 g birth weight. Eur Respir J. 1991;4:188–90.
24. Rosenfeld WN, Davis JM, Parton L, Richter SE, Price A, Flaster E, et al. Safety and pharmacokinetics of recombinant human superoxide dismutase administered intratracheally to premature neonates with respiratory distress syndrome. Pediatrics. 1996;97(6 Part 1):811–7.
25. Davis JM, Parad RB, Michele T, et al. Pulmonary outcome at 1 year corrected age in premature infants treated at birth with recombinant human CuZn superoxide dismutase. Pediatrics. 2003;111:469–76.
26. Pearson E, Bose C, Snidow T, Ransom L, Young T, Bose G, et al. Trial of vitamin A supplementation in very low birth weight infants at risk for bronchopulmonary dysplasia. J Pediatr. 1992;121:420–7.
27. Kennedy KA, Stoll BJ, Ehrenkranz RA, Oh W, Wright LL, Stevenson DK, et al. Vitamin A to prevent bronchopulmonary dysplasia in very-low-birth-weight infants: has the dose been too low? The NICHD Neonatal Research network. Early Hum Dev. 1997;49:19–31.
28. Darlow BA, Graham PJ. Vitamin A supplementation to prevent mortality and short- and long-term morbidity in very low birthweight infants. Cochrane Database Syst Rev. 2011;10:CD000501.

29. Tyson JE, Wright LL, Oh W, Kennedy KA, Mele L, Ehrenkranz RA, et al. Vitamin A supplementation for extremely low birth weight infants. National Institute of Child Health and Human Development Neonatal Research Network. N Engl J Med. 1999;340:1962–8. doi:10.1056/NEJM199906243402505.
30. Poggi C, Dani C. Antioxidant strategies and respiratory disease of the preterm newborn: an update. Oxid Med Cell Longev. 2014;2014:721043.
31. Ramanathan R. Choosing a right surfactant for respiratory distress syndrome treatment. Neonatology. 2008;95(1):1–5.
32. Dani C, Buonocore G, Longini M, et al. Superoxide dismutase and catalase activity in naturally derived commercial surfactants. Pediatr Pulmonol. 2009;44(11):1125–31.
33. Matalon S, Wright JR. Surfactant proteins and inflammation: the Yin and the Yang. Am J Respir Cell Mol Biol. 2004;31(6):585–6.
34. Matalon S, Holm BA, Baker RR, Whitfield MK, Freeman BA. Characterization of antioxidant activities of pulmonary surfactant mixtures. Biochim Biophys Acta. 1990;1035(2):121–7.
35. Merritt TA, Hallman M, Holcomb K. Human surfactant treatment of severe respiratory distress syndrome: pulmonary effluent indicators of lung inflammation. J Pediatr. 1986;108(5):741–8.
36. Haagsman HP, Hogenkamp A, Van Eijk M, Veldhuizen EJA. Surfactant collectins and innate immunity. Neonatology. 2008;93(4):288–94.
37. Matalon S, Shrestha K, Kirk M, et al. Modification of surfactant protein D by reactive oxygen-nitrogen intermediates is accompanied by loss of aggregating activity, in vitro and in vivo. FASEB J. 2009;23(5):1415–30.
38. Wu Y, Adam S, Hamann L, et al. Accumulation of inhibitory κB-α as a mechanism contributing to the anti-inflammatory effects of surfactant protein-A. Am J Respir Cell Mol Biol. 2004;31(6):587–94.
39. Wofford JA, Wright JR. Surfactant protein A regulates IgG-mediated phagocytosis in inflammatory neutrophils. Am J Physiol Lung Cell Mol Physiol. 2007;293(6):L1437–43.
40. Kotecha S, Davies PL, Clark HW, McGreal EP. Increased prevalence of low oligomeric state surfactant protein D with restricted lectin activity in bronchoalveolar lavage fluid from preterm infants. Thorax. 2013;68(5):460–7.
41. Soll RF. Synthetic surfactant for respiratory distress syndrome in preterm infants. Cochrane Database Syst Rev. 2000;2:CD001149.
42. Soll R, Ozek E. Prophylactic protein free synthetic surfactant for preventing morbidity and mortality in preterm infants. Cochrane Database Syst Rev. 2010;1:CD001079.
43. Seger N, Soll R. Animal derived surfactant extract for treatment of respiratory distress syndrome. Cochrane Database Syst Rev. 2009;2:CD007836.
44. Kallapur SG, Jobe AH. Contribution of inflammation to lung injury and development. Arch Dis Child Fetal Neonatal Ed. 2006;91(2):F132–5.
45. Bancalari E, Claure N, Sosenko IR. Bronchopulmonary dysplasia: changes in pathogenesis, epidemiology and definition. Semin Neonatol. 2003;8:63–71.
46. Lahra MM, Beeby PJ, Jeffery HE. Intrauterine inflammation, neonatal sepsis, and chronic lung disease: a 13-year hospital cohort study. Pediatrics. 2009;123(5):1314–9.
47. Fanaroff AA, Korones SB, Wright LL, et al. Incidence, presenting features, risk factors and significance of late onset septicemia in very low birth weight infants. The National Institute of Child Health and Human Development Neonatal Research Network. Pediatr Infect Dis J. 1998;17(7):593–8.
48. Stoll BJ, Hansen N, Fanaroff AA, et al. Late onset sepsis in very low birth weight neonates: the experience of the NICHD neonatal research network. Pediatrics. 2002;110(2 pt 1):285–91.
49. Pugin J. Molecular mechanisms of lung cell activation induced by cyclic stretch. Crit Care Med. 2003;31(4 Suppl):S200–6.
50. Torday JS, Rehan VK. Developmental cell/molecular biologic approach to the etiology and treatment of bronchopulmonary dysplasia. Pediatr Res. 2007;62(1):2–7.

51. Liu Y-Y, Li L-F, Fu J-Y, Kao K-C, Huang C-C, et al. Induced pluripotent stem cell therapy ameliorates hyperoxia-augmented ventilator-induced lung injury through suppressing the Src pathway. PLoS One. 2014;9(10):e109953. doi:10.1371/journal.pone.0109953.
52. Li LF, Kao KC, Yang CT, Huang CC, Liu YY. Ethyl pyruvate reduces ventilation-induced neutrophil infiltration and oxidative stress. Exp Biol Med (Maywood). 2012;237(6):720–7.
53. Li LF, Huang CC, Lin HC, Tsai YH, Quinn DA, Liao SK. Unfractionated heparin and enoxaparin reduce high-stretch ventilation augmented lung injury: a prospective, controlled animal experiment. Crit Care. 2009;13(4):R108.
54. Li LF, Yang CT, Huang CC, Liu YY, Kao KC, Lin HC. Low-molecular-weight heparin reduces hyperoxia-augmented ventilator-induced lung injury via serine/threonine kinase-protein kinase B. Respir Res. 2011;12:90.
55. Stevens TP, Harrington EW, Blennow M, Soll RF. Early surfactant administration with brief ventilation vs. selective surfactant and continued mechanical ventilation for preterm infants with or at risk for respiratory distress syndrome. Cochrane Database Syst Rev. 2007;4:CD003063. pub3.
56. Rojas-Reyes MX, Morley CJ, Soll R. Prophylactic versus selective use of surfactant in preventing morbidity and mortality in preterm infants. Cochrane Database Syst Rev. 2012;3:CD000510.
57. Bhandari V. The potential of non-invasive ventilation to decrease BPD. Semin Perinatol. 2013;37(2):108–14.
58. Meneses J, Bhandari V, Alves JG. Nasal intermittent positive pressure ventilation vs. nasal continuous positive airway pressure for preterm infants with respiratory distress syndrome: a systematic review and meta-analysis. Arch Pediatr Adolesc Med. 2012;166:372–6.
59. Moretti C, Giannini L, Fassi C, Gizzi C, Papoff P, Colarizi P. Nasal flow synchronized intermittent positive pressure ventilation to facilitate weaning in very low birth weight infants: unmasked randomized controlled trial. Pediatr Int. 2008;50:85–91.
60. Kirpalani H, Millar D, Lemyre B, Yoder BA, Chiu A, Roberts R. Nasal intermittent positive pressure (NIPPV) does not confer benefit above nasal CPAP (nCPAP) in extremely low birth weight (ELBW)infants <1000 g BW—the NIPPV International Randomized Controlled Trial. EPAS. 2012;1675.1671.
61. Ramanathan R, Sekar KC, Rasmussen M, Bhatia J, Soll RF. Nasal intermittent positive pressure ventilation after surfactant treatment for respiratory distress syndrome in preterm infants <30 weeks' gestation: a randomized, controlled trial. J Perinatol. 2012;32:336–43.
62. Bhandari A, Bhandari V. Pitfalls, problems, and progress in bronchopulmonary dysplasia. Pediatrics. 2009;123(6):1562–73.
63. Cirino G, Distrutti E, Wallace JL. Nitric oxide and inflammation. Inflamm Allergy Drug Targets. 2006;5(2):115–9.
64. Truog WE, Nelin LD, Das A, et al. Inhaled nitric oxide usage in preterm infants in the NICHD neonatal research network: inter-site variation and propensity evaluation. J Perinatol. 2014;34(11):842–6.
65. Askie LM, Ballard RA, Cutter GR, et al. Inhaled nitric oxide in preterm infants: an individual-patient data meta-analysis of randomized trials. Pediatrics. 2011;128(4):729–39.
66. Barrington KJ, Finer N. Inhaled nitric oxide for respiratory failure in preterm infants. Cochrane Database Syst Rev. 2010;12:CD000509.
67. Kinsella JP, Cutter GR, Steinhorn RH, et al. Noninvasive inhaled nitric oxide does not prevent bronchopulmonary dysplasia in premature newborns. J Pediatr. 2014;165(6):1104–8.e1.
68. Ballard RA, Keller RL, Black DM, Ballard PL, Merrill JD, Eichenwald EC, et al. Randomized trial of late surfactant treatment in ventilated preterm infants receiving inhaled nitric oxide. J Pediatr. 2015 Oct 20. pii:S0022-3476(15)01044-6
69. Aghai ZH, Kode A, Saslow JG, et al. Azithromycin suppresses activation of nuclear factor-kappa B and synthesis of pro-inflammatory cytokines in tracheal aspirate cells from premature infants. Pediatr Res. 2007;62(4):483–8.

70. Ballard HO, Shook LA, Bernard P, et al. Use of azithromycin for the prevention of bronchopulmonary dysplasia in preterm infants: a randomized, double-blind, placebo controlled trial. Pediatr Pulmonol. 2011;46(2):111–8.
71. Nair V, Loganathan P, Soraisham AS. Azithromycin and other macrolides for prevention of bronchopulmonary dysplasia: a systematic review and meta-analysis. Neonatology. 2014;106(4):337–47.
72. Viscardi RM, Othman AA, Hassan HE, et al. Azithromycin to prevent bronchopulmonary dysplasia in ureaplasma-infected preterm infants: pharmacokinetics, safety, microbial response, and clinical outcomes with a 20-milligram-per-kilogram single intravenous dose. Antimicrob Agents Chemother. 2013;57(5):2127–33.
73. Schulzke SM, Kaempfen S, Patole SK. Pentoxifylline for the prevention of bronchopulmonary dysplasia in preterm infants. Cochrane Database Syst Rev. 2014;11:CD010018.
74. Schulzke SM, Deshmukh M, Nathan EA, Doherty DA, Patole SK. Nebulized pentoxifylline for reducing the duration of oxygen supplementation in extremely preterm neonates. J Pediatr. 2015;166(5):1158–62.e2.
75. Roberts D, Dalziel S. Antenatal corticosteroids for accelerating fetal lung maturation for women at risk of preterm birth. Cochrane Database Syst Rev. 2006;3:CD004454.
76. Crowther CA, Mckinlay CJ, Middleton P, Harding JE. Repeat doses of prenatal corticosteroids for women at risk of preterm birth for improving neonatal health outcomes. Cochrane Database Syst Rev. 2011;6:CD003935.
77. Brownfoot FC, Gagliardi DI, Bain E, Middleton P, Crowther CA. Different corticosteroids and regimens for accelerating fetal lung maturation for women at risk of preterm birth. Cochrane Database Syst Rev. 2013;8:CD006764.
78. Doyle LW, Ehrenkranz RA, Halliday HL. Early (<8 days) postnatal corticosteroids for preventing chronic lung disease in preterm infants. Cochrane Database Syst Rev. 2014;5:CD001146. pub4.
79. Doyle LW, Ehrenkranz RA, Halliday HL. Late (>7 days) postnatal corticosteroids for chronic lung disease in preterm infants. Cochrane Database Syst Rev. 2014;5:CD001145.
80. Halliday HL, Ehrenkranz RA, Doyle LW. Early (<8 days) postnatal corticosteroids for preventing chronic lung disease in preterm infants. Cochrane Database Syst Rev. 2010;1:CD001146.
81. Doyle LW, Ehrenkranz RA, Halliday HL. Postnatal hydrocortisone for preventing or treating bronchopulmonary dysplasia in preterm infants: a systematic review. Neonatology. 2010;98(2):111–7.
82. Onland W, Offringa M, van Kaam A. Late (≥ 7 days) inhalation corticosteroids to reduce bronchopulmonary dysplasia in preterm infants. Cochrane Database Syst Rev. 2012;(4):CD002311. doi:10.1002/14651858.CD002311.pub3.
83. Shah VS, Ohlsson A, Halliday HL, Dunn M. Early administration of inhaled corticosteroids for preventing chronic lung disease in ventilated very lowbirth weight preterm neonates. Cochrane Database Syst Rev. 2012;(5):CD001969. doi:10.1002/14651858.CD001969.pub3.
84. Shah SS, Ohlsson A, Halliday HL, Shah VS. Inhaled versus systemic corticosteroids for preventing chronic lung disease in ventilated very low birth weight preterm neonates. Cochrane Database Syst Rev. 2012;(5):CD002058. doi:10.1002/14651858.CD002058.pub2.
85. Iyengar A, Davis JM. Drug therapy for the prevention and treatment of bronchopulmonary dysplasia. Front Pharmacol. 2015;6:12.
86. Bassler D, Plavka R, Shinwell ES, Hallman M, Jarreau PH, Carnielli V, et al. Early inhaled budesonide for the prevention of bronchopulmonary dysplasia. N Engl J Med. 2015;373(16):1497–506. doi:10.1056/NEJMoa1501917.
87. Ma L, Li N, Liu X, et al. Arginyl-glutamine dipeptide or docosahexaenoic acid attenuate hyperoxia-induced lung injury in neonatal mice. Nutrition. 2012;28(11–12):1186–91.
88. Manley BJ, Makrides M, Collins CT, et al. High-dose docosahexaenoic acid supplementation of preterm infants: respiratory and allergy outcomes. Pediatrics. 2011;128(1):e71–7.

89. O'reilly M, Thébaud B. Using cell-based strategies to break the link between bronchopulmonary dysplasia and the development of chronic lung disease in later life. Pulm Med. 2013;2013:874161.
90. Fung ME, Thébaud B. Stem cell-based therapy for neonatal lung disease: it is in the juice. Pediatr Res. 2014;75(1–1):2–7.
91. Chang YS, Ahn SY, Yoo HS, et al. Mesenchymal stem cells for bronchopulmonary dysplasia: phase 1 dose-escalation clinical trial. J Pediatr. 2014;164(5):966–72.e6.
92. Sakurai R, Shin E, Fonseca S, Sakurai T, Litonjua AA, Weiss ST, Torday JS, Rehan VK. 1α,25(OH)2D3 and its 3-epimer promote rat lung alveolar epithelial-mesenchymal interactions and inhibit lipofibroblast apoptosis. Am J Physiol Lung Cell Mol Physiol. 2009;297:L496–505.
93. Nguyen TM, Guillozo H, Marin L, Tordet C, Koite S, Garabedian M. Evidence for a vitamin D paracrine system regulating maturation of developing rat lung epithelium. Am J Physiol Lung Cell Mol Physiol. 1996;271:L392–9.
94. Lykkedegn S, Sorensen GL, Beck-nielsen SS, Christesen HT. The impact of vitamin D on fetal and neonatal lung maturation. A systematic review. Am J Physiol Lung Cell Mol Physiol. 2015;308(7):L587–602.
95. Hollis BW, Wagner CL. Vitamin D deficiency during pregnancy: an ongoing epidemic. Am J Clin Nutr. 2006;84(2):273.
96. Devereux G, Litonjua AA, Turner SW, et al. Maternal vitamin D intake during pregnancy and early childhood wheezing. Am J Clin Nutr. 2007;85(3):853–9.
97. Yurt M, Liu J, Sakurai R, Gong M, Husain SM, Siddiqui MA, Husain M, et al. Vitamin D supplementation blocks pulmonary structural and functional changes in a rat model of perinatal vitamin D deficiency. Am J Physiol Lung Cell Mol Physiol. 2014;307(11):L859–67.
98. Torday JS, Torres E, Rehan VK. The role of fibroblast trans differentiation in lung epithelial cell proliferation, differentiation, and repair in vitro. Pediatr Pathol Mol Med. 2003;22:189–207.
99. Rehan VK, Wang Y, Patel S, Santos J, Torday JS. Rosiglitazone, a peroxisome proliferator-activated receptor-gamma agonist, prevents hyperoxia-induced neonatal rat lung injury in vivo. Pediatr Pulmonol. 2006;41(6):558–69.
100. Morales E, Sakurai R, Husain S, et al. Nebulized PPARγ agonists: a novel approach to augment neonatal lung maturation and injury repair in rats. Pediatr Res. 2014;75(5):631–40.
101. Rehan VK, Sakurai R, Corral J, et al. Antenatally administered PPAR-gamma agonist rosiglitazone prevents hyperoxia-induced neonatal rat lung injury. Am J Physiol Lung Cell Mol Physiol. 2010;299(5):L672–80.
102. Wang Y, Santos J, Sakurai R, et al. Peroxisome proliferator-activated receptor gamma agonists enhance lung maturation in a neonatal rat model. Pediatr Res. 2009;65(2):150–5.
103. Sakurai R, Li Y, Torday JS, Rehan VK. Curcumin augments lung maturation, preventing neonatal lung injury by inhibiting TGF-β signaling. Am J Physiol Lung Cell Mol Physiol. 2011;301(5):L721–30.
104. Sakurai R, Villarreal P, Husain S, et al. Curcumin protects the developing lung against long-term hyperoxic injury. Am J Physiol Lung Cell Mol Physiol. 2013;305(4):L301–11.
105. Zhang Y, Liang D, Dong L, et al. Anti-inflammatory effects of novel curcumin analogs in experimental acute lung injury. Respir Res. 2015;16:43.
106. Farrow KN, Steinhorn RH. Sildenafil therapy for bronchopulmonary dysplasia: not quite yet. J Perinatol. 2012;32(1):1–3.
107. Ladha F, Bonnet S, Eaton F, Hashimoto K, Korbutt G, Thébaud B. Sildenafil improves alveolar growth and pulmonary hypertension in hyperoxia-induced lung injury. Am J Respir Crit Care Med. 2005;172(6):750–6.
108. Rubin LJ, Badesch DB, Fleming TR, Galie N, Simonneau G, Ghofrani HA, et al. Long-term treatment with sildenafil citrate in pulmonary arterial hypertension: SUPER-2. Chest. 2011;140(5):1274–83.

109. De Visser YP, Walther FJ, Laghmani el H, Boersma H, Van der Laarse A, Wagenaar GT. Sildenafil attenuates pulmonary inflammation and fibrin deposition, mortality and right ventricular hypertrophy in neonatal hyperoxic lung injury. Respir Res. 2009;10:30.
110. Park HS, Park JW, Kim HJ, et al. Sildenafil alleviates bronchopulmonary dysplasia in neonatal rats by activating the hypoxia-inducible factor signaling pathway. Am J Respir Cell Mol Biol. 2013;48(1):105–13.
111. Nyp M, Sandritter T, Poppinga N, Simon C, Truog WE. Sildenafil citrate, bronchopulmonary dysplasia and disordered pulmonary gas exchange: any benefits? J Perinatol. 2012;32(1):64–9.
112. Tan K, Krishnamurthy MB, O'heney JL, Paul E, Sehgal A. Sildenafil therapy in bronchopulmonary dysplasia-associated pulmonary hypertension: a retrospective study of efficacy and safety. Eur J Pediatr. 2015;174:1109–15.
113. Chandra S, Davis JM, Drexler S, et al. Safety and efficacy of intratracheal recombinant human Clara cell protein in a newborn piglet model of acute lung injury. Pediatr Res. 2003;54(4):509–15.
114. Wolfson MR, Funanage VL, Kirwin SM, et al. Recombinant human Clara cell secretory protein treatment increases lung mRNA expression of surfactant proteins and vascular endothelial growth factor in a premature lamb model of respiratory distress syndrome. Am J Perinatol. 2008;25(10):637–45.
115. Miller TL, Shashikant BN, Melby JM, Pilon AL, Shaffer TH, Wolfson MR. Recombinant human Clara cell secretory protein in acute lung injury of the rabbit: effect of route of administration. Pediatr Crit Care Med. 2005;6(6):698–706.
116. Levine CR, Gewolb IH, Allen K, et al. The safety, pharmacokinetics, and anti-inflammatory effects of intratracheal recombinant human Clara cell protein in premature infants with respiratory distress syndrome. Pediatr Res. 2005;58(1):15–21.
117. Abdel-latif ME, Osborn DA. Intratracheal Clara cell secretory protein (CCSP) administration in preterm infants with or at risk of respiratory distress syndrome. Cochrane Database Syst Rev. 2011;5:CD008308.
118. Clinical Trials.gov Efficacy of Recombinant Human Clara Cell 10 Protein (rhCC10) Administered to Premature Neonates with Respiratory Distress Syndrome Clinical. Trials.gov identifier: NCT01941745.
119. Schmidt B, Roberts RS, Davis P, et al. Caffeine therapy for apnea of prematurity. N Engl J Med. 2006;354(20):2112–21.
120. Hallman M, Bry K, Hoppu K, Lappi M, Pohjavuori M. Inositol supplementation in premature infants with respiratory distress syndrome. N Engl J Med. 1992;326:1233–9.
121. Howlett A, Ohlsson A. Inositol for respiratory distress syndrome in preterm infants. Cochrane Database Syst Rev. 2003;4:CD000366.
122. Ozdemir R, Erdeve O, Dizdar EA, Oguz SS, Uras N, Saygan S, et al. Clarithromycin in preventing bronchopulmonary dysplasia in urea plasma urealyticum-positive preterm infants. Pediatrics. 2011;128:e1496–501.
123. Beam KS, Aliaga S, Ahlfeld SK, Cohen-Wolkowiez M, Smith PB, Laughon MM. A systematic review of randomized controlled trials for the prevention of bronchopulmonary dysplasia in infants. J Perinatol. 2014;34:705–10.
124. Daniels L, Gibson R, Simmer K. Randomised clinical trial of parenteral selenium supplementation in preterm infants. Arch Dis Child. 1996;74:F158–64.
125. Darlow BA, Winterbourn CC, Inder TE, Graham PJ, Harding JE, Weston PJ, Austin NC, Elder DE, Mogridge N, Buss IH, Sluis KB, The New Zealand Neonatal Study Group. The effect of selenium supplementation on outcome in very low birth weight infants: a randomized controlled trial. J Pediatr. 2000;136:473–80.
126. Huston RK, Jelen BJ, Vidgoff J. Selenium supplementation in low-birthweight premature infants: relationship to trace metals and antioxidant enzymes. J Parent Ent Nutr. 1991;15:556–9.

127. Darlow BA, Austin N. Selenium supplementation to prevent short-term morbidity in preterm neonates. Cochrane Database Syst Rev. 2003;(4):CD003312. doi:10.1002/14651858.CD003312.
128. Trotter A, Maier L, Grill HJ, Kohn T, Heckmann M, Pohlandt F. Effects of postnatal estradiol and progesterone replacement in extremely preterm infants. J Clin Endocrinol Metab. 1999;84:4531–5.
129. Stiskal JA, Dunn MS, Shennan AT, et al. alpha1-Proteinase inhibitor therapy for the prevention of chronic lung disease of prematurity: a randomized, controlled trial. Pediatrics. 1998;101:89–94.
130. Gitto E, Reiter RJ, Amodio A, et al. Early indicators of chronic lung disease in preterm infants with respiratory distress syndrome and their inhibition by melatonin. J Pineal Res. 2004;36(4):250–5.
131. Viscardi RM, Hasday JD, Gumpper KF, et al. Cromolyn sodium prophylaxis inhibits pulmonary proinflammatory cytokines in infants at high risk for bronchopulmonary dysplasia. Am J Respir Crit Care Med. 1997;156:1523–9.
132. Ng GY, Ohlsson A. Cromolyn sodium for the prevention of chronic lung disease in preterm infants. Cochrane Database Syst Rev. 2001;1:CD003059.
133. Watterberg KL, Murphy S. The neonatal cromolyn study group failure of cromolyn sodium to reduce the incidence of bronchopulmonary dysplasia: a pilot study. Pediatrics. 1993;91:803–6.
134. Smith LM, Leake RD, Berman N, et al. Postnatal thyroxine supplementation in infants less than 32 weeks' gestation: effects on pulmonary morbidity. J Perinatol. 2000;20:427–31.
135. Terrin G, Canani RB, Passariello A, Messina F, Conti MG, Caoci S, et al. Zinc supplementation reduces morbidity and mortality in very-lowbirth-weight preterm neonates: a hospital-based randomized, placebo-controlled trial in an industrialized country. Am J Clin Nutr. 2013;98:1468–74.
136. Rush MG, Engelhardt B, Parker RA, Hazinski TA. Double-blind, placebo-controlled trial of alternate-day furosemide therapy in infants with chronic bronchopulmonary dysplasia. J Pediatr. 1990;117(1 Pt 1):112–8.
137. Sahni J, Phelps SJ. Nebulized furosemide in the treatment of bronchopulmonary dysplasia in preterm infants. J Pediatr Pharmacol Ther. 2011;16(1):14–22.
138. Stewart A, Brion LP. Intravenous or enteral loop diuretics for preterm infants with (or developing) chronic lung disease. Cochrane Database Syst Rev. 2011;9:CD001453.
139. Ng G, Da Silva O, Ohlsson A. Bronchodilators for the prevention and treatment of chronic lung disease in preterm infants. Cochrane Database Syst Rev. 2012;6:CD003214.
140. De Boeck K, Smith J, Van Lierde S, Devlieger H. Response to bronchodilators in clinically stable 1-year-old patients with bronchopulmonary dysplasia. Eur J Pediatr. 1998; 157(1):75–9.
141. ClinicalTrials.gov The efficacy and safety of montelukast sodium in the prevention of bronchopulmonary dysplasia (BPD). Clinical.Trials.gov identifier: NCT01717625.
142. Bhandari V. Drug therapy trials for the prevention of bronchopulmonary dysplasia: current and future targets. Front Pediatr. 2014;2:76. doi:10.3389/fped.2014.00076. eCollection 2014.

Index

A
Acute respiratory distress syndrome (ARDS), 282
Adenosine triphosphates (ATPs), 185
Adhesion molecules, 132, 135–136
Adipose tissue (AT), 302
AEC1. *See* Alveolar Type I Epithelial Cells (AEC1)
AECII. *See* Alveolar Type II epithelial cells (AECII)
Aerobic metabolism, 185
Aerobic respiration, 183
Airflow obstruction, 285, 288
Airway and vascular remodeling, 168
Airway obstruction, 168
Alveolar type I epithelial cells (AEC1), 5, 28
Alveolar type II epithelial cells (AECII), 28
Alveolarization, 95, 96
Alveolocapillary gas exchange, 188
American Thoracic Society (ATS) guidelines, 285
Angiopoietin-2, 142
Anti-infective agents, 87–88
Antioxidant (AO)
  capacity, cell resulting, 6
  defense systems, 186, 187
  endogenous enzymes, 6
  low-molecular weight, 7
  mechanisms, 7
Antioxidant enzymes (AOEs), 327
Apoptosis, 188
Arterial oxygen saturation, 176, 178
Arterial partial pressure of O_2 (p_aO_2), 189
ATP-binding cassette, 118
Attention deficit hyperactivity disorder (ADHD), 285
Azithromycin, 87, 88, 330

B
Baboons, 5
BALF. *See* Bronchoalveolar lavage fluid (BALF)
Barotrauma, 59, 60
Bayley III scales, 193
Bi-level CPAP, 210
Biomarkers
  adhesion molecules, 135, 136
  anti-inflammatory cytokines, 140
  CC10, 140, 141
  chemokines, 133
  enzymes, 139
  fetal lung development, 141
  inflammation, 129
  inflammatory process, 130
  limitations, 143
  NAC, 140
  oxidative stress, 139
  preterm infants, 130
  VEGF, 141
Bombesin-like peptide (BLP), 14
Bone marrow (BM), 302
BOOST II trial, 194
Brain oxygenation, 191
Bronchial hyperresponsiveness, 282, 284–288
Bronchoalveolar lavage fluid (BALF), 8, 60, 130
Bronchopulmonary dysplasia (BPD), 3, 79, 167, 223, 259, 281
  acinar development, 156
  adult lungs, 157
  airflow limitations, 282
  airway growth, 160
  alveolar and microvascular remodeling, 149
  alveolar growth abnormalities, 160

V. Bhandari (ed.), *Bronchopulmonary Dysplasia*, Respiratory Medicine,
DOI 10.1007/978-3-319-28486-6

Bronchopulmonary dysplasia (BPD) (*cont.*)
alveolar pathology, 157
alveolar simplification and dysmorphic microvasculature, 157
alveolarization and pulmonary vascular development, 56
alveolarization and vascular development, 69
autopsy findings, 156
bronchial hyperresponsiveness, 282
bronchial lesions or alveolar septal fibrosis, 161
cellularity and fibrosis, 156
characterized, 169
chronic fibroproliferative stage, 154
chronic lung disease, preterm infants, 149, 150
chronic respiratory disease, 281
clinical presentation, 109
CNVs, 111
definition, 283
degree of prematurity, 169, 177
description, 243–247
diagnostic definition, 167, 169–170
elastic fiber architecture, 154
epidemiology of, 168–169
exogenous surfactant, 156
exogenous surfactant and antenatal steroid administration, 149
fetal inflammatory response syndrome, 58–59
fibroproliferative lung injury, 160
fibroproliferative response, 156
genetic association, 112
genetic variants, 111, 113
haplotype, 116
HapMap project, 112
human genome, 111
hyperexpansion and atelectasis, 154
in vitro and in vivo data, 55
incidence of, 176
infection/sepsis, 328
inflammation-induced influx, 326
intra-amniotic infection and inflammation, 55
long-term damage, 154
lung function studies, 159, 160
lung morphogenesis, 149
lung pathology, 55
mechanical ventilation, 149
miRNA, 117
morphometric and biochemical techniques, 157
mycoplasma (*see* Mycoplasma)
neutrophils and macrophages, 68
newborn animal models, 4–5
and nitrogen-free radicals, 188
nutrition (*see* Nutrition)
obstructive bronchiolar lesions, 154
old BPD *vs.* new BPD, 282
and O_2 therapy, 185
oxidative stress, 115
oxidative stress antioxidants, 327
oxygen requirement at postnatal ages, 172–175
oxygen supplementation, 170–172
pathogenesis (*see* Hyperoxia)
pathophysiology, 109
pediatric scientific community, 281
perinatal and neonatal conditions, 161
pharmacological interventions, 56
population at risk, 177–178
postcanalicular lung remodeling, 157
postcanalicular lungs, 161
postnatal factors, 55
pre and postnatal pro-inflammatory conditions, 58, 68
precapillary arteriovenous anastomoses, 157
premature infants, 299
prematurity, 281
prematurity-associated lung injury, 56
prematurity-associated lung pathology, 150
preterm infants, 156, 160
pulmonary arteries and intra-acinar arterioles, 156
pulmonary function in survivors (*see* Preterm birth)
pulmonary hypertension (*see* Pulmonary hypertension (PH))
pulmonary interstitial emphysema, 154
pulmonary microvasculature, 157
RDS, 55, 169, 281
respiratory distress syndrome (RDS), 154
septal interstitium, 154
severe forms of, 168, 169
severity, 288–292
severity classification, 175–176
SPOCK2 gene, 114
surfactant, 149, 327–328
susceptibility, 110
treatment, 336
vascular and airway smooth muscle cell development, 55
vascular hypothesis, 157
Vitamin D, 115
wide spectrum, 150
Brown's meta-analysis, 192

C
Calcium (Ca), 232
Caspases, 10
Cell death
  caspases and components, 10
  and hyperoxia-induced lung cell injury, 9–10
Cell transplantation, 299
  mesenchymal stem cells (MSCs) (*see* MSCs transplantation)
  stem (*see* Stem cell transplantation)
Cerebral palsy, 177
Chemokines, 133–135
Chest radiographs
  bubbly lung, 245
  degree of hyperexpansion, 247
  development of BPD, 247
  differential diagnosis, 249
  digital, 247
  features, 247
  granular pattern, lung parenchyma, 244
  honeycomb or spongelike appearance, 245
  immature lung, 247
  infancy to adulthood, 248–249
  leaky lung syndrome (LLS), 244, 248
  peri- and neonatal care, 247
  premature infants, 248
  scoring of chest CT scan, 250
  scoring systems, 247
  structural changes, lungs, 247
  type 1 and type 2 diseases, 247
Children's Interstitial Lung Disease (ChILD) Research Network, 157
Chorioamnionitis (CA), 79, 85, 86
  adverse pro-inflammatory conditions, 57
  animal experiments, 57
  chronic inflammatory process, 57
  definition, 56
  gestation-independent effect, 57
  lipopolysaccharide (LPS), 57
  maturational effect, 57
  microbial colonization, 57
  microbial invasion/pathological processes, 56
  microorganisms, 56
  pro-inflammatory cytokines, 56
  Ureaplasma spp., 56
  utero infection, 56
Chronic lung disease (CLD), 156, 157, 169, 193
  anti-inflammatory mediators, 326
  infancy, 325
  inflammation-specific cells, 326
  mouse models, 328
  pulmonary infections, 325
Chronic obstructive pulmonary disease
  in adult life, 94
  airway obstruction, 96
  asthma and wheezing, 95
  C/EBPs, 98
  environmental exposures, 100
  lung function, 95
  parental smoking, 100
  pathology, 93
  prevalence, 93
Clara Cell 10 Protein (CC10), 335, 337
Clara cell secretory protein 10 (CC10), 140
Closed-loop FiO_2 control system (CLiO), 194
Continuous positive airway pressure (CPAP), 60, 200
  BPD/death rates, 316
  Bubble, 200
  INSURE technique, 206–207, 316
  intubation group, 315
  modern interfaces, 201
  neonatal ventilators, 200
  observational studies, 203–204
  physiological effects, 200
  post-extubation period, 201
  pressure generation and delivery, 200–201
  pressure-generating devices, 200
  vs. supplemental oxygen, 201–202
  weaning preterm infants, 207
Copy-number variations (CNVs), 111
Cord clamping, 190
CPAP. *See* Continuous positive airway pressure (CPAP)
Curcumin, 334
Cytokine-induced neutrophil chemoattractant-1 (CINC-1), 11
Cytokines, 10, 11, 130

D
Dioxygen, 185
Docosahexaenoic acid (DHA), 332–333
  fetal lung growth, 231
  levels, time of birth, 232
  parenteral lipid administration, 232
  source, 232

E
Early-onset sepsis (EOS), 59
EGFR. *See* Epidermal growth factor receptor (EGFR)
ELBW. *See* Extremely low-birth weight (ELBW)

Endotracheal ventilation, 200, 201, 203
EOS. *See* Early-onset sepsis (EOS)
Epidermal growth factor receptor (EGFR), 35
Erythropoietin (EPO), 188
Eunice Kennedy Shriver National Institute of Child Health and Human Development (NICHD), 169
Extracellular SOD (ecSOD), 7
Extremely low-birth weight (ELBW), 39, 60, 183
Extremely preterm infants, 223
  nutritional support (*see* Nutritional support of extremely preterm infant)
  potential effects of undernutrition, 224

F

FEV_1/forced vital capacity (FVC) ratio, 285, 290, 291
FRC. *See* Functional residual capacity (FRC)
Free radicals, 185
Functional residual capacity (FRC), 33, 200

G

Gene expression, 116
Genetic pathway analyses, 116–117
Genetic susceptibility, 69
Glutathione (GSH), 187

H

Hedgehog interacting protein (HHIP), 98
Hepatocyte growth factor (HGF), 14, 301, 302
Heterodimeric transcription factor, 188
High-flow nasal cannulae (HFNC), 211
  vs. nasal CPAP, 211–214
  vs. NIPPV, 212–213
  for weaning from CPAP, 214–215
High-resolution computed tomography (HRCT)
  adulthood, 254
  BPD patients, 250
  early teenage to adolescence, 246, 253
  evaluation, 249
  infancy and early childhood, 251–253
  lung abnormalities, 249
  multifocal areas, 249
  pulmonary parenchyma, 249
  respiratory dysfunction, 249
  scoring, 252
  scoring systems, 250, 251
  severity of BPD, 249
HIPERSPACE trial, 213
Host immune response, 81–82
Hyaline membrane disease, 153, 154
Hyperoxia, 5–8, 188, 194
  BLP, 14
  CINC-1, 11
  genetic and environmental factors, 3
  HGF, 14
  IFNγ, 12
  IL-1, 10
  IL-10, 11
  IL-6, 10–11
  IL-8, 11
  KGF, 11
  lung injury, mechanism (*see* Lung injury)
  MCP-1, 11
  MIF, 13
  MMP9, 12
  MT, 15
  newborn animal models, 4–5
  pathology of new BPD, 4
  S1P, 15
  SOD, 15–16
  STOP-ROP trial, 3
  TGFβ, 12–13
  TNFα, 13
  VEGF, 13–14
Hypertension, 259
  pulmonary (*see* Pulmonary hypertension (PH))
Hypoxemia, 194
Hypoxia response elements (HREs), 188
Hypoxia-inducible factor 1α (HIF-1α), 6, 184, 189

I

ICAMs. *See* Intercellular adhesion molecules (ICAMs)
IGF. *See* Insulin growth factor (IGF)
Infants, 259, 299, 300, 303–307
Inflammatory cells, 138
Inhaled nitric oxide (iNO), 269, 329
Insulin growth factor (IGF), 41
INSURE technique, 203, 206–207
Intercellular adhesion molecule-1 (ICAM-1), 136
Intercellular adhesion molecules (ICAMs), 62
Interferon gamma (IFNγ), 12
Interleukin-1 (IL-1), 10
Interleukin-10 (IL-10), 11
Interleukin-18 receptor 1 (IL18R1), 114
Interleukin-6 (IL-6), 10–11
Interleukin-6 (IL-6) concentration, 326
Interleukin-8 (IL-8), 11

Intrauterine infection models, 85–87
detection, 88
and lung injury, 81
Intraventricular hemorrhage (IVH), 320
Intubation
BPD, 315
CPAP, 315
and mechanical ventilation, 318
Invasive mechanical ventilation
AEC1, 28
AECII, 28
alveolar development and disruption, 27
alveolar septation, 39–41
alveolar–capillary permeability, 29–31
animal models, 42–43
cell proliferation, differentiation and apoptosis, 41–42
chronic lung disease, 27
EGFR, 41
ELBW, 39
endothelial cells, 29
fibroblasts, 29
lung development, 39
lung inflammation and injury, 27
macrophages, 29
mechanical injury, 28
neutrophils and macrophages, 31–32
saccules, 39
VEGF, 42
VILI, 27

K
Keratinocyte growth factor (KGF), 11
Krebs von den Lungen-6 (KL-6), 142

L
Late-onset sepsis (LOS), 59
Less invasive surfactant administration (LISA)
and BPD, 318–321
death rates, 319
endotracheal tube, 317
Magill forceps, 316
and mechanical ventilation, 317–318
safety, 321
sedation/premedication, 316
VLBW infants, 322
Long-chain polyunsaturated fatty acids (n-3 LCPUFAs), 231, 236
Long-term consequences of preterm birth
ADHD, 292
adulthood, 284
categories of disease severity, 289
clinical characteristics of BPD, 289, 290
dysynaptic/unequal lung growth, 291
early childhood, 283
lung function measurements of BPD subjects, 290, 291
mechanical ventilation and oxygen therapy, 292
mild disease, 289
neonatal respiratory illness, 291
NICHD review, 292
NIH consensus, 289
oxygen dependency, 288
oxygen therapy, 290
pathogenesis, 288
postnatal risk factors, 288
retrospective cohort, 290
retrospective study, 289
supplemental oxygen, 289
LOS. *See* Late-onset sepsis (LOS)
Lung development
alveolar stage, 153
canalicular stage, 151
embryonic stage, 150
fetal, 150, 151
organogenesis, 150
pseudoglandular reflects, 151
pseudoglandular stage, 151
saccular (terminal sac) stage, 152, 153
Lung function, 100
Lung injury, 5–10, 168, 170, 180
hyperoxia
airway epithelial layer thickness and airway smooth muscle area, 8
airway epithelium serves, 8
alveolar type II epithelial cells, 7
cell injury and cell death, 9–10
childhood wheezing disorders, 8
HIF-1α, 6
human neonates, 7
macrophage and PMN infiltration, 8
MnSOD/ecSOD, 7
Nox, 6
Nrf2, 7
O_2, 5
oxidative stress, 6
oxygen-induced injury, 6
P53, 7
pulmonary microvascular endothelial cells, 5
RNS, 5–7
ROS, 5–7
tracheal aspirates and bronchoalveolar lavage (BAL) fluid, 8
VEGF, 6

M

Macrophage migration inhibiting factor (MIF), 13
Macrophages, 134
Magnetic resonance imaging (MRI)
  early changes, emphysema, 255
  lack of radiation exposure, 254
  low-density cyst-like focal abnormalities, 255
  preterm infants, 255
  severe BPD, 256
  T1-weighted and proton density-weighted images, 255
MAPK. *See* Mitogen-activated protein kinase (MAPK)
Matrix metalloproteinase 9 (MMP9), 12
Mechanotransduction
  EGFR, 35
  gene expression, 39
  growth factor receptors, 38
  inflammatory response, 35
  integrins–focal adhesions–cytoskeleton, 37–38
  intracellular signaling pathways, 38
  ion channels, 36, 37
  mechanical deformation, 35
  transcription factors, 38, 39
Medical Research Council (MRC) dyspnea score, 285
Melatonin (MT), 15
Mesenchymal stem cells (MSCs), 305, 333
  adult tissues, 302
  AT, 303
  BM, 302, 303
  characteristics, 302
  donor age, 303
  gestational tissues, 303
  transplantation (*see* MSC transplantation)
  umbilical cord and placental tissue, 303
Migration inhibitory factor (MIF), 137
Mitochondrial manganese SOD (MnSOD), 7
Mitogen-activated protein kinase (MAPK) signaling, 328
Mitogen-activated protein kinases (MAPK), 12, 37
Molecular mechanisms
  alveolar capillary permeability, 65–66
  alveolarization and angiogenesis, 66–67
  cellular and endothelial interaction, 62
  cellular and humoral mediators, 61
  chemotactic and chemokinetic factors, 62
  inflammation, 68
  oxygen radicals and proteolytic mediators, 65
  pro- and anti-inflammatory cytokines, 62–63
  PRRs, 64–65
  repair mechanisms and growth factors, 67
  stem cell therapy, 68
Monocyte chemoattractant protein-1 (MCP-1), 11
MSC transplantation
  long-term safety and outcomes, 306
  optimal dose, 305
  optimal timing, 305–306
  phase I clinical trial, 307
Multiple-banded antigen (MBA)
  size variants, 85
  ureaplasmal cell surface MBA protein, 81
  virulence factors, 80
Mycoplasma, 79, 82–87
  animal models
    human BPD, 82
    intrauterine infection models, 85–87
    mycoplasma infections, 82–84
    pneumonia models, 82–84
    Ureaplasma infection, 82, 85
  anti-infective agents, 87–88
  host immune response, 81–82
  microbiology, 80
  Mycoplasma hominis (*see Mycoplasma hominis*)
  Ureaplasma parvum (*see Ureaplasma parvum*)
  Ureaplasma urealyticum (*see Ureaplasma urealyticum*)
  virulence factors, 80–81
Mycoplasma hominis
  amniotic fluid isolates, 81
  genitourinary tract commensals, 79
  hydrolyzes arginine, 80
  respiratory samples, 79
Myelin basic protein (MBP), 306

N

NAD phosphate (NADP), 185
NADPH oxidase (Nox), 6
Nasal cannula (NC) flow, 178
Nasal continuous positive airway pressure (nCPAP), 195
Nasal intermittent positive pressure ventilation (NIPPV), 204, 329
  history, 208
  in post-extubation period, 209
  physiological effects, 208, 209
  studies, 209–210
National Centre for Biotechnology Information (NCBI), 111
National Institute of Child Health and Human Development (NIHCD), 283

National Institutes of Health (NIH), 170, 175, 289
Necrotizing enterocolitis (NEC), 187, 331
Neonatal European Study of Inhaled Steroids (NEUROSIS), 332
Neonatal intensive care unit (NICU), 183
Neonatal Oxygenation Prospective Meta-analysis Collaboration study (NeOProM), 193
Neonatal ventilators, 200
Neonatal-Onset Respiratory Disease, 117–119
  ABCA3 gene, 118
  SFTPB gene, 118
  SFTPC gene, 119
  TTF1, 119
Neurally adjusted ventilatory assist (NAVA) mode, 209
Newborn animal models
  hyperoxia, 4, 5
Newborns
  lung disease, 13
  mice, 7
  $Nrf2^{-/-}$ mice, 7
  SOD, 16
  with RDS, 15
  treatment, 12
NICHD Neonatal Research Network, 169, 176, 178, 179
Nicotinamide adenine dinucleotide (NAD), 185
Nicotinamide adenine dinucleotide phosphate (NADPH), 328
Nitrogen-free radicals, 188
Nuclear factor kappa B (NF-κB), 187, 327
Nuclear factor-erythroid 2-related factor 2 (Nrf2), 7
Nutrition, 225–228, 235–236
  calcium (Ca), 232–233
  carbohydrates, 230
  degree of critical illness in AGA infants
    energy and fluid intake, 226
    outcome variables, 227
  development of BPD, 224, 225
  extremely preterm infant (*see* Nutritional support of extremely preterm infant)
  fluids usage, 229–230
  guidelines (*see* Standardized feeding guidelines)
  inositol, 230
  magnesium (Mg), 233
  NICU, 223
  phosphorus (P), 233
  post-discharge (*see* Post-discharge nutrition)
  protein, 231
  selenium (Se), 235
  triglycerides and fatty acids, 231–232
  Vitamin A, 233–234
  Vitamin E, 234, 235
Nutritional support of extremely preterm infant
  analysis, 225
  daily energy and fluid intakes, first 3 weeks, 225
  mediation framework, 226
  severity of critical illness for AGA infants, 225
  SGA infants, 226

O

O_2 load, 191
Oxidative phosphorylation, 185
Oxidative stress, 187
Oxidative stress biomarkers, 192
Oxidized glutathione (GSSG), 191
Oxygen
  and mechanical ventilation, 14
  oxygen-induced injury, 6
  ROS, 5
  saturation, 3
  STOP-ROP trial, 3
Oxygen requirement
  at 36 weeks postmenstrual age, 173–175
  at day 28, 172–173
  during first 4 weeks, 170–171
  for more than 28 days, 172
Oxygen Supplementation. *See* Supplemental oxygen

P

Paracrine effects, 301
Paracrine mediators, 301, 302
Patent ductus arteriosus (PDA), 169
Pattern recognition receptors (PRRs), 64, 81
PCNA. *See* Proliferating cell nuclear antigen (PCNA)
Pediatric Academic Societies (PAS) annual meeting, 192
Pentoxifylline, 330–331
Perinatal care, 183
Periventricular leukomalacia (PVL), 187
Peroxisome Proliferator-Activated Receptor gamma Agonists (PPARγ), 334
Phosphodiesterase inhibitors, 335
Phosphorus (P), 233
Pneumonia models, 82–84
Polyunsaturated fatty acids (PUFA), 187
Positive end expiratory pressure (PEEP), 208

Post-discharge nutrition
anthropometric, 235
BPD, 236
management, very low birth weight infants, 235
NICU, 235
planning, 235
preterm infants, 235
primary care pediatrician, 235
Postnatal risk factors
hyperoxia and hypoxia, 60–61
infection, 59
mechanical ventilation, 59–60
Preductal pulse oximetry (SpO_2), 189
Premature, 299, 300, 303, 305, 306
Premature infants, 167, 169, 173, 180
oxygen dependency, 172
with respiratory failure, 168
respiratory control function, 178
supplemental oxygen, 170
Prematurity, 150, 157, 160
consequences, 183
lung development, 183
Prenatal steroid therapy, 168
Prenatal steroids, 4
Preterm, 95, 99
Preterm birth, 283–284
BPD (*see* Bronchopulmonary dysplasia (BPD))
bronchial hyperresponsiveness, 285–288
bronchodilator response, 286
demographic and clinical information, 285, 286
FEV_1/FVC ratio, 285
hospital discharge diagnosis, 284, 285
long-term respiratory outcomes (*see* Long-term consequences of preterm birth)
methacholine challenge, 287
MRC dyspnea score, 285
pulmonary function test, 285
pulmonary lung function, 285, 287
SF-36v2, 285
SGRQ, 285
Preterm infants, 315, 316, 319, 321
chorioamnionitis, 62
lung pathology, 55
oxygen saturation, 60
TNF-α positive macrophages, 63
Proinflammatory cytokines, 136–138
Proliferating cell nuclear antigen (PCNA), 42
Prolyl-hydroxylase enzymes (PHD1–3), 188
Prostacyclin derivatives, 271
PRRs. *See* Pattern recognition receptors (PRRs)
Pulmonary, 259
hypertension (*see* Pulmonary hypertension (PH))
Pulmonary hypertension (PH), 261–264, 269–271
artery pressure measurement, 260
biomarkers, 268
cardiac catheterization, 266, 267
chronic respiratory diseases, childhood, 259
clinical features, 265
development, 262
echocardiographic diagnosis, 266
echocardiography, 265, 266
ELBW infants, 260
heterogeneity and variability, 273
intra- or extra-cardiac shunts, 261
LVDD, infants, 265
management, 271–273
mimic, 265
prevalence, 260
PVD (*see* Pulmonary vascular disease (PVD))
risk, anesthesia, 267
risk, growth-restricted infants, 261
tracheobronchomalacia, 267
treatments, infants and children, 268
vasoconstriction, 268
vasodilators (*see* Pulmonary vasodilators)
vasorelaxation, 269
vein stenosis, 265
VLBW infants, 259
Pulmonary hypertension in infants, 168
Pulmonary vascular disease (PVD), 259
alveolarization, 261
alveologenesis and gas exchange, 264
angiopoietin (ANG)/Tie-2 ligand/receptor system, 263
damage and thickening of pulmonary circulation, 262
endothelial monocyte-activating polypeptide II (EMAP II), 262
endothelial nitric oxide synthase (eNOS), 264
hypoxia-inducible factor-1alpha (HIF-1alpha), 263
low-density lipoprotein receptor-related protein 5 (LRP5, 264
noxious stimuli, 261
nuclear factor kappa B, 263
pathogenesis, 261
Tie2 signaling, 264
vascular endothelial growth factor (VEGF), 262
vasodilation and vasoconstriction, 261

Pulmonary vascularization bed, 184
Pulmonary vasodilators
  endothelin 1 (ET-1), 270
  iNO, 269
  oxygen therapy, 269
  prostacyclin (PGI2, 271
  sildenafil, 270
Pulse oximeter, 194

R

Radiology of BPD, 247, 249, 254
  acute respiratory distress, 243
  adolescence/adulthood, 256
  chest (*see* Chest radiographs)
  chronic disease, 245
  HRCT technique (*see* High-resolution computed tomography (HRCT))
  MRI (*see* Magnetic resonance imaging (MRI))
  period of regeneration, 244
  syndrome, 243
  transition to chronic disease, 244
Randomized controlled trials (RCTs), 207, 329
RDS. *See* Respiratory distress syndrome (RDS)
Reactive nitrogen species (RNS), 186
Reactive oxygen species (ROS), 139–140, 185, 186
receptor for advanced glycation end products (RAGE)., 98
Receptor tyrosine kinase (RTK) receptors, 13
regulated on activation, normal T cell expressed and secreted (RANTES), 135
Respiratory distress syndrome (RDS), 55, 168, 200
Respiratory failure in infants, 167–169
Respiratory health, 285, 287, 288, 292
Respiratory Health Survey, 284
Resuscitation, 189, 190
Retinopathy of prematurity (ROP), 187

S

Saint George's Respiratory (SGRQ) questionnaires, 285
Saugstad's meta-analysis, 193
Secretory leukocyte protease inhibitors (SLPIs), 139
Selenium (Se), 235
SF-36v2, 285
Sildenafil, 270
Single nucleotide polymorphisms (SNPs), 81, 111
Smoking, 93, 100
Solithromycin, 87
Sphingosine kinase 1 (SphK-1), 15
Sphingosine-1-phosphate (S1P), 15
Standardized feeding guidelines
  caloric requirements, 229
  clinical evaluation, 229
  colostrum/donor milk, 228
  development, 228
  enteral nutrition, 229
  evidence-based strategy, 228
  exceptions and non-exceptions, 228
  extremely preterm infants, 228
  implementation, 229
  measurements, growth, 229
  nutritional practices, 228
  parenteral fluid support, 228
  reduction, growth failure, 229
  total parenteral nutrition (TPN), 228
  TPN, 228
StarSync® module, 208
Stem cell therapy, 299
  exogenous administration, 299
  MSCs (*see* Mesenchymal stem cells (MSCs))
  transplantation (*see* Stem cell transplantation)
Stem cell transplantation, 302
  engraftment and differentiation, 300–301
  EPCs, ECFCs, 304
  ESCs, 304
  MSCs (*see* Mesenchymal stem cells (MSCs))
  paracrine effects, 301
  paracrine mediators, 301, 302
  therapeutic potential, 300
  UCB MNCs, 303, 304
Steroids
  hydrocortisone, 332
  inflammation, 331
  intestinal perforation, 331
  neurodevelopmental side effects, 332
  short-term side effects, 331
  treatment, 331
Stretch stress
  animal studies, 328
  hyperoxia, 328
  noninvasive ventilation approach, 328
Superoxide dismutase (SOD), 15–16, 327
Supplemental oxygen, 170, 171, 180
  and premature infants, 170
  cumulative duration, 172
  indicator of lung disease, 176
  need for, 176
Supplemental Therapeutic Oxygen for Prethreshold Retinopathy of Prematurity (STOP-ROP) trial, 3

Surfactant, 202
Surfactant protein-A (SP-A)-deficient mice, 84
surfactant proteins, 118
Synchronized NIPPV (SNIPPV), 208
  vs. NCPAP, 208
  pressure generation and delivery, 208–209

T
The Cochrane Review, 331
Thyroid transcription factor-1 (TTF1), 119
Tissue inhibitor of metalloproteases (TIMPs), 138
TLRs. *See* Toll-like receptors (TLRs)
Toll-like receptors (TLRs), 64
  host immune response, 81
Tracheobronchomalacia, 272
Transforming growth factor (TGF), 141
Transforming growth factor beta (TGFβ), 12–13
Transient receptor potential vanilloids (TRPV), 37
TRPV. *See* Transient receptor potential vanilloids (TRPV)
Tumor necrosis factor alpha (TNFα), 13, 187

U
UCB MNCs, 303, 304
Ureaplasma parvum
  anti-infective agents, 87–88
  genitourinary tract commensals, 79
  intrauterine infection models, 85–87
  pneumonia models, 82–84
  serovar, 80
  wild-type mice, 84
Ureaplasma urealyticum
  anti-infective agents, 87–88
  genitourinary tract commensals, 79
  intrauterine infection models, 85–87
  pneumonia models, 82–84
  serovars, 80

V
Vascular cell adhesion molecules (VCAMs), 62
Vascular endothelial growth factor (VEGF), 13–14, 42, 137, 184, 189, 301, 302
  lung injury, 6
VCAMs. *See* Vascular cell adhesion molecules (VCAMs)
VEGF. *See* Vascular endothelial growth factor (VEGF)
Venous cord blood, 191
Ventilator-induced lung injury (VILI), 27
  air–liquid interfaces, 33
  alveolar epithelial barrier function, 34
  alveolar epithelial plasma membrane stress failure, 34
  atelectrauma, 33
  biotrauma, 33
  calcium, 34
  deformation-induced remodeling, 33
  endothelial and epithelial barriers, 35
  epithelial and endothelial cells, 33
  factors, 33
  FRC, 33
  heterogeneity, 33
  lung volumes, 33
  lysosomes, 34
  mechanical strain, 32
  plasma membrane, 34
  preterm lambs, 33
  shear stress, 32
  surfactant-deficient lung, 33
  vesicular lipid trafficking, 34
  volutrauma, 33
Very low birth weight (VLBW), 192, 282, 284, 288, 289, 325
VILI. *See* Ventilator-induced lung injury (VILI)
Virulence factors
  ammonia, 80
  MBA, 80
  PAMP, 80
  U. parvum serovar 3 clinical strain SV3F4 genome, 80
  Ureaplasma spp., 81
  ureaplasmal, 80
Vitamin A
  administration, 234
  and iNO, 234
  benefits, 234
  deficiency, preterm infants, 233
  prevention, 234
  risk of BPD, 234
  storage and preparation, 234
  supplementation, ELBW infants, 233
Vitamin D (VD), 115, 333
Vitamin E, 234

W
Weaning preterm infants, 207
Wilson–Mikity syndrome, 153
Window of vulnerability, 58, 69

Printed in the United States
By Bookmasters